ADVANCES IN THE ETIOLOGY, PATHOGENESIS AND PATHOLOGY OF VASCULITIS

Edited by **Luis M. Amezcua-Guerra**

Advances in the Etiology, Pathogenesis and Pathology of Vasculitis
Edited by Luis M. Amezcua-Guerra

Published by InTech

Janeza Trdine 9, 51000 Rijeka, Croatia

Publishing Process Manager Dragana Manestar

Technical Editor Teodora Smiljanic

Cover Designer InTech Design Team

Additional hard copies can be obtained from orders@intechopen.com

Advances in the Etiology, Pathogenesis and Pathology of Vasculitis,
Edited by Luis M. Amezcua-Guerra
p. cm.
ISBN 978-953-307-651-5

For EU product safety concerns:
IN TECH d.o.o., Prolaz Marije Krucifikse Kozulić 3, 51000 Rijeka, Croatia,
info@intechopen.com or visit our website at intechopen.com.

Meet the editor

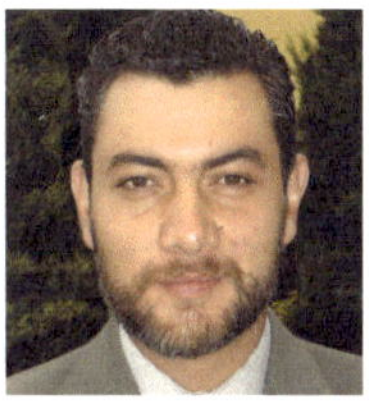

Dr. Luis M. Amezcua-Guerra is a Professor of Rheumatology and Immunology at the Instituto Nacional de Cardiología in Mexico City, Mexico. He is a postgraduate in Rheumatology and Internal Medicine at the School of Medicine, Universidad Nacional Autónoma de México. His work has been seminal to identify and characterize the immune mechanisms that underlie erosive arthritis in systemic lupus erythematosus, especially those related to the abnormal behavior of citrulline and C-reactive protein. He has also been involved in the study of kidney damage in Takayasu's arteritis as well as in the existence of subclinical tissue damage in patients with asymptomatic hyperuricemia. Dr. Amezcua-Guerra teaches immunology to postgraduate students in Rheumatology at the Universidad Nacional Autónoma de México and to undergraduate students at the School of Medicine, La Salle University.

Contents

Preface

"But there were also other fevers, as will be described. Many had their mouths affected with aphthous ulcerations. There were also many defluxions about the genital parts, and ulcerations, boils (phymata), externally and internally, about the groins. Watery ophthalmies of a chronic character, with pains; fungous excrescences of the eyelids, externally and internally, called fig, which destroyed the sight of many persons. There were fungous growths, in many other instances, on ulcers, especially on those seated on the genital organs".

This archetypal description of the Adamantiades-Behçet's disease remains as valid today as when it was detailed by Hippokrates of Kos (460-377 BC) in his *Epidemion*, book III, part 7 (Hipp. Epid. 3.3.7).

Nevertheless, in these last 2500 years we have advanced a lot in the knowledge of vasculitis, a fascinating array of life-threatening and minor diseases caused by inflammatory conditions that affect the blood vessels. Indeed, research in immunology has invigorated the entire field of vasculitis, shaping a rational approach to its etiology, pathogenesis, diagnosis and treatment, which is the matter of the present book.

This is not a textbook on vasculitis, since it was never intended as a compilation of comprehensive reviews. Rather, it represents the view of each author on selected topics related to vasculitis, verifying the scientific evidence with their own expertise. In other words, this book represents the amalgam between an evidence-based medicine to one based on eminence. Only outstanding experts within defined scientific fields of research in vasculitis from all over the world were invited to participate in this publication. This resulted in an exciting combination of original contributions, structured reviews, overviews, state-of the-art articles, and even the proposal of novel etiopathogenetic models of disease.

Organizing this diversity of manuscripts has not been easy, and I am not certain how long will take readers to cover this book from beginning to end, but all the authors have endeavored to draw them into this volume by keeping both the text and the accompanying figures and tables lucid and memorable. This book has been intended to provide a broad base upon which one can build additional knowledge acquired from other sources.

I invite you to read both consecutive but separable books on *Vasculitis* to better understand these fascinating but complex diseases.

Advances in the Etiology, Pathogenesis and Pathology of Vasculitis begins with contributions on the etiology of vasculitis, how some pathogens may interact with the host's immune system to induce autoimmune-mediated tissue injury, how different genes may confer risk for vasculitis and how some antibodies may become pathogenic. The following section deals on the pathology of vasculitis and the potential role of endothelial cells and cytokines in vascular damage and repair. We next find chapters summarizing the latest information on several primary and secondary vasculitis syndromes, to conclude with the coverage of selected topics such as organ-specific vasculitic involvement and quality of life issues in vasculitis.

I am thankful to all the contributing authors. Their expert knowledge and experience has guaranteed a thoughtful and innovative approach for rheumatologists, nephrologists and other specialists interested in the fascinating field of vasculitis. Each author must be certain that their efforts will benefit to all patients suffering from these serious diseases.

I am also grateful to Aleksandar Lazinica for this kind invitation to edit the present book; thank you for your confidence. Off note, this book could not have been edited without the dedicated technical assistance of the publishing process managers, Petra Zobic and Dragana Manestar; thank you for your patience and willingness.

What began for Celsus as *Rubor et tumor cum calore et dolore* and led to Virchow's *Functio laesa* has grown beyond the therapeutic targeting of cytokines. As editor, I hope that some of the enthusiasm and excitement of the contributing authors may be shared by each reader of this book.

Dr. Luis M. Amezcua-Guerra, MD
Department of Immunology
The National Institute of Cardiology "Ignacio Chávez"
Mexico City
Mexico

Part 1

Contributions on the Etiology of Vasculitis

Transcriptome Signature of Nipah Virus Infected Endothelial Cells

Mathieu Cyrille[1], Legras-Lachuer Catherine[2] and Horvat Branka[1]
[1]INSERM, U758; Ecole Normale Supérieure de Lyon, Lyon, F-69007 France; IFR128 BioSciences Lyon-Gerland Lyon-Sud, University of Lyon 1; 69365 Lyon,
[2]University of Lyon 1; 69676 Lyon, France, ProfileExpert, Lyon, France

1. Introduction

The highly pathogenic Nipah virus (NiV) emerged in epidemics in Malaysia in 1998. Regular outbreaks occur since then in Bangladesh and India with the high mortality rate reaching up to 90%. During the first emergence in Malaysia, the only way to contain the outbreak was culling of more than one million pigs leading to major economic issues, estimated at over US$ 100 million (Lee, 2007). Thus, NiV is considered as a potential agent of bioterrorism and is designated as priority pathogens in the National Institute of Allergy and Infectious Diseases (NAID) Biodefense Research Agenda. Neither treatment nor vaccines are available against NiV infection, limiting thus experimentation with live virus to Biosafety level 4 (BSL4) laboratories, which require the highest level of precaution.
Nipah virus infection is often associated to the development of the wide spread vasculitis but molecular basis of its pathogenicity is still largely unknown. To gain insight in the pathogenesis of this highly lethal virus we have performed analysis of virus-induced early transcriptome changes in primary endothelial cells, which are first targets of Nipah infection in humans.

1.1 The virus

Together with the closely related Hendra virus (HeV) that appeared in Australia in 1994, NiV has been classified in the new genus called Henipavirus, in the Paramyxoviridae family. Placed in the order of the Mononegavirales, this family has nonsegmented single stranded negative-sense RNA genome (Lamb & Parks 2007). Henipavirus encodes 6 structural proteins: the nucleocapsid N, phosphoprotein P, the matrix protein M, fusion F, attachment G, and the large polymerase L. The P gene also codes for non-structural protein through two different strategies. First, by mRNA editing, pseudotemplated guanosine residues could be inserted causing a frame shift of either 1 or 2 nucleotides leading to the production of the proteins V and W. The C protein is produced through the initiation of translation of P mRNA at an alternative start codon 20 nucleotides downstream in the +1 ORF (Wang et al., 2001). Because of its short length, the C protein can be produced through P, V and W mRNAs (Fontana et al., 2008).

1.2 Epidemiology

Numerous studies have demonstrated that the natural hosts of NiV are flying foxes in the genera *Pteropus* and *Eidolon* in South-East Asia as well as in Madagascar (Iehlé et al., 2007) and Ghana (Drexler et al., 2009). The emergence of NiV as zoonosis could be due to the fact that large areas of South East Asia have recently been subject to deforestation. Consequently, breeding territories of giant bats have been found in close proximity to people habitation, which has facilitated contact with domesticated animals as well as with humans. Since its emergence in Malaysia in 1998, NiV was shown to be different from the other members of its family by its capacity to cause the most important zoonosis ever observed within Paramyxoviridae. Indeed, during this first outbreak, the virus infected humans, pigs, cats, dogs and horses (Maisner et al., 2009). Among infected people, about 90% were working in pig farms. Serological analysis revealed that pigs were responsible for the transmission of Nipah virus to humans. Therefore, in order to contain this first occurrence, more than 1 million pigs were culled. Although it seems that Nipah outbreaks have been stopped in Malaysia, the virus continues to cause regular outbreaks from 2001 up to nowdays in India and Bangladesh. However, pigs were not involved in those outbreaks, and virus seemed to be transmitted directly form its natural reservoir fruit bats, to humans. Fruit bats from Malaysia, Cambodia, Bangladesh and Thailand were tested and the studies revealed the existence of new strains of NiV (Halpin & Mungall 2007). Even the virus can pass via an intermediate host like pigs, viral transmission occurs during last few years from bats to humans through palm juice (Luby et al., 2006) and has been responsible for reappearance of NiV in 2010 (17 deaths) and 2011 (35 deaths) increasing the total number of NiV outbreaks to 13 since its first appearance (Nahar et al., 2010)(Salah et al., 2011). Finally, human to human transmission has been documented in more than half of the outbreaks (Gurley et al., 2007, Luby et al., 2009).

1.3 NiV tropism

NiV can naturally infect a large panel of mammals suggesting the high conservation of its receptor among them (Eaton et al., 2006). In addition, the glycoproteins G of the Henipavirus show a tropism for a number of different cell types including neural, endothelial, muscular and epithelial cells (Bossart et al., 2002). Ephrin B2 (EFN B2) has been demonstrated as the receptor for both NiV and HeV. Indeed, this highly conserved protein is expressed at the surface of all permissive cell lines. Moreover, the transfection of cells with the gene coding for EFN B2 makes them permissive to the infection (Negrete et al., 2005). EFN B2 is essential to vasculogenesis and neuronal development. This transmembrane protein of 330 aa is expressed by numerous cells, but more particularly at the surface of epithelial, endothelial, smooth muscles and neuronal cells, that show the highest level of viral antigens during infection in patients (Lee, 2007). Finally, despite the high affinity of NiV for EFN B2, its expression at the surface of cells is not always sufficient for the virus entry, suggesting the existence of an additional receptor or intracellular factor necessary for viral replication (Yoneda et al., 2006).

The second entry receptor for NiV and HeV has been identified: Ephrin B3 (EFN B3), with the affinity for NiV 10 times lower than EFN B2 (Negrete et al., 2006). EFN B3 is a transmembrane protein of 340 aa. At the position 121 and 122 of EFN B3 and B2, 2aa appear essential for the virus entry. In contrast to EFN B2, EFN B3 is more expressed at the level of the brainstem, which could be linked with the severity of the neuron dysfunctions during the NiV encephalitis (Negrete et al., 2007).

1.4 The pathology in humans

After incubation period which varies from 4 to 60 days, NiV infection starts similarly to flu. In the large majority of the cases patients present fever, whereas 2/3 of them develop headache, leading frequently to severe acute encephalitis with loss of consciousness. Some of patients develop in addition respiratory symptoms. Death occurs in 40 to 90% within an average time of 10 days post fever, due to the severity of the cerebral damages (Lee, 2007).

The pathology is characterized by a systemic vasculitis with syncytia formation of microvascular endothelial and epithelial cells (Fig. 1). Perivascular cuffing is generally observed. Despite the fact that the virus infects all organs, the microvascularization of central nervous system shows the most severe damages.

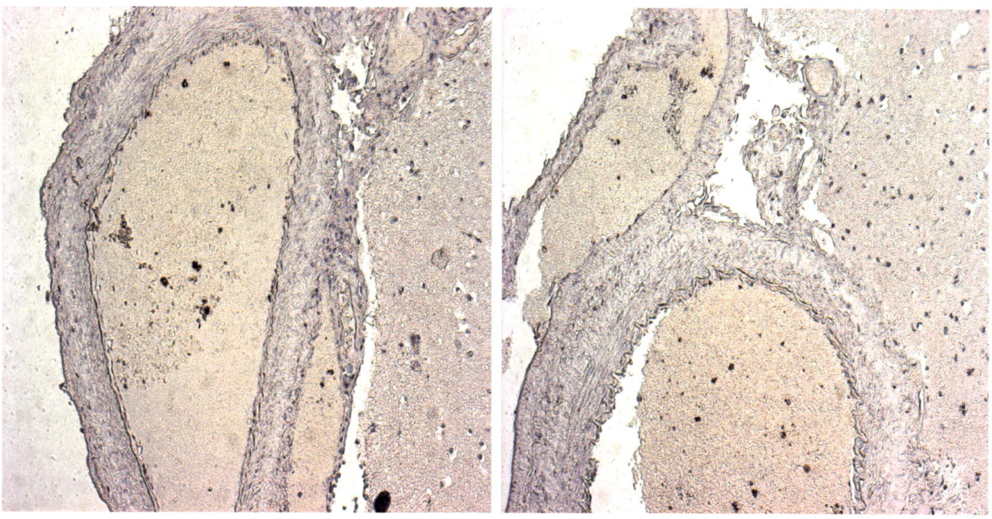

Fig. 1. Photos of hematoxylin staining of cerebral cortex of patients infected with NiV during the first outbreak in Malaysia, showing widespread vasculitis (personal data)

Patients show wide lymphoid necrosis associated to giant multinucleated cells that could be related to the presence of the NiV in this tissue. Virus may propagate initially within the lymphoid tissue, leading to the infection of the endothelial cells, recognized as the first primary targets of NiV. Those cells allow the second cycle of replication of the virus and the viremia.

NiV infection is characterized by the formation of syncytia leading to the endothelial damages, which are thought to be the cause of thrombosis, inflammation, ischemia and finally necrosis. Resulting vascular infarctions and infiltrates lead to extravascular infection and parenchymatous invasion. The invasion of the central nervous system is generally followed by the lethal encephalitis.

Patients who have survived the NiV infection showed severe weakness sometime persisting for several months, and often complicated by neurological and/or motor dysfunctions (Sejvar et al., 2007). Those symptoms appear as a direct consequence of the acute encephalitis. Indeed, those patients develop atrophy of the cerebellum, brainstem lesions, cortical nervous transmission abnormalities and are particularly affected in the white matter (Ng et al., 2004). In Malaysia, about 7,5% of patients who survived the encephalitis had relapsed during the year following their infection without any reexposure to virus. In addition, NiV can cause apparently asymptomatic infection leading to the late onset encephalitis several months to a year after infection (Tan et al., 2002). This fact suggests that the virus can infect more people than those showing clinical symptoms and may stay in latent stage until reactivation under the influence of some still unknown factors.

1.5 Vaccines and treatments

Several studies have been focused on the development of anti-NiV vaccines. The first study has shown that hamsters, vaccinated with vaccinia virus expressing either NiV F or G, were completely protected against NiV. Moreover, this group demonstrated that the naïve animals were also protected by passive transfer of hyperimmune serum prior to challenge (Guillaume et al., 2004). An important advance was next the development of a recombinant vaccine protecting pigs against NiV challenge (Weingartl et al., 2006). The Canarypox virus expressing NiV glycoproteins was shown to be very efficient in pigs and may have a real socio-economic interest in the case of new NiV outbreaks. Recently, one group showed induction of neutralizing antibodies to Henipavirus using an Alphavirus based vaccine (Defang et al., 2010). However, the study has been performed in mice which are not sensitive to NiV infection (Wong et al., 2003), preventing them from testing the efficiency of the vaccination.

Monoclonal antibodies against NiV glycoproteins were shown to protect 50% of infected hamsters even when treatments started 24 h post infection (Guillaume et al., 2006) and anti-NiV F monoclonal antibodies protected hamsters against Hendra virus infection as well (Guillaume et al., 2009). In addition, neutralizing human monoclonal antibody protected ferrets from NiV infection, when given 10 h after oronasal administration of the virus (Bossart et al., 2009).

Treatment of NiV infection was tested using some of known anti-viral chemicals: ribavirin (Chong et al., 2001), chloroquine (Pallister et al., 2009), gliotoxin, gentian violet and brilliant green (Aljofan et al., 2009). Most of those products showed an effect either *in vitro* or *in vivo* but with too low efficiency to consider them as a good treatment for infected patients, even if they were used combined (Freiberg et al., 2010). Finally, anti-fusion peptides were designed that specifically target the entry of Henipavirus (Porotto et al., 2010). To improve the efficiency of this potential treatment, this group has added a cholesterol tag, highly increasing the anti-viral efficiency and allowing peptides to reach brain and limit viral entry into cerebral cells, giving thus very promising results both *in vitro* and *in vivo* in hamsters (Porotto et al., 2010). This new anti-viral approach needs now to be tested in a primate model to consider its potential utilization in humans.

2. Global gene expression analysis of NiV infected endothelial cells, using microarrays

Profound changes are occurring in host cells during viral infections. These pathogen-induced changes are often accompanied by marked changes in gene expression and could be followed through the analysis of the specific RNA fingerprint related to each virus (Glass et al., 2003), (Jenner et al., 2005). For this purpose, microarrays present the essential tool to study global changes in gene expression and better understand which cellular mechanisms are modulated during the viral replication cycle. The aim of this study was to obtain a global overview of NiV effect on endothelial cells, in order to open new perspectives In treatment of this lethal infection.

Very little is known on pathogenesis of NiV infection. To obtain the global insight in different host cell changes during the infection, we have performed gene expression analysis using microarrays. *In vivo*, primary targets of this virus are endothelial cells, smooth muscles and neurons. The infection of microvascular endothelial cells leads to a generalized vasculitis, which is the common symptom diagnosed among all infected animals and humans. This vasculitis usually induces the acute encephalitis that is observed in severe NiV infection. Therefore, primary human endothelial cells were chosen as the most relevant host cell type to analyze the effect of NiV infection on the host cell gene expression.

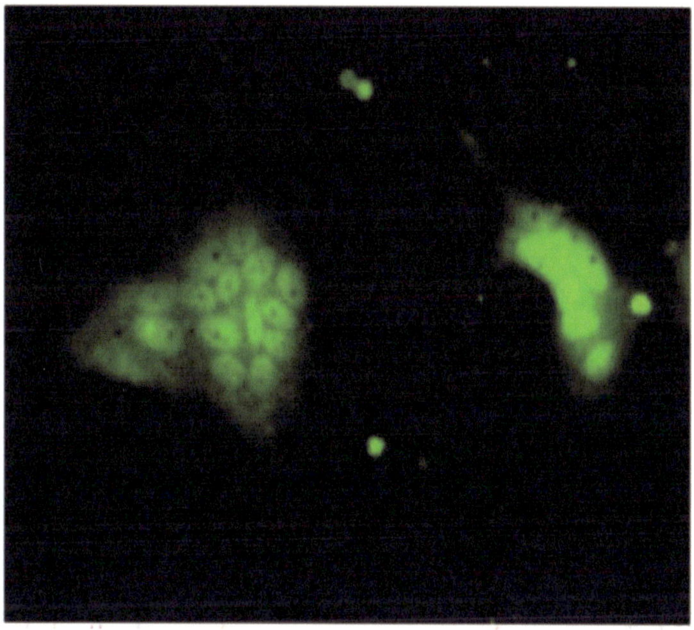

Fig. 2. HUVEC infected with the NiV recombinant strain expressing EGFP (MOI=1) for 24h and presenting a large syncytia, observed under the fluorescent microscope.

2.1 HUVEC culture and NiV infection

We have, thus, analyzed the effect of NiV infection in primary human umbilical vein endothelial cells (HUVEC). These cells are highly permissive to NiV infection and develop large syncytia rapidly after infection, as shown when recombinant NiV expressing the fluorescent green protein EGFP (Yoneda et al., 2006) is used for infection (Fig. 2). Primary HUVEC cells were isolated from umbilical cords of 6 donors (Jaffe et al., 1973). Cells were then transferred in a 75ml flask, precoated with gelatin 0,2% in PBS for 30 min and washed. The following day, cells were trypsinated to eliminate any dead or residual blood cells, and pooled by 2 sets of 3 donors and put in new flasks in order to cover 50% of the surface. After one week of culture, cells were submitted to 16 hours of serum privation just before their infection.

The infection was performed using wild type NiV (isolate UM-MC1, Gene accession N°AY029767) at MOI 1, in 2 sets of 3 different donors, in BSL4 Laboratory Jean Mérieux in Lyon, France.

2.2 Microarray experiments

Early changes associated to initial stages of NiV infection were analyzed by microarray approach (Fig. 3). Total RNAs were extracted from infected cells at 8h post infection and from uninfected cells (mock) cultured in the same conditions. Quality of total RNA was checked on Agilent bioanalyzer 2100. Amplified and biotin-labeled RNAs were obtained from 2µg of total RNA, using the Ambion message Amp kit version II. Different quantities of positive RNA controls (spikes) were added during the first step of reverse transcription of total RNAs. Spikes correspond to 6 bacterial RNAs used to control sensitivity, quality of hybridization and data normalization. Hybridization was performed on Codelink human whole genome bioarray (http://www.codelink bioarrays.com/) that is a 3-D aqueous gel matrix slide surface with 30-base oligonucleotide probes. This 3-D gel matrix provides an aqueous environment that allows an optimal interaction between probe and target and results to higher probe specificity and array sensitivity. Codelink uses a single color system (1 array/sample).

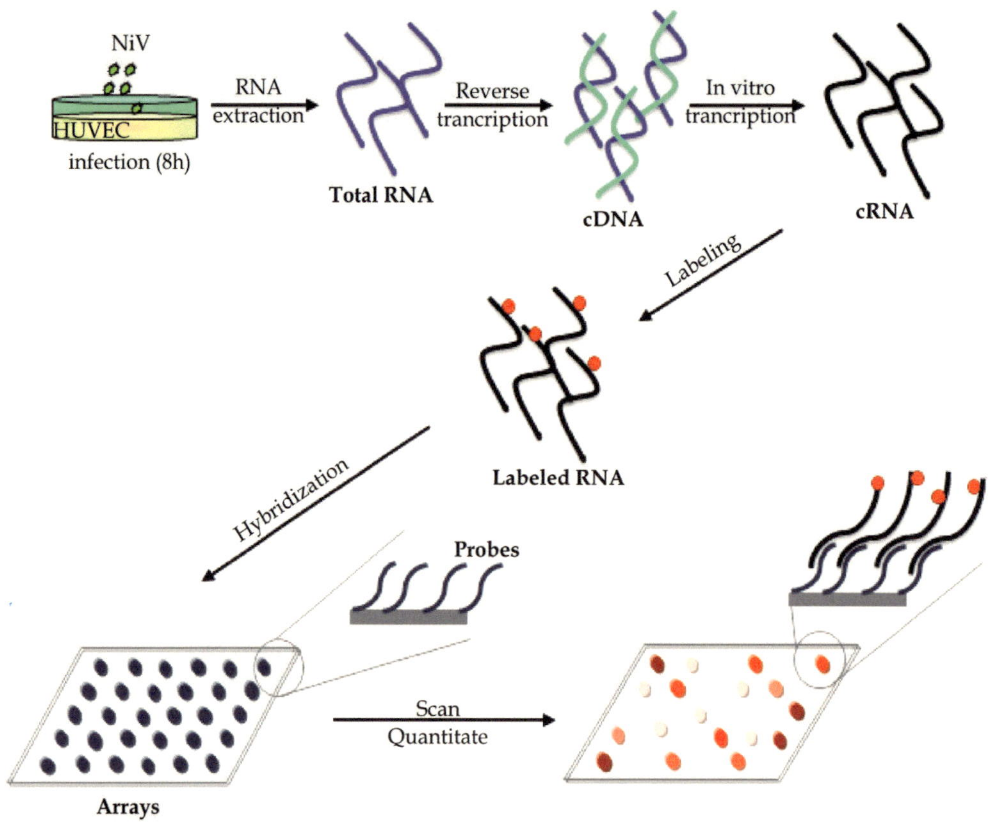

Fig. 3. Representation of the different steps necessary for the microarray analysis, starting from NiV infection of HUVEC cultures up to the analysis of microarrays.

Codelink human whole genome bioarray comprises approximately 55,000 30-mer probes on a single array based on the NCBI/Unigene database that permits the expression analysis of 57,347 transcripts and ESTs. In addition to these 55,000 probes, Codelink human whole genome bioarrays also contain one set of 100 housekeeping genes, 108 positive controls and 384 negative controls (bacterial genes). Hybridization, wash and revelation were performed using Codelink Expression Assay reagent kits. Then, chips were scanned using an Axon Genepix 4000B Scanner. Data extraction and raw data normalization were performed using the CodeLink Gene Expression Analysis v4.0 software. Normalization was performed by the global method. The threshold was calculated using the normalized signal intensity of the negative controls supplemented by 3 times the standard deviation. Spots with signal intensity below this threshold are referred to as "absent". Finally, data are converted to the excel format and data analysis is performed by using the Gene Spring v7.0 software from Agilent.

2.3 Microarray data analysis

The effect of NiV on the modulation of the genes expression was determined by permutation analysis and we considered as pertinent a minimal fold change (FC) of 1,3. Among the 55,000 targeted genes, 1076 genes were found to be differentially expressed in NiV-infected cells in comparison to non infected cells, including 807 up-regulated genes ($1.3 \leq FC \leq 23$) and 269 down-regulated ($-46 \leq FC \leq -1.3$) genes. These 807 up-regulated genes were then classified according to their Gene Ontology (GO) biological processes and their GO molecular functions. This system of clustering takes into account not only the number of genes but also the importance of the modulations in each function. Most of the cellular functions were modified after NiV infection (Fig. 4A). This could be explained by the modulation of some key genes involved in the large majority of the known functions. The most importantly modulated functions were those belonging to "Immune Response" with 37 differentially regulated genes (Table 1A) and to "Organism Abnormalities and Injuries" (22 genes), two functions that are usually altered in case of productive viral infection. Surprisingly, this analysis also revealed changes in the "neurological diseases" function (15 genes) and "nervous dysfunctions" (5 genes). This result could be correlated with the strong involvement of the endothelial cell-induced inflammatory reaction in the development of the encephalitis, as described in the introduction.

To refine the significance of these up-regulated genes, we next investigated the biological functions and interactions of these genes using Ingenuity Pathway Analysis (IPA) software. IPA allows genes that are differentially expressed to be placed in a physiological and biochemical context by grouping them according to canonical pathway and biological network with a statistical probability of validity, based on number of genes being differentially expressed in the respective pathway. This IPA analysis allowed us to identify that the most significantly modulated canonical pathway is the "interferon signaling" pathway ($p=0,01$) (Fig. 4 B). The majority of the top 15 up-regulated genes are related to the Interferon pathway (Table 1B). The involvement of the Interferon pathway has been proposed in the development of the other types of vasculitis, including the post-operative vasculitis (Abe et al., 2008). Four other canonical pathways were significantly found modified during the infection by NiV: "Antigen presentation", "Integrin signaling", "Protein Ubiquitination" and "Nicotinate and Nicotinamide Metabolism" pathways. Finally, IPA allowed us to demonstrate the existence of network of genes involved in the pathway of Gene expression, Cell Death, Connective tissue disorders (Fig. 5). Some of these gene, like TLR3 (Shaw et al., 2005) and CXCL10 (Lo et al., 2010), have been already shown to be associated to NiV infection, while the role of other genes rests to be demonstrated.

A

Gene	Accession number	Fold change
MX1	AF135187	23,253
IFI44L	NM_006820	14,528
CXCL10	NM_001565	10,93
OAS1	AU076579	8,6234
IFI44	NM_006417	5,7188
MX2	NM_002463	5,179
CCL8	NM_005623	4,8824
PLSCR1	AW439730	3,9274
CXCL11	NM_005409	3,538
TAP1	NM_000593	2,9255
TNFSF13B	AI446030	2,8342
STAT1	AK022231	2,5021
PSMB9	NM_002800	2,494
SP140	NM_007237	2,4399
IFI6	NM_002038	2,1447
IRF-1	NM_002198	1,9537
ZC3HAV1	BX108858	1,8427
STAT2	NM_005419	1,803
SECTM1	AA601122	1,7953
MYD88	NM_002468	1,7122
ISG20	NM_002201	1,6514
TRIM22	NM_006074	1,6078
PECAM1	BG739826	1,5874
HSPD1	NM_002156	1,5844
PSMB8	NM_004159	1,5805
TLR3	NM_003265	1,4589
IL15RA	NM_002189	1,4529
CCRL1	NM_016557	1,4023
HLA-E	NM_005516	1,383
CD47	NM_001777	1,3585
REV3L	NM_002912	-1,3367
MAPKAPK2	R97920	-1,36484
ABCA1	NM_005502	-1,40317
IL17RB	NM_018725	-1,55537
FKBP1A	BQ004596	-1,56654
CD1B	NM_001764	-2,1301
NRP1	AI285044	-2,24691

B

Gene	Accession number	Fold change
MX1	AF135187	23,253
IFIT1	NM_001548	19,764
IFIT3	NM_001549	10,793
OAS1	AU076579	8,6234
IFI35	NM_005533	3,3087
TAP1	NM_000593	2,9255
STAT1	AK022231	2,5021
IRF1	NM_002198	1,9537
STAT2	NM_005419	1,803
ISGF3G	NM_006084	1,7891
PSMB8	NM_004159	1,5805

C

CEB1	NM_016323	5,3687
FLJ20637	NM_017912	5,1178
BBAP	NM_138287	4,8868
ISG43	NM_017414	2,9878
TAP1	NM_000593	2,9255
LMP2	NM_002800	2,4940
RIG-B	NM_004223	2,4861
RO52	NM_003141	2,1784
FBG2	NM_018438	1,8813
IFP1	NM_021616	1,8357
IRF9;ISGF3	NM_006084	1,7891
PAD1	NM_005805	1,6306
RNF94	NM_006074	1,6078
MULE	NM_031407	1,5970
LMP7	NM_004159	1,5805
UNPH4	NM_006313	1,5614
EFP	NM_005082	1,5047
TRIM19	NM_033238	1,4574
TRIM5alpha	NM_033034	1,4573
FAT10	NM_006398	1,4544
USP34	BX099597	1,4495
NACSIN	NM_015252	1,4330
PSMA7L	NM_144662	1,4273
ARIH1	AI656728	1,3908
UBE2D3	BQ960542	1,3694
HRCA1	NM_007218	1,3652
APC4	NM_013367	1,3563

Table 1. Genes differentially expressed during NiV infection in the Immune Response (A), Interferon pathway (B), protein ubiquitination pathway (C).

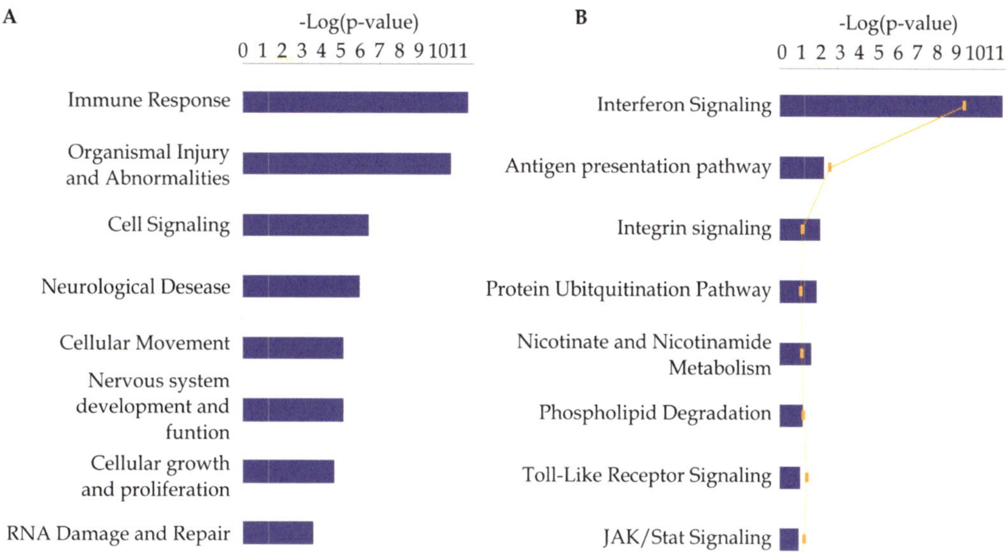

Fig. 4. Impact of NiV infection on biological functions (A) and canonical pathways (B), determined using Ingenuity Pathway Analysis.

Score	Focus Genes	Top Functions
56	35	Gene Expression, Cell Death, Connective Tissue Disorders
24	21	Organismal Injury and Abnormalities, Cellular Movement, Hematological System Development and Function
16	16	Cellular Movement, Hematological System Development and Function, Immune Response
16	16	Immune Response, Cell-To-Cell Signaling and Interaction, Hematological System Development and Function
16	16	Cell Death, Carbohydrate Metabolism, Cellular Assembly and Organization

Table 2. Putative Networks with high score, identified by Ingenuity Pathway Analysis

In addition, this IP analysis revealed that the 2 top putative networks with high score (> 20) were strongly associated with the "Connective Tissue Disorders" and the "Hematological System Development and Function" (Table 2). As microvascular basal lamina plays a critical role in brain injury (Wang & Shuaib, 2007), the loss of basal lamina components may reflect the degradation of proteins by proteolitic enzymes.

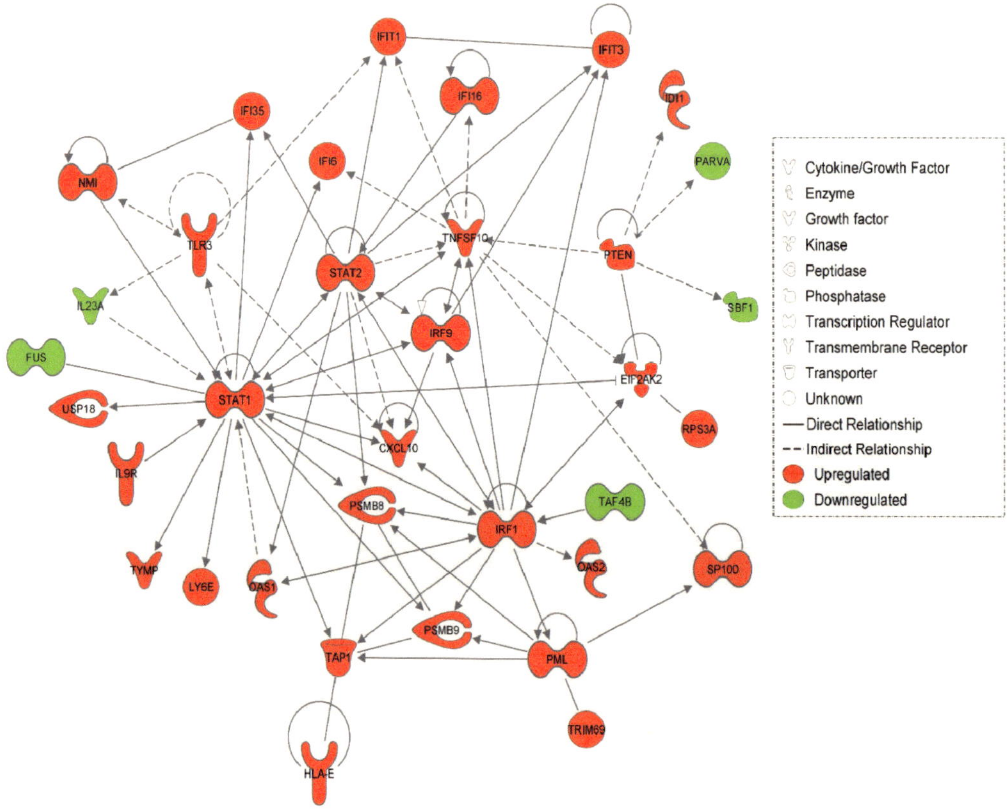

Fig. 5. Gene network identified in NiV infected HUVEC, compared to mock infected controls, reveals involvement of different genes within the pathways of Gene expression, Cell Death and Connective tissue disorders.

2.4 Validation of genes by quantitative real time PCR

To validate data obtained by microarray, we compared mRNA levels of several highest upregulated genes involved in the Immune response, between NiV infected and uninfected cells. These genes included Mx1, OAS1, CXCL10, CXCL11, PSMB9 (also known as LMP2) and RIGB. Total RNA were extracted 8 hours post-infection. Reverse transcriptions were performed on 0,5 µg of total RNA using the iScript cDNA synthesis kit (Bio-Rad) and run in Biometra® T-GRADIENT PCR devise. Obtained cDNAs were diluted 1/10. Quantitative PCR was performed using Platinum® SYBR® Green qPCR SuperMix-UDG with ROX kit (Invitrogen™). qPCR was run on the ABI 7000 PCR system (Applied biosystems) using the following protocol: 95°C 5', and 40 cycles of 95°C 15'', 60°C 1', followed by a melting curve up to 95°C at 0.8°C intervals. All samples were run in duplicate and results were analyzed using ABI Prism 7000 SDS software available in the genetic analysis platform (IFR128 BioSciences Lyon-Gerland). Glyceraldehyde 3-phosphate dehydrogenase (GAPDH) was used as housekeeping gene for viral mRNA quantification and normalization. GAPDH and standard references for the corresponding genes were included in each run to standardize results in respect to RNA integrity, loaded quantity and inter-PCR variations. Primers used were design using Beacon 7.0 software, and validated for their efficacy close to 100%: RiGB for: ATCATCAGCAGTGAGAAC, RiGB rev: GAACTCTTCGGCATTCTT, LMP2 for: GGTCAGGTATATGGAACC, LMP2 rev: CATTGCCCAAGATGACTC, GAPDH for: CACCCACTCCTCCACCTTTGAC, GAPDH rev: GTCCACCACCCTGTTGCTGTAG. The relative expression represents the ratio of the number of copy of mRNA of interest versus mRNA of GAPDH. All calculations were done using the $2^{\Delta\Delta CT}$ model of (Pfaffl, 2001) and experiments were performed according to the MIQE guideline (Bustin et al., 2009).

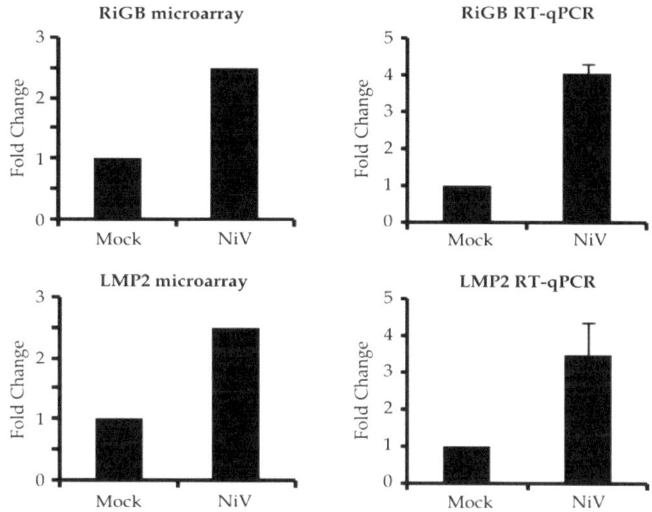

Fig. 6. Example of genes used for the validation of the microarray data. Results obtained from the microarray are shown on the left, whereas RT-qPCR data for the same gene are shown on the right.

2.5 Focus on some genes of interest

Among the cellular pathways activated during the NiV infection, we have particularly focused our attention to the interferon related genes. We have observed that similarly to the other Paramyxoviruses, NiV strongly activates the immune response through the canonical interferon signaling pathway. An over expression of some interferon related genes is known to lead to the activation of several genes related to the proteasome and the ubiquitination pathway. Those genes are involved in loading and expression of the CMH class 1 at the cell surface. In fact, any imbalances in this system can lead to a strong deregulation, resulting in inflammation that could not be controlled by host homeostatic mecahanisms (example: lupus erythematous, (Baechler et al., 2004). TAP1/2 and LMP2 (PSMB9) are the major proteins involved in this system, and both were shown to be up-regulated during NiV infection of endothelial cells (Table 1). The expression of those proteins is regulated by Interferon related proteins called Signal Transducer and Activator of Transcription 1α (STAT1α) and Interferon Regulatory Factor 1 (IRF1) (Chatterjee-Kishore et al., 1998). In normal conditions, TAP1 and 2 are expressed at a basal level in cells, whereas LMP2 is not found (Wright et al., 1995). Our results show that NiV infection increases TAP1 expression without any changes in TAP2. Moreover, LMP2 was also induced. An imbalance in the expression of those proteins that are the major components of the immunoproteasome, are in certain cases responsible for important phenomena of autoimmunity leading to severe

damages on the endothelium, including systemic vasculitis in case of Lupus (Zimmer et al., 1998) and may be therefore involved in the pathogenesis of NiV induced vasculitis.
In addition, our results revealed NiV-induced up regulation of HERC5 (FC=5,37), which belongs to the E3 ubiquitin ligases family. This protein has been shown to be tightly controlled under inflammatory conditions in endothelial cells (Kroismayr et al., 2004). The critical role of Tumor necrosis factor α, Interleukin 1β and NF-KB was suggested in the regulation of this protein. Although we have observed an over expression of TNFSF13b in the NiV infected HUVEC, modulation of IL1β or NF-KB was not found, suggesting another cascade of NiV-induced activation of HERC5.
Virus infection is known to induce a specific chemokine production in infected cells. This chemokine response is often related to the detection of viral genomes by Toll like receptor (TLR) system. Depending on the combination of TLRs involved in this mechanism it will lead to a specific signature of expression. For example, the closely related Measles virus induces several chemokines CCL2, CCL3, CCL4, CCL5 and CXCL10 (Glass et al., 2003). Only CXCL10, CXCL11 and CCL8 were induced by NiV infection in HUVEC (Table 1), suggesting a high capacity of NiV to provoke an imbalance of cell signaling, leading to a miss regulation of inflammation. These results are in accord with demonstrated changes in cytokine production by endothelial cells (Lo et al., 2010). The strong involvement of Interferon related genes in the vasculitis has been described before, but the induction of the monocyte chemoattractant CCL8 remains unclear in the context of a viral infection. Indeed, very few viruses are inducing this protein (Glass et al., 2003). Nevertheless, CCL8 has been shown to be involved in many inflammatory diseases including rheumatoid arthritis (Galligan et al., 2007), (Ockinger et al., 2010) and Graft versus host diseases (Bouazzaoui et al., 2009). The functional importance of CC chemokine ligand genes has been demonstrated in experimental autoimmune encephalomyelitis and multiple sclerosis (Mahad et al., 2004), (Savarin-Vuaillat & Ransohoff 2007). CCL8 is overexpressed by astrocytes and microglia leading to the over recruitment of monocytes and macrophages to the lesions (Vyshkina et al., 2008). This result suggests the importance of regulation of CCL8 either at the genomic level or within the chemokine network, when the virus reaches the brain.
Furthermore, within genes involved in the cellular movement function NiV induced the expression of ADAM 12 (FC=2,38). This protein is a metalloprotease proposed to function as a regulator of fusion of several cell types, including trophoblast and myoblast (Huppertz et al., 2006). This protein also modulates the cell fusion in giant cell tumors of long bones (Meng et al., 2005), by inducing actin cytoskeleton reorganization. This reorganization could be associated to the remodeling of actin induced by NiV binding to its receptor and consequent EFNB2 signaling. In addition to the capacity of ADAM12 to reorganize the extracellular matrix, its over expression in endothelial cells could be related not only to the syncytia formation but also to microvascular basal lamina damages. This phenomenon causes dismantlement of the endothelial wall structure (Wang & Shuaib, 2007). Such microvascular permeability in the brain could compromise the microcirculation by increasing the risk of ischemia and the exposure of this compartment to the immune system, leading thus to an important vascular and perivascular inflammation.

3. Conclusions

NiV is a highly lethal zoonotic pathogen that can cause important socio-economical and health problems. This virus induces a generalized vasculitis leading to the disruption of the endothelial microvascular tissue in brain and inducing severe damages in the CNS. Micorarray analysis of NiV infected primary endothelial cells allowed us to obtain a global overview of the host cell responses to NiV early during the infection. This global approach revealed that NiV infection has an important impact in several pathways and functions that are directly related to the pathogenesis observed in patients and animals. The analysis revealed a high induction of the immune response through the important modulation of genes in the Interferon signaling pathway, Antigen presentation pathway and the Protein ubiquitination pathway. We focused our analysis on several highly induced genes which could be involved in the control of the vascular inflammation and disruption of endothelium, allowing the passage of the virus in the organs. The early NiV infection of endothelial cells importantly upregulated the chemokines TNFSF13B, CXCL10, CXCL11 and CCL8 that are involved in many processes of autoimmune diseases as well as proteins belonging to the ubiquitination pathway. More precisely, TAP1 and LMP2 were overexpressed during the infection. NiV-induced sustained inflammatory conditions and modified regulation of the immunoproteasome expression could lead to an imbalance of the MHC class 1 exposure at the surface of cells, inducing haemostatic disturbance during NiV infection. This study presents the first comprehensive analysis of global host transcriptional response to NiV infection. Obtained results shed new light to early stage of NiV pathogenesis and should help in understanding the host response to this virus and open perspectives for design of treatment for this emerging lethal infectious disease.

4. Acknowledgements

The authors are grateful to the members of ProfileXpert plateform (IFR19, Lyon), especially to Dr. J. Lachuer and N. Nazareth for the technical help in the microarray analysis. In addition, we thank Drs A. Sabine and V. Guillaume (INSERM U758) for the help in the generation of HUVEC and initial viral infections and K.T. Wong (University of Malaya, Malaysia) for providing the histological samples from NiV patients. The work was supported by INSERM, University Claude Bernard Lyon1, Cluster 10 of Infectiology, ANR MIME and ANR-09-MIEN-018-01.

5. References

Abe, T., Kenji S., Masaki M., Kouhei O, Keisuke I., Tohru K., Takamitsu H., & al. 2008. Possible involvement of interferon beta in post-operative vasculitis restricted to the tumour bed: a case report ». *Neurosurgical Review* 31 (4): 447-450; discussion 450. doi:10.1007/s10143-008-0149-1.

Aljofan, M., M. L., Sganga, M. K Lo, C. L Rootes, M. Porotto, A. G Meyer, S. Saubern, A. Moscona, & BA Mungall. 2009. « Antiviral activity of gliotoxin, gentian violet and brilliant green against Nipah and Hendra virus in vitro ». *Virology Journal* 6: 187. doi:10.1186/1743-422X-6-187.

Baechler, E. C, P. K Gregersen, & T. W Behrens. 2004. « The emerging role of interferon in human systemic lupus erythematosus ». *Current Opinion in Immunology* 16 (6): 801-807. doi:10.1016/j.coi.2004.09.014.

Bossart, K. N, L-F Wang, M. N Flora, K. B. Chua, S. K. Lam, B. T Eaton, & C. C Broder. 2002. « Membrane fusion tropism and heterotypic functional activities of the Nipah virus and Hendra virus envelope glycoproteins ». *Journal of Virology* 76 (22): 11186-11198.

Bossart, K. N, Z. Zhu, D. Middleton, J. Klippel, G. Crameri, J. Bingham, J. A McEachern, & al. 2009. « A neutralizing human monoclonal antibody protects against lethal disease in a new ferret model of acute nipah virus infection ». *PLoS Pathogens* 5 (10): e1000642. doi:10.1371/journal.ppat.1000642.

Bouazzaoui, A, E Spacenko, G Mueller, S M., E Huber, E Holler, R Andreesen, & G C Hildebrandt. 2009. « Chemokine and chemokine receptor expression analysis in target organs of acute graft-versus-host disease ». *Genes and Immunity* 10 (8): 687-701. doi:10.1038/gene.2009.49.

Bustin, S. A, V. Benes, J. A Garson, J. Hellemans, J. Huggett, M. Kubista, R Mueller, & al. 2009. « The MIQE guidelines: minimum information for publication of quantitative real-time PCR experiments ». *Clinical Chemistry* 55 (4): 611-622. doi:10.1373/clinchem.2008.112797.

Chatterjee-Kishore, M, R Kishore, D J Hicklin, F M Marincola, & S Ferrone. 1998. « Different requirements for signal transducer and activator of transcription 1alpha and interferon regulatory factor 1 in the regulation of low molecular mass polypeptide 2 and transporter associated with antigen processing 1 gene expression ». *The Journal of Biological Chemistry* 273 (26): 16177-16183.

Chong, H T, A Kamarulzaman, C T Tan, K J Goh, T Thayaparan, S R Kunjapan, N K Chew, K B Chua, & S K Lam. 2001. « Treatment of acute Nipah encephalitis with ribavirin ». *Annals of Neurology* 49 (6): 810-813.

Defang, G., N, D., Khetawat, C Broder, & G. V., Quinnan. 2010. « Induction of neutralizing antibodies to Hendra and Nipah glycoproteins using a Venezuelan equine encephalitis virus in vivo expression system ». *Vaccine* 29 (2): 212-220. doi:10.1016/j.vaccine.2010.10.053.

Drexler, J F, V M Corman, F Gloza-Rausch, A Seebens, A Annan, A Ipsen, T Kruppa, et al. 2009. « Henipavirus RNA in African bats ». *PloS One* 4 (7): e6367. doi:10.1371/journal.pone.0006367.

Eaton, B T, C C Broder, D Middleton, & L-F Wang. 2006. « Hendra and Nipah viruses: different and dangerous ». *Nature Reviews. Microbiology* 4 (1): 23-35. doi:10.1038/nrmicro1323.

Fontana, J M, B Bankamp, & P A Rota. 2008. « Inhibition of interferon induction and signaling by paramyxoviruses ». *Immunological Reviews* 225: 46-67. doi:10.1111/j.1600-065X.2008.00669.x.

Freiberg, A N, M N Worthy, B Lee, & M R Holbrook. 2010. « Combined chloroquine and ribavirin treatment does not prevent death in a hamster model of Nipah and Hendra virus infection ». *The Journal of General Virology* 91 (Pt 3): 765-772. doi:10.1099/vir.0.017269-0.

Galligan, C L, E Baig, V Bykerk, E C Keystone, & E N Fish. 2007. « Distinctive gene expression signatures in rheumatoid arthritis synovial tissue fibroblast cells: correlates with disease activity ». *Genes and Immunity* 8 (6): 480-491. doi:10.1038/sj.gene.6364400.

Glass, W G, H F Rosenberg, & P M Murphy. 2003. « Chemokine regulation of inflammation during acute viral infection ». *Current Opinion in Allergy and Clinical Immunology* 3 (6): 467-473. doi:10.1097/01.all.0000104448.09202.91.

Guillaume, V, H Contamin, P Loth, M-C Georges-Courbot, A Lefeuvre, P Marianneau, K B Chua, et al. 2004. « Nipah virus: vaccination and passive protection studies in a hamster model ». *Journal of Virology* 78 (2): 834-840.

Guillaume, V, H Contamin, P Loth, I Grosjean, M C Georges Courbot, V Deubel, R Buckland, & T F Wild. 2006. « Antibody prophylaxis and therapy against Nipah virus infection in hamsters ». *Journal of Virology* 80 (4): 1972-1978. doi:10.1128/JVI.80.4.1972-1978.2006.

Guillaume, V, K T Wong, R Y Looi, M-C Georges-Courbot, L Barrot, R Buckland, T F Wild, & B Horvat. 2009. « Acute Hendra virus infection: Analysis of the pathogenesis and passive antibody protection in the hamster model ». *Virology* 387 (2): 459-465. doi:10.1016/j.virol.2009.03.001.

Gurley, E., J. Montgomery, M. J. Hossain, M. Bell, A. K. Azad, M. R. Islam, M. A. Molla, D. S. Carroll, T. G. Ksiazek, P. A. Rota, L. Lowe, J. A. Comer, P. Rollin, M. Czub, A. Grolla, H. Feldmann, S. P. Luby, J. L. Woodward, & R. F. Breiman. 2007. «Person-to-person transmission of Nipah virus in a Bangladeshi community«. *Emerging Infectious Diseases* 13:1031-7.

Halpin, Kim, & BA Mungall. 2007. « Recent progress in henipavirus research ». *Comparative Immunology, Microbiology and Infectious Diseases* 30 (5-6): 287-307. doi:10.1016/j.cimid.2007.05.008.

Huppertz, B, C Bartz, & M Kokozidou. 2006. « Trophoblast fusion: fusogenic proteins, syncytins and ADAMs, and other prerequisites for syncytial fusion ». *Micron (Oxford, England: 1993)* 37 (6): 509-517. doi:10.1016/j.micron.2005.12.011.

Iehlé, C, G Razafitrimo, J Razainirina, N Andriaholinirina, S M Goodman, C Faure, M-C Georges-Courbot, D Rousset, & J-M Reynes. 2007. « Henipavirus and Tioman virus antibodies in pteropodid bats, Madagascar ». *Emerging Infectious Diseases* 13 (1): 159-161.

Jaffe, E A, R L Nachman, C G Becker, & C R Minick. 1973. « Culture of human endothelial cells derived from umbilical veins. Identification by morphologic and immunologic criteria ». *The Journal of Clinical Investigation* 52 (11): 2745-2756. doi:10.1172/JCI107470.

Jenner, R G., & R A. Young. 2005. « Insights into host responses against pathogens from transcriptional profiling ». *Nat Rev Micro* 3 (4): 281-294. doi:10.1038/nrmicro1126.

Kroismayr, R, U Baranyi, C Stehlik, A Dorfleutner, B R Binder, & J Lipp. 2004. « HERC5, a HECT E3 ubiquitin ligase tightly regulated in LPS activated endothelial cells ». *Journal of Cell Science* 117 (Pt 20): 4749-4756. doi:10.1242/jcs.01338.

Lamb, RA, & GD Parks. 2007. Paramyxoviridae: the viruses and their replication. *Fields virology*, 1449-1496. 5e éd. Philadelphia: Lippincott Williams & Wilkins.

Lee, B. 2007. « Envelope-receptor interactions in Nipah virus pathobiology ». *Annals of the New York Academy of Sciences* 1102: 51-65. doi:10.1196/annals.1408.004.

Lo, M K, D Miller, M Aljofan, BA Mungall, P E Rollin, W J Bellini, & P A Rota. 2010. « Characterization of the antiviral and inflammatory responses against Nipah virus in endothelial cells and neurons ». *Virology* 404 (1): 78-88.

Luby, S P, M Rahman, MJ Hossain, L S Blum, M M Husain, E Gurley, R Khan, et al. 2006. « Foodborne transmission of Nipah virus, Bangladesh ». *Emerging Infectious Diseases* 12 (12): 1888-1894.

Luby, S. P., E. S. Gurley, & M. J. Hossain. 2009. «Transmission of human infection with Nipah virus«. *Clinical Infectious Diseases* 49:1743-8.

Mahad, D J, C Trebst, P Kivisäkk, S M Staugaitis, B Tucky, T Wei, C F Lucchinetti, H Lassmann, & R M Ransohoff. 2004. « Expression of chemokine receptors CCR1 and CCR5 reflects differential activation of mononuclear phagocytes in pattern II and pattern III multiple sclerosis lesions ». *Journal of Neuropathology and Experimental Neurology* 63 (3): 262-273.

Maisner, A, J Neufeld, & H Weingartl. 2009. « Organ- and endotheliotropism of Nipah virus infections in vivo and in vitro ». *Thrombosis and Haemostasis* 102 (6): 1014-1023. doi:10.1160/TH09-05-0310.

Meng, Xue-mei, S-feng Yu, Min Lu, Jie Zheng, & Zhi-hui Han. 2005. « [Expression of macrophage inflammatory protein-1alpha, a disintegrin-like and metalloproteinase 8 and 12, and CD68 protein in giant cell lesions of jaw and giant cell tumors of long bone] ». *Zhonghua Bing Li Xue Za Zhi Chinese Journal of Pathology* 34 (7): 393-396.

Nahar, N, R Sultana, ES Gurley, MJ Hossain, & S P Luby. 2010. « Date palm sap collection: exploring opportunities to prevent Nipah transmission ». *EcoHealth* 7 (2): 196-203. doi:10.1007/s10393-010-0320-3.

Negrete, O A, D Chu, Hr C Aguilar, & B Lee. 2007. « Single amino acid changes in the Nipah and Hendra virus attachment glycoproteins distinguish ephrinB2 from ephrinB3 usage ». *Journal of Virology* 81 (19): 10804-10814. doi:10.1128/JVI.00999-07.

Negrete, O A, E L Levroney, H C Aguilar, A Bertolotti-Ciarlet, R Nazarian, S Tajyar, & B Lee. 2005. « EphrinB2 is the entry receptor for Nipah virus, an emergent deadly paramyxovirus ». *Nature* 436 (7049): 401-405. doi:10.1038/nature03838.

Negrete, O A, M C Wolf, H C Aguilar, S Enterlein, W Wang, E Mühlberger, S V Su, A Bertolotti-Ciarlet, R Flick, & B Lee. 2006. « Two key residues in ephrinB3 are critical for its use as an alternative receptor for Nipah virus ». *PLoS Pathogens* 2 (2): e7. doi:10.1371/journal.ppat.0020007.

Ng, B-Y, C C Tchoyoson Lim, A Yeoh, & WL Lee. 2004. « Neuropsychiatric sequelae of Nipah virus encephalitis ». *The Journal of Neuropsychiatry and Clinical Neurosciences* 16 (4): 500-504. doi:10.1176/appi.neuropsych.16.4.500.

Ockinger, J, P Stridh, A D Beyeen, F Lundmark, M Seddighzadeh, A Oturai, P S Sørensen, et al. 2010. « Genetic variants of CC chemokine genes in experimental autoimmune encephalomyelitis, multiple sclerosis and rheumatoid arthritis ». *Genes and Immunity* 11 (2): 142-154. doi:10.1038/gene.2009.82.

Pallister, J, D Middleton, G Crameri, M Yamada, R Klein, T J Hancock, A Foord, et al. 2009. « Chloroquine administration does not prevent Nipah virus infection and disease in ferrets ». *Journal of Virology* 83 (22): 11979-11982. doi:10.1128/JVI.01847-09.

Pfaffl, M W. 2001. « A new mathematical model for relative quantification in real-time RT-PCR ». *Nucleic Acids Research* 29 (9): e45.

Porotto, M, B Rockx, CC Yokoyama, A Talekar, I Devito, L M Palermo, J Liu, et al. 2010. « Inhibition of Nipah virus infection in vivo: targeting an early stage of paramyxovirus fusion activation during viral entry ». *PLoS Pathogens* 6 (10): e1001168. doi:10.1371/journal.ppat.1001168.

Porotto, M, CC Yokoyama, L M Palermo, B Mungall, M Aljofan, R Cortese, A Pessi, & Anne Moscona. 2010. « Viral entry inhibitors targeted to the membrane site of action ». *Journal of Virology* 84 (13): 6760-6768. doi:10.1128/JVI.00135-10.

Salah Uddin Khan, M, J Hossain, ES Gurley, N Nahar, R Sultana, & S P Luby. 2011. « Use of Infrared Camera to Understand Bats' Access to Date Palm Sap: Implications for Preventing Nipah Virus Transmission ». *EcoHealth*. doi:10.1007/s10393-010-0366-2. http://www.ncbi.nlm.nih.gov.gate2.inist.fr/pubmed/21207105.

Sato, H, R Honma, M Yoneda, R Miura, K Tsukiyama-Kohara, F Ikeda, T Seki, S Watanabe, & C Kai. 2008. « Measles virus induces cell-type specific changes in gene expression ». *Virology* 375 (2): 321-330. doi:10.1016/j.virol.2008.02.015.

Savarin-Vuaillat, C, & R M Ransohoff. 2007. « Chemokines and chemokine receptors in neurological disease: raise, retain, or reduce? » *Neurotherapeutics: The Journal of the American Society for Experimental NeuroTherapeutics* 4 (4): 590-601. doi:10.1016/j.nurt.2007.07.004.

Sejvar, J J, J Hossain, S K Saha, ES Gurley, S Banu, J D Hamadani, M A Faiz, et al. 2007. « Long-term neurological and functional outcome in Nipah virus infection ». *Annals of Neurology* 62 (3): 235-242. doi:10.1002/ana.21178.

Shaw ML, Cardenas WB, Zamarin D, Palese P, Basler CF. 2005 « Nuclear localization of the Nipah virus W protein allows for inhibition of both virus- and toll-like receptor 3-triggered signaling pathways ». *Journal of Virolology* 79 (10): 6078-6088.

Tan, C T, K J Goh, K T Wong, S A Sarji, K B Chua, N K Chew, Paramsothy Murugasu, et al. 2002. « Relapsed and late-onset Nipah encephalitis ». *Annals of Neurology* 51 (6): 703-708. doi:10.1002/ana.10212.

Vyshkina, T, A Sylvester, S Sadiq, E Bonilla, A Perl, & B Kalman. 2008. « CCL genes in multiple sclerosis and systemic lupus erythematosus ». *Journal of Neuroimmunology* 200 (1-2): 145-152. doi:10.1016/j.jneuroim.2008.05.016.

Wang, CX, & A Shuaib. 2007. « Critical role of microvasculature basal lamina in ischemic brain injury ». *Progress in Neurobiology* 83 (3): 140-148. doi:10.1016/j.pneurobio.2007.07.006.

Wang, L, B H Harcourt, M Yu, A Tamin, P A Rota, W J Bellini, & B T Eaton. 2001. « Molecular biology of Hendra and Nipah viruses ». *Microbes and Infection / Institut Pasteur* 3 (4): 279-287.

Weingartl, HM, Y Berhane, J L Caswell, S Loosmore, J-C Audonnet, J A Roth, & M Czub. 2006. « Recombinant nipah virus vaccines protect pigs against challenge ». *Journal of Virology* 80 (16): 7929-7938. doi:10.1128/JVI.00263-06.

Wong, K T, I Grosjean, C Brisson, B Blanquier, M Fevre-Montange, A Bernard, P Loth, et al. 2003. « A golden hamster model for human acute Nipah virus infection ». *The American Journal of Pathology* 163 (5): 2127-2137. doi:10.1016/S0002-9440(10)63569-9.

Wright, K L, L C White, A Kelly, S Beck, J Trowsdale, & J P Ting. 1995. « Coordinate regulation of the human TAP1 and LMP2 genes from a shared bidirectional promoter ». *The Journal of Experimental Medicine* 181 (4): 1459-1471.

Yoneda, M, V Guillaume, Fusako Ikeda, Y Sakuma, H Sato, T F Wild, & C Kai. 2006. « Establishment of a Nipah virus rescue system ». *Proceedings of the National Academy of Sciences of the United States of America* 103 (44): 16508-16513. doi:10.1073/pnas.0606972103.

Zimmer, J, L Donato, D Hanau, J P Cazenave, M M Tongio, A Moretta, & H de la Salle. 1998. « Activity and phenotype of natural killer cells in peptide transporter (TAP)-deficient patients (type I bare lymphocyte syndrome) ». *The Journal of Experimental Medicine* 187 (1): 117-122.

2

Takayasu's Arteritis and Its Potential Pathogenic Association with *Mycobacterium tuberculosis*

Luis M. Amezcua-Guerra[1,2] and Diana Castillo-Martínez[3]
[1]*Department of Immunology, Instituto Nacional de Cardiología Ignacio Chávez*
[2]*La Salle University School of Medicine*
[3]*Department of Dermatology, Hospital General de Zona 2-A, Instituto Mexicano del Seguro Social*
Mexico

1. Introduction

Takayasu's arteritis is an idiopathic, inflammatory disease which involves large- and medium-sized arteries, specially the aorta, its major branches and the pulmonary arteries. In contrast to other vasculitides, Takayasu's arteritis is restricted to certain geographical areas. Initially thought to be confined to Japan and Korea, it has now been reported with increased frequency in Mexico, India, China, South America, South Africa, and the Mediterranean basin; while, the disease continues to be exceptionally described in individuals from the United States, North and Central Europe and other high-income regions.

The etiology of Takayasu's arteritis is unclear and attempts to clarify it are still limited. There are clinical and laboratory features suggesting an autoimmune basis, while others raise a question that aortitis may be the expression of delayed-type hypersensitivity reaction to tuberculin or other sensitizers. Finally, the occurrence of Takayasu's arteritis in homozygotic twins suggests a genetic background for predisposition.

A possible relationship between Takayasu's arteritis with both latent and active tuberculosis was suggested long time ago. Both diseases show similar chronic inflammatory lesions on histology, with occasional granuloma formation into the arterial walls. Delayed hypersensitivity to tuberculin is frequently found to be increased in patients with Takayasu's arteritis from almost all ethnicities. Isolated cases of Takayasu's arteritis coexisting with both latent and active tuberculosis, and improvement of arteritis after antituberculous treatment have been occasionally described. Finally, there are studies showing increased humoral and cellular immune responses directed toward mycobacterial 65 kDa heat shock protein (HSP) and its human homolog 60 kDa HSP. All these indirect evidences support that *Mycobacterium tuberculosis* and probably other mycobacteria may play a role in the immunopathogenesis of Takayasu's arteritis, possibly through molecular mimicry mechanisms; however, results of several recent studies are challenging this old but still valid etiopathogenic hypothesis of association. Analyzing this possible link is not futile because the potential risk of using anti-tumour necrosis factor (TNF) therapies in the treatment of patients with Takayasu's arteritis and the increasing use of Bacille Calmette-Guérin (BCG) for vaccination purposes around the world.

In this chapter we will discuss the main epidemiological, immunological and genetic evidence supporting and rejecting the existence of a pathogenic link between Takayasu's arteritis and *Mycobacterium tuberculosis*, to conclude hypothesizing on a novel, unifying pathogenic model that may explain the intricate relationship between tuberculosis and Takayasu's arteritis.

2. Overview on the history of Takayasu's arteritis

In 1830, Rokushu Yamamoto described a 45-year-old man with fever, pulselessness, loss of weight and breathlessness, who finally died after 11 years of follow-up and probably represents the first patient case reported in the literature. In 1905, Mikito Takayasu described a 21-year-old woman with ocular changes consisting of a peculiar capillary flush in the ocular fundi, a wreathlike arteriovenous anastomosis around the papillae, and blindness due to cataracts; even though, Professor Takayasu did not indicate if other arteries were involved. However, in the discussion of that case, Onishi and Kagoshima pointed out in two additional cases with similar ocular findings along the absence of the radial pulses. In 1948, Shimizu and Sano detailed the clinical features of the disorder, which was termed Takayasu's arteritis by first time in 1954 (Tann et al., 2008; Lupi-Herrera et al., 1977). Nowadays, both clinical manifestations and imaging findings typical of Takayasu's arteritis are adequately outlined, and different sets of classification criteria have been proposed and validated (Amezcua-Guerra & Pineda, 2007).

3. What is the Takayasu's arteritis?

Takayasu's arteritis is an idiopathic, chronic inflammatory disease which involves large- and medium-sized arteries, specially the aorta, its major branches and the pulmonary arteries, although virtually any arterial territory may be involved (Lupi et al., 1975; de Pablo et al., 2007; Pineda et al., 2003).

On the histological study, aortic sections reveal thickening of the adventitia, leukocyte infiltration of the tunica media and hyperplasia of the intimae. It has been postulated that *vasa vasorum* may act as the portal of entry for infiltrating inflammatory cells, which are mainly constituted by activated dendritic cells, several subsets of T lymphocytes, B lymphocytes, macrophages and multinucleated giant cells (Weyand & Goronzy, 2003). Hyperplasia of the intimae results from myofibroblast proliferation driven by growth factors such as the platelet-derived growth factor, which ultimately leads to fibrosis and to the development of arterial stenosis and occlusions typical of the late-stage disease. Occasionally, interstitial release of matrix metalloproteases and reactive oxygen species may induce arterial wall damage with formation of local aneurysms (Mason, 2010).

4. Influence of geography and ethnicity on the clinical expression of Takayasu's arteritis

In contrast to other vasculitides, Takayasu's arteritis is restricted to certain geographical areas around the world. Initially it was thought to be confined to Japan and Korea, but Takayasu's arteritis has been reported with increased frequency in Mexico, India, China, South America, South Africa, Israel, and the Mediterranean basin (specially in Iberian and

Italic Peninsulas); while, the disease continues to be exceptionally described in individuals from the United States, North and Central Europe and other high-income regions (Pantell & Goodman, 1981).

In essence, Takayasu's arteritis is a disease of childhood and early adulthood, with three quarters of patients initiating before the age of 20 years (Lupi-Herrera et al., 1977); nonetheless, there is a wide range of presenting age with anecdotal cases initiating as early as 2 years old (Ladhani et al., 2001). To date, Takayasu's arteritis is the third commonest vasculitis during childhood worldwide, and is responsible for more than half of cases with renovascular hypertension in young individuals (Tann et al., 2008; Kumar et al., 2003).

As regards to gender distribution, almost all available reports agree that the disease is more common in women, although the ratio varies by geographical affiliation of each population. While in Mexico it is reported that up to 84% of patients with Takayasu's arteritis are women (female/male ratio, 8.5 to 1) (Lupi-Herrera et al., 1977), the disease seems to occur almost equally in both genders (female/male ratio, 1.58 to 1) in patients from India (Chhetri et al., 1974).

Mortality rates associated with Takayasu's arteritis are high and also vary geographically. In Mexico, a retrospective analysis showed that 16 of the 107 cases died (overall mortality 14%) from causes directly related to arteritis (heart and renal failure, myocardial infarction, stroke, rupture of aneurysms) over 19-year follow-up period (Lupi-Herrera et al., 1977). Accordingly, 10-year survival is described to be around 85% in India (Subramanyan et al., 1989), with a similar figure reported from Korean patients (Park et al., 2005). In contrast, a clinical series including 75 patients from the United States showed 3% mortality by causes directly related with arteritis over 12-year follow-up period (Maksimowicz-McKinnon et al., 2007). The higher mortality rates observed in Mexican and Asian cohorts compared with North American patients may have several explanations, including differences in the treatment approaches as well as in the access to medical and surgical therapy in each country. This notion is supported by data from a Japanese cohort, which showed that 15-year survival rates have dramatically improved from 80% (1957 to 1975 period) to 96.5% (1976 to 1990 period), apparently in association with standardization of better health care protocols (Ishikawa & Maetani, 1994). However, these differences may also have been related to ethnic differences influencing both disease phenotypes and severity of disease expression (Maksimowicz-McKinnon et al., 2007). In this regard, there are severe manifestations of Takayasu's arteritis commonly found in Latin American and Asian patients whose presence has been barely reported in patients from the United States and Europe. A recent study focused on the renal microscopic changes in Takayasu's arteritis found that more than half of biopsy specimens from Mexican patients (14 of 25, 56%) showed high-grade inflammatory cell infiltrates in the glomerular microvasculature, diffuse mesangial proliferative glomerulonephritis and other associated glomerulopathies (de Pablo et al., 2007); similarly, it has been found that the patients with Mexican/mestizo ethnicity often develop uveitis and arteritis of the ophthalmic arteries (Pineda et al., 2003).

It is noteworthy that, in addition to geographical and ethnic differences, the prognosis of patients with Takayasu's arteritis is strongly affected by complications such as retinopathy, secondary hypertension, aortic regurgitation and arterial aneurysms. Data from an Indian cohort showed that, while five-year survival rate from diagnosis is 100% for patients with not any complication this figure drops to 70 to 80% for those with one or more complications (Subramanyan et al., 1989).

5. Insights suggesting an association between Takayasu's arteritis and tuberculosis

Cumulative data support a central role for the immune system in the pathogenesis of Takayasu's arteritis, with both B and T lymphocytes as key culprits in mediation of aortitis; however, the primary cause of Takayasu's arteritis remains unclear and attempts to clarify it are still limited. As regards to etiology, there are clinical and laboratory data suggesting an autoimmune basis, while others suggest that aortitis may be an expression of delayed-type hypersensitivity reaction to tuberculin or other sensitizers. Moreover, the association of Takayasu's arteritis with specific human leukocyte antigen (HLA) haplotypes and the anecdotal occurrence of Takayasu's arteritis in identical twins suggest the existence of a genetic background for predisposition. Additionally, it is clear that exogenous factors such as environment and infectious agents are crucial to the development of Takayasu's arteritis.

A possible relationship between Takayasu's arteritis and both latent and active tuberculosis was first pointed out in 1948 by Shimizu and Sano (Shimizu & Sano, 1948). They suggested this hypothesis because the presence of Langhans giant-cell granulomas on arterial specimens from patients with Takayasu's arteritis, which morphologically resembled those found in tuberculous lesions. This was further supported by the finding of occlusive lesions in the arterial walls from patients with advanced pulmonary tuberculosis (Cicero & Celis, 1955). After that, several cases about the unquestionable coexistence of pulmonary and extra-pulmonary tuberculous foci in patients with Takayasu's arteritis have been published (Duzova et al., 2000, Kontogiannis et al., 2000; Lupi-Herrera et al., 1977). Moreover, there are anecdotal cases of patients with tuberculosis and concomitant Takayasu's arteritis showing complete symptomatic remission including return of pulses after successful antituberculous therapy (Baumgarten & Cantor, 1933; Owens & Bass, 1944; Pantell & Goodman, 1981). These inconclusive findings were pivotal for the exploration about a possibly causal, not coincidental association between tuberculosis and Takayasu's arteritis.

Epidemiological data show that past or present tuberculosis infection is over-represented in Takayasu's arteritis, with prevalence rates ranging from 21.8% to 70%. In a case series from India, patients with Takayasu's arteritis were 46.6 times as likely to have had active tuberculosis compared with general population (70% versus 1.5%) (Kinare, 1970). While, data from Mexico indicate that this ratio could be exceeded. From a clinical study including 107 cases with Takayasu's arteritis, 48% of patients were positive for a previous tuberculous infection such as pulmonary tuberculosis, tuberculous adenopathy, and Bazin's erythema induratum; in sharply contrast, the prevalence of active tuberculosis was reported to be 0.028% in the general population from Mexico (Lupi-Herrera et al., 1977).

6. Bacille Calmette-Guérin (BCG) vaccination and tuberculin skin tests in Takayasu's arteritis

Mantoux screening test is the main tuberculin reaction used in the world. It consists of an intradermal injection of a standard dose of 5 Tuberculin (purified protein derivative –PPD-) units; the reaction is assessed by measuring the diameter of induration after 48 to 72 hours. An individual who has been exposed to *Mycobacterium tuberculosis* is expected to mount an immune response in the skin containing the mycobacterial proteins; however, positive results may be caused by non-tuberculous mycobacteria as well as previous administration of Bacille Calmette-Guérin (BCG) vaccine.

PPD skin test is found to be positive in 81% of Mexican patients with Takayasu's arteritis, as compared with 66% in the normal controls; interestingly, intradermal reactions with specific antigens of *Mycobacterium kansasii* (84%) and *Mycobacterium avium* (78%) are also more commonly positive in patients with Takayasu's arteritis than in average population with no arteritis (11 to 15% for both non-tuberculous mycobacteria) (Lupi et al., 1972). Of note, BCG vaccination is routinely administrated at birth in Mexico. Recently, it was showed that skin delayed hypersensitivity to PPD with induration over 10 mm may be as frequent (92.5% versus 89%) in Takayasu's arteritis as in patients with extra-pulmonary tuberculosis (Soto et al., 2007). Higher frequencies of positive tuberculin tests in Takayasu's patients than in general population also are described in series from Japan (85-92% versus 0.3%) and Korea (90% versus 4.2%) (Ueda et al., 1968 & Keun-Soo et al., 1967, as cited in Pantell & Goodman, 1981). Notably, the age of presentation does not appear to be a factor influencing sensitivity to intradermal reaction against mycobacterium; it has been showed that PPD test is positive in 73% of children with Takayasu's arteritis compared with 22% reported in healthy children (Morales et al., 1991).

In the context that BCG vaccine is routinely administrated at birth or during the infancy in almost all countries with high incidence of Takayasu's arteritis, a role for BCG vaccination as causative has been suggested (Kothari, 1995). However, the nearly worldwide coverage of BCG vaccination (including countries in which Takayasu's arteritis is exceptional) as well as the intricate relationship between mycobacterial infection and the immune system of the host maintains this provocative thesis as a merely speculative issue.

7. Loss of self tolerance to heat shock proteins

Heat shock proteins (HSP) are a family of phylogenetically conserved proteins found in a wide range of species extending from bacteria to humans. HSP form an ancient, primary system for intracellular self-defense with scavenger activities that are also involved in the correct folding of newly synthesized proteins. These molecules are known to be synthesized in response to a large variety of stimuli besides heat shock itself. Environmental stresses leading to the expression of HSP and other stress proteins include ultra-violet radiation, alcohol, heavy metal ions, oxidation/reduction cell imbalance, calcium influx inside the cell, overload of the endoplasmic reticulum, increased blood pressure, viral and bacterial infections, and unspecific inflammation (Quintana & Cohen, 2011).

Normal function of HSP is necessary for the homeostasis of the living cells, and becomes especially important in disease, when our cells have to cope with a stressful environment (Tiroli-Cepeda & Ramos, 2011). Of note, loss of self tolerance to diverse stress-induced cell proteins including human HSP and its consequent cross-reactivity against HSP from infectious agents is believed to be partially responsible for various rheumatic diseases such as rheumatoid arthritis and Behçet disease (Direskeneli & Saruhan-Direskeneli, 2003; Huang et al., 2010).

8. Role of humoral immune responses against heat shock proteins

Growing evidence points to a critical role of HSP in the pathogenesis of Takayasu's arteritis. In this regard, it is interesting that the main immunogenic component of BCG vaccine 65 kDa HSP is also a major immunoreactive protein antigen present in *Mycobacterium tuberculosis* and other mycobateria (Shinnick et al., 1987). Hernandez-Pando and colleagues have reported that Mexican patients with Takayasu's arteritis have an enhanced immune response against the mycobacterial antigens 65 kDa HSP and in a lesser extent, 38 kDa HSP (Hernandez-Pando et al., 1994). In this study, anti-65 kDa HSP IgG antibody titers were higher in patients with Takayasu's arteritis than in controls, and similar to those found in patients with pulmonary tuberculosis. Notably, serum antibody titers were higher in patients with active than in those with inactive arteritis. In contrast, Aggarwal and colleagues were unable to find differences in the positivity of anti-65 kDa HSP IgG antibodies between patients and healthy controls from India; however, they found a heightened immune response mediated by antibodies of IgM and IgA isotypes directed against the 65 kDa HSP (Aggarwal et al., 1996).

Recently, humoral immune responses against mycobacterial 65 kDa HSP and its human homologue 60 kDa HSP were investigated in 26 Indian patients with Takayasu's arteritis (Kumar Chauhan et al., 2004). Kumar Chauhan and colleagues found a significantly higher prevalence of IgG isotype reactive to both mycobacterial 65 kDa HSP (92% versus 11%, $P<0.0001$) and human 60 kDa HSP (84% versus 22%, $P<0.001$) in patients with Takayasu's arteritis compared with healthy controls. Moreover, a strongly positive correlation between anti-65 kDa HSP IgG and anti-60 kDa HSP IgG antibodies (*r* coefficient=0.814, $P<0.001$) was observed in patients with Takayasu's arteritis.

In support to an infection-induced autoimmunity through molecular mimicry mechanisms, 65 kDa HSP is over-expressed in the aortic tissue from patients with Takayasu's arteritis (Seko et al., 1994). However, this notion has been challenged by the finding of a similar increased cell expression of 65 kDa HSP in aortic tissue from patients with advanced atherosclerotic lesions; moreover, this expression is associated with elevated titers of circulating IgG antibodies against the 65 kDa HSP molecule (Xu et al., 1993).

9. Phenotypic analyses of infiltrating T cells in the arterial tissue with Takayasu's arteritis

Chronic inflammatory cell infiltration and its resulting injury to vessel wall suggest that diverse cell-mediated immunological mechanisms play an important pathogenic role in Takayasu's arteritis. A seminal report analyzing the phenotypes of infiltrating cells demonstrated a marked infiltration of T lymphocytes CD3+ CD8+, and absence of CD4+ T cells in aortic tissue from a single patient with Takayasu's arteritis (Scott et al., 1986). Subsequently, a more exhaustive study from Japan compared the immunological phenotypes of infiltrating cells among aortic specimens from patients with either Takayasu's arteritis or atherosclerotic aneurysms (Seko et al., 1994). In this study, it was found that infiltrating cells in Takayasu's arteritis consisted of CD4+ (14% of total cells) and CD8+ (15%) T lymphocytes displaying T-cell receptor $\alpha\beta$, CD14+ macrophages (13%), CD16+ natural killer cells (20%), and CD4- CD8- T lymphocytes displaying T-cell receptor $\gamma\delta$ (31%). In contrast, aortic sections from atherosclerotic aneurysms showed infiltration by CD4+ $\alpha\beta$ T lymphocytes (6%), CD8+$\alpha\beta$ T lymphocytes (12%), macrophages (31%), natural killer cells (29%), and just few numbers of $\gamma\delta$ T cells. As can be noted, the percentage of infiltrating macrophages and $\gamma\delta$ T lymphocytes are quite different between diseases, with $\gamma\delta$ T cells representing the main infiltrating lymphocytic phenotype in Takayasu's arteritis.

In addition to natural killer and cytotoxic CD8+ T cells, T lymphocytes bearing γδ T-cell receptor are recognized to play a critical role in cytolysis. These killer cells exert cytotoxicity through different two major pro-apoptotic pathways. One is the perforin-dependent colloid-osmotic lysis of target cell membrane; the other is Fas/Fas ligand (L)-mediated apoptosis signal induction. In support to a pathogenic role for cytotoxicity in the vascular damage seen in Takayasu's arteritis, Seko and colleagues found an increased expression of perforin in peripheral cytoplasmic granules of natural killer cells, CD8+ and γδ T lymphocytes, and demonstrated that numerous perforin molecules are released from these infiltrating cells directly onto the surface of aortic vascular cells (Seko et al., 1994). These authors also explore the expression of both Fas-L in infiltrating cells and Fas in aortic vascular cells from Takayasu's arteritis (Seko, 2000). They found that Fas was strongly expressed in vascular cells of *vasa vasorum*, while its ligand Fas-L was expressed in most of the infiltrating cells. However, aortic vascular cells seemed not to have undergone apoptosis, while some of the infiltrating cells underwent activation-induced cell death. These data suggest that perforin-mediated necrosis but not Fas/Fas-L apoptosis may play a major role in the mechanism of vascular injury in Takayasu's arteritis.

Perhaps the utmost demonstration for a main role for γδ T lymphocytes is the finding that infiltrating cells in Takayasu´s arteritis have restricted usage of T-cell receptor genes. In an elegant experiment, Seko and colleagues analyzed T-cell receptor Vγ and Vδ gene utilization by infiltrating γδ T lymphocytes in arterial specimens from a single patient with Takayasu's arteritis, and found that almost all T-cell receptor Vγ (Vγ1 to Vγ4) as well as Vδ (Vδ1 to Vδ5, with exception of Vδ4) genes were expressed in peripheral blood lymphocytes, whereas only Vγ3, Vγ4, and Vδ1 were preferentially rearranged and transcribed in infiltrating cells, indicating a tissue-specific oligoclonal accumulation of Vδ1+ T lymphocytes. Interestingly, this selective accumulation apparently is guided by over-expression of co-stimulatory molecules such as CD80, CD86, CD40, CD27L, and OX40L into the inflamed arterial tissue (Seko et al., 2000).

Studies focused on T lymphocytes displaying T-cell receptor αβ also have demonstrated that a limited number of Vα as well as Vβ genes are preferentially rearranged and transcribed in infiltrating cells from aortic tissue with Takayasu's arteritis. In contrast, almost all Vα as well as Vβ genes are expressed in peripheral blood lymphocytes from patients with Takayasu's arteritis as well as in aortic infiltrating cells from individuals with atherosclerotic aortic aneurysms (Seko et al., 1996; Swanson et al., 1994).

Restricted utilization of T-cell receptor Vα as well as Vβ genes or Vγ as well as Vδ genes by infiltrating T lymphocytes in Takayasu's arteritis indicate that at least one specific antigen located in the aortic tissue is targeted. Even when the exact nature of this antigen (or antigens) remains unknown, recently it was demonstrated that γδ T lymphocytes present in patients with Takayasu's arteritis are reactive to human 60 kDa HSP, and these T cells possess spontaneous cytotoxicity to aortic endothelial cells. Moreover, direct stimulation of these γδ T lymphocytes with 60 kDa HSP results in further enhancement of their cytotoxic potential. These cellular effects were found in γδ T lymphocytes from Takayasu's arteritis patients, while were absent in cells from patients with systemic lupus erythematosus and healthy controls (Chauhan et al., 2007).

Co-localization of 60 kDa and 65 kDa HSP over-expression and activated γδ T lymphocytes reactive to self-HSP into the arterial lesions as well as the restricted T-cell receptor gene usage of infiltrating αβ and γδ T cells in patients with Takayasu's arteritis suggest the existence of a 60 kDa HSP driven expansion and infiltration of these cytotoxic cells in the arterial wall, which in turn may cause arterial damage mediated through both the perforin and Fas/Fas-L pathways.

10. Role of genetic factors in the immunopathology of Takayasu's arteritis

Both geographical incidence and occasional familiar occurrence suggest a role for genetic factors in the immunopathology of the disease. This autoimmune susceptibility arises from allelic variants or mutants in genes encoding a variety of relevant proteins of immune function. Several studies have proposed an association between Takayasu's arteritis and specific human leukocyte antigen (HLA) haplotypes.

As regards to major histocompatibility complex (MHC) it is described that susceptibility may be related with both class I and class II molecules. Specifically, alleles HLA-B52, DRB1*1502, DRB5*0102, DQA1*0103, DQB1*0601 as well as the extended haplotype HLA-Bw52-DRB1*1502-DRB5*0102-DQA1*0103-DQB1*0601 -DPA1*02-DPB1*0901 may confer susceptibility to Takayasu's arteritis in Japanese patients; whereas the combination HLA-Bw54-DRB1*0405-DRB4*0101-DQA1*0301-DQB1*0401 seems to confer resistance (Dong et al., 1992). While, studies based on Mexican cohorts show that Takayasu's arteritis is associated with higher frequencies of alleles HLA-B39, -B52, and –B39 class I molecules, as well as allele HLA-DRB1*1301 class II molecule (Girona et al., 1996; Soto et al., 2007; Vargas-Alarcón et al., 2008). In Indian patients, an association with alleles HLA-B5 and –B21 has been described (Rose et al., 1991).

Interestingly, some clinical forms of tuberculosis have been related with specific alleles of class II and class I molecules. An association with HLA-DR2 and particularly with its subtype DR15 in linkage disequilibrium with DQ5 has been found in patients with smear-positive pulmonary tuberculosis (Bellamy, 1998). This observation has been refined using DNA based HLA typing and it was confirmed a link with genes *DRB1*1501* and *DQB1*0502* (Meyer et al., 1998). Similarly, a higher frequency distribution of class I HLA-B60 antigen is seen in patients with smear-positive pulmonary tuberculosis than in non-infected, exposed controls (Bothamley, 1999).

Similar class I and class II MHC molecules have been described in association with Takayasu's arteritis and active tuberculosis, suggesting a possible genetic relationship between diseases. While, it may support a biological plausibility to PPD delayed-type hypersensitivity intradermal reactions commonly seen in both diseases. Unfortunately, available results from few studies focused on HLA-B alleles do not support this attractive thesis (Soto et al., 2007; Vargas-Alarcón et al., 2008).

Alternatively, there is a group of innate immune molecules whose genes are located near the HLA-B gene region; these molecules are termed MHC class I chain-related A (MIC-A) and may have a crucial role in the pathogenesis of Takayasu's arteritis. *MIC-A* genes are polymorphic and divergent from classical MHC class I genes. After different stimuli inducing cellular stress, *MIC-A* genes are rapidly over-expressed and their resulting proteins are deployed in membrane; then, MIC-A molecules may be recognized by NKG2D receptors expressed on the γδ T lymphocytes and natural killer cells. On cytotoxic cells, engagement of NKG2D receptors results in activation of cytolytic responses directed against targeted-cells expressing MIC-A (Bauer et al., 1999). In this regard, Kimura and colleagues have reported that *MIC-A-1.2* polymorphism is associated with Takayasu's arteritis in absence of *HLA-B52* gene, suggesting that a part of the HLA-linked genetic susceptibility to Takayasu's arteritis may be mapped near the *MIC-A* gene region (Kimura et al., 1998). To further investigate the role of these cytotoxicity-mediated mechanisms, Seko and colleagues analyzed the expression of MIC-A and some co-stimulatory molecules in the aortic tissue as well as their counterpart ligands in the infiltrating cells from patients with Takayasu's arteritis. They found that MIC-A molecules are strongly expressed in the aortic tissue, along with over-expression of co-stimulatory molecules 4-1BBL and Fas; while, most of the infiltrating cells express NKG2D receptors as well as 4-1BB and FasL (Seko et al., 2004). These findings suggest that γδ T lymphocytes and other killer cells may recognize stressed aortic cells expressing MIC-A throughout NKG2D receptors. Over-expression of co-stimulatory molecules may facilitate further recognition and activation of cytotoxic cells, leading to an increase in the cellular stress of aorta and self-maintenance of chronic inflammation.

11. Absence of *Mycobacterium tuberculosis* in arterial tissue from Takayasu's arteritis

Despite clinical and laboratory studies supporting that *Mycobacterium tuberculosis* could be involved in the pathogenesis of Takayasu's arteritis, the pathogen has not been detected directly in the arterial tissue. Recently, Arnaud and colleagues looked for the presence of *Mycobacterium tuberculosis* by acid-fast and auramine-fluorochrome staining, mycobacterial cultures on Lowenstein-Jensen culture media, and nucleic acid -16S ribosomal RNA-amplification in arterial specimens (aorta and carotid arteries) from 10 patients with Takayasu's arteritis underwent surgery (Arnaud et al., 2009). Of note, no patient had evidence of active tuberculosis at the time of surgery and patients were Caucasians or North Africans; histological examination showed five active and five inactive arterial lesions. *Mycobacterium tuberculosis* was not detected in arterial specimens of either active or inactive Takayasu's arteritis by any of the methods used. Although these results almost exclude a direct arterial infection, do not exclude a latent, extra-arterial infection with anti-mycobacterial immune responses triggering a cross-reaction against antigens located in the arterial wall.

Diagnosis of latent infection by *Mycobacterium tuberculosis* has dramatically improved with the arrival of Quantiferon-TB Gold test. Quantiferon-TB Gold test identifies latent and active tuberculosis infection by measuring the *in vitro* interferon-γ release from T lymphocytes in response to three unique antigens highly specific for *Mycobacterium tuberculosis*, which are absent in almost all non-tuberculous mycobacteria including BCG vaccine. This test has been particularly helpful in countries in which the interpretation of PPD intradermal reaction is confounded because routinely early application of BCG vaccine (Lalvani, 2007). Recently, Karadag and colleagues assess the possibility of latent tuberculosis infection in ninety-four Turkish patients with Takayasu's arteritis using tuberculin test and Quantiferon-TB Gold test and compare it with healthy controls (Karadag et al., 2010). Even when tuberculin test positivity was higher in patients with Takayasu's arteritis than in controls (62.5% versus 41.4%; $P=0.008$), Quantiferon-TB Gold test positivity was equal between groups (22.3% versus 22.4%; $P>0.05$), suggesting that latent tuberculosis is similar in patients with Takayasu's arteritis and in healthy controls.

12. Proposal for a novel unifying model of pathogenesis

Previous model of pathogenesis has been supported on the premise that the arteritis results from delayed hypersensitivity to active or latent tuberculosis infection, through cross-reactivity mechanisms against vascular peptides mimicking antigens constituents of *Mycobacterium tuberculosis* and other mycobacteria. This model has fascinated researchers and clinicians for more than a half century; however, recent studies showing absence of mycobacteria into the arterial tissue as well as absence of latent *Mycobacterium tuberculosis* infection by highly-specific *ex vivo* functional assays have knocked out this attractive hypothesis. Nevertheless, it is irrefutable the vast evidence showing indirect associations between Takayasu's arteritis and *Mycobacterium tuberculosis*; hence, we will hypothesize on a novel, unifying pathogenic model that may explain this relationship.

We speculate that, in a first step (non self-reactive phase), unspecific injuries such as infections, increased blood pressure, and other non-specific inflammatory stimuli may induce cellular stress in endothelial vascular cells, which in turn result in the production of large amounts of 60 kDa HSP and other stress-induced proteins. These "warning of danger" molecules may be sensed by innate cytotoxic cells through pattern-recognition receptors (PRR's) such as Toll-like (TLR) and Nucleotide-binding and oligomerisation domain (NOD)-like (NLR) receptors. After recognition, cytotoxic cells become activated and may promote apoptosis of vascular endothelial cells through perforin and Fas/Fas-L pathways, thus enhancing the stressed cellular environment.

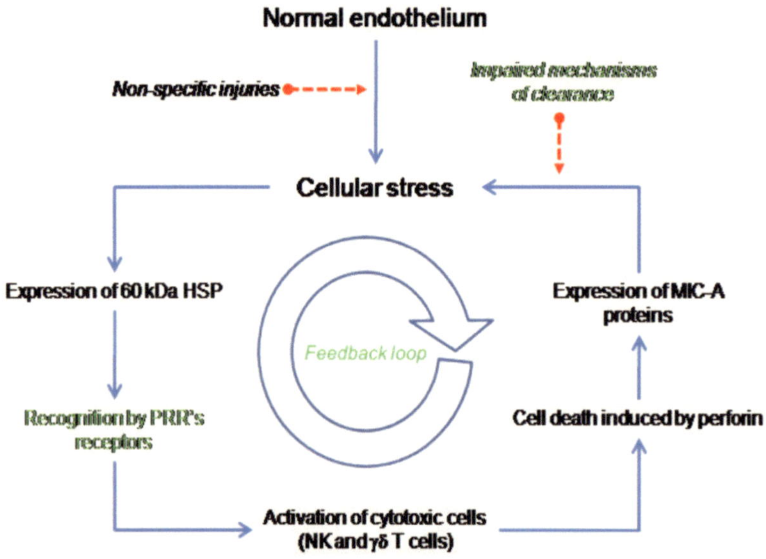

Fig. 1. A novel pathogenic model in Takayasu's arteritis. Non self-reactive phase. Unspecific damage factors induce stress in endothelial cells, which results in the expression of several stress-induced proteins, including 60 kDa heat shock protein (HSP). These stress-induced proteins are engaged by innate cytotoxic cells through pattern-recognition receptors (PPR's) and become activated, promoting apoptosis of vascular endothelial cells and enhancing the stressed cellular environment.

In a second step (self-reactive, innate immune phase), stressed vascular cells may rapidly activate *MIC-A* gene transcription (for instance, *MIC-A-1.2* polymorphism). Then, MIC-A molecules on endothelium may be recognized by NKG2D receptors on infiltrating Vδ1+ γδ T lymphocytes and natural killer cells, which in turn result in cytolytic responses against endothelial targeted-cells expressing MIC-A. Vascular infiltration of oligoclonally expanded γδ T cells producing interferon-γ may amplify the expression of HLA class II and class I molecules (*i.e.* HLA-Bw52-DRB1*1502-DRB5*0102-DQA1*0103-DQB1*0601 -DPA1*02-DPB1*0901) and co-stimulatory molecules. Co-expression of MHC proteins and vascular antigens (muted or misfolded self-antigens?) may lead to massive aortic infiltration by oligoclonally expanded self-reactive αβ CD4+and CD8+ T lymphocytes.

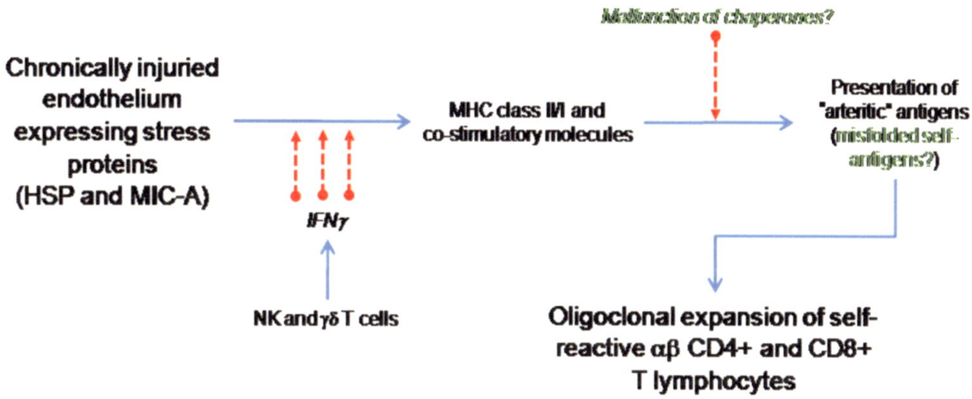

Fig. 2. A novel pathogenic model in Takayasu's arteritis. Self-reactive, innate immune phase. MIC-A molecules are over-expressed on vascular endothelial cells and may be recognized by infiltrating natural killer (NK) and γδ T cells, which amplify the interferon (IFN)γ-dependent expression of HLA class II and class I molecules and co-stimulatory molecules. Co-expression of MHC proteins and vascular antigens (muted or misfolded self-antigens?) lead to aortic infiltration by oligoclonally expanded self-reactive αβ CD4+and CD8+ T cells.

In a third phase (self-reactive, adaptive immune phase), self-reactive αβ CD4+ T lymphocytes may play central and multiple roles in the amplification and progression of the inflammatory response in Takayasu's arteritis. Different T cell subsets may provide help for B cell production of "arteritic" auto-antibodies such as anti-endothelial cells and anti-60 kDa HSP antibodies as well as antigen-driven T cell-dependent IgG isotype switching. T cells subsets also may modulate expansion and effector functions by infiltrating macrophages, directing their transformation into Langhans multinucleated giant cells and granuloma formation. Finally, infiltrating CD4+ and CD8+T cell subsets may promote the progression and maintenance of granuloma as well as the recruitment of fibroblasts; late in the process of tissue injury, massive deposition of collagen and matrix proteins may lead to fibrosis of arterial walls, which characterizes the pulseless stage of chronic Takayasu's arteritis.
In addition to better explain arterial tissue damage, this novel pathogenic model also may explain the common positive reaction to PPD (and other mycobacterial antigens) observed in patients with Takayasu's arteritis. Intradermal deposition of mycobacterial antigens may trigger both recruitment and activation of several subsets of T lymphocytes self-reactive against human 60 kDa HSP. These T cells may also mediate cross-reacting responses with the mycobacterial homologue 65 kDa HSP and, in a lesser extent, 38 kDa HSP, thus explaining the delayed hypersensitivity that underlies the Mantoux test as just an epiphenomenon.

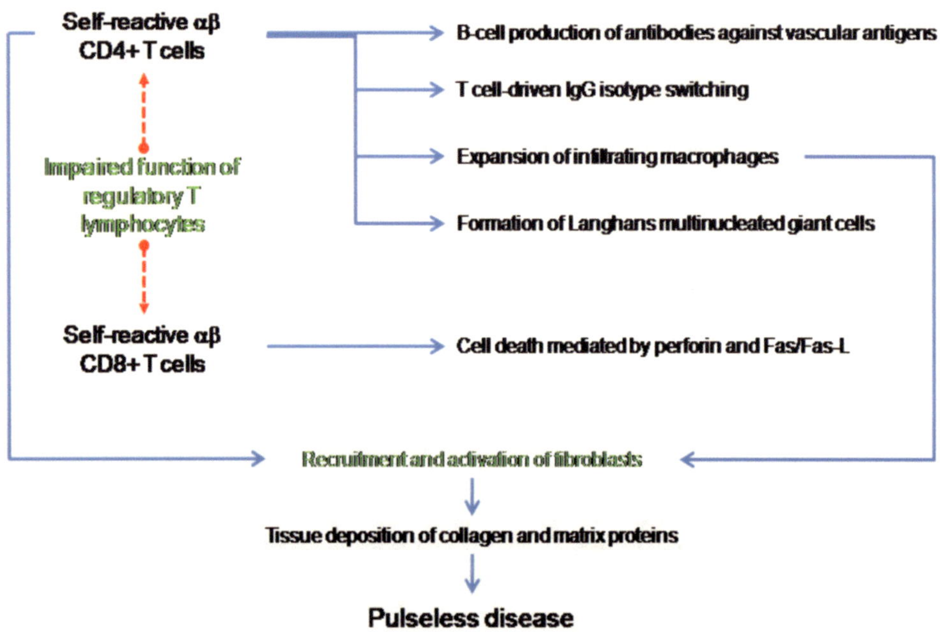

Fig. 3. A novel pathogenic model in Takayasu's arteritis. Self-reactive, adaptive immune phase. Self-reactive αβ CD4+ T lymphocytes play central roles in the inflammatory response seen in Takayasu's arteritis. Helper T cell subsets provide help for B cell production of antibodies against vascular antigens and IgG isotype switching. Helper T cell subsets also may modulate effector functions by infiltrating macrophages.

Finally, CD4+ and CD8+T cells may promote recruitment of fibroblasts and deposition of collagen and matrix proteins leading to fibrosis of arterial vessels (pulseless stage of Takayasu's arteritis).

13. Conclusion

A relationship between Takayasu's arteritis and both latent and active tuberculosis has been discussed for more than a half century. Indirect evidence had suggested that *Mycobacterium tuberculosis* and probably other mycobacteria could play a role in the immunopathogenesis of Takayasu's arteritis, possibly through molecular mimicry mechanisms. However, recent studies showing absence of mycobacteria directly into the arterial tissue as well as absence of latent *Mycobacterium tuberculosis* infection by highly-specific *ex vivo* functional assays have knocked out this attractive hypothesis.

Supported on currently available data, we speculate on a novel model of pathogenesis which may explain the intricate relationship between Takayasu's arteritis and *Mycobacterium tuberculosis*. This model is based in the loss of self-tolerance against stress-induced cellular molecules, with the innate immune system as key culprit in the initiation, amplification and progression of inflammatory response observed in Takayasu's arteritis.

14. Acknowledgements

Of utmost importance, a substantial part of data presented in this review has been generated by several generations of cardiologists, immunologists and rheumatologists from the

Instituto Nacional de Cardiología Ignacio Chávez at Mexico City, Mexico. We wish that the present compilation serves as a humble tribute to all them.
We are indebted with Dr. Angélica Vargas for her critical review and comments to this manuscript.

15. References

Aggarwal, A., Chag, M., Sinha, N. & Naik, S. (1996). Takayasu's arteritis: role of Mycobacterium tuberculosis and its 65 kDa heat shock protein. *International Journal of Cardiology*, 55, 1, 49-55.

Amezcua-Guerra, L.M. & Pineda, C. (2007). Imaging studies in the diagnosis and management of vasculitis. *Current Rheumatology Reports*, 9, 4, 320-327.

Arnaud, L., Cambau, E., Brocheriou, I., Koskas, F., Piette, J.C. & Amoura, Z. (2009). Absence of Mycobacterium tuberculosis in arterial lesions from patients with Takayasu's arteritis. *The Journal of Rheumatology*, 36, 8, 1682-1685.

Bauer, S., Groh, V., Wu, J., Steinle, A., Phillips, J.H., Lanier, L.L. & Spies, T. (1999). Activation of NK cells and T cells by NKG2D, a receptor for stress-inducible MICA. *Science*, 285, 5428, 727-729.

Baumgarten, E.C. & Cantor, M.O. (1933). Tuberculous mesarteritis with aneurysm of the femoral artery: report of a case. *The Journal of the American Medical Association*, 100, 24, 1918-1920.

Bellamy, R. (1998). Genetics and pulmonary medicine. 3. Genetic susceptibility to tuberculosis in human populations. *Thorax*, 53, 7, 588-593.

Bothamley, G.H. (1999). Differences between HLA-B44 and HLA-B60 in patients with smear-positive pulmonary tuberculosis and exposed controls. *The Journal of Infectious Diseases*, 179, 4, 1051-1052.

Chauhan, S.K., Singh, M. & Nityanand, S. (2007) Reactivity of gamma/delta T cells to human 60-kd heat-shock protein and their cytotoxicity to aortic endothelial cells in Takayasu arteritis. *Arthritis and Rheumatism*, 56, 8, 2798-2802.

Chhetri, M.K., Raychaudhuri, B., Neelakantan, C., Basu, J., Chaki, S. & Saha, A.K. (1974). A profile of non-specific arteritis as observed in Eastern India. *The Journal of the Association of Physicians of India*, 22, 11, 839-847.

Cicero, R. & Celis, A. (1955). Ante-mortem and post-mortem angiography of the pulmonary arterial tree in advanced tuberculosis. *American Review of Tuberculosis*, 71, 6, 810-821.

de Pablo, P., García-Torres, R., Uribe, N., Ramón, G., Nava, A., Silveira, L.H., Amezcua-Guerra, L.M., Martínez-Lavín, M. & Pineda, C. (2007). Kidney involvement in Takayasu arteritis. *Clinical and Experimental Rheumatology*, 25, 1 Suppl 44, S10-S14.

Direskeneli, H. & Saruhan-Direskeneli, G. (2003). The role of heat shock proteins in Behcet's disease. *Clinical and Experimental Rheumatology*, 21, 4 Suppl 30, S44-S48.

Dong, R.P., Kimura, A., Numano, F., Yajima, M., Hashimoto, Y., Kishi, Y., Nishimura, Y. & Sasazuki, T. (1992). HLA-DP antigen and Takayasu arteritis. *Tissue Antigens*, 39, 3, 106-110.

Duzova, A., Turkmen, O., Cinar, A., Cekirge, S., Saatci, U. & Ozen, S. (2000). Takayasu's arteritis and tuberculosis: a case report. *Clinical Rheumatology*, 19, 6, 486-489.

Girona, E., Yamamoto-Furusho, J.K., Cutiño, T., Reyes, P., Vargas-Alarcón, G., Granados, J. & Alarcón-Segovia, D. (1996). HLA-DR6 (possibly DRB1*1301) is associated with susceptibility to Takayasu arteritis in Mexicans. *Heart and Vessels*, 11, 6, 277-280.

Hernández-Pando, R., Reyes, P., Espitia, C., Wang, Y., Rook, G. & Mancilla, R. (1994). Raised agalactosyl IgG and antimycobacterial humoral immunity in Takayasu's arteritis. *The Journal of Rheumatology*, 21, 10, 1870-1876.

Huang, M.N., Yu, H. & Moudgil, K.D. (2010). The involvement of heat-shock proteins in the pathogenesis of autoimmune arthritis: a critical appraisal. *Seminars in Arthritis and Rheumatism*, 40, 2, 164-175.

Ishikawa, K. & Maetani, S. (1994). Long-term outcome for 120 Japanese patients with Takayasu's disease. Clinical and statistical analyses of related prognostic factors. *Circulation*, 90, 4, 1855-1860.

Karadag, O., Aksu, K., Sahin, A., Zihni, F.Y., Sener, B., Inanc, N., Kalyoncu, U., Aydin, S.Z., Ascioglu, S., Ocakci, P.T., Bilgen, S.A., Keser, G., Inal, V., Direskeneli, H., Calguneri, M., Ertenli, I. & Kiraz, S. (2010). Assessment of latent tuberculosis infection in Takayasu arteritis with tuberculin skin test and Quantiferon-TB gold test. *Rheumatology International*, 30, 11, 1483-1487.

Kimura, A., Kobayashi, Y., Takahashi, M., Ohbuchi, N., Kitamura, H., Nakamura, T., Satoh, M., Sasaoka, T., Hiroi, S., Arimura, T., Akai, J., Aerbajinai, W., Yasukochi, Y. & Numano, F. (1998). MICA gene polymorphism in Takayasu's arteritis and Buerguer's disease. *International Journal of Cardiology*, 66, Suppl 1, S107-S113, discussion S115.

Kinare, S.G. (1970). Aortitis in early life in India and its association with tuberculosis. *The Journal of Pathology*, 100, 1, 69-76.

Kontogiannis, V., Dalziel, K.L. & Powell, R.J. (2000). Papulonecrotic tuberculide and stenosis of the abdominal aorta. *Rheumatology (Oxford)*, 39, 2, 205-208.

Kothari, S.S. (1995). Aetiopathogenesis of Takayasu's arteritis and BCG vaccination: the missing link?. *Medical Hypotheses*, 45, 3, 227-230.

Kumar, A., Dubey, D., Bansal, P., Sanjeevan, K.V., Gulati, S., Jain, S. & Sharma, K. (2003). Surgical and radiological management of renovascular hypertension in a developing country. *The Journal of Urology*, 170, 3, 727-730.

Kumar Chauhan, S., Kumar Tripathy, N., Sinha, N., Singh, M. & Nityanand, S. (2004). Cellular and humoral immune responses to mycobacterial heat shock protein-65 and its human homologue in Takayasu's arteritis. *Clinical and Experimental Immunology*, 138, 3, 547-553.

Ladhani, S., Tulloh, R. & Anderson, D. (2001). Takayasu disease masquerading as interruption of the aortic arch in a 2-year-old child. *Cardiology in the Young*, 11, 2, 244-246.

Lalvani, A. (2007). Diagnosing tuberculosis infection in the 21st century: new tools to tackle and old enemy. *Chest*, 131, 6, 1898-1906.

Lupi, E., Sánchez, G., Horwitz, S. & Gutierrez, E. (1975). Pulmonary artery involvement in Takayasu's arteritis. *Chest*, 67, 1, 69-74.

Lupi, H.E., Sanchez-Torres, G. & Castillo P.U. (1972). Reactividad cutánea al PPD a los antígenos de micobacterias atípicas (Kansasii, avium y fortuitum) en pacientes con arteritis inespecífica. *Archivos del Instituto de Cardiología de México*, 42:717.

Lupi-Herrera, E., Sánchez-Torres, G., Marcushamer, J., Mispireta, J., Horwitz, S. & Vela, J.E. (1977). Takayasu's arteritis. Clinical study of 107 cases. *American Heart Journal*, 93, 1, 94-103.

Maksimowicz-McKinnon, K., Clark, T.M. & Hoffman, G.S. (2007). Limitations of therapy and a guarded prognosis in an American cohort of Takayasu arteritis patients. *Arthritis and Rheumatism*, 56, 3, 1000-1009.

Mason, J.C. (2010). Takayasu arteritis - advances in diagnosis and management. *Nature Reviews Rheumatology*, 6, 7, 406-415.

Meyer, C.G., May, J. & Stark, K. (1998). Human leukocyte antigens in tuberculosis and leprosy. *Trends in Microbiology*, 6, 4, 148-154.

Morales, E., Pineda, C. & Martínez-Lavín, M. (1991). Takayasu's arteritis in children. *The Journal of Rheumatology*, 18, 7, 1081-1084.

Owens, J.N. Jr. & Bass, A.D. (1944). Tuberculous aneurysm of the abdominal aorta: report of a case. *Archives of Internal Medicine*, 74, 413-415.

Pantell, R.H. & Goodman, B.W. Jr. (1981). Takayasu's arteritis: the relationship with tuberculosis. *Pediatrics*, 67, 1, 84-88.

Park, M.C., Lee, S.W., Park, Y.B., Chung, N.S. & Lee, S.K. (2005). Clinical characteristics and outcomes of Takayasu's arteritis: analysis of 108 patients using standardized criteria for diagnosis, activity assessment, and angiographic classification. *Scandinavian Journal of Rheumatology*, 34, 4, 284-292.

Pineda, C., Rivera, M., Soto, M.E., Castañón, C., Cantú, C., Amezcua-Guerra, L., Nava, A., Reyes, P. & Martínez-Lavín, M. (2003). Uveitis: a forgotten manifestation of Takayasu arteritis. *Arthritis & Rheumatism*, 48, Suppl, S202.

Quintana, F.J. & Cohen, I.R. (2011). The HSP60 immune system network. *Trends in Immunology*, 32, 2, 89-95.

Rose, S., Mehra, N.K., Kumar, R. & Vaidya, M.C. (1991). HLA-B5 and B21 antigens in aortoarteritis. Indian Journal of Pediatrics, 58, 1, 85-89.

Scott, D.G., Salmon, M., Scott, D.L., Blann, A., Bacon, P.A., Walton, K.W., Oakland, C.D. & Slaney, G.F. (1986). Takayasu's arteritis: a pathogenetic role for cytotoxic T lymphocytes?. *Clinical Rheumatology*, 5, 4, 517-522.

Seko, Y., Minota, S., Kawasaki, A., Shinkai, Y., Maeda, K., Yagita, H., Okumura, K., Sato, A., Takagi, A. & Tada, Y. (1994). Perforin-secreting killer cell infiltration and expression of a 65-kD heat-shock protein in aortic tissue of patients with Takayasu's arteritis. *The Journal of Clinical Investigation*, 93, 2, 750-758.

Seko, Y., Sato, O., Takagi, A., Tada, Y., Matsuo, H., Yagita, H., Okumura, K. & Yazaki, Y. (1996). Restricted usage of T-cell receptor Valpha-Vbeta genes in infiltrating cells in aortic tissue of patients with Takayasu's arteritis. *Circulation*, 93, 10, 1788-1790.

Seko, Y., Takahashi, N., Tada, Y., Yagita, H., Okumura, K. & Nagai, R. (2000). Restricted usage of T-cell receptor Vgamma-Vdelta genes and expression of costimulatory molecules in Takayasu's arteritis. *International Journal of Cardiology*, 75, Suppl 1, S77-S83, discussion S85-S87.

Seko, Y. (2000). Takayasu arteritis: insights into immunopathology. *Japanese Heart Journal*, 41, 1, 15-26.

Seko, Y., Sugishita, K., Sato, O., Takagi, A., Tada, Y., Matsuo, H., Yagita, H., Okumura, K. & Nagai, R. (2004). Expression of costimulatory molecules (4-1BBL and Fas) and major histocompatibility class I chain-related A (MICA) in aortic tissue with Takayasu's arteritis. *Journal of Vascular Research*, 41, 1, 84-90.

Shimizu, K. & Sano, K. (1948). Pulseless disease. *Clinical Surgery*, 3, 337.

Shinnick, T.M., Sweetser, D., Thole, J., van Embden, J. & Young, R.A. (1987). The etiologic agents of leprosy and tuberculosis share an immunoreactive protein antigen with the vaccine strain Mycobacterium bovis BCG. Infection and Immunity, 55, 8, 1932-1935.

Soto, M.E., Vargas-Alarcón, G., Cicero-Sabido, R., Ramírez, E., Alvarez-León, E. & Reyes, P.A. (2007). Comparison distribution of HLA-B alleles in Mexican patients with Takayasu artereitis and tuberculosis. *Human Immunology*, 68, 5, 449-453.

Subramanyan, R., Joy, J. & Balakrishnan, K.G. (1989). Natural history of aortoarteritis (Takayasu's disease). *Circulation*, 80, 3, 429-437.

Swanson, S.J., Rosenzweig, A., Seidman, J.G. & Libby, P. (1994). Diversity of T-cell antigen receptor V beta gene utilization in advanced human atheroma. *Arteriosclerosis and Thrombosis*, 14, 7, 1210-1214.

Tann, O.R., Tulloh, R.M. & Hamilton, M.C. (2008). Takayasu's disease: a review. *Cardiology in the Young*, 18, 3, 250-259.

Tiroli-Cepeda, A.O. & Ramos, C.H. (2011). An overview of the role of molecular chaperones in protein homeostasis. *Protein and Peptide Letters*, 18, 2, 101-109.

Vargas-Alarcón, G., Soto, M.E., Pérez-Hernández, N., Cicero-Sabido, R., Ramírez, E., Alvarez-León, E. & Reyes, P.A. (2008). Comparative study of the residues 63 and 67 on the HLA-B molecule in patients with Takayasu's arteritis and tuberculosis. *Cell Biochemistry and Function*, 26, 7, 820-823.

Weyand, C.M. & Goronzy, J.J. (2003). Medium- and large-vessel vasculitis. *The New England Journal of Medicine*, 349, 2, 160-169.

Xu, Q., Willeit, J., Marosi, M., Kleindienst, R., Oberhollenzer, F., Kiechl, S., Stulniq, T., Luef, G. & Wick, G. (1993). Association of serum antibodies to heat-shock protein 65 with carotid atherosclerosis. *Lancet*, 341, 8840, 255-259.

3

Mycoplasma pneumoniae as an Under- Recognized Agent of Vasculitic Disorders

Mitsuo Narita
Department of Pediatrics, Sapporo Tokushukai Hospital
Japan

1. Introduction

Mycoplasma pneumoniae, commonly known as a major causative agent of primary atypical pneumonia, also causes various kinds of extrapulmonary manifestations involving almost all the organs of the human body. The author has classified the extrapulmonary manifestations due to *M. pneumoniae* infection into three categories: the first is a direct type in which locally induced cytokines play a role, the second is an indirect type in which immune modulation such as autoimmunity plays a role, and the third is a vascular occlusion type in which vasculitis and/or thrombosis with or without systemic hypercoagulable state plays a role [Narita, 2009, 2010]. This classification system is intended to facilitate the understanding of the pathogenesis of extrapulmonary manifestations due to *M. pneumoniae* infection. A diagram depicting the possible ways in which *M. pneumoniae* can induce these three types of extrapulmonary manifestations in relation to the possible pathomechanism of pneumonia is shown in Fig 1. Further concrete explanations of each mechanism, based on the accumulated in-vitro and in-vivo data, are provided in the following sections. Of particular interest is the fact that *M. pneumoniae* can cause many kinds of vasculitic/thrombotic disorders. *Mycoplasma pneumoniae* may locally affect a vascular wall by inducing cytokines and chemokines such as tumor necrosis factor-α and interleukin-8, which cause local vasculitic and/or thrombotic vascular occlusion without systemic hypercoagulable state. Alternatively, generalized thrombotic vascular occlusion can occur as a result of a systemic hypercoagulable state which is in turn a consequence of immune modulation leading to the activation of chemical mediators such as complements and fibrin D-dimer.

Although it is already well known that *M. pneumoniae* can cause a few coagulation abnormality disorders such as disseminated intravascular coagulation and stroke, *M. pneumoniae* remains under-recognized as a causative agent for many other vasculitic/thrombotic disorders involving various organs of the human body. One reason for this must be that the ability of *M. pneumoniae* to cause vasculitic/thrombotic vascular disorders through the local operation of chemical mediators such as cytokines in the absence of an apparent systemic hypercoagulable state is not yet widely known.

In this chapter, the author presents organ-specific and systemic manifestations of vasculitic/thrombotic disorders that may be associated with *M. pneumoniae* infection.

Comments are made principally on the etiology by which *M. pneumoniae* acts as a pathogenic agent for each disease.

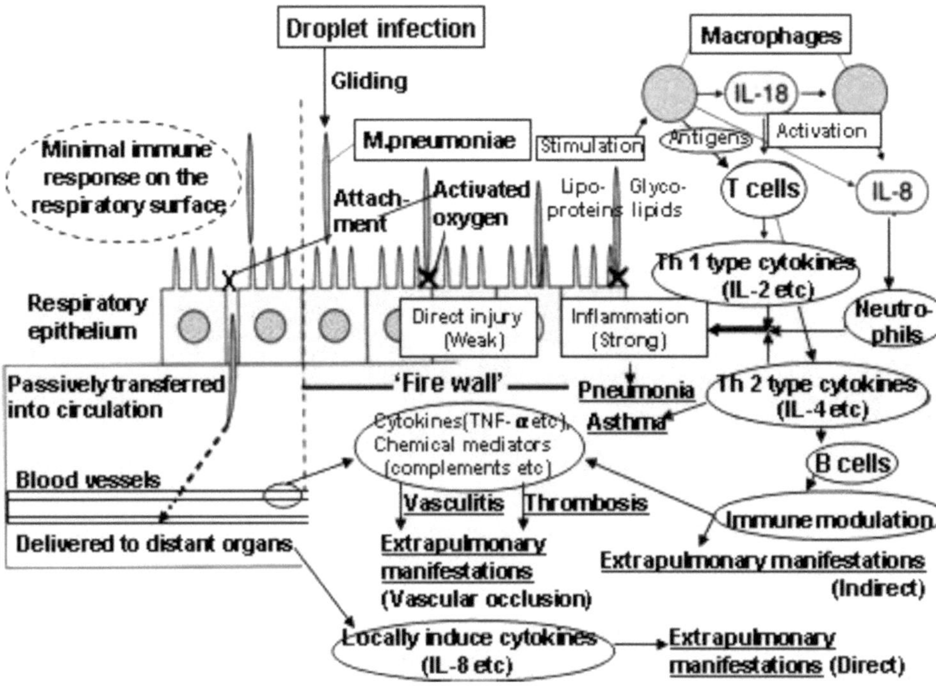

Fig. 1. Pathomechanism of vasculitic/thrombotic disorders caused by *M. pneumoniae* infection (Modified from ref. Narita, 2009. For details, see text).

2. Mechanism of vasculitic disorders due to *M. pneumoniae* infection

2.1 Respiratory infection and hematogenous dissemination

Mycoplasma pneumoniae is one of the smallest free-living bacteria. It possesses only a minor ability to injure respiratory epithelial cells by producing an excess of activated oxygen within the infected cells [for review, see Waites & Talkington, 2004]. Recent evidence has shown that *M. pneumoniae* produces the community acquired respiratory distress syndrome toxin, but its pathogenic role in human illness still remains to be elucidated [Hardy et al., 2009; Kannan & Baseman, 2006]. Nevertheless, *M. pneumoniae* is a major pathogen of primary atypical pneumonia as well as a number of extrapulmonary diseases. In this context, many previous works have disclosed that the cell membrane of *M. pneumoniae* contains lipoproteins which are potent inducers of cytokines equivalent to bacterial lipopolysaccharides [for review, see Sánchez-Vargas & Gómez-Duarte, 2008; Yang et al., 2004]. Thus it is currently understood that *M. pneumoniae* pneumonia results from the operation of the host immune system, specifically of various kinds of cytokines, rather than from direct injury by the organism itself; in other words, *M. pneumoniae* pneumonia develops via immune pathogenesis.

Following an initial droplet infection to the lower respiratory tract below the larynx, *M. pneumoniae* begins to propagate on the respiratory surface with ciliated epithelium [Krunkosky et al., 2007]. This event facilitates non-specific recognition of the organism by the innate immunity of the host through Toll-like receptors 1, 2, and 6, among which Toll-like receptor 2 plays a major role in initiating intracellular signal transmission [Shimizu, 2005]. *Mycoplasma pneumoniae* infection then leads to pneumonia by inducing various kinds of cytokines. Among a number of cytokines reported to be associated with the pathomechanism of *M. pneumoniae* pneumonia, the author and coworkers have demonstrated that the macrophage-derived cytokines interleukin-18 and interleukin-8 play significant roles in the development of pneumonia and are directly related to disease severity [Narita et al., 2000, 2001a; Tanaka et al., 2002]. Interleukin-18 is an immune regulatory cytokine that functions as an activator of T cells and a subsequent cascade of T helper-1 and T helper-2 type cytokines [Tanaka et al., 1996]. Interleulin-8 is an inflammatory cytokine and functions as an activator of neutrophils. Several lines of recent in-vitro evidence have supported the pathogenic importance of interleukin-8 in the development of the clinical picture of *M. pneumoniae* respiratory infection [Chmura et al., 2008; Sohn et al., 2005; Yang et al., 2002]. From this perspective, the activation of interleukin-8 by *M. pneumoniae* is one of the key steps in inducing the vasculitic disorders which are the main subject of this chapter.

As regards the presence of pneumonia in relation to the development of extrapulmonary diseases, the author and coworkers have found, using polymerase chain reaction methodology [Narita et al., 1992], that the genome of *M. pneumoniae* can be detected more frequently in serum from patients without pneumonia than in serum from patients with pneumonia [Narita et al., 1996]. This means that pneumonia, which is a consequence of the local host immune response occurring on the respiratory surface, plays an important role as a kind of fire-wall preventing dissemination of the organism beyond the respiratory tract [Cartner et al., 1998; Tanaka et al., 1996]. In this regard, it is important to note that direct-type extrapulmonary manifestations not infrequently occur in the absence of pneumonia, which is a hallmark of mycoplasmal infection. This must be another reason why *M. pneumoniae* is under-recognized as a vasculitic agent: in the absence of pneumonia, mycoplasmal infection is not suspected and the patient is not further tested for *M. pneumoniae* serology.

2.2 Direct mechanisms of vasculitic/thrombotic vascular occlusion

M. pneumoniae, following its passive transfer into the circulation through the gaps that result from direct yet modest injury to the respiratory epithelial cells, is delivered to the distant vessels and organs, where it activates various inflammatory substances which then elicit vasculitis. These inflammatory substances include interleukin-8, tumor necrosis factor-α, macrophage inflammatory peptide-1α [Hardy et al., 2001], intercellular adhesion molecule-1 [Krunkosky et al., 2007], and regulated upon activation, normal T cells expression and secreted [Dakhama et al., 2003], among others. Tumor necrosis factor-α has been observed to be induced by *M. pneumoniae* in vitro from an early period of investigation [Arai et al., 1990; Kita et al., 1992]. This cytokine, along with interleukin-8, must play a pivotal role in eliciting vasculitic/thrombotic vascular occlusion. In this context, it is of some interest that the community acquired respiratory distress syndrome toxin can also induce the production of interleukin-8, macrophage inflammatory peptide-1α, and regulated upon activation, normal T cells expression and secreted [Hardy et al., 2009]. This toxin also might play some role in the development of vascular disorders. As regards the vascular occlusion-type manifestations with direct mechanisms, only occasionally has *M. pneumoniae* been found by culture or by polymerase chain reaction at the site of disease manifestation, typically, in the cerebrospinal fluid from patients with central nervous system manifestations.

2.3 Indirect mechanisms of vasculitic/thrombotic vascular occlusion

Mycoplasma pneumoniae contains potent immunogenic substances such as glycolipids, glycoproteins, and phospholipids within its cytoplasm. Macrophages, following phagocytosis of the organism, present these various kinds of mycoplasmal antigens to immunocompetent cells causing immune modulation which subsequently elicits autoimmunity through these antigens' molecular mimicry of various human cell components [for review, see Yang et al., 2004; Waites & Talkington, 2004]. From the perspective of vasculopathy due to *M. pneumoniae*, the most important aspect of this process must be the production of antiphospholipid (anticardiolipin) antibodies [Graw-Panzer et al., 2009; Nagashima et al., 2010; Snowden et al., 1990; Witmer et al., 2007]. Production of these antibodies is well known to occur during the course of autoimmune disorders such as systemic lupus erythematosus and to induce hypercoagulable state resulting in vasculopathy. As mentioned in the following sections, this ability of *M. pneumoniae* to induce antiphospholipid (anticardiolipin) antibodies is an important key in unraveling the indirect pathomechanisms of the vasculitic disorders caused by *M. pneumoniae*.
Mycoplasma pneumoniae can also form immune complexes [Biberfeld & Norberg, 1974; Mizutani & Mizutani, 1984], which activate complements and platelets, inducing coagulopathy, or affect the vascular epithelium, eliciting vasculitis. This ability of *M. pneumoniae* to form immune complexes is another important key to understanding the pathomechanisms of the vasculitic disorders caused by *M. pneumoniae*. To summarize, the immune modulations mentioned in this section can in several ways activate platelets, complements, and coagulation factors, leading to systemic or local hypercoagulable state. In vascular occlusion-type manifestations with indirect mechanisms, *M. pneumoniae* itself cannot typically be found at disease manifestation sites, though this is not the case in disease manifestations with direct mechanisms.

3. Vasculitic/thrombotic disorders due to *M. pneumoniae* infection

In Table 1, vascular occlusion-type extrapulmonary manifestations due to *M. pneumoniae* infection are classified according to type of pathomechanism, that is, direct or indirect, and according to the organ system which is mainly affected. Kawasaki disease, which involves multiple-organs in its manifestations, which include skin rash, lymphadenitis, and coronary aneurysm, is included in the cardiovascular category because of its disease severity.
In the following sections, comments are made on how these disorders can be considered consequences of *M. pneumoniae* infection. Since *M. pneumoniae* is a ubiquitous agent in the general population, the possibility of accidental coinfection by *M. pneumoniae* during the course of an unassociated disease should always be taken into account. One must remember to distinguish clearly between what *M. pneumoniae* can do and what it cannot do on the basis of its biological abilities. This chapter preferentially includes papers reporting vasculitic/thrombotic disorders for which at least one possible pathomechanism could reasonably be considered.

System	Direct mechanism	Indirect mechanism
Cardiovascular		Kawasaki disease, Cardiac thrombus, Temporal arteritis
Dermatological		Anaphylactoid purpura, Cutaneous vasculitis
Digestive		Pancreatitis
Hematological/ Hematopoietic		Disseminated intravascular coagulation, Thrombocytopenia, Splenic infarct
Musculoskeletal	Arthritis/Arthropathy*, Rhabdomyolysis*	Arthritis/Arthropathy*, Rhabdomyolysis*
Nervous	Stroke*, Striatal necrosis, Psychological disorders, Acute disseminated encephalomyelitis*, Transverse myelitis*	Stroke*, Acute disseminated encephalomyelitis*, Transverse myelitis*, Facial nerve palsy
Respiratory		Pulmonary embolism
Sensory	Sudden hearing loss	
Urogenital	Priapism	

* Mechanisms of both types (direct and indirect) can be postulated for these disorders.

Table 1. Vasculitic/thrombotic disorders caused by *M. pneumoniae* infection

3.1 Cardiovascular system

Although the existence of a link between acute or chronic *M. pneumoniae* infection and the development of atherosclerosis or coronary heart disease has been a matter for debate in the past, a connection between these conditions now seems less likely on the basis of recent evidence [Barski et al., 2010; Weiss et al., 2006] and is not included in this chapter. This question must be answered with certainty through future research.

3.1.1 Kawasaki disease

Kawasaki disease is a febrile illness mainly affecting infants and younger children; it is characterized by persistent fever (lasting longer than 5 days) that is nonresponsive to antibiotics; bilateral ocular conjunctivitis; redness of the lips, tongue (strawberry tongue) and oral cavity; changes in the peripheral extremities (indurative edema and desquamation); polymorphous exanthema of the body; and nonpurulent cervical lymph node swelling. It has been considered a systemic vasculitic disease with a predilection for the coronary arteries, resulting in the development of coronary aneurysm in the most severe cases [for review, see Pinna et al., 2008; Wood & Tulloh, 2009]. Though only a very small number of cases have been reported from Western countries [Leen & Ling, 1996; Vitale et al., 2010], reports of Kawasaki disease in association with *M. pneumoniae* infection are not infrequent in the Japanese literature. Kawasaki disease was first described from Japan [Kawasaki et al., 1974] and must have an inclination to the Asian ethnicity. Based on this assumption, there may be some inherent difference in genetic background in terms of the link between *M. pneumoniae* infection and susceptibility to Kawasaki disease. Although the pathomechanism of Kawasaki disease itself is not yet fully understood, the disease is generally believed to be immune-mediated [Pinna et al., 2008; Wood & Tulloh, 2009]. *Mycoplasma pneumoniae* has several arrays for immunomodulation, including cytokine production and T cell/B cell activation, and thereby could be a trigger of Kawasaki disease.

According to the previous case reports, which are mostly from Japan, pneumonia may or may not be present in *M. pneumoniae* infection-associated Kawasaki disease. Thus, even in the absence of pneumonia, *M. pneumoniae* infection must be considered in Kawasaki disease particularly when it is encountered during an epidemic of *M. pneumoniae* infection. Coronary arteries are not severely affected in most cases [Leen & Ling, 1996; Narita et al., 2001a; Sakai et al., 2007]; there has been only one exception, namely, an aneurysm in a single case reported from Taiwan [Wang et al., 2001].

3.1.2 Cardiac thrombus

Although it is only a single case to date, a large cardiac thrombus in the right ventricle has recently been reported in association with *M. pneumoniae* infection; it was successfully removed through cardiac surgery [Nagashima et al., 2010]. In this case, antiphospholipid antibodies (anticardiolipin IgM) were detected in the acute phase of infection but disappeared subsequently during convalescence; this observation supports the idea of a causal relation between *M. pneumoniae* infection and the production of antiphospholipid antibodies.

3.1.3 Temporal arteritis

One epidemiological study in Denmark has shown a close link between distinct peak incidences of temporal arteritis and two epidemics of *M. pneumoniae* infection [Elling et al., 1996]. Although neither additional case reports nor subsequent further clinical studies seem to exist, it is highly possible given the ability of *M. pneumoniae* to elicit vasculitis that *M. pneumoniae* is also a triggering agent for temporal arteritis.

3.2 Dermatological system

3.2.1 Anaphylactoid purpura

Anaphylactoid purpura, also called allergic purpura or Schönlein-Henoch purpura, is an allergic inflammation of the systemic capillary vessels most commonly affecting children, which is characterized by nonthrombocytopenic purpura, most remarkably on the bilateral lower extremities. This systemic disorder of the capillary vessels is not restricted to the skin; rather it also leads to microvascular bleeding manifesting as arthropathy (pain, swelling), gastrointestinal symptoms (severe abdominal pain, intestinal bleeding), and renal involvement (hematuria, nephritis) etc. It is possible that several infections can elicit these allergic reactions, and *M. pneumoniae*-infection-associated anaphylactoid purpura has sporadically been reported [Ghosh & Clements, 1992; Kano et al., 2007]. Considering the immunomodulatory properties of *M. pneumoniae*, it is reasonable to assume that *M. pneumoniae* can cause anaphylactoid purpura.

3.2.2 Cutaneous vasculitis

A few cases of cutaneous vasculitis, which is characterized by skin manifestations represented by erythematous macropapular rash resembling that observed in erythema multiforme, and by histological findings compatible with vasculitis such as leukocytoclastic vasculitis, have been reported in association with *M. pneumoniae* infection. Interestingly, cutaneous vasculitis due to *M. pneumoniae* was always accompanied by involvement of other organs; specifically, retinal vasculitis [Greco et al., 2007], polyarthritis [Perez et al., 1997], encephalitis [Perez & Montes, 2002], and acute respiratory distress syndrome, erythema multiforme, and pancreatitis [Van Bever et al., 1992]. This suggests either that skin biopsy, which is essential for the diagnosis of cutaneous vasculitis, is not likely to be performed unless other systemic diseases are present, or that cutaneous vasculitis occurs inherently as a part of systemic inflammation. In fact, immune complex-mediated activation of platelets has been postulated as an etiology for it [Perez & Montes, 2002].

3.3 Digestive system

3.3.1 Pancreatitis

Pancreatitis, which is often accompanied by other diseases affecting multiple organs [Daxböck et al., 2002; Van Bever et al., 1992], has been included among the extrapulmonary manifestations of *M. pneumoniae* infection, but its exact etiology when associated with *M. pneumoniae* infection remains unknown. Although an autoimmune-mediated mechanism has been postulated, no concrete evidence supporting this has been obtained. Van Bever et al. have suggested that pancreatitis is a consequence of ischemia, that is, persistent shock [Van Bever et al., 1992], in which case it could in a broad sense be classified as a vascular occlusion (cessation of blood supply)-type extrapulmonary manifestation.

3.4 Hematological/Hematopoietic system

3.4.1 Disseminated intravascular coagulation

Disseminated intravascular coagulation is a representative vascular occlusion-type extrapulmonary manifestation [Chryssanthopoulos et al., 2001; De Vos et al., 1974; Koletsky & Weinstein, 1980; Kountouras et al., 2003; Maisel et al., 1967; Nilsson et al; 1971]. Although the exact mechanism of this disorder when it occurs in association with *M. pneumoniae* infection remains unclear, it must be a consequence of some kind of immune dysregulation, perhaps of the release of coagulative substances (i.e. thromboplastin) from damaged lung tissue [Maisel et al., 1967; Nilsson et al; 1971], immune complex-mediated activation of complements [Chryssanthopoulos et al., 2001; De Vos et al., 1974], or stimulation of procoagulant activity among mononuclear cells, which can be induced by lipoglycans of *M. pneumoniae* [Fumarola, 1997]. Among those disorders that arise due to *M. pneumoniae* infection but are fundamentally benign in nature, disseminated intravascular coagulation is one of the most serious conditions, as it can lead to multiorgan failure with an occasional fatal outcome.

3.4.2 Thrombocytopenia/Thrombocytopenic purpura

Enough cases of thrombocytopenia with or without purpura due to *M. pneumoniae* infection have been reported that literature reviews have been published on this subject [Okoli et al., 2009; Venkatesan et al., 1996]. In one case, isolated thrombocytopenia preceded disseminated intravascular coagulation [Chiou et al., 1997]. Several immune-mediated etiologies have been considered, including the production of cross-reactive antibodies between mycoplasmal antigens and the von Willebrand factor-cleaving metalloprotease [Bar

Meir et al., 2000], microvascular platelet thrombosis [Cameron et al., 1992], the production of anti-platelet antibodies of some kind [Chen et al., 2004; Venkatesan et al., 1996], and the production of autoantibodies to the I antigen, which is expressed not only on erythrocytes but also on platelet surfaces [Gursel et al., 2009]. The formation of immune complexes may also play a role in the pathomechanism [Veenhoven et al., 1990].
Hemophagocytic syndrome, which is characterized by erythrophagocytosis in the bone marrow and believed to be a consequence of immune dysregulation, has been reported in association with *M. pneumoniae* infection. Although hemophagocytic syndrome in itself is not a vasculitic disease, this disorder predisposes patients to thrombocytopenia through thrombophagocytosis with hyperactivation of cytokines [Mizukane et al., 2001] or through formation of microthrombi [Bruch et al., 2001].

3.4.3 Splenic infarct

One reported case of splenic infarct occurred during the course of *M. pneumoniae* infection and was associated with the production of antiphospholipid antibodies [Witmer et al., 2007]. It must be emphasized that although an autoimmune etiology of this type occurring in association with *M. pneumoniae* infection has been undetectable to date, so that the possibility of its existence has been overlooked, such an etiology might underlie several thrombotic disorders involving various organs other than the spleen.

3.5 Musculoskeletal system

3.5.1 Arthritis/arthropathy

Arthropathy is frequently encountered during the course of systemic diseases which affect the microvasculature of large joints such as anaphylactoid purpura or thrombocytopenic purpura, both of which have been mentioned in preceding sections. Apart from this, arthritis is a common manifestation of *M. pneumoniae* infection [Sánchez-Vargas & Gómez-Duarte, 2008; Waites & Talkington, 2004]. Both monoarthritis and polyarthritis have been reported. It is possible that local inflammation elicited by *M. pneumoniae* through the function of cytokines contributes to the disease manifestation affecting the microvasculature of joints.

3.5.2 Rhabdomyolysis

Rhabdomyolysis is characterized by swollen, painful muscles, elevated serum creatine phosphokinase concentrations, hyperkalaemia, hypocalcaemia, and myoglobinuria occasionally leading to renal dysfunction. Infections have been included in the panel of causes, and *M. pneumoniae* infection-associated rhabdomyolysis has not infrequently been reported [Berger & Wadowksy, 2000; Daxböck et al., 2002; Decaux et al., 1980; Minami et al., 2003, Rothstein & Kenny, 1979; Weng et al., 2009]. A central role in the development of this disease condition has been assigned to tumor necrosis factor-α, which can cause acute proteolysis [Knochel, 1993] and which can be induced by *M. pneumoniae*. Microthrombosis has also been identified as a possible contributing factor to disease progression [Knochel, 1993]. On an interesting related note, rhabdomyolysis due to *M. pneumoniae* infection has occasionally been accompanied by neurological manifestations, in one case with acute disseminated encephalomyelitis [Decaux et al., 1980] and in two cases with transverse myelitis [Rothstein & Kenny, 1979; Weng et al., 2009]; the etiology of both of these neurological manifestations are presumed to involve vasculopathy (see next section). Regardless of whether they have an etiological link with *M. pneumoniae*-associated rhabdomyolysis, these neurological manifestations deserve further study on the assumption that there are common pathogenetic factors leading to vascular damage.

3.6 Nervous system

Nervous system manifestations are the most frequently reported type of extrapulmonary manifestations due to *M. pneumoniae* infection. *Mycoplasma pneumoniae* can cause neurologic symptoms through vasculitis or vascular occlusion with or without systemic hypercoagulative state. With regard to direct mechanisms, the author and coworkers have demonstrated that interleukin-6 and interleukin-8 play a significant role in the development of neurologic manifestations [Narita et al., 2005]. Moreover, interleukin-6 and interleukin-8 must be produced intrathecally, because elevated levels of these cytokines were observed in acute-phase cerebrospinal fluids without concomitant elevation in sera [Narita et al., 2005]. Rather unexpectedly, tumor necrosis factor-α and interferon-γ, which are the key cytokines in the development of neurologic diseases associated with bacterial or viral infections, were not elevated at all in acute-phase cerebrospinal fluids from patients with *M. pneumoniae* infection. These observations suggest that the pathomechanisms involved in mycoplasmal central nervous system manifestations are distinct from those involved in central nervous system diseases due to bacterial or viral infections.

3.6.1 Stroke

Stroke can occur in children [Fu et al., 1998; Lee et al., 2009; Leonardi et al., 2005; Ovetchkine et al., 2002; Parker et al., 1981; Tanir et al., 2006; Visudhiphan et al., 1992] as well as in adults [Mulder & Spierings, 1987; Padovan et al., 2001; Senda et al., 2010; Snowden et al., 1990; Sočan et al., 2001; Sotgiu et al., 2003]. The middle cerebral arteries are most often affected [Fu et al., 1998; Leonardi et al., 2005; Mulder & Spierings, 1987; Parker et al., 1981; Senda et al., 2010; Sotgiu et al., 2003], though the internal carotid arteries are affected in a few cases [Lee et al., 2009; Tanir et al., 2006; Visudhiphan et al., 1992]. Although the presence of systemic hypercoagulable state has been reported in a few cases, evidenced by disseminated intravascular coagulation [Mulder & Spierings, 1987] or by the production of antiphospholipid (anticardiolipin) antibodies [Senda et al., 2010; Snowden et al., 1990; Tanir et al., 2006], most cases occur in the absence of such conditions. Accordingly, many authors have suggested the presence of local vasculitis leading to vascular occlusion as an etiology. In fact, *M. pneumoniae* was isolated from the cerebrospinal fluid of a stroke patient [Sočan et al., 2001], and its genome has been detected in the cerebrospinal fluid as well [Padovan et al., 2001], reinforcing the theory of a direct mechanism. In addition, a case of multiple stenosis in the entire right Sylvian territory, suggesting the presence of vasculitis, has been reported [Ovetchkine et al., 2002]. Hematogenously-transferred *M. pneumoniae* must elicit cerebral vasculitis through the operation of inflammatory cytokines such as interleukin-8.

3.6.2 Striatal necrosis

Striatal necrosis is a peculiar central nervous system disease characterized by alteration of consciousness, extrapyramidal symptoms, and magnetic resonance imaging abnormality of the bilateral striata (the caudate and putamen nuclei). It has been reported in association with *M. pneumoniae* infection [Sakoulas, 2001; Saitoh et al., 1993; van Buiren & Uhl, 2003; Zambrino et al., 2000]. Chorea or choreiform movements may be a neurological consequence of striatal damage [Al-Mateen et al., 1988; Decaux et al, 1980; Zambrino et al., 2000]. Concerning its etiology, it has been reported that no patients with *M. pneumoniae*-associated striatal necrosis have also exhibited systemic hypercoagulative state. A similar disease called acute necrotizing encephalopathy affecting the bilateral thalami is believed to stem from vascular injury in the absence of a thrombotic mechanism [Mizuguchi et al., 1995], and a few cases of bilateral thalamic necrosis strongly resembling acute necrotizing encephalopathy have been reported in association with *M. pneumoniae* infection [Ashtekar et al., 2003; Perez et al., 2002]. It can reasonably be postulated that the pathomechanism underlying striatal necrosis must be local vasculitis induced by *M. pneumoniae* through the operation of cytokines and chemokines and leading eventually to vascular occlusion. In fact, cerebrospinal fluid from a patient with this disease was found to contain the genome of *M. pneumoniae* [Saitoh et al., 1993], which suggested a direct mechanism. Moreover, two reported cases of the involuntary movement disorder Tourette syndrome have been accompanied by the detectable presence of the *M. pneumoniae* genome in cerebrospinal fluid [Müller et al., 2000]. This strongly suggests that Tourette syndrome associated with *M. pneumoniae* infection is a result of vasculopathy in the basal ganglia resulting from a direct type mechanism inducing vascular occlusion. The accumulated evidence strongly suggests a vasculitic vascular occlusion mechanism for extrapyramidal diseases with involuntary movements as common manifestations.

3.6.3 Psychological disorders

Kluver-Bucy syndrome is a rare neurobehavioral syndrome which has been described in association with several neurologic disorders that cause destruction or dysfunction of the temporal lobe(s). It is characterized by psychic blindness, a strong urge to examine all subjects by mouth, and altered sexual behavior, among others. One case has been reported in association with M. pneumoniae infection [Auvichayapat et al., 2006]. This disorder was originally reported in rhesus monkeys following temporal lobectomy. It can reasonably be assumed that the transient interruption of blood supply to the temporal lobe caused by M. pneumoniae infection elicits the clinical manifestation of Kluver-Bucy syndrome.

3.6.4 Acute disseminated encephalomyelitis

Acute disseminated encephalomyelitis is a life-threatening disease which involves extensive lesions spreading over the brain and spinal cord. Because of its diverse distribution of affected areas, an indirect mechanism has been postulated, namely, immune complex-mediated vasculopathy [Behan et al., 1986; Guleria et al., 2005; Gupta et al., 2009]. On the other hand, recent studies on patients with acute disseminated encephalomyelitis have demonstrated the presence of M. pneumoniae genome in the cerebrospinal fluid [Matsumoto et al., 2009; Riedel et al., 2001; Yiş et al., 2008], or the presence of M. pneumoniae antigens inside the macrophages in the brain tissue [Stamm et al., 2008]. Thus it is highly possible that a direct mechanism, namely, vasculitis as a consequence of cytokine activation by M. pneumoniae, is responsible for some instances of acute disseminated encephalomyelitis.

3.6.5 Transverse myelitis

As in the case of acute disseminated encephalomyelitis, indirect immunological mechanisms such as immune complex-mediated injury leading to vasculopathy have been postulated as etiologies for transverse myelitis [Behan et al., 1986; Tsiodras et al., 2006]. As in acute disseminated encephalomyelitis, recent studies using polymerase chain reaction have reported the successful detection of the genome of *M. pneumoniae* in cerebrospinal fluid from patients with transverse myelitis [Abele-Horn et al., 1998; Goebels et al., 2001]. The possibility that vasculitis as a consequence of local cytokine activation at the site of inflammation by *M. pneumoniae* is an etiology of transverse myelitis must not be ignored.

3.6.6 Facial nerve palsy

A single case of facial nerve palsy in association with *M. pneumoniae* infection with production of antiphospholipid antibodies has been reported [Snowden et al., 1990]. This suggests that vasculopathy of the peripheral vessels resulting from the production of these autoantibodies leading to neural damage can be a cause of cranial, and possibly also peripheral, nerve palsies.

3.7 Respiratory system

3.7.1 Pulmonary embolism

A few cases of pulmonary embolism have been reported in association with *M. pneumoniae* infection [Graw-Panzer et al., 2009; Sterner and Biberfeld, 1969]. In one case with a documented popliteal venous thrombosis, the production of antiphospholipid (anticardiolipin) antibodies was demonstrated to be an underlying mechanism [Graw-Panzer et al., 2009]. As this chapter has repeatedly mentioned, the production of such antibodies must play a crucial role in many aspects of *M. pneumoniae* infection.

3.8 Sensory system

3.8.1 Sudden hearing loss

A possible link between sudden hearing loss and *M. pneumoniae* infection [García Berrocal et al., 2000] is interesting in terms of what it can tell us about pathomechanisms. Sudden hearing loss has two major etiologies; direct neural damage as in the case of infection with the mumps virus, and vascular damage leading to neural dysfunction. García Berrocal et al. have reported that, although the mumps virus is the most frequent of the infectious causes implicated in sudden hearing loss, *M. pneumoniae* is the second. Assuming the vascular etiology of sudden hearing loss, it is highly possible that vasculitis or thrombosis caused by *M. pneumoniae* infection occurring within cochlear branches of a labyrinthine artery could cause neural dysfunction that would lead to sudden hearing loss. Not a few cases of sudden hearing loss due to *M. pneumoniae* infection might have been overlooked.

3.9 Urogenital system

3.9.1 Priapism

Priapism as a consequence of obstruction of the outflow of blood through the dorsal vein of the penis may be a unique, vascular occlusion-type extrapulmonary manifestation of *M. pneumoniae* infection. Although there has only been a single case report [Hirshberg et al., 1996], it is highly possible that *M. pneumoniae* can cause this disease, considering the ability of *M. pneumoniae* to elicit vascular occlusion not only within arteries but also within veins.

4. Diagnosis and treatment of vasculitic disorders due to *M. pneumoniae* infection

4.1 Diagnosis of vasculitic disorders due to *M. pneumoniae* infection

Diagnosis of vasculitic disorders due to *M. pneumoniae* infection should be made primarily by serologically rather than molecular detection methodologies, for two major reasons. Firstly, *M. pneumoniae* is not always present at the site of vascular damage, except in conditions associated with direct vascular occlusion such as striatal necrosis and stroke, where a tiny amount of *M. pneumoniae* may be detected in cerebrospinal fluid by culture [Sočan et al., 2001] or by polymerase chain reaction [Padovan et al., 2001; Saitoh et al., 1993]. Secondly, respiratory samples such as oropharyngeal swabs, which are routinely utilized for molecular detection of infectious organisms, are not always adequate for the diagnosis of extrapulmonary manifestations with very little or no respiratory symptoms such as cough and sputa. It must be remembered that extrapulmonary manifestations due to *M. pneumoniae* infection occur not infrequently in the absence of pneumonia or even in the absence of respiratory symptoms.

In the serological diagnosis of *M. pneumoniae* infection, it is important to recall that antibodies to *M. pneumoniae* (that is, both the IgM- and IgG-class antibodies which are available for serological testing in routine clinical practice) can persist at detectable levels in the serum for several months or even years after the acute phase of infection [Eun et al., 2008; Lind & Bentzon, 1991]. In addition, given that the human can be infected with *M. pneumoniae* several times during his or her lifetime with or without clinical symptoms, it seems likely that there are many asymptomatic antibody carriers in the general population [Foy, 1993], assuming the fact that antibody responses are evoked during each instance of infection [Eun et al., 2008; Ito et al., 2001; Kung et al., 2007]. Thus, testing paired acute- and convalescent- phase sera using quantitative methods such as the complement fixation test, the particle agglutination test, and the enzyme-linked immunosorbent assay to show a significant increase in antibody titers is required for the precise diagnosis of a current, rather than a recent past, *M. pneumoniae* infection [Gnarpe et al., 1992]. Diagnosis by a single high titer of antibodies to *M. pneumoniae* alone, or by a single positive IgM test result alone, would be misleading because either of these tests can respond to evidence of a recent past infection and may return positive results when there is no current infection.

4.2 Treatment of vasculitic disorders due to *M. pneumoniae* infection

A strategy for the treatment of *M. pneumoniae* infection-associated vascular disorders has unfortunately not yet been established. Therapy is fundamentally palliative and may or may not include anticoagulative or fibrinolytic treatment. Treatments specific to particular diseases, such as high-dose intravenous immunoglobulin infusions for Kawasaki disease, have been administered when indicated. The use of macrolide antibiotics, which have not only antibiotic effects against *M. pneumoniae* but also immunomodulatory effects [for review, see Amsden, 2005], is reasonable considering the likelihood of an immune pathogenesis of the extrapulmonary manifestations of *M. pneumoniae* infection. In this context, steroid therapy in combination with antibiotic therapy is also recommended, and appears promising as a treatment for the extrapulmonary manifestations of *M. pneumoniae* because of its immunomodulatory effects [Cimolai, 2006]; it has been shown to have beneficial effects on experimental respiratory infection by *M. pneumoniae* [Tagliabue et al., 2008].

The successful practical application of immunomodulatory agents such as steroids or immunoglobulins in the treatment of vascular occlusion-type extrapulmonary manifestations of *M. pneumoniae* infection has been reported in not a few instances. In these cases, neurological disorders such as acute disseminated encephalomyelitis or transverse myelitis and thrombocytopenic disorders such as disseminated intravascular coagulation or thrombocytopenic purpura are most often treated by immunomodulatory agents because of the severity of these diseases. Some authors have reported that therapy with immunomodulatory agents was very effective, while others have reported that the effects are uncertain. Although it cannot be expected that immunomodulatory agents will affect thrombotic disorders that are already established, it is clear that they must have some beneficial effects on vasculitic disorders during ongoing inflammation. Additional accumulation of data will be necessary to construct a therapeutic strategy for the treatment of vascular occlusion-type extrapulmonary manifestations of *M. pneumoniae* infection.

4.3 Prognosis of vasculitic disorders due to *M. pneumoniae* infection

Prognosis of vasculitic disorders due to *M. pneumoniae* infection is variable depending on the disease manifestations. While the clinical symptoms of *M. pneumoniae* infection are immune-mediated, and can therefore generally be considered self-limiting toward a favorable outcome, some cases with fatal outcomes have been reported. Most of these were cases with neurological and hematological manifestations; disseminated intravascular coagulation was particularly strongly associated with fatal outcome. Delay in the diagnosis of *M. pneumoniae* infection might be a devastating factor in severe cases. Therefore, it must always be recalled that *M. pneumoniae* infection cause vasculitic disorders even in the absence of pneumonia, particularly when these vasculitic disorders are encountered during an epidemic of *M. pneumoniae* infection.

5. Conclusion

This chapter has discussed the ability of *M. pneumoniae* to cause various kinds of vascular occlusion-type extrapulmonary manifestations as a consequence of immune modulations such as cytokine production, lymphocyte proliferation, and immune complex formation. Such cases probably occur far more frequently than they are recognized. These vascular diseases may occur in the absence of pneumonia or even in the absence of respiratory symptoms, with or without systemic hypercoagulable state. With this in mind, the possibility of *M. pneumoniae* infection must be considered in diagnosing vasculitic/thrombotic disorders, particularly when such disorders are encountered during an epidemic period or within an endemic region of *M. pneumoniae* infection. Mycoplasmal infections are strictly species-specific. For example, rodents are natural hosts of *M. pulmonis* but not of *M. pneumoniae*, and although they can serve as a model for respiratory infection they do not develop extrapulmonary manifestations. To date, the only versatile animal models that permit the study of the extrapulmonary manifestations seen in humans are exceptional cases such as chimpanzee models [Barile et al., 1994]. For this reason, the continued accumulation of human case reports is crucially important to ensure further progress in this field.

6. References

Abele-Horn, M, Franck, W, Busch, U, Nitschko, H, Roos, R, Heesemann, J. (1998). Transverse myelitis associated with *Mycoplasma pneumoniae* infection. *Clin Infect Dis*, 26 (4), 909-912.

Al-Mateen, M, Gibbs, M, Dietrich, R, Mitchell, WG, Menkes, JH. (1988). Encephalitis lethargica-like illness in a girl with mycoplasma infection. *Neurology*, 38 (7), 1155-1158.

Amsden, GW. (2005). Anti-inflammatory effects of macrolides- an underappreciated benefit in the treatment of community-acquired respiratory tract infections and chronic inflammatory pulmonary conditions? *J Antimicrob Chemother*, 55 (1), 10-21.

Arai, S, Furukawa, M, Munakata, T, Kuwano, K, Inoue, H, Miyazaki, T. (1990). Enhancement of cytotoxicity of active macrophages by Mycoplasma: role of Mycoplasma-associated induction of tumor necrosis factor-α (TNF-α) in macrophages. *Microbiol Immunol*, 34 (3), 231-243.

Ashtekar, CS, Jaspan, T, Thomas, D, Weston, V, Gayatri, NA, Whitehouse, WP. (2003). Acute bilateral thalamic necrosis in a child with *Mycoplasma pneumoniae*. *Dev Med Child Neurol*, 45 (9), 634-637.

Auvichayapat, N, Auvichayapat, P, Watanatorn, J, Thamaroj, J, Jitpimolmard, S. (2006). Kluver-Bucy syndrome after mycoplasmal bronchitis. *Epilep Behav*, 8 (1), 320-322.

Bar Meir, E, Amital, H, Levy, Y, Kneller, A, Bar-Dayan, Y, Schoenfeld, Y. (2000). *Mycoplasma-pneumoniae*-induced thrombotic thrombocytopenic purpura. *Acta Haematol*, 103 (2), 112-115.

Barile, MF, Kapatais-Zoumbos, K, Snoy, P, Grabowski, MW, Sneller, M, Miller, L, Chandler, DKF. (1994). Experimentally induced septic arthritis in chimpanzees infected with *Mycoplasma hominis, Mycoplasma pneumoniae*, and *Ureaplasma urealyticum*. *Clin Infect Dis*, 18 (5), 694-703.

Barski, L, Nevzorov, R, Horowitz, J, Horowitz, S. (2010). Antibodies to various mycoplasmas in patients with coronary heart disease. *Isr Med Assoc J*, 12 (7), 396-399.

Behan, PO, Feldman, RG, Segerra, JM, Draper, IT. (1986). Neurological aspects of mycoplasmal infection. *Acta Neurol Scand* 74 (4), 314-322.

Berger, RP, Wadowksy, RM. (2000). Rhabdomyolysis associated with infection by *Mycoplasma pneumoniae*: a case report. *Pediatrics*, 105 (2), 433-436.

Biberfeld, G, Norberg, R. (1974). Circulating immune complexes in *Mycoplasma pneumoniae* infection. *J Immunol*, 112 (1), 413-415.

Bruch, LA, Jefferson, RJ, Pike, MG, Gould, SJ, Squier, W. (2001). *Mycoplasma pneumoniae* infection, meningoencephalitis, and hemophagocytosis. *Pediatr Neurol*, 25 (1), 67-70.

Cameron, D, Welsby, P, Turner, M. (1992). Thrombotic thrombocytopenic purpura due to *Mycoplasma pneumoniae*. *Postgrad Med J*, 68 (799), 393-394.

Cartner, SC, Lindsey, JR, Gibbs-Erwin, J, Cassell, GH, Simecka, JW. (1998). Roles of innate and adaptive immunity in respiratory mycoplasmosis. *Infect Immun*, 66 (8), 3485-3591.

Chen, CJ, Juan, CJ, Hsu, ML, Lai, YS, Lin, SP, Cheng, SN. (2004). *Mycoplasma pneumoniae* infection presenting as neutropenia, thrombocytopenia, and acute hepatitis in a child. *J Microbiol Immunol Infect*, 37 (2), 128-130.

Chiou, C-C, Liu, Y-C, Lin, H-H, Hsieh, K-S. (1997). *Mycoplasma pneumoniae* infection complicated by lung abscess, pleural effusion, thrombocytopenia and disseminated intravascular coagulation. *Pediatr Infect Dis J*, 16 (3), 327-329.

Chmura, K, Bai, X, Nakamura, M, Kandasamy, P, McGibney, M, Kuronuma, K, Mitsuzawa, H, Voelker, DR, Chan, ED. (2008). Induction of IL-8 by *Mycoplasma pneumoniae* membrane in BEAS-2B cells. Am J Physiol Lung *Cell Mol Physiol*, 295 (1), L220-230.

Chryssanthopoulos, C, Eboriadou, M, Monti, K, Soubassi, V, Sava, K. (2001). Fatal disseminated intravascular coagulation caused by *Mycoplasma pneumoniae. Pediatr Infect Dis J*, 20 (6), 634-635.

Cimolai, N. (2006). Corticosteroids and complicated *Mycoplasma pneumoniae* infection. *Pediatr Pulmonol*, 41 (10), 1008-1009.

Dakhama, A, Kraft M, Martin, RJ, Gelfand, EW. (2003). Induction of regulated upon activation, normal T cells expression and secreted (RANTES) and transforming growth factor-β1 in airway epithelial cells by *Mycoplasma pneumoniae. Am J Respir Cell Mol Biol*, 29 (3 Pt 1), 344-351.

Daxböck, F, Brunner, G, Popper, H, Krause R, Schmid, K, Krejs, GJ, Wenisch, C. (2002). A case of lung transplantation following *Mycoplasma pneumoniae* infection. *Eur J Clin Microbiol Infect Dis*, 21 (4), 318-322.

De Vos, M, Van Nimmen, L, Baele, G. (1974). Disseminated intravascular coagulation during a fatal *Mycoplasma pneumoniae* infection. *Acta Haemat*, 52 (2), 120-125.

Decaux, G, Szyper, M, Ectors, M, Cornil, A, Franken, L. (1980). Central nervous system complications of mycoplasma pneumoniae. *J Neurol Neurosurg Psychiatry*, 43 (10), 883-887.

Elling, P, Olsson, AT, Elling, H. (1996). Synchronous variation of the incidence of temporal arteritis and polymyalgia rheumatica in different regions of Denmark; association with epidemics of *Mycoplasma pneumoniae* infection. *J Rheumatol*, 23 (1), 112-119.

Eun, BW, Kim, NH, Choi, EH, Lee, HJ. (2008). *Mycoplasma pneumoniae* in Korean children: the epidemiology of pneumonia over an 18-year period. *J Infect*, 56 (5), 326-331.

Foy, HM. (1993). Infections caused by *Mycoplasma pneumoniae* and possible carrier state in different populations of patients. *Clin Infect Dis*, 17(Suppl 1), S37-46.

Fu, M, Wong, KS, Lam, WWM, Wong, GWK. (1998). Middle cerebral artery occlusion after recent *Mycoplasma pneumoniae* infection. *J Neurol Sci*, 157 (1), 113-115.

Fumarola, D. (1997). Intravascular coagulation and *Mycoplasma pneumoniae* infection. *Pediatr Infect Dis J*, 16 (10), 1012-1013.

García Berrocal, JR, Ramírez-Camacho, R, Portero, F, Vargas, JA. (2000). Role of viral and *Mycoplasma pneumoniae* infection in idiopathic sudden sensorineural hearing loss. *Acta Otolaryngol*, 120 (7), 835-839.

Ghosh, K, Clements, GB. (1992). Surveillance of *Mycoplasma pneumoniae* infections in Scotland 1986-1991. *J Infect*, 25 (2), 221-227.

Gnarpe, J, Lundbäck, A, Sundelöf, B, Gnarpe, H. (1992). Prevalence of *Mycoplasma pneumoniae* in subjectively healthy individuals. *Scand J Infect Dis*, 24 (2), 161-164.

Goebels, N, Helmchen, C, Abele-Horn, M, Gasser, T, Pfister, H-W. (2001). Extensive myelitis associated with *Mycoplasma pneumoniae* infection: magnetic resonance imaging and clinical long-term follow-up. *J Neurol*, 248 (3), 204-208.

Graw-Panzer, KD, Verma, S, Rao, S, Miller, ST, Lee, H. (2009). Venous thrombosis and pulmonary embolism in a child with pneumonia due to *Mycoplasma pneumoniae. J Natl Med Assoc,* 101 (9), 956-958.

Greco, F, Sorge, A, Salvo, V, Sorge, G. (2007). Cutaneous vasculitis associated with *Mycoplasma pneumoniae* infection: case report and literature review. *Clin Pediatr (Phila),* 46 (5), 451-453.

Guleria, R, Nisar, N, Chawla, TC, Biswas, NR. (2005). *Mycoplasma pneumoniae* and central nervous system complications: a review. *J Lab Clin Med,* 146 (2), 55-63.

Gupta, A, Kimber, T, Crompton, JL, Karagiannis, A. (2009). Acute disseminated encephalomyelitis secondary to *Mycoplasma pneumoniae. Intern Med J,* 39 (1), 68-69.

Gursel, O, Altun, D, Atay, AA, Bedir, O, Kurekci, AE. (2009). *Mycoplasma pneumoniae* infection associated with pancytopenia. A case report. *J Pediatr Hematol Oncol,* 31 (10), 760-762.

Hardy, RD, Jafri, HS, Olsen, K, Wordemann, M, Hatfield, J, Rogers, BB, Patel, P, Duffy, L, Cassell, G, McCracken, GH, Ramilo, O. (2001). Elevated cytokine and chemokine levels and prolonged pulmonary airflow resistance in a murine *Mycoplasma pneumoniae* pneumonia model: a microbiologic, histologic, immunologic, and respiratory plethysmographic profile. *Infect Immun,* 69 (6), 3869-3876.

Hardy, RD, Coalson, JJ, Peters, J, Chaparro, A, Techasaensiri, C, Cantwell, AM, Kannan, TR, Basemann, JB, Dube, PH. (2009). Analysis of pulmonary inflammation and function in the mouse and baboon after exposure to *Mycoplasma pneumoniae* CARDS toxin. *PLoS ONE,* 4 (10), e7562.

Hirshberg, SJ, Charles, RS, Ettinger, JB. (1996). Pediatric priapism associated with *Mycoplasma pneumoniae. Urology* 47 (5), 745-746.

Ito, I, Ishida, T, Osawa, M, Arita, M, Hashimoto, T, Hongo, T, Mishima, M. (2001). Culturally verified *Mycoplasma pneumoniae* pneumonia in Japan: a long-term observation from 1979-99. *Epidemiol Infect,* 127 (2), 365-367.

Kannan, TR, Baseman, JB. (2006). ADP-ribosylating and vacuolating cytotoxin of *Mycoplasma pneumoniae* represents unique virulence determinant among bacterial pathogens. *Proc Natl Acad Sci,* 103 (17), 6724-6729.

Kano, Y, Mitsuyama, Y, Hirahara, K, Shiohara, T. (2007). *Mycoplasma pneumoniae* infection-induced erythema nodosum, anaphylactoid purpura, and acute urticaria in 3 people in a single family. *J Am Acad Dermatol,* 57 (2 Suppl), S33-35.

Kawasaki, T, Kosaki, F, Okawa S, Shigematsu, I, Yanagawa, H. (1974). A new infantile acute febrile mucocutaneous lymph node syndrome (MLNS) prevailing in Japan. *Pediatrics,* 54 (3), 271-276.

Kita, M, Ohmoto, Y, Hirai, Y, Yamaguchi, N, Imanishi, J. (1992). Induction of cytokines in human peripheral blood mononuclear cells by Mycoplasmas. *Microbiol Immunol,* 36 (5), 507-516.

Knochel, JP. (1993). Mechanisms of rhabdomyolysis. *Curr Opin Rheumatol,* 5 (6), 725-731.

Koletsky, RJ, Weinstein, AJ. (1980). Fulminant *Mycoplasma pneumoniae* infection. *Am Rev Respir Dis,* 122 (3), 491-496.

Kountouras, D, Deutsch, M, Emmanuel, T, Georgiadis, G, Koskinas, J. (2003). Fulminant *Mycoplasma pneumoniae* infection with multi-organ involvement: a case report. *Eur J Int Med,* 14 (5), 329-331.

Krunkosky, TM, Jordan, JL, Chambers, E, Krause, DC. (2007). *Mycoplasma pneumoniae* host-pathogen studies in an air-liquid culture of differentiated human airway epithelial cells. *Microb Pathog*, 42 (2-3), 98-103.

Kung, C-M, Wang, H-L. (2007). Seroprevalence of *Mycoplasma pneumoniae* in healthy adolescents in Taiwan. (2007). *Jpn J Infect Dis*, 60 (6), 352-354.

Lee, C-Y, Huang, Y-Y, Huang, F-L, Liu, F-C, Chen, P-Y. (2009). *Mycoplasma pneumoniae*-associated cerebral infarction in a child. *J Trop Pediatr*, 55 (4), 272-275.

Leen, C, Ling, S. (1996). Mycoplasma infection and Kawasaki disease. *Arch Dis Child*, 75 (3), 266-267.

Leonardi, S, Pavone, P, Rotolo, N, La Rosa, M. (2005). Stroke in two children with *Mycoplasma pneumoniae* infection. A causal or casual relationship? *Pediatr Infect Dis J*, 24 (9), 843-845.

Lind, K, Bentzon, MW. (1991). Ten and a half years seroepidemiology of *Mycoplasma pneumoniae* infection in Denmark. *Epidemiol Infect*, 107 (1), 189-199.

Maisel, JC, Babbitt, LH, John, TJ. (1967). Fatal *Mycoplasma pneumoniae* infection with isolation of organisms from lung. *J Am Med Assoc*, 202 (4), 139-142.

Matsumoto, N, Takahashi, S, Toriumi, N, Sarashina, T, Makita, Y, Tachibana, Y, Fujieda, K. (2009). Acute disseminated encephalomyelitis in an infant with incontinentia pigmenti. *Brain Dev*, 31 (8), 625-628.

Minami, K, Maeda, H, Yanagawa, T, Suzuki, H, Izumi, G, Yoshikawa, N. (2003). Rhabdomyolysis associated with *Mycoplasma pneumoniae* infection. *Pediatr Infect Dis J*, 22 (3), 291-293.

Mizuguchi, M, Abe, J, Mikkaichi, K, Noma, S, Yoshida, K, Yamanaka, T, Kamoshita, S. (1995). Acute necrotizing encephalopathy of childhood: a new syndrome presenting with multifocal, symmetric brain lesions. *J Neurol Neurosurg Psychiatry*, 58 (5), 555-561.

Mizukane, R, Kadota, J, Yamaguchi, T, Kiya, T, Fukushima, H, Nakatomi, M, Kohno, S. (2002). An elderly patient with hemophagocytic syndrome due to severe *Mycoplasma* pneumonia with marked hypercytokinemia. *Respiration*, 69 (1), 87-91.

Mizutani, H, Mizutani, H. (1984). Circulating immune complexes in patients with mycoplasmal pneumonia. *Am Rev Respir Dis*, 130 (4), 627-629.

Mulder, LJMM, Spierings, ELH. (1987). Stroke in a young adult with *Mycoplasma pneumoniae* infection complicated by intravascular coagulation. *Neurology*, 37 (8), 1430-1431.

Müller, N, Riedel, M, Förderreuther, S, Blendinger, C, Abele-Horn, M. (2000). Tourette's syndrome and *Mycoplasma pneumoniae* infection. *Am J Psychiatry*, 157 (3), 481-482.

Nagashima, M, Higaki, T, Satoh, H, Nakano, T. (2010). Cardiac thrombus associated with *Mycoplasma pneumoniae* infection. *Interact Cardiovasc Thoracic Surg*, 11 (6), 849-851.

Narita, M, Matsuzono, Y, Togashi, T, Kajii, N. (1992). DNA diagnosis of central nervous system infection by *Mycoplasma pneumoniae*. *Pediatrics*, 90 (2), 250-253.

Narita, M, Matsuzono, Y, Itakura, O, Togashi, T, Kikuta, H. (1996). Survey of mycoplasmal bacteremia detected in children by polymerase chain reaction. *Clin Infect Dis*, 23 (3), 522-525.

Narita, M, Tanaka, H, Abe, S, Yamada, S, Kubota, M, Togashi, T. (2000). Close association between pulmonary disease manifestation in *Mycoplasma pneumoniae* infection and enhanced local production of interleukin-18 in the lung, independent of gamma interferon. *Clin Diagn Lab Immunol*, 7 (6), 909-914.

Narita, M, Yamada, S, Nakayama, T, Sawada, H, Nakajima, M, Sageshima, S. (2001a). Two cases of lymphadenopathy with liver dysfunction due to *Mycoplasma pneumoniae* infection with mycoplasmal bacteraemia without pneumonia. *J Infect*, 42 (2), 154-156.

Narita, M, Tanaka, H, Yamada, S, Abe, S, Ariga, T, Sakiyama, Y. (2001b). Significant role of interleukin-8 in pathogenesis of pulmonary disease due to *Mycoplasma pneumoniae* infection. *Clin Diagn Lab Immunol*, 8 (5), 1028-1030.

Narita, M, Tanaka, H, Togashi, T Abe, S. (2005). Cytokines involved in CNS manifestations caused by *Mycoplasma pneumoniae*. *Pediatr Neurol*, 33 (2), 105-109.

Narita, M. (2009). Pathogenesis of neurologic manifestations of *Mycoplasma pneumoniae* infection. *Pediatr Neurol*, 41 (3), 159-66.

Narita, M. (2010). Pathogenesis of extrapulmonary manifestations of *Mycoplasma pneumoniae* infection with special reference to pneumonia. *J Infect Chemother*, 16 (3), 162-169.

Nilsson, IM, Rausing, A, Denneberg, T, Christensson, P. (1971). Intravascular coagulation and acute renal failure in a child with mycoplasma infection. *Acta Med Scand*, 189 (5), 359-365.

Okoli, K, Gupta, A, Irani, F, Kasmani, R. (2009). Immune thrombocytopenia associated with *Mycoplasma pneumoniae* infection: a case report and review of literature. *Blood Coagul Fibrinolysis*, 20 (7), 595-598.

Ovetchkine, P, Brugières, P, Seradj, A, Reinert, P, Cohen, R. (2002). An 8-y-old boy with acute stroke and radiological signs of cerebral vasculitis after recent *Mycoplasma pneumoniae* infection. *Scand J Infect Dis*, 34 (4), 307-309.

Padovan, CS, Pfister, H-W, Bense, S, Fingerle, V, Abele-Horn, M. (2001). Detection of *Mycoplasma pneumoniae* DNA in cerebrospinal fluid of a patient with *M. pneumoniae* infection- "associated" stroke. *Clin Infect Dis*, 33 (10), e119-121.

Parker, P, Puck, J, Fernandez, F. (1981). Cerebral infarction associated with Mycoplasma *pneumoniae*. *Pediatrics*, 67 (3), 373-375.

Perez, C, Mendoza, H, Hernandez, R, Valcayo, A, Guarch, R. (1997). Leukocytoclastic vasculitis and polyarthritis associated with *Mycoplasma pneumoniae* infection. *Clin Infect Dis*, 25 (1) 154-155.

Perez, C, Montes, M. (2002). Cutaneous leukocytoclastic vasculitis and encephalitis associated with *Mycoplasma pneumoniae* infection. *Arch Intern Med*, 162 (3), 352-354.

Pinna, GS, Kafetzis, DA, Tselkas, OI, Skevaki, CL. (2008). Kawasaki disease: an overview. *Curr Opin Infect Dis*, 21 (3), 263-270.

Riedel, K, Kempf, VAJ, Bechtold, A, Klimmer, M. (2001). Acute disseminated encephalomyelitis (ADEM) due to *Mycoplasma pneumoniae* infection in an adolescent. *Infection*, 29 (4), 240-242.

Rothstein, TL, Kenny, GE. (1979). Cranial neuropathy, myeloradiculopathy, and myositis. Complications of *Mycoplasma pneumoniae* infection. *Arch Neurol*, 36 (8), 476-477.

Saitoh, S, Wada, T, Narita, M, Kohsaka, S, Mizukami, S, Togashi, T, Kajii, N. (1993). *Mycoplasma pneumoniae* infection may cause striatal lesions leading to acute neurologic dysfunction. *Neurology*, 43 (10), 2150-2151.

Sakai, R, Sakaguchi, S, Oguchi S, Aoyanagi, Y, Suzuki, K, Wada, M, Kuriya, T, Watanabe, H, Takada, M. (2007). Three cases of Kawasaki disease complicated by *Mycoplasma pneumoniae* infection. *Shonika Rinsho*, 60 (7), 1591-1596 (Japanese with English abstract).

Sakoulas, G. (2001). Brainstem and striatal encephalitis complicating *Mycoplasma pneumoniae* pneumonia: possible benefit of intravenous immunoglobulin. *Pediatr Infect Dis J*, 20 (5), 543-545.

Sánchez-Vargas, FM, Gómez-Duarte, OG. (2008). *Mycoplasma pneumoniae*- an emerging extra-pulmonary pathogen. *Clin Microbiol Infect*, 14 (2), 105-115.

Senda, J, Ito, M, Atsuta, N, Watanabe, H, Hattori, N, Kawai, H, Sobue, G. (2010). Paradoxical brain embolism induced by *Mycoplasma pneumoniae* infection with deep venous thrombus. *Inter Med*, 49 (18), 2003-2005.

Shimizu, T, Kida, Y, Kuwano, K. (2005). A dipalmitoylated lipoprotein from *Mycoplasma pneumoniae* activates NF-κB through TLR1, TLR2, and TLR6. *J Immunol*, 175 (7), 4641-4646.

Snowden, N, Wilson, PB, Longson, M, Pumphrey, RSH. (1990). Antiphospholipid antibodies and *Mycoplasma pneumoniae* infection. *Postgrad Med J*, 66 (775), 356-362.

Počan, M, Ravnik, I, Benčina, D, Dovč, P, Zakotnik, B, Jazbec, J. (2001). Neurological symptoms in patients whose cerebrospinal fluid is culture- and/or polymerase chain reaction-positive for *Mycoplasma pneumoniae*. *Clin Infect Dis*, 32 (2), e31-35.

Sohn, MH, Lee, KE, Choi, SY, Kwon, BC, Chang, MW, Kim, K-E. (2005). Effect of *Mycoplasma pneumoniae* lysate on interleukin-8 gene expression in human respiratory epithelial cells. *Chest*, 128 (1), 322-326.

Sotgiu, S, Pugliatti, M, Rosati, G, Deiana, GA, Sechi, GP. (2003). Neurological disorders associated with *Mycoplasma pneumoniae* infection. *Eur J Neurol*, 10 (2), 165-168.

Stamm, B, Moschopulos, M, Hungerbuehler, H, Guarner, J, Genrich, GL, Zaki, SR. (2008). Neuroinvasion by *Mycoplasma pneumoniae* in acute disseminated encephalomyelitis. *Emerg Infect Dis*, 14 (4), 641-643.

Sterner, G, Biberfeld, G. (1969). Central nervous system complications of *Mycoplasma pneumoniae* infection. *Scand J Infect Dis*, 1 (3), 203-208.

Tagliabue, C, Salvatore, CM, Techasaensiri, C, Mejias, A, Torres, JP, Katz, K, Gomez, AM, Esposito, S, Principi, N, Hardy, RD. (2008). The impact of steroids given with macrolide therapy on experimental *Mycoplasma pneumoniae* respiratory infection. *J Infect Dis*, 198 (8), 1180-1188.

Tanaka, H, Honma, S, Abe, S, Tamura, H. (1996). Effects of interleukin-2 and cyclosporin A on pathologic features in *Mycoplasma* pneumonia. *Am J Respir Crit Care Med*, 154 (6), 1908-1912.

Tanaka, H, Narita, M, Teramoto, S, Saikai, T, Oashi, K, Igarashi, T, Abe, S. (2002). Role of interleukin-18 and T-helper type 1 cytokines in the development of *Mycoplasma pneumoniae* pneumonia in adults. *Chest*, 121 (5), 1493-1497.

Tanir, G, Aydemir, C, Yilmaz, D, Tuygun, N. (2006). Internal carotid artery occlusion associated with *Mycoplasma pneumoniae* infection in a child. *Turk J Pediatr*, 48 (2), 166-171.

Tsiodras, S, Kelesidis, Th, Kelesidis, I, Voumbourakis, K Giamarellou, H. (2006). *Mycoplasma pneumoniae*-associated myelitis: a comprehensive review. *Eur J Neurol*, 13 (2), 112-124.

Van Bever, HP, Van Doorn, JWD, Demey, HE. (1992). Adult respiratory distress syndrome associated with *Mycoplasma pneumoniae* infection. *Eur J Pediatr*, 151 (3), 227-228.

van Buiren, M, Uhl, M. (2003). Bilateral striatal necrosis associated with *Mycoplasma pneumoniae* infection. *New Engl J Med*, 348 (8), 720.

Veenhoven, WA, Smithuis, RH, Kerst, AJ. (1990). Thrombocytopenia associated with *Mycoplasma pneumoniae* infection. *Neth J Med*, 37 (1-2), 75-76.

Venkatesan, P, Patel, V, Collingham, KE, Ellis, CJ. (1996). Fatal thrombocytopenia associated with *Mycoplasma pneumoniae* infection. *J Infect*, 33 (2), 115-117.

Visudhiphan, P, Chiemchanya, S, Sirinavin, S. (1992). Internal carotid artery occlusion associated with *Mycoplasma pneumoniae* infection. *Pediatr Neurol*, 8 (3), 237-239.

Vitale, EA, La Torre, F, Calcagno, G, Infricciori, G, Fede, C, Conti, G, Chimenz, R, Falcini, F. (2010). *Mycoplasma pneumoniae*: a possible trigger of Kawasaki disease or a mere coincidental association? Report of the first four Italian cases. *Minerva Pediatr*, 62 (6), 605-607.

Waites, KB, Talkington, DF. (2004). *Mycoplasma pneumoniae* and its role as a human pathogen. *Clin Microbiol Rev*, 17 (4), 697-728.

Wang, JN, Wang, SM, Liu, CC, Wu, JM. (2001). *Mycoplasma pneumoniae* infection associated with Kawasaki disease. *Acta Paediatr*, 90 (5), 594-595.

Weiss, TW, Kvakan, H, Kaun, C, Prager, M, Speidl, WS, Zorn, G, Pfaffenberger, S, Huk, I, Maurer, G, Huber, K, Wojta, J. (2006). No evidence for a direct role of *Helicobacter pylori* and *Mycoplasma pneumoniae* in carotid artery atherosclerosis. *J Clin Pathol*, 59 (11), 1186-1190.

Weng, W-C, Peng, SS-F, Wang, S-B, Chou, Y-T, Lee, W-T. (2009). *Mycoplasma pneumoniae*-associated transverse myelitis and rhabdomyolysis. *Pediatr Neurol*, 40 (2), 128-130.

Witmer, CM, Steenhoff, AP, Shah, SS, Raffini, LJ. (2007). *Mycoplasma pneumoniae*, splenic infarct, and transient antiphospholipid antibodies: a new association? *Pediatrics*, 119 (1), e292-295.

Wood, LE, Tulloh, RM. (2009). Kawasaki disease in children. *Heart*, 95 (10), 787-792.

Yang, J, Hooper, WC, Phillips, DJ, Talkington, DF (2002). Regulation of proinflammatory cytokines in human lung epithelial cells infected with *Mycoplasma pneumoniae*. *Infect Immun*, 70 (7), 3649-3655.

Yang, J, Hooper, WC, Phillips, DJ, Talkington, DF. (2004). Cytokines in *Mycoplasma pneumoniae* infections. *Cytokine Growth Fac Rev*, 15 (2-3), 157-168.

Yiş, U, Kurul, SH, Çakmakçi, H, Dirik, E. (2008). *Mycoplasma pneumoniae*: nervous system complications in childhood and review of the literature. *Eur J Pediatr*, 167 (9), 973-978.

Zambrino, CA, Zorzi, G, Lanzi, G, Uggetti, C, Egitto, MG. (2000). Bilateral striatal necrosis associated with *Mycoplasma pneumoniae* infection in an adolescent: clinical and neuroradiologic follow up. *Mov Disord*, 15 (5), 1023-1026.

4

Vasculitis: Endothelial Dysfunction During Rickettsial Infection

Yassina Bechah, Christian Capo and Jean-Louis Mege
Unité de Recherche sur les Maladies Infectieuses Transmissibles et Emergentes (URMITE), UMR CNRS 6236, IRD 3R198, Institut Fédératif de Recherche 48, Université de la Méditerranée, Faculté de Médecine, 13385 Marseille, France

1. Introduction

Rickettsial infections cause irreversible damage to the human host and are associated with a high morbidity and high mortality. The mortality rate can be as high as 20 % for Rocky Mountain spotted fever and 30 % for epidemic typhus, which are both diseases that are caused by rickettsiae. Some rickettsiae species, such as *Rickettsia prowazekii* and *Rickettsia rickettsii*, are currently considered bioterrorism agents. The study of rickettsiae organisms is fascinating due to the nature of these pathogens, which are obligate intracellular bacteria, and to their tropism for the endothelium. The endothelium plays a key role in numerous physiological processes, such as vascular homeostasis, the regulation of blood flow and vascular tone, coagulation, angiogenesis and inflammation. In this chapter, we give a general overview of rickettsial diseases, the endothelium, and how rickettsial infection impacts endothelial function. Specifically, we focus on the endothelial cell response to rickettsial infections and emphasize the role of the endothelial cells in the clinical symptoms and tissue injury caused by rickettsioses.

2. Rickettsioses

Rickettsioses are infectious diseases that are caused by heterogeneous, gram-negative, obligate intracellular bacteria (figure 1). The *Rickettsiaceae* bacterial family contains the genus *Orientia*, which has only one species (*Orientia tsutsugamushi*), and the genus *Rickettsia*. The *Rickettsia* genus contains two major groups: the spotted fever group (SFG) and the typhus group (TG). The SFG group includes *Rickettsia conorii*, which causes Mediterranean spotted fever, and *R. rickettsii*, which causes Rocky Mountain spotted fever, as well as several other species. The TG group (TG) includes only two species: *Rickettsia typhi*, which causes murine typhus, and *R. prowazekii*, which causes epidemic typhus. Rickettsioses may lead to irreversible damage in the host and ultimately patient death, especially with *R. rickettsii* and *R. prowazekii* infections. The mortality rates of *R. rickettsii* and *R. prowazekii* infection are estimated to be 20 and 30 %, respectively, in the absence of antibiotic treatment [Azad, 2007]. Rickettsiae are typically transmitted to humans and animals by infected arthropods, including ticks, mite, fleas and lice. However, several studies have shown that inhalation of contaminated aerosols or blood transfusions with contaminated samples may also transmit these diseases [Oster et al., 1977; Bechah et al., 2011; Wells et al., 1978]. Arthropods are the main reservoirs of rickettsiae, with the exception of *R. prowazekii* that kills lice some days after infection [Houhamdi et al., 2002].

Currently, the risk of contracting a rickettsiosis is increasing throughout the world, and the risk of outbreaks is especially high in countries at war or impacted by natural disasters. In addition, some rickettsiae, such as *R. prowazekii,* can survive within infected individuals for the lifetime of the host. Under intense stress, these latent bacteria can become active and cause Brill-Zinsser disease, which is a relapsing form of epidemic typhus [Saah, 2000]. This form of infection may be the source of new epidemic typhus outbreaks, especially if louse infestation is prevalent.

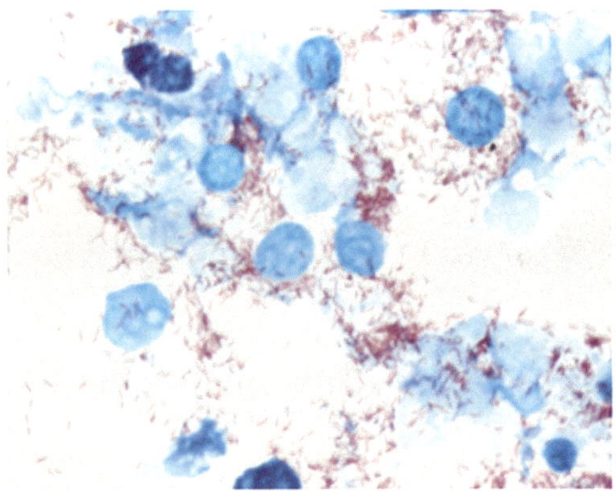

Fig. 1. Gimenez staining of *R. prowazekii* (red) in the cytoplasm of L929 cells (blue).

R. prowazekii and *R. rickettsii* have been classified as biological weapons according to the Centers for Disease Control and Prevention. Rickettsiae pathogens are often stable in an environment outside the host, are infectious at low doses, may be transmitted to humans or animals through aerosols and may persist in infected individuals for the rest of their life, becoming re-active and infectious at any moment.

The rickettsial genome size is small and ranges from 1.1 Mb for TG rickettsiae to 1.5 Mb for *R. bellii* [Merhej et al., 2009; Blanc et al., 2007; Andersson & Andersson S. G. E., 1999]. Because of their reduced genomes, rickettsiae depend on interactions with the infected host eukaryotic cells for survival. In humans, rickettsioses are associated with a large spectrum of clinical symptoms, including fever, rash, headache, myalgia and arthromyalgia. Rickettsiae tend to target and replicate in the vascular endothelium, especially within small vessels. Bacterial infection and replication in the endothelium often results in vasculitis (figure 2A), and the morbidity and mortality caused by rickettsioses appear to be a consequence of vascular injury, inflammation and thrombotic complications.

3. Endothelium

The endothelium is a monolayer of cells that line the interior of the blood and lymphatic vessels. This cellular layer is attached to the basal membrane and participates in the exchange of materials between the blood and tissues. The endothelium consists of about 10^{13} cells [Augustin et al., 1994] and weighs approximately 1 kg in humans [Ait-Oufella et al.,

2010; Sumpio et al., 2002]. Endothelial cells are approximately 100 x 10 μm in size and are tightly connected to each other, which helps to maintain the vascular integrity. Endothelial cells exhibit a large degree of plasticity and heterogeneity, and their morphology is influenced by their environment [Davies, 1995; Allaire and Clowes A. W., 1997; Steinsiepe and Weibel E. R., 1970; Ishii et al., 1986; Tse and Stan R. V., 2010]. For example, arterial endothelial cell morphology is different from venous endothelial cell morphology; interestingly, venous endothelial cells that are subjected to increased shear flow elongate and resemble endothelial cells from arteries [Allaire and Clowes A. W., 1997].

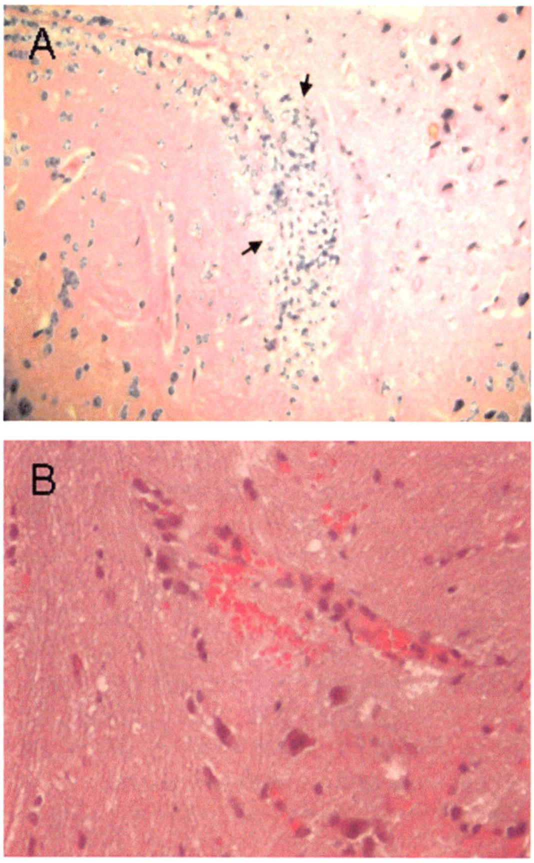

Fig. 2. Brain lesions induced by *R. prowazekii* Mice are infected with *R. prowazekii* for 7 days. Sections (5 μm) of paraffin-embedded brain are stained with hematoxylin-eosin to assess the presence of lesions. A. Note vasculitis composed mainly of mononuclear cell infiltrates. B. Note hemorrhage in the brain parenchyma. Original magnifications, X 200.

Endothelial cells release a multitude of biological mediators, such as growth factors (e.g., transforming growth factor, basic fibroblast growth factor), vasoactive mediators (e.g., prostacyclin, nitric oxide (NO), endothelin and angiotensin), coagulation and fibrinolysis proteins (e.g., thrombomodulin, heparin, tissue factor, plasminogen activator inhibitor, platelet activating factor, von Willebrand factor) and immune factors, including cytokines, chemokines and adhesion molecules [Ait-Oufella et al., 2010]. Because the endothelium controls the release of these molecules, endothelial cells have been implicated in numerous processes, including vascular homeostasis, coagulation, fibrinolysis, the regulation of blood flow and vasomotor tone, angiogenesis, the regulation of leukocyte adhesion/migration and inflammation [McGettrick et al., 2007]. In addition to their implied role in the innate immune response, endothelial cells express major histocompatibility complex class I and class II molecules and co-stimulation molecules, such as CD86 and CD58, which allow endothelial cells to directly interact with $CD8^+$ and $CD4^+$ T lymphocytes [Pober et al., 1996; Marelli-Berg et al., 1996; Ait-Oufella et al., 2006].

4. Rickettsia-endothelial cell interactions

In vertebrate hosts, rickettsiae typically target the microvascular endothelium (figure 3) and damage the endothelial cells. Studies have shown that rickettsiae bind to the membrane receptor Ku70, which is a component of the DNA-dependent protein kinase that is present at the surface of endothelial cells. The molecular nature of the rickettsial ligands of Ku70 has been determined; they include OmpB, which is expressed by both SFG and TG rickettsiae [Uchiyama, 2003], and OmpA, which is only expressed by SFG [Li and Walker D. H., 1998]. OmpB and OmpA are outer membrane proteins that belong to a large rickettsial surface cell antigen family (*sca*) [Blanc et al., 2005]. Studies have shown that monoclonal antibodies against OmpB and/or OmpA significantly decrease rickettsial infection of endothelial cells both *in vitro* and *in vivo*, and administration of these antibodies protects mice from death [Li and Walker D. H., 1998; Feng et al., 2004]. Additional rickettsial adhesion proteins that play a role in host cell entry have been recently identified, they include the proteins RC1281 and RP828 identified in *R. conorii* and *R. prowazekii*, respectively [Renesto et al., 2005a; Renesto et al., 2006]. After binding to endothelial cells, rickettsiae are actively internalized by the endothelial cells [Walker, 1984; Li and Walker D. H., 1992].
To avoid destruction within the phagosome, rickettsiae have developed a strategy to rapidly escape from phagosomes and relocate to the cytosol prior to phagolysosomal fusion [Teysseire et al., 1995]. Phagosome escape appears to be mediated by the hemolysin C (Tly C) and phospholipase D (PLD) proteins, as demonstrated by the complementation of *Salmonella enterica* by the genes encoding Tly C and PLD [Whitworth et al., 2005; Renesto et al., 2003]. Moreover, a *R. prowazekii* Evir strain *pld* mutant has decreased virulence in a guinea pig model. Interestingly, immunization of the guinea pigs with this mutant protects them from infection with subsequent challenges with a virulent strain of *R. prowazekii* (Breinl strain) [Driskell et al., 2009].
Once in the cytoplasm, rickettsiae acquire nutrients from their host cells through transmembrane exchange proteins that are encoded by genes present in the rickettsial genome in multiple copies [Andersson et al., 1998; McLeod et al., 2004; Renesto et al., 2005b]. The intracellular spreading mechanisms of SFG rickettsiae and TG rickettsiae are different. SFG rickettsiae induce actin polymerization and move within host cells, which allows them to invade the neighboring cells without cell damaging the initially infected cells [Heinzen et al., 1993; Jeng et al., 2004; Gouin et al., 2004]. In contrast, TG rickettsiae are not motile within the cells and can only infect adjacent cells when the bacterial load increases (5-8 times greater than that observed for SFG) and induces host cell lysis [Hackstadt, 1996]. Interestingly, the intracellular motility of *Rickettsia* species is not associated with virulence, unlike *Shigella flexneri* [Heindl et al., 2010] and *Listeria monocytogenes* [Vazquez-Boland et al., 2001]. Avirulent rickettsiae (*Rickettsia montana* and avirulent strains of *R. rickettsii*) also

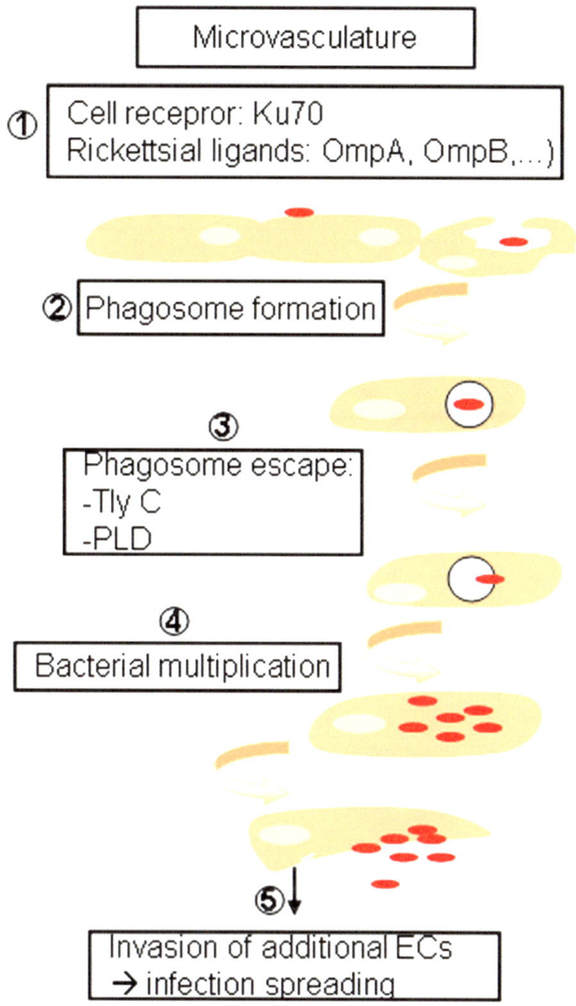

Fig. 3. Hypothetical *Rickettsia*-endothelial cell interactions After attachment to the endothelial cell receptors Ku70 using adhesins proteins (1), rickettsiae are ingested (2) but rapidly escape from phagosomes using PLD and Tly C proteins (3) and replicate in the cytoplasm (4). SFG rickettsiae spread directly to neighbouring cells via actin polymerization without cell damages. TG rickettsiae are released in the extracellular space after damages of infected cells; they infect adjacent cells leading to infection widespread.

induce actin tails [Heinzen et al., 1993], which indicates that other factors mediate rickettsial virulence. Previous studies have suggested that actin polymerization is dependent upon expression of the Rick A protein, although additional data suggest that Rick A is not the sole protein involved in rickettsial motility. For example, *R. typhi* induces the formation of short actin tails even in the absence of Rick A [Heinzen et al., 1993]. In addition, *Rickettsia raoultii*, which belongs to the SFG, expresses Rick A but is unable to mobilize actin [Balraj et al., 2008]. The Sca 2 (surface cell antigen 2) protein may also be involved in the actin-based motility of *R. rickettsii* [Kleba et al., 2010]; however, *Rickettsia peacockii*, which is a member of the SFG that does not exhibit actin-based motility, expresses an apparently intact Sca 2 ortholog and does not express Rick A [Simser et al., 2005]. Thus, the data indicate that the actin-based motility of rickettsiae is a complex process that involves the Rick A and Sca 2 proteins, as well as other unidentified proteins. A large fraction of the rickettsial genome encodes proteins with unknown functions, and no known homologs of these proteins exist in the current databases.

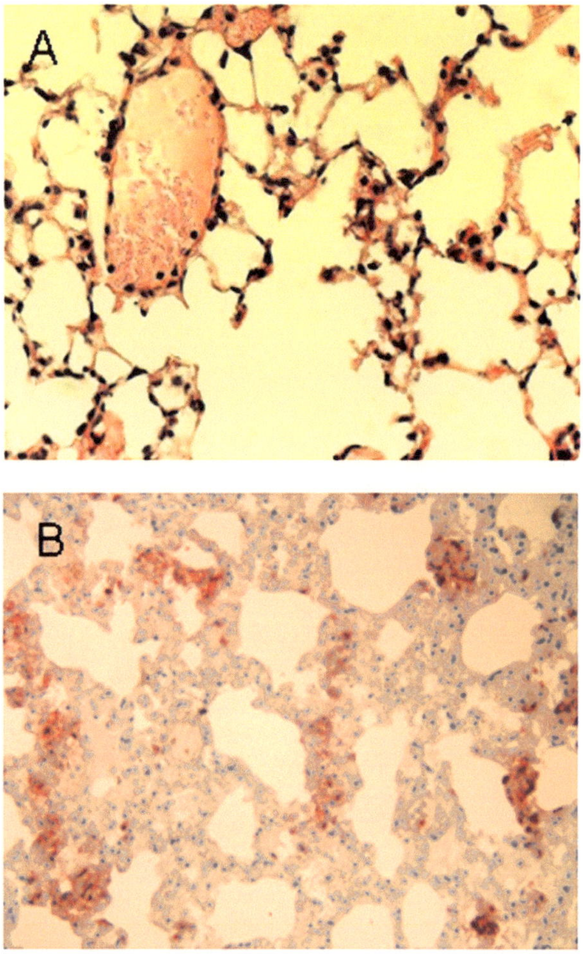

Fig. 4. Lung lesions induced by *R. prowazekii* Mice are infected with *R. prowazekii* for 7 days. Sections (5 µm) of paraffin-embedded lungs are stained with hematoxylin-eosin to assess the presence of lesions. They are also incubated with rabbit anti-*R. prowazekii* polyclonal antibodies, and bacteria are revealed using biotin-conjugated antibodies and peroxidase-labeled streptavidin. A. Edema in the airways. B. massive *R. prowazekii* infection (red brown staining) is shown in the inflammatory infiltrates. A, B: original magnifications, X 250.

5. Endothelium and pathophysiology of rickettsioses

As endothelial infection progresses endothelial dysfunction progressively increases, which results in the associated disease symptoms. Endothelial cell dysfunction in vital organs such as the lungs and brain may cause the high morbidity and the mortality associated with rickettsioses. Microscopic endothelial injury includes increased vascular permeability; infiltration of plasma fluid, plasma proteins and mononuclear cells into the surrounding tissues; the formation of hemorrhagic foci (figure 2B); edema (figure 4A); and inflammatory lesions (figure 4B).

Several mechanisms may explain the increased permeability of blood vessels during rickettsial infections. During the early stages of infection, the endothelial cells demonstrate increased permeability, although they do not die. Rickettsiae binding to the endothelial cells may stimulate signal transduction pathways in the endothelial cells, which results in remodeling of the actin cytoskeleton and changes in the junction proteins. The cellular junctions maintain the vascular integrity and mediate anchorage to the actin microfilaments through the vascular endothelial cadherin and catenin proteins [Dejana et al., 1999; Bazzoni and Dejana E., 2004]. A previous study has shown that within 24 hours after *R. rickettsii* infection the vascular permeability is increased, and the β and p120 catenin proteins dissociate from the inter-endothelial cellular junctions [Woods and Olano J. P., 2008].

One parameter to measure endothelial damage is to quantify the number of circulating endothelial cells [Brevetti et al., 2008]. A previous study has shown that the number of circulating endothelial cells increases in individuals infected with rickettsiae because the infected endothelial cells detach [George et al., 1993]. Endothelial cell detachment is not observed at the beginning of the disease because at this stage rickettsiae, as other strictly intracellular organisms, are within the cells and do not induce host cell death. One major strategy employed by rickettsiae to survive and replicate within their host cells is to inhibit endothelial cell apoptosis via NF-κB activation [Sahni et al., 1998; Joshi et al., 2003; Sporn et al., 1997]. NF-κB is a transcription factor that triggers an inflammatory response during rickettsial infection of the endothelial cells. Interestingly, in an *in vitro* system where endothelial cells were infected with a virulent *R. prowazekii* strain, the expression of pro-apoptotic genes, such as *Bcl* 2, caspase 8 and *Naip* was decreased; moreover, expression of the interferon type I (IFN-I)-inducible genes was inhibited [Bechah et al., 2010]. This response suggests that the survival of rickettsiae within their host cells depends on a combination of several mechanisms. The death and the subsequent detachment of infected endothelial cells in the later stages of infection may be caused by a marked increased in the bacterial load, especially with the TG rickettsiae; previous studies have also shown that apoptotic/necrotic cell death may be mediated by $CD8^+$ cytotoxic T lymphocytes [Feng et al., 1997; Walker et al., 1994].

The increased vascular permeability during rickettsial infection may also be mediated by the production of cytokines and chemokines. *In vivo* and *in vitro* studies have shown that rickettsial infection of endothelial cells stimulates the release of proinflammatory cytokines, such as IL-1α, IL-6 and IL-8 [Sporn and Marder V. J., 1996; Oristrell et al., 2004; Damas et al., 2009], as well as the secretion of chemokines, such as CCL-2, CCL-5, CXCL-9, CXCL-10 and CX3CL-1 [Bechah et al., 2008; Bechah et al., 2007; Valbuena et al., 2003; Valbuena and Walker D. H., 2005]. Additional *in vitro* and *in vivo* studies have also shown that infection increases the expression of adhesive molecules, such as E-selectin, intercellular adhesion molecule-1 (ICAM-1) and vascular cell adhesion molecule-1 (VCAM-1) [Dignat-George et al., 1997; Damas et al., 2009]; these adhesive molecules regulate leukocyte movement between the circulation and the surrounding tissues.

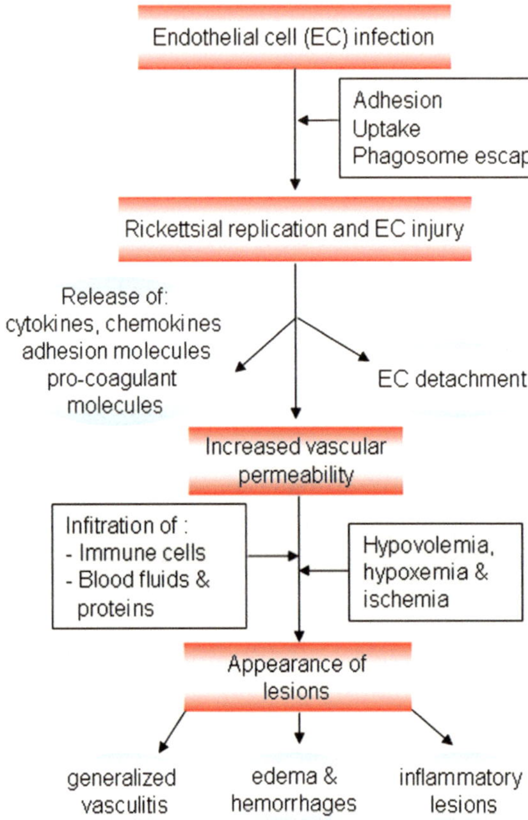

Fig. 5. Schematic representation of the natural history of rickettsial infections This representation of rickettsial infections is based on both *in vitro* and *in vivo* data. Infection of endothelial cells is followed by endothelial dysfunction. Several phenotypic and physiological disorders occur: expression and release of adhesion molecules, cytokines, chemokines as well as procoagulant molecules. These disorders lead to increased vascular permeability and the passage of blood molecules and inflammatory cells from vessels to interstitial space. They also lead to the alteration of coagulation pathway. Consequently, edema, microhemorrhages and inflammatory lesions appear as well as hypovolemia, shock with multiple organ dysfunctions as major manifestations.

In addition, rickettsial infection of the endothelial cells induces the secretion of prostaglandins, leukotrienes and nitric oxide (NO) [Walker et al., 1990; Rydkina et al., 2006; Woods et al., 2005], which are vasoactive mediators that increase vascular permeability. Prostaglandins and leukotrienes are generated from arachidonic acid by the cyclooxygenase (COX) enzymes, which are controlled by heme oxygenase (HO-1) [Haider et al., 2002; Rydkina et al., 2002]. *In vitro* and *in vivo* studies of rickettsial infection have shown that increased COX-2 expression in endothelial cells is related to increased prostaglandin secretion, which may explain some of the clinical manifestations of rickettsioses, such as pain, fever and inflammation. NO is synthesized from L-arginine by endothelial NO synthase (eNOS), and the expression level of eNOS rapidly increases after rickettsial infection [Walker et al., 1997]. NO increases the vascular permeability of endothelial cells

[Woods et al., 2005] and plays a role in inducing rickettsial death [Feng and Walker D. H., 2000; Walker et al., 1997]. Correspondingly, the inhibition of NO generation increases the rickettsial burden in infected endothelial cells [Walker et al., 1997].

In addition to stimulating the release of cytokines/chemokines and vasoactive mediators, rickettsial endothelial cell infection also induces the release of pro-coagulant proteins, such as thrombomodulin, tissue factor, plasminogen activator inhibitor, platelet activating factor and von Willebrand factor both *in vitro* and *in vivo* [Elghetany and Walker D. H., 1999; Schmaier et al., 2001; Teysseire et al., 1992; Shi et al., 1996; Bechah et al., 2008; Lorant et al., 1995; Schmaier et al., 2001]. The release of pro-coagulant proteins may explain why thrombosis is associated with severe forms of rickettsioses.

Collectively, these changes to be in the endothelium during infection induce massive transmigration and infiltration of blood components and immune cells into the interstitial space. The subsequent hypovolemia contributes to shock and decreases the supply of nutrients and oxygen (perfusion) to various organs; as a consequence, multiple organ dysfunction, such as renal and cardiac failure, may be observed. The infiltration of blood components and inflammatory cells into the interstitial space leads to edema, microhemorrhages and inflammatory lesions that are mainly composed of infiltrating mononuclear cells; all of these symptoms are characteristic for rickettsial infection (figure 5). The increased transmigration of leukocytes may further increase tissue damage because these cells release proteases and oxygen radicals. We have recently shown that leukocytes that migrate throughout *R. prowazekii*-infected endothelial cells secrete increased levels of inflammatory and procoagulant mediators and may subsequently recruit additional immune cells [Bechah et al., 2008].

6. Conclusions

Rickettsioses are infectious diseases that target endothelial cells and cause endothelial dysfunction. The hallmark of rickettsial infections is widespread vascular injury that results in increased permeability of the endothelium and the escape of fluids and cells from the blood vessels into the interstitial space. This leakage ultimately results in edema, microhemorrhages, rashes and mononuclear cell infiltration around vessels and into surrounding tissues that form the characteristic lesions of rickettsioses (vasculitis). Changes in vital organs, such as the brain and lungs, induce hypoxemia, compression and increase oxidative stress, which result in a high morbidity and mortality. The leakage of blood fluids induces hypovolemia and ischemia in the affected organs, whereas other organs may be affected as a result of poor blood perfusion. Finally, cell death and an exaggerated host response with pro-coagulant activity in small vessels may lead to the development of occlusive thrombosis. We believe that understanding the endothelial cell dysfunction caused by rickettsioses may provide new insights to prevent the severity and the progression of rickettsial diseases. Finally, the treatment of vasculitis induced by rickettsiae depends on the bacterial control by antibiotics. However, as vasculitis may also be exacerbated in patients through excessive host response, the understanding of the mechanisms governing inflammatory responses could improve patient follow-up and avoid any squeals.

7. References

Ait-Oufella H, Maury E, Lehoux S, Guidet B, Offenstadt G. (2010). The endothelium: physiological functions and role in microcirculatory failure during severe sepsis. *Intensive Care Med.* 36 1286-1298.

Ait-Oufella H, Salomon B L, Potteaux S, Robertson A K, Gourdy P, Zoll J, Merval R, Esposito B, Cohen J L, Fisson S, Flavell R A, Hansson G K, Klatzmann D, Tedgui A, Mallat Z. (2006). Natural regulatory T cells control the development of atherosclerosis in mice. *Nat. Med.* 12 178-180.

Allaire E, Clowes A W. (1997). Endothelial cell injury in cardiovascular surgery: the intimal hyperplastic response. *Ann. Thorac. Surg.* 63 582-591.

Andersson JO, Andersson S G E. (1999). Genome degradation is an ongoing process in *Rickettsia*. *Mol. Biol. Evol.* 16 1178-1191.

Andersson SG, Zomorodipour A, Andersson J O, Sicheritz-Ponten T, Alsmark U C, Podowski R M, Naslund A K, Eriksson A S, Winkler H H, Kurland C G. (1998). The genome sequence of *Rickettsia prowazekii* and the origin of mitochondria. *Nature* 396 133-140.

Augustin HG, Kozian D H, Johnson R C. (1994). Differentiation of endothelial cells: analysis of the constitutive and activated endothelial cell phenotypes. *Bioessays.* 16 901-906.

Azad AF. (2007). Pathogenic rickettsiae as bioterrorism agents. *Clin. Infect. Dis.* 45 Suppl 1 S52-S55.

Balraj P, El K K, Vestris G, Espinosa L, Raoult D, Renesto P. (2008). *Rick*A expression is not sufficient to promote actin-based motility of *Rickettsia raoultii*. *PLoS. One* 3 e2582.

Bazzoni G, Dejana E. (2004). Endothelial cell-to-cell junctions: molecular organization and role in vascular homeostasis. *Physiol. Rev.* 84 869-901.

Bechah Y, Capo C, Grau G E, Raoult D, Mege J L. (2007). A murine model of infection with *Rickettsia prowazekii*: implications for pathogenesis of epidemic typhus. *Microbes. Infect.* 9 898-906.

Bechah Y, Capo C, Raoult D, Mege J L. (2008). Infection of endothelial cells with virulent *Rickettsia prowazekii* increases the transmigration of leukocytes. *J. Infect. Dis.* 197 142-147.

Bechah Y, El Karkouri K, Mediannikov O, Leroy Q, Pelletier N, Robert C, Medigue C, Mege J L, Raoult D. (2010). Genomic, proteomic, and transcriptomic analysis of virulent and avirulent *Rickettsia prowazekii* reveals its adaptive mutation capabilities. *Genome Res.* 20 655-663.

Bechah Y, Socolovschi C, Raoult D. (2011). Identification of rickettsial infections by using cutaneous swab specimens and PCR. *Emerg. Infect. Dis.* 17 83-86.

Blanc G, Ngwamidiba M, Ogata H, Fournier P E, Claverie J M, Raoult D. (2005). Molecular evolution of *Rickettsia* surface antigens: evidence of positive selection. *Mol. Biol. Evol.* 22 2073-2083.

Blanc G, Ogata H, Robert C, Audic S, Suhre K, Vestris G, Claverie J M, Raoult D. (2007). Reductive Genome Evolution from the Mother of Rickettsia. *PLoS. Genet.* 3 e14.

Brevetti G, Schiano V, Chiariello M. (2008). Endothelial dysfunction: a key to the pathophysiology and natural history of peripheral *Atherosclerosis.* 197 1-11.

Damas JK, Davi G, Jensenius M, Santilli F, Otterdal K, Ueland T, Flo T H, Lien E, Espevik T, Froland S S, Vitale G, Raoult D, Aukrust P. (2009). Relative chemokine and adhesion molecule expression in Mediterranean spotted fever and African tick bite fever. *J. Infect.* 58 68-75.

Davies PF. (1995). Flow-mediated endothelial mechanotransduction. *Physiol. Rev.* 75 519-560.

Dejana E, Bazzoni G, Lampugnani M G. (1999). Vascular endothelial (VE)-cadherin: only an intercellular glue? *Exp. Cell Res.* 252 13-19.

Dignat-George F, Teysseire N, Mutin M, Bardin N, Lesaule G, Raoult D, Sampol J. (1997). *Rickettsia conorii* infection enhances vascular cell adhesion molecule-1- and intercellular adhesion molecule-1- dependent mononuclear cell adherence to endothelial cells. *J. Infect. Dis.* 175 1142-1152.

Driskell LO, Yu X J, Zhang L, Liu Y, Popov V L, Walker D H, Tucker A M, Wood D O. (2009). Directed mutagenesis of the *Rickettsia prowazekii* pld gene encoding phospholipase D. *Infect. Immun.* 77 3244-3248.

Elghetany MT, Walker D H. (1999). Hemostatic changes in Rocky Mountain spotted fever and Mediterranean spotted fever. *Am. J. Clin. Pathol.* 112 159-168.

Feng H, Popov V L, Yuoh G, Walker D H. (1997). Role of T lymphocyte subsets in immunity to spotted fever group Rickettsiae. *J. Immunol.* 158 5314-5320.

Feng HM, Walker D H. (2000). Mechanisms of intracellular killing of *Rickettsia conorii* in infected human endothelial cells, hepatocytes, and macrophages. *Infect. Immun.* 68 6729-6736.

Feng HM, Whitworth T, Popov V, Walker D H. (2004). Effect of antibody on the rickettsia-host cell interaction. *Infect. Immun.* 72 3524-3530.

George F, Brouqui P, Boffa M C, Mutin M, Drancourt M, Brisson C, Raoult D, Sampol J. (1993). Demonstration of *Rickettsia conorii*-induced endothelial injury in vivo by measuring circulating endothelial cells, thrombomodulin and Von Willebrand factor in patients with mediterranean spotted fever. *Blood.* 82 2109-2116.

Gouin E, Egile C, Dehoux P, Villiers V, Adams J, Gertler F, Li R, Cossart P. (2004). The RickA protein of *Rickettsia conorii* activates the Arp2/3 complex. *Nature.* 427 457-461.

Hackstadt T. (1996). The biology of rickettsiae. *Inf. Agents Dis.* 5 127-143.

Haider A, Olszanecki R, Gryglewski R, Schwartzman M L, Lianos E, Kappas A, Nasjletti A, Abraham N G. (2002). Regulation of cyclooxygenase by the heme-heme oxygenase system in microvessel endothelial cells. *J. Pharmacol. Exp. Ther.* 300 188-194.

Heindl JE, Saran I, Yi C R, Lesser C F, Goldberg M B. (2010). Requirement for formin-induced actin polymerization during spread of *Shigella flexneri*. *Infect. Immun.* 78 193-203.

Heinzen RA, Hayes S F, Peacock M G, Hackstad T. (1993). Directional actin polymerization associated with spotted fever group rickettsia infection of Vero cells. *Infect. Immun.* 61 1926-1935.

Houhamdi L, Fournier P E, Fang R, Lepidi H, Raoult D. (2002). An experimental model of human body louse infection with *Rickettsia prowazekii*. *J. Infect. Dis.* 186 1639-1646.

Ishii H, Salem H H, Bell C E, Laposata E A, Majerus P W. (1986). Thrombomodulin, an endothelial anticoagulant protein, is absent from the human brain. *Blood.* 67 362-365.

Jeng RL, Goley E D, D'Alessio J A, Chaga O Y, Svitkina T M, Borisy G G, Heinzen R A, Welch M D. (2004). A *Rickettsia* WASP-like protein activates the Arp2/3 complex and mediates actin-based motility. *Cell. Microbiol.* 6 761-769.

Joshi SG, Francis C W, Silverman D J, Sahni S K. (2003). Nuclear factor kappa B protects against host cell apoptosis during *Rickettsia rickettsii* infection by inhibiting activation of apical and effector caspases and maintaining mitochondrial integrity. *Infect. Immun.* 71 4127-4136.

Kleba B, Clark T R, Lutter E I, Ellison D W, Hackstadt T. (2010). Disruption of the *Rickettsia rickettsii* Sca2 autotransporter inhibits actin-based motility. *Infect. Immun.* 78 2240-2247.

Li H, Walker D H. (1992). Characterization of rickettsial attachment to host cells by flow cytometry. *Infect. Immun.* 60 2030-2035.

Li H, Walker D H. (1998). RompA is a critical protein for the adhesion of *Rickettsia rickettsii* to host cells. *Microbial. Pathogenesis.* 24 289-298.

Lorant DE, Zimmerman G A, McIntyre T M, Prescott S M. (1995). Platelet-activating factor mediates procoagulant activity on the surface of endothelial cells by promoting leukocyte adhesion. *Semin. Cell Biol.* 6 295-303.

Marelli-Berg FM, Hargreaves R E, Carmichael P, Dorling A, Lombardi G, Lechler R I. (1996). Major histocompatibility complex class II-expressing endothelial cells induce allospecific nonresponsiveness in naive T cells. *J. Exp. Med.* 183 1603-1612.

McGettrick HM, Filer A, Rainger G E, Buckley C D, Nash G B. (2007). Modulation of endothelial responses by the stromal microenvironment: effects on leucocyte recruitment. *Biochem. Soc. Trans.* 35 1161-1162.

McLeod MP, Qin X, Karpathy S E, Gioia J, Highlander S K, Fox G E, McNeill T Z, Jiang H, Muzny D, Jacob L S, Hawes A C, Sodergren E, Gill R, Hume J, Morgan M, Fan G, Amin A G, Gibbs R A, Hong C, Yu X J, Walker D H, Weinstock G M. (2004). Complete genome sequence of *Rickettsia typhi* and comparison with sequences of other rickettsiae. *J. Bacteriol.* 186 5842-5855.

Merhej V, Royer-Carenzi M, Pontarotti P, Raoult D. (2009). Massive comparative genomic analysis reveals convergent evolution of specialized bacteria. *Biol. Direct.* 4 13.

Oristrell J, Sampere M, Amengual M J, Font B, Segura F. (2004). Plasma interleukin-6 levels in Mediterranean spotted fever. *Eur. J. Clin. Microbiol. Infect. Dis.* 23 417-418.

Oster CN, Burke D S, Kenyon R H, Ascher M S, Harber P, Pedersen C E, Jr. (1977). Laboratory-acquired Rocky Mountain spotted fever. The hazard of aerosol transmission. *N. Engl. J. Med.* 297 859-863.

Pober JS, Orosz C G, Rose M L, Savage C O. (1996). Can graft endothelial cells initiate a host anti-graft immune response? *Transplantation.* 61 343-349.

Renesto P, Azza S, Dolla A, Fourquet P, Vestris G, Gorvel J P, Raoult D. (2005a). *Rickettsia conorii* and *R. prowazekii* proteome analysis by 2DE-MS: a step toward functional analysis of *Rickettsial* genomes. *Ann. N Y Acad. Sci.* 1063 90-93.

Renesto P, Dehoux P, Gouin E, Touqui L, Cossart P, Raoult D. (2003). Identification and characterization of a phospholipase D-superfamily gene in rickettsiae. *J. Infect. Dis.* 188 1276-1283.

Renesto P, Ogata H, Audic S, Claverie J M, Raoult D. (2005b). Some lessons from *Rickettsia* genomics. *FEMS. Microbiol. Rev.* 29 99-117.

Renesto P, Samson L, Ogata H, Azza S, Fourquet P, Gorvel J P, Heinzen R A, Raoult D. (2006). Identification of two putative rickettsial adhesins by proteomic analysis. *Res. Microbiol.* 157 605-612.

Rydkina E, Sahni A, Baggs R B, Silverman D J, Sahni S K. (2006). Infection of human endothelial cells with spotted Fever group rickettsiae stimulates cyclooxygenase 2 expression and release of vasoactive prostaglandins. *Infect. Immun.* 74 5067-5074.

Rydkina E, Sahni A, Silverman D J, Sahni S K. (2002). *Rickettsia rickettsii* infection of cultured human endothelial cells induces heme oxygenase 1 expression. *Infect. Immun.* 70 4045-4052.

Saah AJ. (2000). *Rickettsia prowazekii* (Epidemic or louse-borne typhus). In: *Principles and Practice of Infectious Diseases.* Mandell GL, Bennett JE, Dolin R, eds. Philadelphia, PA: Churchill Livingstone; pp 2050-2053.

Sahni SK, Vanantwerp D J, Eremeeva M E, Silverman D J, Marder V J, Sporn L A. (1998). Proteasome-independent activation of nuclear factor kappa-B in cytoplasmic extracts from human endothelial cells by *Rickettsia rickettsii. Infect. Immun.* 66 1827-1833.

Schmaier AH, Srikanth S, Elghetany M T, Normolle D, Gokhale S, Feng H M, Walker D H. (2001). Hemostatic/fibrinolytic protein changes in C3H/HeN mice infected with *Rickettsia conorii*--a model for Rocky Mountain spotted fever. *Thromb. Haemost.* 86 871-879.

Shi RJ, Simpsonhaidaris P J, Marder V J, Silverman D J, Sporn L A. (1996). Increased expression of plasminogen activator inhibitor-1 in *R- rickettsii*-infected endothelial cells. *Thromb. Haemost.* 75 600-606.

Simser JA, Rahman M S, Dreher-Lesnick S M, Azad A F. (2005). A novel and naturally occurring transposon, ISRpe1 in the *Rickettsia peacockii* genome disrupting the rickA gene involved in actin-based motility. *Mol. Microbiol.* 58 71-79.

Sporn LA, Marder V J. (1996). Interleukin-1 alpha production during *Rickettsia rickettsii* infection of cultured endothelial cells: Potential role in autocrine cell stimulation. *Infect. Immun.* 64 1609-1613.

Sporn LA, Sahni S K, Lerner N B, Marder V J, Silverman D J, Turpin L C, Schwab A L. (1997). *Rickettsia rickettsii* infection of cultured human endothelial cells induces NF-κB activation. *Infect. Immun.* 65 2786-2791.

Steinsiepe KF, Weibel E R. (1970). [Electron microscopic studies on specific organelles of endothelial cells in the frog (Rana temporaria)]. *Z. Zellforsch. Mikrosk. Anat.* 108 105-126.

Sumpio BE, Riley J T, Dardik A. (2002). Cells in focus: endothelial cell. *Int. J. Biochem. Cell Biol.* 34 1508-1512.

Teysseire N, Arnoux D, George F, Sampol J, Raoult D. (1992). Von Willebrand factor release, thrombomodulin and tissue factor expression in *Rickettsia conorii* infected endothelial cells. *Infect. Immun.* 60 4388-4393.

Teysseire N, Boudier J A, Raoult D. (1995). *Rickettsia conorii* entry into vero cells. *Infect. Immun.* 63 366-374.

Tse D, Stan R V. (2010). Morphological heterogeneity of endothelium. *Semin. Thromb. Hemost.* 36 236-245.

Uchiyama T. (2003). Adherence to and invasion of Vero cells by recombinant *Escherichia coli* expressing the outer membrane protein rOmpB of *Rickettsia japonica. Ann. N. Y. Acad. Sci.* 990 585-590.

Valbuena G, Bradford W, Walker D H. (2003). Expression analysis of the T-cell-targeting chemokines CXCL-9 and CXCL-10 in mice and humans with endothelial infections caused by rickettsiae of the spotted fever group. *Am. J Pathol.* 163 1357-1369.

Valbuena G, Walker D H. (2005). Expression of CX3CL1 (fractalkine) in mice with endothelial-target rickettsial infection of the spotted-fever group. *Virchows Arch.* 446 21-27.

Vazquez-Boland JA, Kuhn M, Berche P, Chakraborty T, Dominguez-Bernal G, Goebel W, Gonzalez-Zorn B, Wehland J, Kreft J. (2001). Listeria pathogenesis and molecular virulence determinants. *Clin. Microbiol. Rev.* 14 584-640.

Walker DH, Popov V L, Crocquet-Valdes P A, Welsh C J, Feng H M. (1997). Cytokine-induced, nitric oxide-dependent, intracellular antirickettsial activity of mouse endothelial cells. *Lab. Invest.* 76 129-138.

Walker DH, Popov V L, Wen J, Feng H M. (1994). *Rickettsia conorii* infection of C3H/HeN mice. *Lab. Invest.* 70 358-368.

Walker TS. (1984). Rickettsial interactions with human endothelial cells in vitro: adherence and entry. *Infect. Immun.* 44 205-210.

Walker TS, Brown J S, Hoover C S, Morgan D A. (1990). Endothelial prostaglandin secretion: effects of typhus rickettsiae. *J. Infect. Dis.* 162 1136-1144.

Wells GM, Woodward T E, Fiset P, Hornick R B. (1978). Rocky mountain spotted fever caused by blood transfusion. *J. Amer. Med. Assoc.* 239 2763-2765.

Whitworth T, Popov V L, Yu X J, Walker D H, Bouyer D H. (2005). Expression of the *Rickettsia prowazekii* pld or tlyC gene in *Salmonella enterica* serovar Typhimurium mediates phagosomal escape. *Infect. Immun.* 73 6668-6673.

Woods ME, Olano J P. (2008). Host defenses to *Rickettsia rickettsii* infection contribute to increased microvascular permeability in human cerebral endothelial cells. *J. Clin. Immunol.* 28 174-185.

Woods ME, Wen G, Olano J P. (2005). Nitric oxide as a mediator of increased microvascular permeability during acute rickettsioses. *Ann. N. Y. Acad. Sci.* 1063 239-245.

5

Responsible Genetic Factors for Vasculitis in Kawasaki Disease

Yoshihiro Onouchi and Akira Hata
RIKEN & Chiba University
Japan

1. Introduction

Kawasaki disease (KD) is an acute febrile illness of early childhood that is characterized by high fever, bilateral conjunctivitis, redness of the oral mucosa, polymorphous skin rash, indurative edema of the hands and feet, and cervical lymphadenopathy (Kawasaki, 1967). The major pathological lesion of KD is vasculitis of small and medium-sized arteries (Amano et al., 1979). The coronary arteries are the most severely affected and coronary artery lesions (CALs) occur in 15-25% of untreated patients (Kato et al., 1975), making KD a leading cause of childhood acquired heart disease in developed countries. The fact that the peak incidence of KD is at 9–11 months of age, which coincides with the waning of maternal immunity, indicates that infections could contribute to the pathogenesis of KD. However, despite more than 40 years of intensive research, the causative microorganism of KD remains unknown. On the other hand, epidemiological studies have revealed a significant role of genetic components in host susceptibility to KD pathogenesis.

2. Epidemiological features of KD suggesting a genetic predisposition

Since the first description of KD (Kawasaki, 1967) more than four decades ago, biannual epidemiological surveys conducted in Japan and epidemiological studies performed in almost all ethnic groups during this period have highlighted the contribution of genetic factors in the pathogenesis of KD.

2.1 Ethnic differences in the incidence of KD

KD is much more prevalent in East Asia than in any other countries of the world. In Japan, its incidence was 218.6 per 100,000 children younger than 4 years old in 2008 and continues to rise (Nakamura et al., 2010). Its incidence in Korea and Taiwan, the neighboring countries to Japan, are the second (113.1) and third (69.0) highest, respectively (Huang et al., 2009; Park et al., 2011). The incidence of KD in Western countries is 10–20 times lower than in Japan. Recent surveillance of KD in Hawaii revealed that Asian children, especially those of Japanese ancestry, had the highest incidence (210.5), and that the incidence among Caucasian children in Hawaii (13.7) was similar to that of the continental United States (Holman et al., 2010). These facts indicate that the high incidence of KD in East Asian countries is due to the racial/ethnic genetic background rather than to geographic factors.

2.2 Individual susceptibility to KD

In Japan, a total of 20 nationwide biannual continued surveillances of KD have been carried out since 1970. Epidemiological evidence collected from these surveys suggested individual susceptibility to KD, which was mainly composed of multiple genetic factors. For example, sibling cases of KD have a ≥10 times higher incidence than expected (Fujita et al., 1989). In addition, parents of KD patients, who were affected by KD during their childhood, were observed 2 times more often than expected (Uehara et al., 2003).

3. Genetic studies of KD

KD is considered to be a multifactorial disease that is caused by the interplay of external and personal factors (Fig. 1). Thus, identification of the responsible genetic factors, which presumably determine an individual's susceptibility to KD, should provide clues to the pathogenesis of the disease. Furthermore, it could contribute to the development of novel clinical applications, such as a severity prediction method and new therapeutic measures.

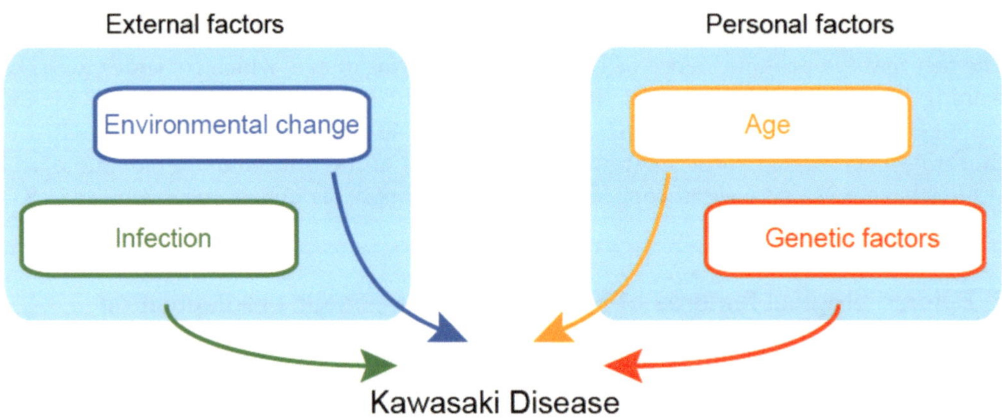

Fig. 1. Multiple factors that are linked to KD.

3.1 Candidate gene studies

KD is an immune-mediated vasculitis syndrome; therefore, genes encoding proteins related to innate and acquired immune function or to vascular remodeling could be involved in its pathogenesis, response to treatment, and prognosis. Variations within such "candidate genes" have been extensively studied.

3.1.1 Human leukocyte antigen (HLA) genes

Genetic studies of KD were initially conducted by focusing on the HLA class I genes, and several serotypes of the HLA-B locus have been associated with KD in different ethnic groups (Table 1).

Recently, significant associations of single nucleotide polymorphisms (SNPs) within the HLA-G and HLA-E genes were reported (J.J. Kim et al., 2008; Y.J. Lin et al., 2009). However, most of the previous studies, including those describing negative association results, were conducted by analyzing a relatively small number of cases and controls, while replication studies with larger cohorts have not been performed yet.

Locus	Haplotype /SNP	Method	Ethnicity (cases/controls)	Reference
HLA-B	Bw22J	Serotyping	Japanese (32/76)	Matsuda et al., 1977
HLA-B	Bw22J2	Serotyping	Japanese (205/500)	Kato et al., 1978
HLA-B	Bw15			
HLA-B	Bw51	Serotyping	Caucasian (23/244)	Krensky et al., 1981
HLA-B	Bw51	Serotyping	Jewish (12/90)	Keren et al., 1982
HLA-B	Bw44	Serotyping	Caucasian (23/246)	Krensky et al., 1983
HLA-B	Bw44	Serotyping	Caucasian (16/608)	Kaslow et al., 1985
HLA-B	B35	Genotyping	Korean (74/159)	Oh et al., 2008
HLA-B	B75			
HLA-C	Cw09			
HLA-DRB3	DRB3*0301	Genotyping	Caucasian (21/200)	Barron et al., 1992
HLA-G	rs12722477 C/A A allele	Genotyping	Korean (92/90)	J.J. Kim et al., 2008
HLA-E	rs2844724 C/T C allele	Genotyping	Taiwanese (680/3312)	Y.J. Lin et al., 2009

Table 1. Association studies between HLA genes and KD.

3.1.2 Non-HLA genes

Advances from the Human Genome and Hapmap projects have dramatically reduced the effort and cost of conducting genetic association studies of complex diseases, leading to a recent increase in the number of candidate gene studies, especially since 2005 (Table 2). Among the genes studied, tumor necrosis factor (TNF), which is a proinflammatory cytokine deeply related to the pathogenesis of KD, has been most frequently analyzed. Although many of these studies have failed to identify a statistically significant association, a systematic meta-analysis revealed a trend of association between the G allele of rs180629, which is located 308 bases upstream of the TNF gene, and KD (Ari-Ong et al., 2010).

Gene	Chromosomal region	Reference	
		Associated	Not associated
Cytokines, chemokines, and their receptors			
IL-10	1q31-q32	Hsueh et al., 2009	Jin et al., 2007 Weng et al., 2010a
TGFB2	1q41	Shimizu et al., 2011	
IL-1α	2q14		Weng et al., 2010b S.K. Kim et al., 2011
IL-1β	2q14		S.F. Wu et al., 2005 Weng et al., 2010b S.K. Kim et al., 2011
IL-1Ra	2q14.2	S.F. Wu et al., 2005	Weng et al., 2010b S.K. Kim et al., 2011
CXCR2	2q35		Breunis et al., 2007
CXCR1	2q35		Breunis et al., 2007
TGFBR2	3p22	Shimizu et al., 2011	
CX3CR1	3p21.3		Breunis et al., 2007
CCR3	3p21	Breunis et al., 2007	
CCR2	3p21	Breunis et al., 2007	
CCR5	3p21	Burns et al., 2005 Jhang et al., 2009 Breunis et al., 2007	Mamtani et al., 2010 Chaudhuri et al., 2011
IL-8	4q13-q21		Weng et al., 2010b
IL-4	5q31.1	Burns et al., 2005	S.F. Wu et al., 2005 F.Y. Huang et al., 2008a Weng et al., 2010b
LTA	6p21.3	Quasney et al., 2001	
TNF-α	6p21.3	Cheung et al., 2008	Kamizono et al., 1999 Quasney et al., 2001 Ahn et al., 2003 Chien et al., 2003 Weng et al., 2010b
IL-6	7p21		Sohn et al., 2001 Weng et al., 2010b
IL-18	11q22.2-q22.3	Hsueh et al., 2008a Chen et al., 2009	
TNFRSF1A	12p13.2	Wang et al., 2011	
MCP1	17q11.2-q12		Jibiki et al., 2001
CCL5	17q11.2-q12		Chaundhuri et al., 2011
CCL3L1	17q11.2	Burns et al., 2005 Mamtani et al., 2010	
TGFB1	19q13.1		Weng et al., 2010b
MIF	22q11.2		Simonini et al., 2009
Vasoactive molecules or molecules related to vascular remodeling			
AGTR1	3q21-q25		Fukazawa et al., 2004
TIMP4	3p25		Ban et al., 2009
VEGFR2	4q12		Kariyazono et al., 2004
VEGFA	6p12	Breunis et al., 2006 Hsueh et al., 2008b	Kariyazono et al., 2004 F.Y. Huang et al., 2008b
eNOS	7q36		Khajoee et al., 2003

MMP26	11p15		Ban et al., 2010
MMP7	11q21-22		Ban et al., 2010
MMP3	11q22.3		J.A. Park et al., 2005 Ikeda et al., 2008 Hong et al., 2008
MMP12	11q22.3		Ikeda et al., 2008 Ban et al., 2010
MMP13	11q22.3		Ikeda et al., 2008
MMP2	16q13-q21		Ikeda et al., 2008
iNOS	17q11.2-q12		Khajoee et al., 2003
ACE	17q23	S.F. Wu et al., 2004 Shim et al., 2006	Fukazawa et al., 2004
TIMP2	17q25		Furuno et al., 2007
MMP9	20q11.2-q13		J.A. Park et al., 2005 Ikeda et al., 2008
MMP11	22q11.2	Ban et al., 2010	
Molecules related to innate immune functions			
CRP	1q21-q23	Cheung et al., 2008	
SLC11A1	2q35	Ouchi et al., 2003	
CD14	5q31.1		Nishimura et al., 2003
MBL	10q11.2-q21	Biezeveld et al., 2003	Cheung et al., 2004
Molecules related to acquired immune functions			
FCGR2A	1q23		Taniuchi et al., 2005 Biezeveld et al., 2007
FCGR2B	1q23		Biezeveld et al., 2007
FCGR3A	1q23	Taniuchi et al., 2005	Biezeveld et al., 2007
FCGR3B	1q23		Taniuchi et al., 2005 Biezeveld et al., 2007
CTLA4	2q33		Kuo et al., 2010
PD-1	2q37.3	Chun et al., 2010	
MICA	6p21.3	F.Y. Huang et al., 2000	
BTNL2	6p21.3	Hsueh et al., 2010	
CD40L	Xq26		Y. Onouchi et al., 2004 F.Y. Huang et al., 2008c
Others			
MTHFR	1p36.3	Tsukahara et al., 2000	
UGT1A1	2q37		Kanai et al., 2003
BAT2, 3, 5	6p21.3	Hsieh et al., 2010	
NOTCH4	6p21.3		Kang et al., 2011
COL11A2	6p21.3	Shue et al., 2010	
ITPR3			Y.C. Huang et al., 2010
PAFAH	6p21.2-p12		Minami et al., 2005
TPH2	12q21.1		S.W. Park et al., 2010
SMAD3	15q22.33	Shimizu et al., 2011	
MEFV	16p13		Yamaguchi et al., 2009
HMOX1	22q12		Kanai et al., 2003

Table 2. Association studies between polymorphisms of candidate genes and KD.

The association of these candidate SNPs and patient response to intravenous immunoglobulin (IVIG) therapy and the development of CALs has also been studied (Table 3).

Gene	Phenotype	Reference	
		Association	No association
MTHFR	CAL	Tsukahara et al., 2000	
CRP	CAL		Cheung et al., 2008
	Intima-media thickness	Cheung et al., 2008	
	Arterial stiffness	Cheung et al., 2008	
IL-10	CAL	Jin et al., 2007	Hseuh et al., 2009
	Serum albumin	Jin et al., 2007	
FCGR2A	CAL	Taniuchi et al., 2005	Biezeveld et al., 2007
FCGR2B	CAL		Biezeveld et al., 2007
FCGR3A	CAL		Taniuchi et al., 2005 Biezeveld et al., 2007
FCGR3B	CAL		Taniuchi et al., 2005 Biezeveld et al., 2007
TGFB2	CAL/ coronary z score	Shimizu et al., 2011	
	Diameter of aortic root	Shimizu et al., 2011	
	Response to IVIG	Shimizu et al., 2011	
IL-1α	CAL		S.K. Kim et al., 2011
IL-1β	Response to IVIG	Weng et al., 2010	S.K. Kim et al., 2011
IL-1Ra	CAL		S.K. Kim et al., 2011
CTLA4	CAL	Kuo et al., 2010	
PD-1	CAL		Chun et al., 2010
TIMP4	CAL	Ban et al., 2009	
TGFBR2	CAL/ coronary z score	Shimizu et al., 2011	
	Diameter of aortic root	Shimizu et al., 2011	
	Response to IVIG	Shimizu et al., 2011	
CCR5	CAL	Mamtani et al., 2010 Chaudhuri et al., 2011	Jhang et al., 2009
AGTR1	Coronary stenosis	Fukazawa et al., 2004	
VEGFR2	CAL	Kariyazono et al., 2003	
IL-4	CAL		Burns et al., 2005 F.Y.Huang et al., 2008a
CD14	CAL	Nishimura et al., 2003	
VEGFA	CAL	Kariyazono et al., 2003	Hsueh et al., 2008b F.Y.Huang et al., 2008b
MICA	CAL	F.Y. Huang et al., 2000	
LTA	CAL		Quasney et al., 2001
TNF-α	CAL	Quasney et al., 2001	Cheung et al., 2008

	Arterial stiffness	Cheung et al., 2008	
BAT2, 3, 5	CAL	Hsieh et al., 2010	
NOTCH4	CAL		Kang et al., 2011
BTNL2	CAL	Hsueh et al., 2010	
COL11A2	CAL	Shue et al., 2010	
ITPR3	CAL	Y.C. Huang et al., 2010	
	CRP	Y.C. Huang et al., 2010	
PAFAH	CAL		Minami et al., 2005
PAFAH	Response to IVIG	Minami et al., 2005	
eNOS	CAL		Khajoee et al., 2003
MBL	CAL	Biezeveld et al., 2003 Biezeveld et al., 2006	Cheung et al., 2004
	Arterial stiffness	Cheung et al., 2004	
MMP26	CAL		Ban et al., 2010
IL-18	CAL		Hsueh et al., 2008a
MMP7	CAL		Ban et al., 2010
MMP3	CAL	J.A. Park et al., 2005	Ikeda et al., 2008 Hong et al., 2008
MMP12	CAL		Ikeda et al., 2008 Ban et al., 2010
MMP13	CAL	Ikeda et al., 2008	
TPH2	CAL	S.W. Park et al., 2010	
SMAD3	CAL/ coronary z score	Shimizu et al., 2010	
	Diameter of aortic root	Shimizu et al., 2010	
	Response to IVIG	Shimizu et al., 2010	
MEFV	CAL		Yamaguchi et al., 2009
MMP2	CAL		Ikeda et al., 2008
iNOS	CAL		Khajoee et al., 2003
CCL3L1	CAL		Mamtani et al., 2010
	Response to IVIG	Mamtani et al., 2010	
CCL%	CAL		Chaundhuri et al., 2011
ACE	CAL	Takeuchi et al., 1997	S.F. Wu et al., 2004 Shim et al., 2006
	Coronary stenosis	Fukazawa et al., 2004	
TIMP2	CAL	Furuno et al., 2007	
MMP9	CAL		J.A. Park et al., 2005 Ikeda et al., 2008
MIF	CAL	Simonini et al., 2009	
MMP11	CAL		Ban et al., 2010
CD40L	CAL	Y. Onouchi et al., 2004	Huang et al., 2008c

Table 3. Association studies between candidate gene polymorphisms and KD-related phenotypes.

3.2 Genome-wide studies

In contrast to candidate gene studies, which are based on an assumption of the underlying cause of the disease, a strategy to identify disease-causing mutations or variations from the whole genome relies solely on positional information and was originally developed to map and identify the genes for Mendelian disorders. This genome-wide strategy has been adapted for complex diseases and has become the most reliable tool to identify disease-related genes following the completion of the Human Genome Project.

3.2.1 Linkage study

The first genome-wide study for KD was conducted by our group (Y. Onouchi et al., 2007). In this study, 399 microsatellite marker alleles that were shared identical by descent between 78 affected KD sib-pairs were analyzed, and 10 chromosomal regions linked with the disease were identified (Fig. 2).

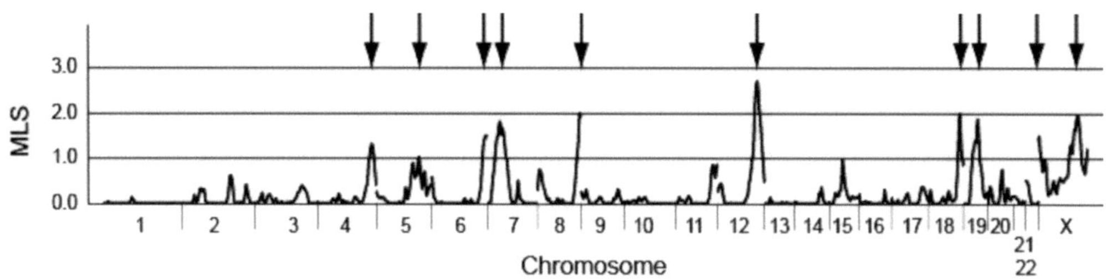

Fig. 2. Results from an affected sib-pair study (Y. Onouchi et al., 2007). Arrows indicate those chromosomal regions with a maximum LOD score (MLS) >1.0.

3.2.1.1 Linkage disequilibrium mapping

We narrowed down the candidate regions identified in the sib-pair study with a case-control association study using "tagging" SNPs. Chunks of genomic regions containing the associated tagging SNPs were extensively analyzed by re-sequencing and a further association study. We identified a SNP that was associated with KD in both the Japanese and US populations (Y. Onouchi et al., 2008) (Table 4). The SNP, rs28493229, is located in intron 1 of the inositol 1,4,5-trisphosphate 3-kinase C (ITPKC) gene, which catalyzes the phosphorylation of inositol 1,4,5-trisphosphate (IP3).

Alleles[1]	Japanese Case-control study			USA TDT		
	Risk allele frequency		OR (95% CI)[2] P value[2]	No. of families	T:U[3]	OR (95% CI) P value
	KD n=637	Control n=1034				
G/C	0.23	0.15	1.89 (1.53 - 2.33) 2.2x10^{-9}	209	64:30	2.13 (1.38 - 3.29) 0.00045

Table 4. Association of rs28493229 with KD. [1]Risk allele is underlined. [2]Dominant inheritance model. [3]Transmitted:untransmitted ratio. TDT: transmission disequilibrium test, OR: odds ratio, CI: confidence interval.

The at-risk allele of rs28493229 (C) reduces the splicing efficiency of ITPKC (Fig. 3). Transcripts with an unspliced intron are not properly translated because of premature termination. An increase in the number of such immature transcripts might lead to reduced ITPKC activity. IP3 is a second messenger molecule of the Ca^{2+}/NFAT pathway in a wide variety of cells and, in mammals, 3 iso-enzymes (ITPKA, ITPKB, and ITPKC) have been identified with the same enzyme activity.

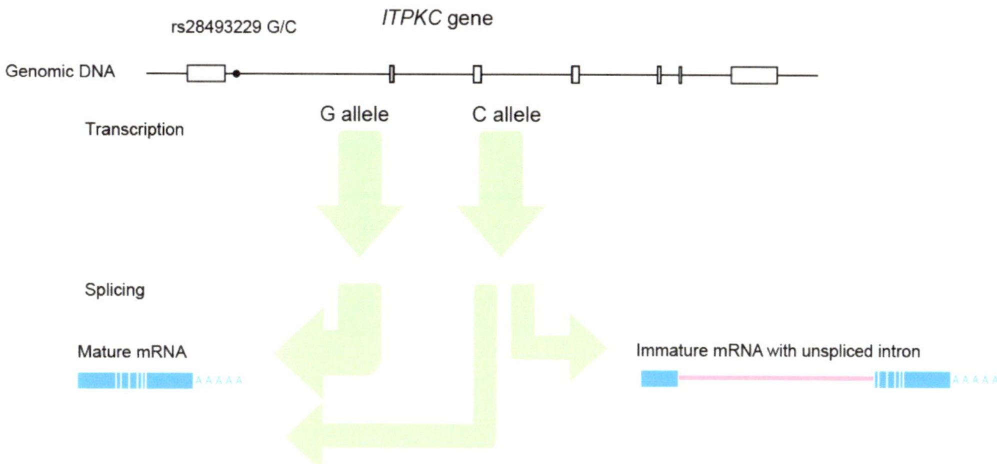

Fig. 3. Functional significance of rs28493229 on ITPKC mRNA.

Knockdown and overexpression experiments of ITPKC in the Jurkat cell line result in increased and decreased NFAT activity, respectively, as well as the expression of interleukin 2 mRNA. These findings highlighted the importance of the Ca^{2+}/NFAT pathway in the pathogenesis of KD. The association with the at-risk SNP allele was higher in KD patients with CAL than in those without CAL in both the Japanese and US populations. The same trend was also observed in KD patients in the US who responded poorly to intravenous immunoglobulin (IVIG) therapy. Two replication studies for the association of this SNP to KD, one negative and one positive, have been reported in the Taiwanese population (Chi et al., 2010; M.T. Lin et al., 2011). In the positive report, the SNP was also associated with the reactivation of previous BCG inoculation sites (M.T. Lin et al., 2011).

3.2.1.2 Positional candidate gene analysis

From the candidate region of chromosome 4, we identified the susceptibility gene via a different approach. The caspase-3 gene, which is located at 185.8 Mb, close to the linkage peak at 184.9 Mb, was focused on and studied as a positional candidate gene (Y. Onouchi et al. 2010). Multiple SNPs around the gene in linkage disequilibrium were associated with KD in the Japanese and US Caucasian populations. The functional SNP (rs72689236 G/A) was located in the 5'-untranslated region of the gene, and the risk allele (A) reduces the enhancer activity around the SNP to which NFATc2 is related (Table 5, Fig. 4).

Caspase-3 is an effector caspase with a central role in apoptosis. T cells from caspase-3-deficient mice have a reduced susceptibility to activation-induced cell death (Woo et al, 1998). It was also reported that caspase-3 cleaves Nfatc2 as a substrate (W. Wu et al, 2006). Transient anergy of peripheral T cells in the convalescent phase of KD, which has been documented in a couple of reports, is suggestive because the NFAT-driven expression of caspase-3 in T cells is related to T cell anergy (Macián et al., 2002). Currently, only one replication study has examined the association between rs72689236 and KD (Kuo et al, 2011). Although not statistically significant, the same trend of association was observed in the Taiwanese population. Notably, in this report, the SNP was associated with increased risk for IVIG resistance and CAL formation.

Alleles[1]	Japanese case-control study			United States TDT		
	Risk allele frequency		OR (95% CI)[2] P value[2]	No. of families	T:U[3]	OR (95% CI) P value
	KD n=920	Control n=1,409				
G/A	0.45	0.37	1.40 (1.24–1.57) 4.2×10^{-9}	249	120:79	1.54 (1.16–2.05) 0.0037

Table 5. Association of rs72689236 with KD. [1]Risk allele is underlined. [2]Allelic model. [3]Transmitted:untransmitted ratio. TDT: transmission disequilibrium test, OR: odds ratio, CI: confidence interval.

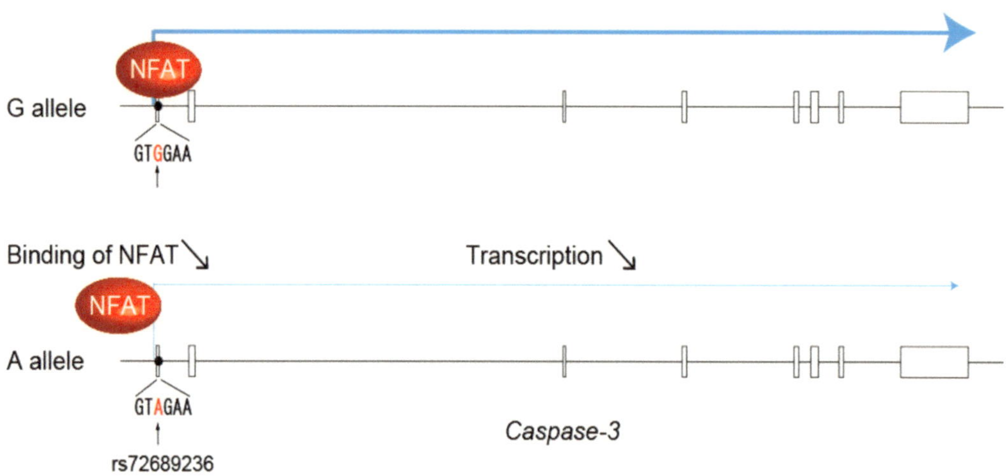

Fig. 4. Functional significance of rs72689236 on caspase-3 mRNA.

3.2.2 Genome-wide association studies (GWAS)

Today, GWAS using platforms by which 5.0×10^5 to 1×10^6 SNPs can be genotyped at a time have become commonplace for the analysis of complex disorders. GWAS for KD have been performed in 3 different ethnic groups: Caucasian, Korean, and Taiwanese (Burgner et al., 2009; J.J. Kim et al., 2011; Tsai et al., 2011). The number of subjects and SNPs analyzed in each study are summarized in Table 6.

Although many candidate SNPs were identified, no locus was repeatedly associated with KD in these studies (Table 7). Considering that none of these associations fulfilled the genome-wide level significance threshold, further validation of the association at each locus within the same populations is essential.

Ethnic group	Number of subjects KD/controls		No. of SNPs	Reference
	GWAS	Follow-up		
Caucasian	119/135	583/1357[1]	223,922	Burgner et al., 2009
Korean	186/600	266/600	641,760	J.J. Kim et al., 2011
Korean	63/600[2]	86/600[2]	641,760	J.J. Kim et al., 2011
Taiwanese	250/446	208/366	723,638	Tsai et al., 2011

Table 6. Summary of GWAS for KD (I). [1]583 KD patients and their unaffected siblings and biological parents. [2]KD patients with coronary artery lesions and healthy controls.

SNP	Chr	Position	P value	Gene	Reference
rs527409	1	58,757,915	1.5×10^{-6}	*DAB1*	J.J. Kim et al., 2011
rs952354	1	63,549,282	3.1×10^{-5}	-*	J.J. Kim et al., 2011
rs7604693	2	64,349,202	2.0×10^{-6}	*PELI1**	J.J. Kim et al., 2011
rs10183521	2	123,762,542	9.5×10^{-5}	-	Burgner et al., 2009
rs16849083	3	139,184,279	2.2×10^{-5}	*MRPS22, COPB2, RBP2*	Tsai et al., 2011
rs9834548	3	165,139,947	9.8×10^{-6}	-	Burgner et al., 2009
rs17531088	3	174,893,775	1.1×10^{-6}	*NAALADL2*	Burgner et al., 2009
rs3773986	3	190,278,915	6.2×10^{-5}	*IL1RAP**	J.J. Kim et al., 2011
rs4864471	4	54,426,184	3.4×10^{-5}	*LNX1, LOC441016*	Burgner et al., 2009
rs13128867	4	138,840,995	2.2×10^{-5}	*SLC7A11*	Tsai et al., 2011
rs149481	5	96,114,346	4.6×10^{-5}	*ERAP1*	Tsai et al., 2011
rs9392158	6	7,427,350	8.5×10^{-5}	*RIOK1*	Burgner et al., 2009
rs9364166	6	72,106,622	9.8×10^{-5}	*OGFRL1, C6orf155*	J.J. Kim et al., 2011
rs362794	7	103,201,263	3.0×10^{-5}	*RELN*	Tsai et al., 2011
rs6469101	8	108,252,238	5.4×10^{-5}	*ANGPT1*	Burgner et al., 2009
rs328879	9	107,789,252	1.2×10^{-5}	-	Burgner et al., 2009
rs10984642	9	122,450,340	2.6×10^{-5}	-	Burgner et al., 2009
rs10984642	9	122,450,340	5.8×10^{-5}	-	Burgner et al., 2009
rs4918458	10	111,505,407	9.8×10^{-5}	-*	J.J. Kim et al., 2011
rs285032	13	98,786,532	1.7×10^{-5}	*FARP1*	Burgner et al., 2009
rs34246750	14	52,868,757	4.8×10^{-5}	*PTGER2, TXNDC16*	J.J. Kim et al., 2011
rs10129255	14	107,176,213	6.8×10^{-6}	*IGHV*	Tsai et al., 2011
rs1568657	15	83,726,179	6.6×10^{-6}	*BTBD1*	Tsai et al., 2011
rs7199343	16	73,009,024	2.4×10^{-6}	*ZFHX3*	Burgner et al., 2009
rs8059315	16	74,506,447	8.5×10^{-5}	*GLG1*	Burgner et al., 2009
rs2270133	17	61,473,325	4.6×10^{-5}	*TANC2**	J.J. Kim et al., 2011

Table 7. Summary of GWAS for KD (II). * Association was observed between KD patients with CAL and healthy controls. Chr: chromosome.

4. Clinical implementation of genetic findings

The standard treatment for KD is a combination of oral aspirin and high-dose IVIG (Z. Onouchi & Kawasaki, 1999). While the majority of patients respond to this therapy, around 15% are resistant and require additional IVIG or alternative drugs to prevent the development of CAL. As the etiology and pathophysiology of KD are largely unknown, the mechanism of action of these therapies on the disease is not fully understood. The identification of genetic factors that influence patient response to therapy might provide an insight to this problem.

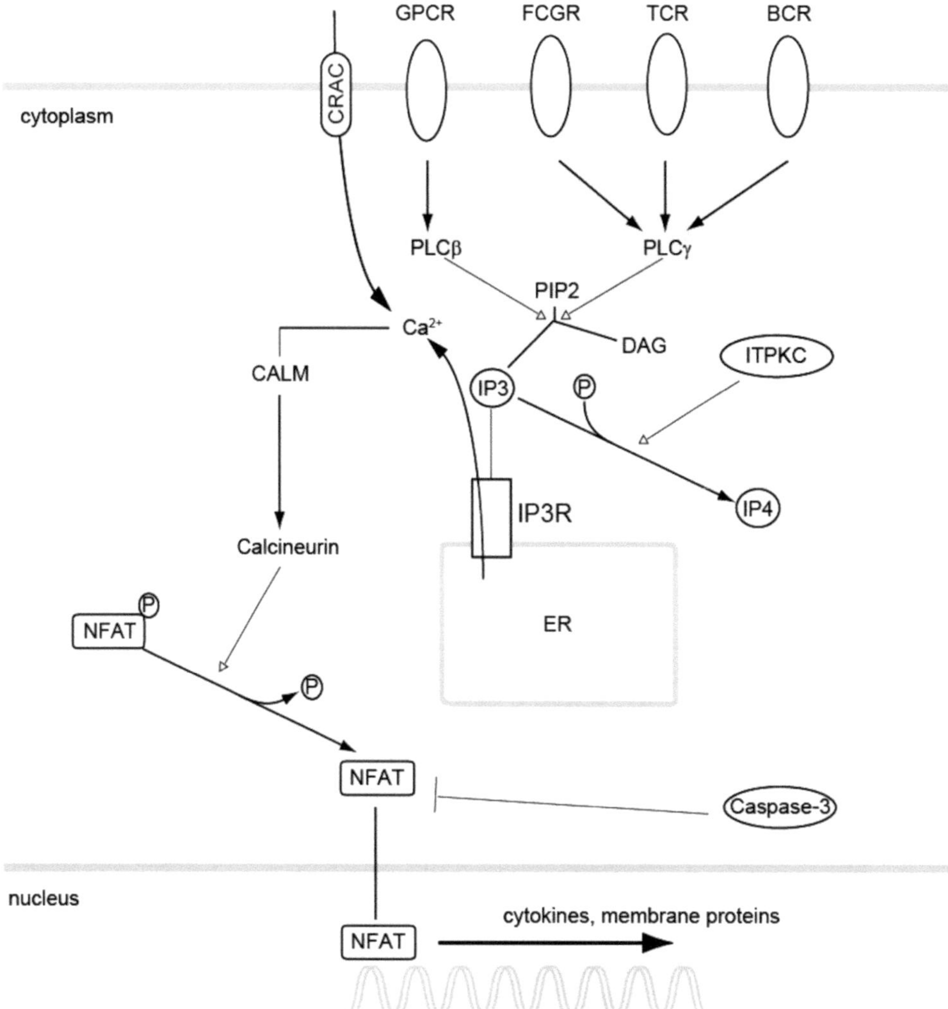

Fig. 5. Possible role of ITPKC and caspase-3 in the immune response.

CRAC: calcium release-activated calcium channel, GPCR: G-protein-coupled receptor, FCGR: Fc gamma receptor, BCR: B cell receptor, TCR: T cell receptor, NFAT: nuclear factor of activated T cells, PLC: phospholipase, PIP2: phosphatidylinositol 4,5-bisphosphate, DAG: diacylglycerol, CALM: calmodulin, IP3R: IP3 receptor, ER: endoplasmic reticulum.

We investigated the association between the functional SNPs in the ITPKC and caspase-3 genes with IVIG unresponsiveness and CAL formation, and found that patients with at least 1 susceptible allele at both SNPs had 2.7–2.9 times higher risk for these unfavorable events (manuscript submitted). Considering that ITPKC and caspase-3 are possibly negative regulators of the Ca^{2+}/NFAT pathway (Fig. 5), hyperactivation of the pathway might underlie a more severe clinical manifestation of the disease.

From this point of view, Cyclosporine A, an immunosuppressant drug which potently suppresses the activity of T cells by targeting calcineurin, a key molecule of the Ca^{2+}/NFAT pathway (Fig. 5), may be a good option for refractory cases of KD. In Japan, a study to investigate the tolerability, safety, and efficacy of Cyclosporine A for KD has been started.

5. Conclusion

Many candidate variations for susceptibility to KD have been reported from candidate gene and genome-wide studies; however, most of the findings from these studies are not robust and have yet to be confirmed by replication studies. Considering the modest odds ratios observed in recent GWAS for complex disorders, discovery studies should be conducted with much larger cohorts. Replication studies in different ethnic groups should be designed with careful attention to their power to detect a significant association and, most importantly, to the difference in the linkage disequilibrium structure. As the majority of KD patients are infants and children and the disease incidence is low, especially in countries outside East Asia, there are limitations in collecting subjects. In an attempt to overcome this difficulty, several consortia have been formed. Those engaged in KD research hope to unravel the mystery of this vasculitis and save these children from damage to their heart. We wish to contribute to this important mission by identifying the underlying genetic components of this disease.

6. References

Ahn, SY.; Jang, GC.; Shin, JS.; Shin, KM. & Kim DS. (2003). Tumor necrosis factor-alpha levels and promoter polymorphism in patients with Kawasaki disease in Korea. *Yonsei Medical Journal*, Vol.44, No.6, pp. 1021-1026, (December 2003). ISSN 0513-5796

Amano, S.; Hazama, F. & Hamashima Y. (1979). Pathology of Kawasaki disease: II. Distribution and incidence of the vascular lesions. *Japanese Circulation Journal*, Vol.43, No.8, pp. 741-748, (August 1979), ISSN 0047-1828

Ari-Ong, S.; Thakkinstian, A.; McEvoy, M. & Attia, J. (2010). A systematic review and meta-analysis of tumor necrosis factor a-308 polymorphism and Kawasaki disease. *Pediatrics International*, Vol.52, No.4, pp. 527-532, (February 2010), ISSN 1328-8067

Ban, JY.; Yoon, KL.; Kim, SK.; Kang, S. & Chung, JH. (2009). Promoter polymorphism (rs3755724, -55C/T) of tissue inhibitor of metalloproteinase 4 (TIMP4) as a risk factor for Kawasaki disease with coronary artery lesions in a Korean population. *Pediatric Cardiology*, Vol.30, No.3, pp. 331-335, (April 2009). ISSN 0172-0643

Ban, JY.; Kim, SK.; Kang, SW.; Yoon, KL. & Chung, JH. (2010). Association between polymorphisms of matrix metalloproteinase 11 (MMP-11) and Kawasaki disease in the Korean population. *Life Sciences*, Vol.86, No.19-20, pp. 756-759, (May 2010). ISSN 0024-3205

Biezeveld, MH.; Kuipers, IM.; Geissler, J.; Lam, J.; Ottenkamp, JJ.; Hack, CE. & Kuijpers, TW. (2003). Association of mannose-binding lectin genotype with cardiovascular abnormalities in Kawasaki disease. *The Lancet*, Vol.361, No.9365, pp. 1268-1270, (April 2003). ISSN 0140-6736

Biezeveld, MH.; Geissler, J.; Weverling, GJ.; Kuipers, IM.; Lam, J.; Ottenkamp, J. & Kuijpers, TW. (2006). Polymorphisms in the mannose-binding lectin gene as determinants of age-defined risk of coronary artery lesions in Kawasaki disease. *Arthritis & Rheumatism*, Vol.54, No.1, pp. 369-376, (January 2006). ISSN 0004-3591

Biezeveld, M.; Geissler, J.; Merkus, M.; Kuipers, IM.; Ottenkamp, J. & Kuijpers, T. (2007). The inVolvement of Fc gamma receptor gene polymorphisms in Kawasaki disease. *Clinical & Experimental Immunology*, Vol.147, No.1, pp. 106-111, (January 2007). ISSN 0009-9104

Breunis, WB.; Biezeveld, MH.; Geissler, J.; Ottenkamp, J.; Kuipers, IM.; Lam, J.; Hutchinson, A.; Welch, R.; Chanock, SJ. & Kuijpers, TW. (2006). Vascular endothelial growth factor gene haplotypes in Kawasaki disease. *Arthritis & Rheumatism*, Vol.54, No.5, pp. 1588-1594, (May 2006). ISSN 0004-3591

Breunis, WB.; Biezeveld, MH.; Geissler, J.; Kuipers, IM.; Lam, J.; Ottenkamp, J.; Hutchinson, A.; Welch, R.; Chanock, SJ. & Kuijpers, TW. (2007). Polymorphisms in chemokine receptor genes and susceptibility to Kawasaki disease. *Clinical & Experimental Immunology*, Vol.150, No.1, pp. 83-90, (October 2007). ISSN 0009-9104

Burgner, D.; Davila, S.; Breunis, WB.; Ng, SB.; Li, Y.; Bonnard, C.; Ling, L.; Wright, VJ.; Thalamuthu, A.; Odam, M.; Shimizu, C.; Burns, JC.; Levin, M.; Kuijpers, TW. & Hibberd, ML; International Kawasaki Disease Genetics Consortium. (2009). A genome-wide association study identifies novel and functionally related susceptibility Loci for Kawasaki disease. *PLoS Genetics*, Vol.5, No.1, pp. e1000319, (January 2009). ISSN 1553-7404

Burns, JC.; Shimizu, C.; Gonzalez, E.; Kulkarni, H.; Patel, S.; Shike, H.; Sundel, RS.; Newburger, JW. & Ahuja SK. (2005). Genetic variations in the receptor-ligand pair CCR5 and CCL3L1 are important determinants of susceptibility to Kawasaki disease. *The Journal of Infectious Diseases*, Vol.192, No.2, pp. 344-349. (July 2005). ISSN 0022-1899

Burns, JC.; Shimizu, C.; Shike, H.; Newburger, JW.; Sundel, RP.; Baker, AL.; Matsubara, T.; Ishikawa, Y.; Brophy, VA.; Cheng, S.; Grow, MA.; Steiner, LL.; Kono, N. & Cantor RM. (2005). Family-based association analysis implicates IL-4 in susceptibility to Kawasaki disease. *Genes & Immunity*, Vol.6, No.5, pp. 438-444, (August 2005). ISSN 1466-4879

Chaudhuri, K.; Singh, Ahluwalia, T.; Singh, S.; Binepal, G. & Khullar, M. (2011). Polymorphism in the promoter of the CCL5 gene (CCL5G-403A) in a cohort of North Indian children with Kawasaki disease. A preliminary study. *Clinical & Experimental Rheumatology*, Vol.29, No.1, pp. 126-130, (May 2011). ISSN 0392-856X

Chen, SY.; Wan, L.; Huang, YC.; Sheu, JJ.; Lan, YC.; Lai, CH.; Lin, CW.; Chang, JS.; Tsai, Y.; Liu, SP.; Lin, YJ. & Tsai, FJ. (2009). Interleukin-18 gene 105A/C genetic polymorphism is associated with the susceptibility of Kawasaki disease. *Journal of Clinical Laboratory Analysis*, Vol.23, No.2, pp. 71-76. (n.d. 2009). ISSN 0887-8013

Cheung, YF.; Ho, MH.; Ip, WK.; Fok, SF.; Yung, TC. & Lau, YL. (2004). Modulating effects of mannose binding lectin genotype on arterial stiffness in children after Kawasaki disease. *Pediatric Research*, Vol.56, No.4, pp. 591-596, (October 2004).ISSN 0031-3998

Cheung, YF.; Huang, GY.; Chen, SB.; Liu, XQ.; Xi, L.; Liang, XC.; Huang, MR.; Chen, S.; Huang, LS.; Liu, XQ.; Chan, KW. & Lau, YL. (2008). Inflammatory gene polymorphisms and susceptibility to kawasaki disease and its arterial sequelae. *Pediatrics*, Vol. 122, No.3, pp. e608-614, (September 2008). ISSN 0031-4005

Chi, H.; Huang, FY.; Chen, MR.; Chiu, NC.; Lee, HC.; Lin, SP.; Chen, WF.; Lin, CL.; Chan, HW.; Liu, HF.; Huang, LM. & Lee, YJ. (2010). ITPKC gene SNP rs28493229 and Kawasaki disease in Taiwanese children. *Human Molecular Genetics*, Vol.15, No.6, pp. 1147-1151, (March 2010). ISSN 1434-5161

Chien, YH.; Chang, KW.; Yang, YH.; Lu, MY.; Lin, YT. & Chiang BL. (2003). Association between levels of TNF-alpha and TNF-alpha promoter -308 A/A polymorphism in children with Kawasaki disease. *Journal of the Formosan Medical Association*, Vol.102, No. 3, pp. 147-150, (March 2003). ISSN 0929-6646

Chun, JK.; Kang, DW.; Yoo, BW.; Shin, JS. & Kim, DS. (2010). Programmed death-1 (PD-1) gene polymorphisms lodged in the genetic predispositions of Kawasaki Disease. *European Journal of Pediatrics*, Vol.169, No.2, pp. 181-185, (February 2010). ISSN 0340-6199

Fujita, Y.; Nakamura, Y,; Sakata, K,; Hara, N,; Kobayashi, M,; Nagai, M,; Yanagawa, H. & Kawasaki, T. (1989). Kawasaki disease in families. *Pediatrics*, Vol.84, No.4, pp. 666-669, (October 1989). ISSN 1098-4275

Fukazawa, R.; Sonobe, T.; Hamamoto, K.; Hamaoka, K.; Sakata, K.; Asano, T.; Imai, T.; Kamisago, M.; Ohkubo, T.; Uchikoba, Y.; Ikegami, E.; Watanabe, M. & Ogawa, S. (2004). Possible synergic effect of angiotensin-I converting enzyme gene insertion/deletion polymorphism and angiotensin-II type-1 receptor 1166A/C gene polymorphism on ischemic heart disease in patients with Kawasaki disease. *Pediatric Research*, Vol.56, No.4, pp. 597-601, (October 2004). ISSN 0031-3998

Furuno, K.; Takada, H.; Yamamoto, K.; Ikeda, K.; Ohno, T.; Khajoee, V.; Mizuno, Y. & Hara T. (2007). Tissue inhibitor of metalloproteinase 2 and coronary artery lesions in Kawasaki disease. *The Journal of Pediatrics*, Vol.151, No.2, pp. 155-160, (August 2007). ISSN 1085-8695

Holman, RC.; Christensen, KY.; Belay, ED.; Steiner, CA.; Effler, PV.; Miyamura, J.; Forbes, S.; Schonberger, LB. & Melish, M. (2010). Racial/ethnic differences in the incidence of Kawasaki syndrome among children in Hawaii. *Hawaii Medical Journal*, Vol.69, No.8, pp. 194-197, (August 2010). ISSN 0017-8594

Hong, YM.; Jin, HS.; Park, IS. & Hong, SJ. Association of the matrix metalloproteinase-3 (-439C/G) promoter polymorphism with Kawasaki disease in Korean children. *Heart and Vessels*, Vol.23, No.5, pp. 341-347, (September 2008). ISSN 0910-8327

Hsieh, YY.; Lin, YJ.; Chang, CC.; Chen, DY.; Hsu, CM.; Wang, YK.; Hsu, KH. & Tsai FJ. (2010). Human lymphocyte antigen B-associated transcript 2, 3, and 5 polymorphisms and haplotypes are associated with susceptibility of Kawasaki disease and coronary artery aneurysm. *Journal of Clinical Laboratory Analysis*, Vol.24, No.4, pp. 262-268, (n.d. 2010). ISSN 0887-8013

Hsueh, KC.; Lin, YJ.; Chang, JS.; Wan, L.; Tsai, YH.; Tsai, CH.; Chen, CP. & Tsai FJ. (2008). Association of vascular endothelial growth factor C-634 G polymorphism in Taiwanese children with Kawasaki disease. *Pediatric Cardiology*, Vol.29, No.2, pp. 292-296, (March 2008). ISSN 0172-0643

Hsueh, KC.; Lin, YJ.; Chang, JS.; Wan, L.; Tsai, YH.; Tsai, CH. & Tsai, FJ. (2008). Influence of interleukin 18 promoter polymorphisms in susceptibility to Kawasaki disease in Taiwan. *The Journal of Rheumatology*, Vol.35, No.7, pp. 1408-1413, (July 2008). ISSN 0315-162X

Hsueh, KC.; Lin, YJ.; Chang, JS.; Wan, L.; Tsai, YH.; Tsai, CH.; Chen, CP. & Tsai, FJ. (2009). Association of interleukin-10 A-592C polymorphism in Taiwanese children with Kawasaki disease. *Journal of Korean Medical Science*, Vol.24, No.3, pp. 438-442, (June 2009). ISSN: 1011-8934

Hsueh, KC.; Lin, YJ.; Chang, JS.; Wan, L. & Tsai, FJ. (2010). BTNL2 gene polymorphisms may be associated with susceptibility to Kawasaki disease and formation of coronary artery lesions in Taiwanese children. *European Journal of Pediatrics*, Vol.169, No.6, pp. 713-719, (June 2010). ISSN 0340-6199

Huang, FY.; Lee, YJ.; Chen, MR.; Hsu, CH.; Lin, SP.; Sung, TC.; Chang, SC. & Chang, JG. (2000). Polymorphism of transmembrane region of MICA gene and Kawasaki disease. *Experimental and Clinical Immunogenetics*, Vol.17, No. 3, pp. 130-137, (June 2000). ISSN 0254-9670

Huang, FY.; Chang, TY.; Chen, MR.; Lee, HC.; Chiu, NC.; Chi, H.; Hsu, CH.; Lin, SP.; Liu, HF.; Chen, WF.; Chu, CC.; Lin, M. & Lee, YJ. (2008). The -590 C/T and 8375 A/G interleukin-4 polymorphisms are not associated with Kawasaki disease in Taiwanese children. *Human Immunology*, Vol.69, No.1, pp. 52-57, (January 2008). ISSN 0198-8859

Huang, FY.; Chang, TY.; Chen, MR.; Lee, HC.; Chi, H.; Chiu, NC.; Hsu, CH.; Lin, SP.; Kao, HA.; Chen, WF.; Chan, HW.; Liu, HF.; Chu, CC.; Lin, M. & Lee, YJ. (2008). Lack of association of the vascular endothelial growth factor gene polymorphisms with Kawasaki disease in Taiwanese children. *Journal of Clinical Immunology*, Vol.28, No.4, pp. 322-328, (July 2008). ISSN 0271-9142

Huang, FY.; Chang, TY.; Chen, MR.; Chiu, NC.; Chi, H.; Lee, HC.; Lin, SP.; Chen, CK.; Chan, HW.; Chen, WF.; Liu, HF.; Chu, CC.; Lin, M. & Lee, YJ. (2008). Genetic polymorphisms in the CD40 ligand gene and Kawasaki disease. *Journal of Clinical Immunology*, Vol.28, No.5, pp. 405-410, (September 2008). ISSN 0271-9142

Huang, WC.; Huang, LM.; Chang, IS.; Chang, LY.; Chiang, BL.; Chen, PJ.; Wu, MH.; Lue, HC.; & Lee, CY.; Kawasaki Disease Research Group. (2009). Epidemiologic features of Kawasaki disease in Taiwan, 2003-2006. *Pediatrics*, Vol.123, No.3, pp. e401-405, (Mar 2009), ISSN 1098-4275

Huang, YC.; Lin, YJ.; Chang, JS.; Chen, SY.; Wan, L.; Sheu, JJ.; Lai, CH.; Lin, CW.; Liu, SP.; Chen, CP. & Tsai FJ. (2010). Single nucleotide polymorphism rs2229634 in the ITPR3 gene is associated with the risk of developing coronary artery aneurysm in children with Kawasaki disease. *International Journal of Immunogenetics*, Vol.37, No.6, pp. 439-443, (December 2010). ISSN 1744-3121

Ikeda, K.; Ihara, K.; Yamaguchi, K.; Muneuchi, J.; Ohno, T.; Mizuno, Y. & Hara, T. (2008). Genetic analysis of MMP gene polymorphisms in patients with Kawasaki disease. *Pediatric Research*, Vol.63, No.2, pp. 182-185, (February 2008). ISSN 0031-3998

Jhang, WK.; Kang, MJ.; Jin, HS.; Yu, J.; Kim, BJ.; Kim, BS.; Lee, JK.; Seo, EJ.; Yoo, HW.; Park, IS.; Hong, YM. & Hong, SJ. (2009). The CCR5 (-2135C/T) polymorphism may be associated with the development of Kawasaki disease in Korean children. *Journal of Clinical Immunology*, Vol.29, No.1, pp. 22-28, (January 2009). ISSN 0271-9142

Jibiki, T.; Terai, M.; Shima, M.; Ogawa, A.; Hamada, H.; Kanazawa, M.; Yamamoto, S.; Oana, S. & Kohno, Y. (2001). Monocyte chemoattractant protein 1 gene regulatory region polymorphism and serum levels of monocyte chemoattractant protein 1 in Japanese patients with Kawasaki disease. *Arthritis & Rheumatism*, Vol.44, No. 9, pp. 2211-2212, (September 2001). ISSN 0004-3591

Jin, HS.; Kim, HB.; Kim, BS.; Lee, JK.; Seo, EJ.; Yoo, HW.; Park, IS.; Hong, YM. & Hong, SJ. (2007). The IL-10 (-627 A/C) promoter polymorphism may be associated with coronary aneurysms and low serum albumin in Korean children with Kawasaki disease. *Pediatric Research*, Vol.61, No.5, pp. 584-587, (May 2007). ISSN 0031-3998

Kamizono, S.; Yamada, A.; Higuchi, T.; Kato, H. & Itoh, K. (1999). Analysis of tumor necrosis factor-alpha production and polymorphisms of the tumor necrosis factor-alpha gene in individuals with a history of Kawasaki disease. *Pediatrics International*, Vol.41, No.4, pp. 341-345, (August 1999). ISSN 0179-0358

Kanai, M.; Tanabe, S.; Okada, M.; Suzuki, H.; Niki, T.; Katsuura, M.; Akiba, T. & Hayasaka, K. (2003). Polymorphisms of heme oxygenase-1 and bilirubin UDP-glucuronosyltransferase genes are not associated with Kawasaki disease susceptibility. *The Tohoku Journal of Experimental Medicine*, Vol.200, No.3, pp. 155-159, (July 2003). ISSN 0040-8727

Kang, SW.; Ban, JY.; Yoon, KL.; Kim, SK.; Kang, SW.; Chung, JH. & Cho, J. (2011). Notch Homolog 4 Polymorphism and Kawasaki Disease. *Indian Journal of Pediatrics*, in press. ISSN 0019-5456

Kariyazono, H.; Ohno, T.; Khajoee, V.; Ihara, K.; Kusuhara, K.; Kinukawa, N.; Mizuno, Y. & Hara, T. (2004). Association of vascular endothelial growth factor (VEGF) and VEGF receptor gene polymorphisms with coronary artery lesions of Kawasaki disease. *Pediatric Research*, Vol.56, No.6, pp. 953-959, (December 2004). ISSN 0031-3998

Kaslow, RA.; Bailowitz, A.; Lin, FY.; Koslowe, P.; Simonis, T. & Israel, E. (1985). Association of epidemic Kawasaki syndrome with the HLA-A2, B44, Cw5 antigen combination. *Arthritis & Rheumatism*, Vol.28, No.8, pp. 938-940, (August 1985). ISSN 0004-3591

Kato, H.; Koike, S.; Yamamoto, M.; Ito, Y. & Yano, E. (1975). Coronary aneurysms in infants and young children with acute febrile mucocutaneous lymph node syndrome. *The Journal of Pediatrics*, Vol.86, No.6, pp. 892-898, (June 1975), ISSN 1085-8695

Kato, S.; Kimura, M.; Tsuji, K.; Kusakawa, S.; Asai, T., Juji, T. & Kawasaki, T. (1978). HLA antigens in Kawasaki disease. *Pediatrics*, Vol.61, No.2, pp. 252-255, (February 1978). ISSN 1098-4275

Kawasaki, T. (1967), Acute febrile mucocutaneous syndrome with lymphoid inVolvement with specific desquamation of the fingers and toes in children. *Arerugi,* Vol.16, No.3, pp. 178-222, (March 1967), ISSN 0021-4884

Keren, G.; Danon, YL.; Orgad, S.; Kalt, R. & Gazit, E. (1982). HLA Bw51 is increased in mucocutaneous lymph node syndrome in Israeli patients. *Tissue Antigens,* Vol.20, No.2, pp. 144-146, (August 1982). ISSN 0001-2815

Khajoee, V.; Kariyazono, H.; Ohno, T.; Ihara, K.; Mizuno, Y.; Kusuhara, K. & Hara T. (2003). Inducible and endothelial constitutive nitric oxide synthase gene polymorphisms in Kawasaki disease. *Pediatrics International,* Vol.45, No.2, pp. 130-134, (April 2003). ISSN 0179-0358

Kim, JJ.; Hong, SJ.; Hong, YM.; Kim, S.; Kang, MJ.; Kim, KJ.; Seo, EJ.; Yoo, HW.; Cheong, HS.; Shin, HD.; Park, IS & Lee, JK. (2008). Genetic variants in the HLA-G region are associated with Kawasaki disease. *Human Immunology,* Vol.69, No.12, pp.867-871, (December 2008). ISSN 0198-8859

Kim, JJ.; Hong, YM.; Sohn, S.; Jang, GY.; Ha, KS.; Yun, SW.; Han, MK.; Lee, KY.; Song, MS.; Lee, HD.; Kim, DS.; Lee, JE.; Shin, ES.; Jang, JH.; Lee, YS.; Kim, SY.; Lee, JY.; Han, BG.; Wu, JY.; Kim, KJ.; Park, YM.; Seo, EJ.; Park, IS. & Lee, JK.; Korean Kawasaki Disease Genetics Consortium. (2011). A genome-wide association analysis reveals 1p31 and 2p13.3 as susceptibility loci for Kawasaki disease. *Human Genetics,* Vol.129, No.5, pp. 487-495, (May 2011). ISSN 0340-6717

Kim, SK.; Kang, SW.; Chung, JH.; Lee, JS.; Park, HK.; Yoon, KL. & Kim, SC. (2011). Coding single-nucleotide polymorphisms of interleukin-1 gene cluster are not associated with Kawasaki disease in the Korean population. *Pediatric Cardiology,* Vol.32, No.4, pp. 381-385, (April 2011). ISSN 0172-0643

Krensky, AM.; Berenberg, W.; Shanley, K. & Yunis, EJ. (1981). HLA antigens in mucocutaneous lymph node syndrome in New England. *Pediatrics,* Vol.67, No.5, pp. 741-743, (May 1981). ISSN 1098-4275

Krensky, AM.; Grady, S.; Shanley, KM.; Berenberg, W. & Yunis, EJ. (1983). Epidemic and endemic HLA-B and DR associations in mucocutaneous lymph node syndrome. *Human Immunology,* Vol.6, No.2, pp. 75-77, (February 1983). ISSN 0198-8859

Kuo, HC.; Liang, CD.; Yu, HR.; Wang, CL.; Lin, IC.; Liu, CA.; Chang, JC.; Lee, CP.; Chang, WC. & Yang, KD. (2010). CTLA-4, Position 49 A/G Polymorphism Associated with Coronary Artery Lesions in Kawasaki Disease. *Journal of Clinical Immunology,* in press. ISSN 0271-9142

Kuo, HC.; Yu, HR.; Juo, SH.; Yang, KD.; Wang, YS.; Liang, CD.; Chen, WC.; Chang, WP.; Huang, CF.; Lee, CP.; Lin, LY.; Liu, YC.; Guo, YC.; Chiu, CC & Chang, WC. (2011). CASP3 gene single-nucleotide polymorphism (rs72689236) and Kawasaki disease in Taiwanese children. *Journal of Human Genetics,* Vol.56, No.2 pp. 161-165, (February 2011). ISSN 1434-5161

Lin, YJ.; Wan, L.; Wu, JY.; Sheu, JJ.; Lin, CW.; Lan, YC.; Lai, CH.; Hung, CH.; Tsai, Y.; Tsai, CH.; Lin, TH.; Lin, JG.; Hsueh, KC.; Huang, YM.; Chang, JS & Tsai, FJ. (2009). HLA-E gene polymorphism associated with susceptibility to Kawasaki disease and formation of coronary artery aneurysms. *Arthritis & Rheumatism,* Vol.60, No.2, pp. 604-610, (February 2009). ISSN 0004-3591

Lin, MT.; Wang, JK.; Yeh, JI.; Sun, LC.; Chen, PL.; Wu, JF.; Chang, CC.; Lee, WL.; Shen, CT.; Wang, NK.; Wu, CS.; Yeh, SZ.; Chen, CA.; Chiu, SN & Wu, MH. (2011). Clinical Implication of the C Allele of the ITPKC Gene SNP rs28493229 in Kawasaki Disease: Association with Disease Susceptibility and BCG Scar Reactivation. *The Pediatric Infectious Disease Journal*, Vol.30, No.2, pp. 148-152, (February 2011). ISSN 0891-3668

Macián, F.; García-Cózar, F.; Im, SH.; Horton, HF.; Byrne, MC. & Rao, A. (2002). Transcriptional mechanisms underlying lymphocyte tolerance. Cell, Vol.109, No.6, pp. 719-731, (June 2002). ISSN 0092-8674

Mamtani, M.; Matsubara, T.; Shimizu, C.; Furukawa, S.; Akagi, T.; Onouchi, Y.; Hata, A.; Fujino, A.; He, W.; Ahuja, SK. & Burns, JC. (2010). Association of CCR2-CCR5 haplotypes and CCL3L1 copy number with Kawasaki Disease, coronary artery lesions, and IVIG responses in Japanese children. *PLoS One*, Vol.5, No.7, pp. e11458, (July 2010). ISSN 1932-6203

Minami, T.; Suzuki, H.; Takeuchi, T.; Uemura, S.; Sugatani, J. & Yoshikawa N. (2005). A polymorphism in plasma platelet-activating factor acetylhydrolase is inVolved in resistance to immunoglobulin treatment in Kawasaki disease. *Journal of Pediatrics*, Vol.147, No.1, pp. 78-83, (July 2005). ISSN 0022-3476

Matsuda, I.; Hattori, S.; Nagata, N.; Fruse, A. & Nambu, H. (1977). HLA antigens in mucocutaneous lymph node syndrome. *American Journal of Diseases of Children*, Vol.131, No.12, pp. 1417-1418, (December 1977). ISSN 0002-922X

Nakamura, Y.; Yashiro, M.; Uehara, R.; Sadakane, A.; Chihara, I.; Aoyama, Y.; Kotani, K. & Yanagawa, H. (2010). Epidemiologic features of Kawasaki disease in Japan: results of the 2007-2008 nationwide survey. Journal of Epidemiology, Vol. 20, No. 4, pp. 302-307, (July 2010), ISSN 0917-5040

Nishimura, S.; Zaitsu, M.; Hara, M.; Yokota, G.; Watanabe, M.; Ueda, Y.; Imayoshi, M.; Ishii, E.; Tasaki, H. & Hamasaki, Y. (2003). A polymorphism in the promoter of the CD14 gene (CD14/-159) is associated with the development of coronary artery lesions in patients with Kawasaki disease. *The Journal of Pediatrics*, Vol.143, No.3, pp. 357-362, (September 2003). ISSN 1085-8695

Onouchi, Y.; Onoue, S.; Tamari, M.; Wakui, K.; Fukushima, Y.; Yashiro, M.; Nakamura, Y.; Yanagawa, H.; Kishi, F.; Ouchi, K.; Terai, M.; Hamamoto, K.; Kudo, F.; Aotsuka, H.; Sato, Y.; Nariai, A.; Kaburagi, Y.; Miura, M.; Saji, T.; Kawasaki, T.; Nakamura, Y. & Hata, A. (2004). CD40 ligand gene and Kawasaki disease. *European Journal of Human Genetics*, Vol.12, No.12, pp. 1062-1068, (December 2004). ISSN 1018-4813

Onouchi, Y.; Tamari, M.; Takahashi, A.; Tsunoda, T.; Yashiro, M.; Nakamura, Y.; Yanagawa, H.; Wakui, K.; Fukushima, Y.; Kawasaki, T.; Nakamura, Y. & Hata, A. (2007). A genomewide linkage analysis of Kawasaki disease: evidence for linkage to chromosome 12. *Journal of Human Genetics*, Vol.52, No.2, pp. 179-190, (February 2007), ISSN 1434-5161

Onouchi, Y.; Gunji, T.; Burns, JC.; Shimizu, C.; Newburger, JW.; Yashiro, M.; Nakamura, Y.; Wakui, K.; Fukushima, Y.; Kishi, F.; Hamamoto, K.; Terai, M.; Sato, Y.; Ouchi, K.; Saji, T.; Nariai, A.; Kaburagi, Y.; Yoshikawa, T.; Suzuki, K.; Tanaka, T.; Nagai, T.; Cho, H.; Fujino, A.; Sekine, A.; Nakamichi, R.; Tsunoda, T.; Kawasaki, T.;

Nakamura, Y. & Hata, A. (2008). ITPKC functional polymorphism associated with Kawasaki disease susceptibility and formation of coronary artery aneurysms. *Nature Genetics*, Vol.40, No.1, pp. 35-42, (January 2008), ISSN 1061-4036

Onouchi, Y.; Ozaki, K.; Burns, JC.; Shimizu, C.; Hamada, H.; Honda, T.; Terai, M.; Honda, A.; Takeuchi, T.; Shibuta, S.; Suenaga, T.; Suzuki, H.; Higashi, K.; Yasukawa, K.; Suzuki, Y.; Sasago, K.; Kemmotsu, Y.; Takatsuki, S.; Saji, T.; Yoshikawa, T.; Nagai, T.; Hamamoto, K.; Kishi, F.; Ouchi, K.; Sato, Y.; Newburger, JW.; Baker, AL.; Shulman, ST.; Rowley, AH.; Yashiro, M.; Nakamura, Y.; Wakui, K.; Fukushima, Y.; Fujino, A.; Tsunoda, T.; Kawasaki, T.; Hata, A.; Nakamuram, Y. & Tanaka, T. (2010). Common variants in CASP3 confer susceptibility to Kawasaki disease. *Human Molecular Genetics*, Vol.19, No.14, pp. 2898-2906, (July 2010), ISSN 0964-6906

Onouchi, Z & Kawasaki, T. (1999). Overview of pharmacological treatment of Kawasaki disease. Drugs, vol.58, No.5, pp. 813-822, (November 1999). ISSN 0012-6667

Ouchi, K.; Suzuki, Y.; Shirakawa, T. & Kishi, F. (2003). Polymorphism of SLC11A1 (formerly NRAMP1) gene confers susceptibility to Kawasaki disease. *The Journal of Infectious Diseases*, Vol.187, No.2, pp. 326-329, (January 2003). ISSN 0022-1899

Park, JA.; Shin, KS. & Kim, YW. (2005). Polymorphism of matrix metalloproteinase-3 promoter gene as a risk factor for coronary artery lesions in Kawasaki disease. *Journal of Korean Medical Science*, Vol.20, No.4, pp. 607-611, (August 2005). ISSN 1011-8934

Park, SW.; Ban, JY.; Yoon, KL.; Kim, HJ.; Chung, JY.; Yi, JW.; Lee, BJ. & Chung, JH. (2010). InVolvement of tryptophan hydroxylase 2 (TPH2) gene polymorphisms in susceptibility to coronary artery lesions in Korean children with Kawasaki disease. *European Journal of Pediatrics*, Vol.169, No.4, pp. 457-461, (April 2010). ISSN 0340-6199

Park, YW.; Han, JW.; Hong, YM.; Ma, JS.; Cha, SH.; Kwon, TC.; Lee, SB.; Kim, CH.; Lee, JS.; & Kim, CH. (2011). Epidemiological features of Kawasaki disease in Korea, 2006-2008. *Pediatrics International*, Vol.53, No.1, pp. 36-39, (February 2011), ISSN 1328-8067

Quasney, MW.; Bronstein, DE.; Cantor, RM.; Zhang, Q.; Stroupe, C.; Shike, H.; Bastian, JF.; Matsubara, T.; Fujiwara, M.; Akimoto, K.; Newburger, JW. & Burns, JC. (2001). Increased frequency of alleles associated with elevated tumor necrosis factor-alpha levels in children with Kawasaki disease. *Pediatric Research*, Vol.49, No.5, pp. 686-690, (May 2001). ISSN 0031-3998

Sheu, JJ.; Lin, YJ.; Chang, JS.; Wan, L.; Chen, SY.; Huang, YC.; Chan, C.; Chiu, IW. & Tsai FJ. (2010). Association of COL11A2 polymorphism with susceptibility to Kawasaki disease and development of coronary artery lesions. *International Journal of Immunogenetics*, Vol.37, No.6, pp. 487-492, (December 2010). ISSN 1744-3121

Shim, YH.; Kim, HS.; Sohn, S. & Hong, YM. (2006). Insertion/deletion polymorphism of angiotensin converting enzyme gene in Kawasaki disease. *Journal of Korean Medical Science*, Vol.21, No.2, pp. 208-211, (April 2006). ISSN 1011-8934

Shimizu, C.; Jain, S.; Davila, S.; Hibberd, ML.; Lin, KO.; Molkara, D.; Frazer, JR.; Sun, S.; Baker, AL.; Newburger, JW.; Rowley, AH.; Shulman, ST.; Davila, S.; Burgner, D.; Breunis, WB.; Kuijpers, TW.; Wright, VJ.; Levin, M.; Eleftherohorinou, H.; Coin, L.;

Popper, SJ.; Relman, DA.; Fury, W.; Lin, C.; Mellis, S.; Tremoulet, AH. & Burns JC. (2011). Transforming growth factor-beta signaling pathway in patients with Kawasaki disease. *Circulation: Cardiovascular Genetics*, Vol.4, No.1, pp. 16-25, (February 2011). ISSN 1942-325X

Simonini, G.; Corinaldesi, E.; Massai, C.; Falcini, F.; Fanti, F.; De Martino, M. & Cimaz, R. (2009). Macrophage migration inhibitory factor -173 polymorphism and risk of coronary alterations in children with Kawasaki disease. *Clinical & Experimental Rheumatology*, Vol.27, No. 6, pp. 1026-1030, (2009 November-December). ISSN 0392-856X

Sohn, MH.; Hur, MW. & Kim DS. (2001). Interleukin 6 gene promoter polymorphism is not associated with Kawasaki disease. Genes & Immunity, Vol.2, No.7, pp. 357-362, (October 2001). ISSN 1466-4879

Takeuchi, K.; Yamamoto, K.; Kataoka, S.; Kakihara, T.; Tanaka, A.; Sato, S. & Uchiyama, M. (1997). High incidence of angiotensin I converting enzyme genotype II in Kawasaki disease patients with coronary aneurysm. *European Journal of Pediatrics*, Vol.156, No.4, pp. 266-268, (April 1997). ISSN 0340-6199

Taniuchi, S.; Masuda, M.; Teraguchi, M.; Ikemoto, Y.; Komiyama, Y.; Takahashi, H.; Kino, M. & Kobayashi, Y. (2005). Polymorphism of Fc gamma RIIa may affect the efficacy of gamma-globulin therapy in Kawasaki disease. *Journal of Clinical Immunology*, Vol.25, No.4, pp. 309-313, (July 2005). ISSN 0271-9142

Tsai, FJ.; Lee, YC.; Chang, JS.; Huang, LM.; Huang, FY.; Chiu, NC.; Chen, MR.; Chi, H.; Lee, YJ.; Chang, LC.; Liu, YM.; Wang, HH.; Chen, CH.; Chen, YT. & Wu, JY. (2011). Identification of novel susceptibility Loci for Kawasaki disease in a Han Chinese population by a genome-wide association study. *PLoS One*. Vol.6, No.2, pp. e16853, (February 2011). ISSN 1817-101X

Tsukahara, H.; Hiraoka, M.; Saito, M.; Nishida, K.; Kobata, R.; Tsuchida, S.; Toyooka, M.; Kimura, H.; Gejyo, F. & Mayumi, M. (2000). Methylenetetrahydrofolate reductase polymorphism in Kawasaki disease. *Pediatrics International*, Vol.42, No.3, pp. 236-240, (June 2000). ISSN 1328-8067

Uehara, R.; Yashiro, M.; Nakamura, Y. & Yanagawa, H. (2003). Kawasaki disease in parents and children. *Acta Paediatrica*, Vol.92, No. 6, pp. 694-697, (June 2003). ISSN 0803-5253

Wang, GB.; Li, CR.; Yang, J.; Wen, PQ. & Jia, SL. (2011). A regulatory polymorphism in promoter region of TNFR1 gene is associated with Kawasaki disease in Chinese individuals. *Human Immunology*, Vol.72, No.5, pp. 451-457, (May 2011). ISSN 0198-8859

Weng, KP.; Hsieh, KS.; Hwang, YT.; Huang, SH.; Lai, TJ.; Yuh, YS.; Hou, YY.; Lin, CC.; Huang, SC.; Chang, CK.; Lin, MW. & Ger, LP. (2010). IL-10 polymorphisms are associated with coronary artery lesions in acute stage of Kawasaki disease. *Circulation Journal*, Vol.74, No.5, pp. 983-989, (May 2010). ISSN 1346-9843

Weng, KP.; Ho, TY.; Chiao, YH.; Cheng, JT.; Hsieh, KS.; Huang, SH.; Ou, SF.; Liu, KH.; Hsu, CJ.; Lu, PJ.; Hsiao, M. & Ger LP. (2010). Cytokine genetic polymorphisms and susceptibility to Kawasaki disease in Taiwanese children. *Circulation Journal*, Vol.74, No.12, pp. 2726-2733, (November 2010). ISSN 1346-9843

Woo, M.; Hakem, R.; Soengas, MS.; Duncan, GS.; Shahinian, A.; Kägi, D.; Hakem, A.; McCurrach, M.; Khoo, W.; Kaufman, SA.; Senaldi, G.; Howard, T.; Lowe, SW & Mak, TW. (1998). Essential contribution of caspase 3/CPP32 to apoptosis and its associated nuclear changes. *Genes & Development* Vol.12, No.6, pp. 806-819, (March 1998). ISSN 0890-9369

Wu, SF.; Chang, JS.; Peng, CT.; Shi, YR. & Tsai FJ. (2004). Polymorphism of angiotensin-1 converting enzyme gene and Kawasaki disease. *Pediatric Cardiology*, Vol.25, No.5, pp. 529-533, (September-October 2004). ISSN 0172-0643

Wu, SF.; Chang, JS.; Wan, L.; Tsai, CH. & Tsai, FJ. (2005). Association of IL-1Ra gene polymorphism.; but no association of IL-1beta and IL-4 gene polymorphisms.; with Kawasaki disease. *Journal of Clinical Laboratory Analysis*, Vol.19, No.3, pp. 99-102, (n.d. 2005). ISSN 0887-8013

Wu, W., Misra, R.S., Russell, J.Q., Flavell, R.A., Rinco´n, M. & Budd, R.C. (2006) Proteolytic regulation of nuclear factor of activated T (NFAT) c2 cells and NFAT activity by caspase-3. *The Journal of Biological Chemistry*, Vol.281, No.16, pp. 10682–10690, (April 2006). ISSN 0021-9258

Yamaguchi, K.; Ikeda, K.; Ihara, K.; Takada, H.; Kusuhara, K. & Hara, T. (2009). Lack of association between E148Q MEFV variant and Kawasaki disease. *Human Immunology*, Vol.70, No.6, pp. 468-471, (January 2009). ISSN 0198-8859

6

The Role of Proteinase 3 and Neutrophils in ANCA-Associated Systemic Vasculitis

Mohamed Abdgawad
Lund University, Lund
Sweden

1. Introduction

Systemic vasculitides are a group of disorders characterized by vascular inflammation, leading to vessel occlusion and consequent necrosis or ischemia. Depending on site and extent of inflammation, vasculitis has a varied presentation and prognosis. The classification of systemic vasculitides is based on the dominant vessel involved. They are also classified as idiopathic, primary and secondary to connective tissue diseases (rheumatoid arthritis, systemic lupus erythematosis), infections (infective endocarditis) and drugs (Firestein GS, 2008; Watts R, 1995). AASV (ANCA-Associated Systemic Vasculitis) is the most common primary small-vessel vasculitis that occurs in adults, and recent data indicates that the incidence has shown an up-swing. As per recent reports, the annual incidence of AASV varies from 12.4 to 19.8 per million. In two recent studies by our group, we found an incidence for AASV of 20.9/million, with a point prevalence of 268/million inhabitants in southern Sweden (Knight, 2006; Mohammad, 2007; Mohammad, 2009).

ANCA (anti neutrophil cytoplasmic antibodies)-associated Vasculitis is a term that refers to a group of disorders marked by multi-organ system involvement, small vessel vasculitis and the presence of ANCA. These include Wegener's granulomatosis (WG), Churg-Strauss syndrome (CSS) and Microscopic polyangiitis (MPA). The two most important ANCA antigens are PR3 and MPO. The vast majority of anti-PR3 antibodies yield a c-ANCA (cytoplasmic) pattern on IIF, while most anti- MPO antibodies produce a p-ANCA (perinuclear) pattern, with some exceptions (Segelmark, 1994). As per an international consensus document from 1999, anti-MPO and anti-PR3 antibodies are referred to as MPO-ANCA and PR3-ANCA. AASV is characterized histologically by leukocytoclasis, infiltration and accumulation of apoptotic and necrotic neutrophils in tissues, and fibrinoid necrosis of the vessel walls. The histological lesions in AASV are also termed pauci-immune, as only a few or no immunoglobulins/ complement components are detected in the vasculitic lesions. AASV is associated with significant morbidity and mortality (median survival of five months, in the absence of treatment), with almost all patients requiring long term and aggressive immunosuppressive treatment (Booth, 2003).

The etiology of AASV remains largely unknown. Genetic predisposition (PIZ allele of α1-AT, CTLA-4, PTPN22, HLA DR1-DQw1) and environmental factors including exposure to silica and asbestos, drugs (anti-thyroid medications), and various infections (bacterial endocarditis, hepatitis C virus) have been demonstrated to either predispose to, or correlate with ANCA and development of vasculitis (Beaudreuil, 2005; Choi, 2000; Elzouki, 1994;

Hay, 1991). The pathophysiological processes underlying the development of AASV are not fully understood; data suggests that neutrophils and lymphocytes play key roles. Intriguingly, though the association between ANCA and pauci-immune small vessel vasculitides is well established, the exact role of ANCA in the pathogenesis of AASV remains an enigma. This review focuses on the role of proteinase 3 and neutrophil apoptosis in AASV.

2. Proteinase 3

Proteinase 3 (PR3), also called myeloblastin and proteinase 4, was originally identified by Ohlsson, and later characterized by Baggiolini et al (Baggiolini, 1978; K. Ohlsson & I. Olsson 1973). PR3 is a neutral serine protease found in the azurophilic granules of neutrophils and peroxidase-positive lysosomes of monocyte. It is also present in specific granules and in secretory vesicles, and is expressed on the plasma membrane of normal blood neutrophils (Csernok, 1994; Rao, 1991; Witko-Sarsat, 1999). The PR3 gene maps to chromosome 19p13.3, in a cluster with HLE and azurocidin (AZU); it spans 6570 base pairs and consists of five exons and four introns (Sturrock, 1993). Introns I and IV include regions with repeating motifs, which may cause chromosomal instability and a predisposition to genetic rearrangements and deletions. A bi-allelic restriction fragment length polymorphism (RFLP) has been described in the PR3 gene. The gene is transcribed in the promyelocytic stage. Allelic variations in PR3 may be associated with quantitative/qualitative differences in the expression and/or function of PR3 (Gencik, 2000). PR3-mRNA is detected in early cells of the myeloid lineage and is down-regulated during myeloid differentiation. The mechanisms that promote high level transcription of PR3 in myeloid cells committed to granulocyte differentiation are not completely understood, although it is known that two transcriptional factors are needed for the expression of PR3, PU.1 and CG element (Sturrock, 1996).

PR3 is synthesized as a prepro-enzyme, which is processed in four consecutive steps into a mature form consisting of 222 amino acids. Following removal of signal peptide, it is transported into the endoplasmic reticulum (ER), where it is glycosylated with high-mannose oligosaccharides. Glycosylation of PR3 may influence its subcellular localization, with certain glycosylated isoforms being designated for granular cells and others for secretion or expression on the plasma membrane. The propeptide of PR3 is removed in the post-Golgi organelle, after which a seven-amino-acid carboxy-terminal extension is removed, possibly by a trypsin-like proteinase. During this process, small amounts of the pro-form of PR3 escape granular targeting and are secreted. These molecules may play a role in negative feedback regulation of granulopoiesis.

2.1 Membrane expression of PR3

PR3 is expressed on the plasma membrane (mPR3) of a subpopulation of resting neutrophils. Halbwachs-Mecarelli et al. noted the existence of two distinct neutrophil subpopulations, mPR3+ and mPR3-negative, in normal healthy individuals, termed as the bimodal expression of PR3 (Halbwachs-Mecarelli, 1995), Figure 1. Despite the high variability in the proportion of PR3-expressing cells among individuals, the proportion is highly stable in a given individual over long periods of time, suggesting genetic control of mPR3 expression (Schreiber, 2003). This is supported by twin studies demonstrating that the proportion of mPR3 expressing neutrophils in monozygotic twins is highly concordant. The intracellular levels of PR3 do not correlate with mPR3 levels. mPR3 is released from and recruited to the plasma membrane on a continuous on- going basis, such that the amount of mPR3 on the surface of mPR3+ neutrophils remains relatively constant (Bauer, 2007).

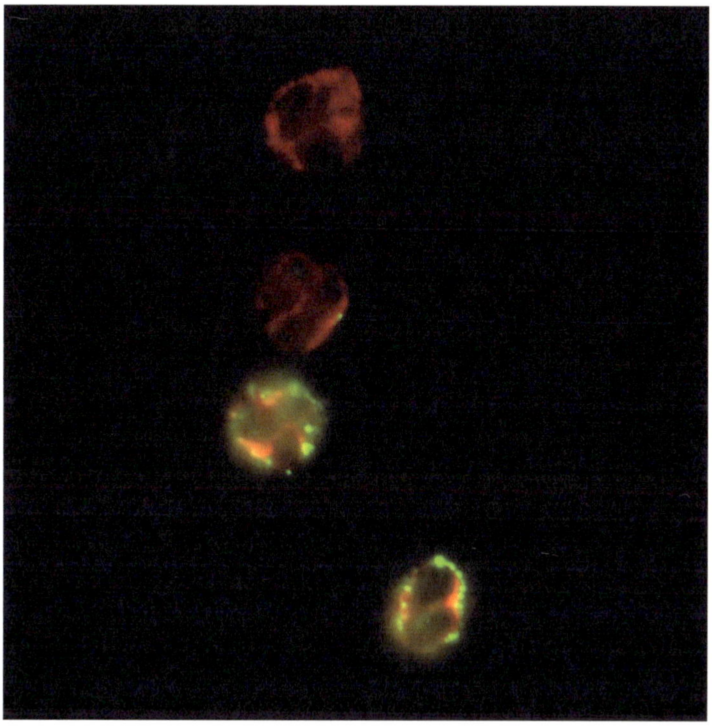

Fig. 1. Bimodal expression of PR3. A Fluorescent micrograph showing four neutrophils, the lower two cells express PR3 (represented with green colour, Alexa Fluor 488), while the upper two neutrophils do not express PR3 on their membrane. All neutrophils contain PR3 intracellularly shown in red (Alexa 594).

Expression of PR3 on the membrane of neutrophils is upregulated by multiple proinflammatory mediators including TNF-α, PMA, IL-18, LPS, IL-8, PAF, fMLP and GM-CSF, and by one anti-inflammatory cytokine: TGF-β (Campbell, 2000; Csernok, 1996; Hellmich, 2000). Membrane PR3 is active and quite resistant to inhibition by naturally occurring proteinase inhibitors including α1-AT, possibly due to steric hindrance of the membrane-embedded protease. PR3 can be eluted from the membrane of PMN following cellular activation; ionic interactions are important in the binding of PR3 to the plasma membrane. It is a cationic protein (isoelectric point 9.1), can bind stably to anionic and neutral membranes, but binds more strongly to negatively-charged bilayers. It has been suggested that PR3 membrane binding is possibly mediated by protein partners such as FcγRIIIb (CD16b), or β2 itegrin (CD11b/CD18). Fridlich et al. showed that cleavage of neutrophil glycosylphosphatidylinositol (GPI) anchors by phosphatidyl inositol-specific phospholipase C (PI-PLC) reduces the level of mPR3, indicating that a GPI protein, possibly FcγRIIIb, (or another yet unidentified GPI-anchored protein) attaches PR3 to the membrane (Fridlich, 2006). PR3 is also expressed on the plasma membrane of apoptotic cells, independent of degranulation, and this is associated with phosphatidylserine (PS) externalization. Kantari et al. demonstrated that phospholipid scramblase- 1 (PLSCR1) interacts with PR3 and may promote its translocation to the plasma membrane during apoptosis (Kantari, 2007).

2.2 PR3 functions

PR3 is an autoantigen, possesses catalytic activity, is a hematopoietic regulator and has apoptosis inducing capabilities. mPR3 shows enzymatic activity; it degrades fibronectin, elastin, laminin, collagen type IV and heparan sulfate proteoglycans in the subendothelial matrix (Campbell, 2000). The soluble form of PR3 cleaves and activates cytokine precursors, including IL-8, IL-1β, and TNFα. PR3 also induces detachment and cytolysis of endothelial cells in vitro (Ballieux, 1994). A secreted proform of PR3 (retaining an amino terminal dipeptide) can downregulate DNA synthesis in normal CD34+ hematopoietic progenitor cells (S phase reduction); thus, PR3 may act as a negative feedback regulator of granulopoiesis in the bone marrow (Skold, 1999). Interestingly, this inhibitory effect of pro-PR3 is reversible; it can be abrogated by G-CSF or GM-CSF. PR3 actions are inhibited by α1-AT. MPO protects the enzymatic activity of PR3 by oxidizing a histidine residue on α1-AT, which tilts the protease anti-protease balance at sites of inflammation.

A recombinant cellular model has been used to demonstrate that PR3 plays a role in neutrophil survival. In particular, PR3 activates procaspase-3 into a specific 22-kDa fragment localized to the membrane compartment of neutrophils, but lacking from apoptotic neutrophils. This PR3-activated caspase-3 is restricted to the plasma membrane-enriched compartment, and segregated from its target proteins that mediate apoptosis from downstream components of the caspase-3 cleavage cascade. Thus in this model, PR3 can cause activation of caspase 3, but not apoptosis. Vong et al. devised a novel assay for PR3-protease activity using double-tagged recombinant annexin A1 (AnxA1) as substrate. This substrate was cleaved by recombinant PR3 or the membrane fraction of cells stably-transfected with PR3 in vitro and in vivo, suggesting that AnxA1 may be a physiologically-relevant substrate for PR3. AnxA1 has counter-regulatory inhibitory properties, and functions as an anti-inflammatory protein as well as inducer of neutrophil apoptosis. In activated neutrophils, AnxA1 translocates to the membrane, and becomes available for PR3. It is likely that cleavage of AnxA1 by PR3 decreases its innate inhibitory function, and promotes a pro-inflammatory response (Pederzoli, 2005; Vong, 2007). All these studies, together with the observation of high levels of PR3 within fibrinoid necrotic lesions in vasculitis, provide strong evidence that PR3 promotes a pro-inflammatory response.

2.3 mPR3 and CD177

CD177, also known as Polycythemia Vera protein-1 (PRV-1), is a glycoprotein that was first discovered in 1970 in connection with studies of Polycythemia Vera (Lalezari, 1971). It belongs to the Leukocyte Antigen 6 (Ly-6) supergene family and is the best characterized member of this family (Caruccio, 2006). As with PR3, CD177 has the unique distinction of being expressed on a subset/ fraction of the neutrophil population (Stroncek, 2004). In neutrophils that express CD177, CD177-mRNA levels are increased by exposure to G-CSF and by inflammatory states (sepsis, burns) associated with increased neutrophil production (Bux J, 2002; Gohring, 2004). CD177-mRNA is more abundant in CD177+ neutrophils than in CD177– PMNs (Wolff, 2003). Complete CD177-mRNA is not detected in CD177– neutrophils, suggesting a defect in transcription or splicing of CD177 mRNA. The functions of CD177 are not known, although there is evidence that it may play a role in adhesion of neutrophils to endothelial cells. CD177 can directly bind to PECAM-1 (CD31), expressed at the junctions of the endothelial cells, on the membrane of neutrophils, monocytes and platelets, enhancing transendothelial migration of CD177+ neutrophils (Goldschmeding, 1992; Sachs, 2007). Also, CD177 is thought to be a marker of increased granulopoiesis.

We have shown that mPR3 and CD177 are co-expressed on the same subset of circulating neutrophils in AASV patients (Bauer, 2007), Figure 2. Also, we found that both CD177 and mPR3 are up-regulated in parallel, and to a similar extent, in this neutrophil subset. Following stimulation of cells with PMA or with CyB/fMLP, mPR3 and CD177 expression are co-induced approximately five-fold on the membrane of mPR3+/CD177+ cells and also converted the mPR3-negative/CD177-negative cells to mPR3/CD177-expressing cells, Figure 3.

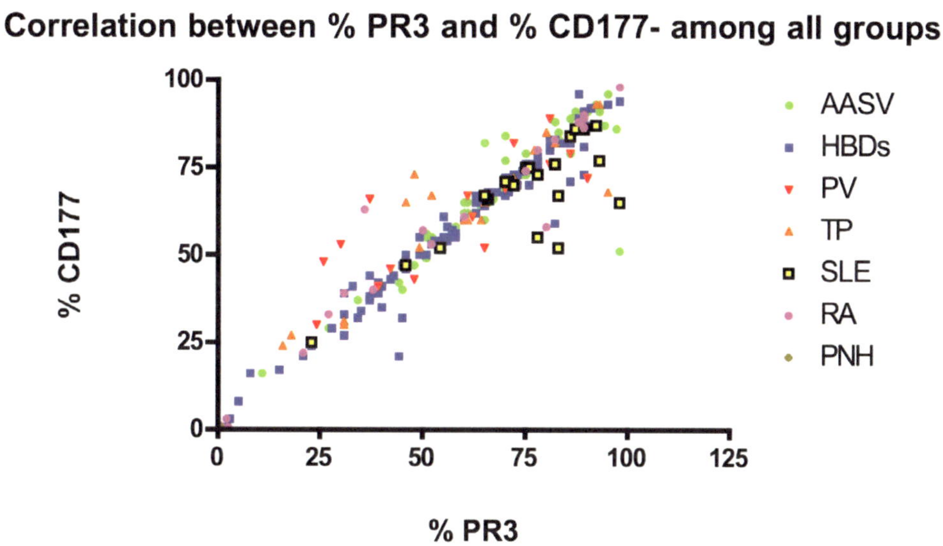

Fig. 2. Correlation between mPR3 and CD177 among all the groups. Shows the results of 91 HBDs, 52 AASV patients, 17 PV patients, 20 TP, 21 SLE patients, and 17 RA patients and one patient with PNH. There was a strong correlation between % of mPR3-positive neutrophils and % of CD177-positive neutrophils among all the groups, i.e. they define the same population of neutrophils (mPR3- and CD177-positive population). AASV= ANCA-associated Systemic Vasculitis. HBD= healthy blood donors. PV= Polycythemia Vera. TP= renal transplant recipients. SLE= Systemic Lupus Erythematosus. RA= Rheumatoid Arthritis. PNH= Paroxysmal Nocturnal Hemoglobinuria.

The bimodal expression of mPR3 in neutrophils is not explained by binding of mPR3 to CD16 and CD18 as CD16 and CD18 are expressed on all neutrophils. It may be that certain adaptor/transport proteins, possibly CD177 itself, that are expressed primarily in mPR3-positive cells, play a role in the expression of mPR3 on a subset of neutrophils. Von Vietinghoff et al. have provided evidence of direct binding between PR3 and CD177. Because the concentration of intracellular PR3 is similar in all cells, these putative adaptor proteins would be required to selectively facilitate PR3 localization to the plasma membrane in CD177-positive cells. It can also be postulated that a subset of cells, in which large amounts of PR3 and CD177 are stored in secondary and secretory vesicles during granulopoiesis, are precursors to the mPR3+/CD177+ circulating neutrophils. This would argue for the existence of a genetic mechanism, whereby the genes encoding PR3 and CD177 are co-regulated during the later stages of granulopoiesis. The fact that only 4% of cells express only one of the two markers favours this hypothesis, and suggests that a similar mechanism is involved in mobilizing PR3 and CD177 from a common intracellular storage site to the plasma membrane (Bauer, 2007).

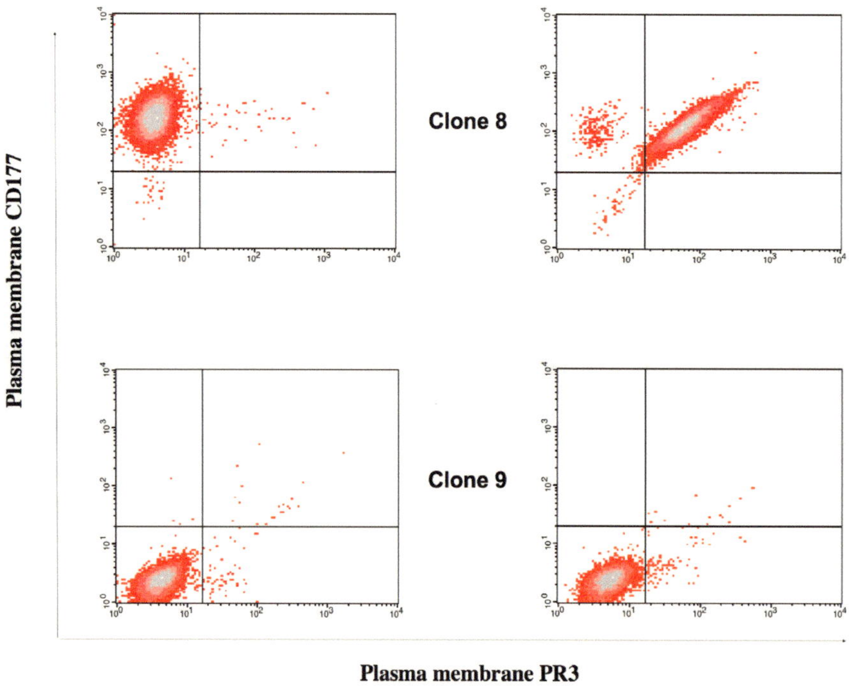

Fig. 3. U937 and exogenous PR3 binding. The left panel shows the membrane expression of U937-clone 8-cells (express CD177 but not PR3 on their plasma membrane), and U937-clone 9-cells (do not express PR3 or CD177 on their plasma membrane), measured by FACS. In the right panel, membrane expression of PR3 and CD177 was measured again on the same cells after incubation with mature PR3 for two hours. Clone 8 cells expressed the PR3 on their plasma membrane (upper right), while clone 9 cells did not express any PR3 or CD177 on their membranes (lower right).

2.4 PR3 and AASV

An A/G single nucleotide polymorphism (SNP) at coordinate -564 in the PR3 promoter has been identified, and it has been suggested that it was associated with WG. However, Pieters et al. showed that the -564 A/G polymorphism did not increase activity of the PR3 promoter, arguing against the possibility that the polymorphism results in an increased transcription/production of PR3 in WG patients (Pieters, 2004). In experiments performed by our group, the G allele of the -564 A/G polymorphism in the promoter of PR3 was not associated with WG (60% WG versus 69% HBD) or the mPR3^{high} phenotype in AASV patients (Abdgawad, 2006). We did find a significant correlation between high plasma PR3 and the A allele of the -564 A/G polymorphism in HBD and in AASV patients, indicating that the -564 A/G polymorphism might influence plasma PR3 levels.The fact that heterozygocity for deficiency alleles of α1-AT are associated with WG suggests that defects in the enzymatic function of PR3 may have functional effects. It has also been reported that presence of the PiZ allele correlates with poor prognosis (Segelmark, 1995).

Patients with systemic small vessel vasculitis exhibit higher plasma levels of PR3 than healthy persons and disease controls. This holds true also during stable remission and shows no relation to general inflammation, medical treatment or decreased renal function (Henshaw, 1994; Ohlsson, 2003). Studies by our group have shown that the levels of plasma PR3, mPR3 and pro-PR3 are all elevated in patients with AASV (Abdgawad, 2010). Also, it was observed that mPR3+ neutrophils are more abundant in AASV compared to healthy donors, which agrees with previous studies suggesting that a high percentage of mPR3+ cells may be a risk factor for vasculitis. Circulating neutrophils and monocytes from patients with AASV display upregulated transcription of the PR3 gene. It is likely that aberrant PR3/mPR3 expression may reflect, or be a marker of a specific functional defect in neutrophils. A possible origin of high plasma levels is shedding of membrane PR3. Witko-Sarsat et al. reported that the $mPR3^{high}$ phenotype was more frequent in vasculitis patients than in controls, independent of the ANCA antigen specificity (Witko-Sarsat, 1999). We have reported a weak but significant correlation between plasma PR3 and mPR3-MFI in MPO-ANCA-positive patients, which suggests that shedding of PR3 from the membrane may be at least partly responsible for increasing the plasma level of PR3. However, this correlation was not seen in PR3-ANCA patients. It is possible that PR3-ANCA either enhances clearance of plasma PR3 from the circulation, or interferes with detection of PR3 by ELISA. In support of this hypothesis, a significant negative correlation between plasma ANCA levels and plasma PR3 levels in the subgroup of PR3-ANCA patients was observed, while this was not seen in the MPO-ANCA patients.

Rarok et al. found that the length of time between diagnosis and relapse was significantly shorter in WG patients with high mPR3 expression (total level of mPR3 expression), and that individuals with high total mPR3 expression were more likely to have a relapse than patients with low mPR3 (Rarok, 2002). Csernok et al. showed that PR3 induces maturation of a fraction of blood monocyte derived dendritic cells (DC) in vitro (Csernok, 2006). In this context, they also observed that PR3 activates PAR-2 receptor-dependent signaling, which in turn up-regulates HLA-DR, CD80, CD83 and CD86 and down-regulates CD14. These PR3-activated DCs stimulate autoreactive Th1-type PR3-specific CD4+T cells.

Our group has demonstrated that the mPR3+/CD177+ neutrophil subpopulation was larger in AASV patients as compared to healthy controls, which suggests a distinct pathophysiological basis (Abdgawad, 2010). mPR3 and CD177 exhibit a parallel dynamic membrane expression with rapid internalization and re-expression. Interestingly, higher CD177-mRNA, but not PR3-mRNA was found to correlate with a higher proportion of mPR3+/CD177+ cells, suggesting that overproduction of CD177 could lead to an increase in the proportion of mPR3+/CD177+ neutrophils. Consistent with this, CD177 mRNA was significantly higher in mPR3- positive than in mPR3-negative human neutrophils, while PR3 mRNA was not.

3. Neutrophils and neutrophil apoptosis

Neutrophils represent 60 to 70% of the total circulating leukocytes and are the major phagocytes of the body's defense system against infections. Mature neutrophils are nonproliferating, non-dividing cells with a segmented nucleus, mixed granular populations (staining pink or purple-blue following treatment with a neutral dye), small Golgi regions and accumulation of glycogen particles. On an average, a neutrophil contains 200 to 300 granules, one third of which are peroxidase positive (azurophilic), while the rest are peroxidase-negative (specific and tertiary). Azurophilic granules are spherical, appear at the pro-myelocytic stage and contain MPO, serine proteases and antibiotic proteins, and form the microbicidal compartment of neutrophils.

C/EBPα and PU.1 are both key regulators of granulopoiesis and myelopoiesis. Neutrophil development requires co-expression of C/EBPα and low amounts of PU.1 (Ward, 2000; Lenny, 1997). While GM-CSF is important for the growth of neutrophil progenitors in early stages, G-CSF is necessary for their terminal differentiation into mature neutrophilic granulocytes. G-CSF increases the rate of production of neutrophils by reducing their maturation time in bone marrow, while the half-life of circulating neutrophils is mainly unaffected. In contrast, GM-CSF markedly increases the half-life of the neutrophils in circulation, while the production rate is only slightly increased (Lord, 1992). Skold et al. have shown that a secreted proform of Proteinase 3 (PR3) acts as a negative feedback regulator of granulopoiesis, and counters the effect of G-CSF (Skold, 1999). It is interesting that this feedback regulation by PR3 is reversible and abrogated by GCSF and GM-CSF.

Neutrophils contribute to immune surveillance and participate in elimination of micro-organisms and cell debris. This major function of neutrophils can be divided into 5 step functions; (1) adhesion. (2) trans-endothelial migration/diapedesis, (3) Interstitial migration/locomotion, (4) phagocytosis of bacteria and/or degranulation, and (5) apoptosis. Neutrophils are activated via two steps, priming and full activation. Multiple agents including bacterial products, cytokines such as TNF-α, GM-CSF, IL-8 and IFN-γ can prime neutrophils. Neutrophils are then mobilized to the site of infection/ inflammation by the help of chemoattractants where they encounter a second stimulus by which they become fully activated and kill bacteria or ingest cell debris. Migration of neutrophils from the circulation to the site of infection/inflammation is controlled by interactions with the vascular endothelium. L-selectins expressed on neutrophils allow rolling and loose adhesion of neutrophils to ligands expressed on the endothelial cell membrane (like E- and P-selectins). This loose adhesion leads to conformational changes in the leukocyte integrins of the β2 subfamily (CD11a, CD11b, CD11c/CD18), leading to engagement of other adhesion molecules on the membrane of endothelial cells such as intercellular adhesion molecule-1 (ICAM-1), ICAM-2, vascular cell-adhesion molecule-1 (VCAM-1) and mucosal vascular cell adhesion molecule-1 (MDAM-1), leading to high affinity ligand binding and firm adherence (Ley, 2007). Then, binding of chemoattractants such as IL-8, released from the endothelial cells, to neutrophil receptors lead to arrest of the neutrophil rolling. At the site of infection, membrane receptors recognize and bind opsonized bacteria leading to the formation of pseudopodia, phagocytosis of the pathogen in a phagosome that fuses with protease-rich granules leading to the destruction of the pathogen within the intracellular phagosome. Neutrophil phagocytosis of bacteria and cell debris involves the Fcγ-Receptors (FcγRIIa/ CD32 and FcγRIIIb/ CD16) and the complement receptors (CR1/ CD35 and CR3 or CD11b/CD18 integrin) (Witko-Sarsat, 2000).

Neutrophils express an array of proteases, contained in their granules, and can generate reactive oxygen species (ROS) in order to rapidly kill phagocytosed bacteria (Spitznagel, 1990). Once activated, they attack the invading pathogens by a combination of three mechanisms: phagocytosis, degranulation, and extracellular traps. During phagocytosis, the neutrophils ingest the pathogen forming a phagosome; while at the same time secrete ROS (reactive oxygen species) and hydrolytic enzymes to destroy it. Degranulation refers to the process by which various cytotoxic molecules residing in cytoplasmic granules are released. Examples include myeloperoxidase (MPO), an enzyme that is responsible for converting hydrogen peroxide to hypochlorous acid, a highly effective bactericide. Most recently, a novel extracellular mechanism (NETosis) of destroying pathogens has been described by Brinkmann et al (Brinkmann, 2004). Activation of neutrophils causes the release of chromatin fibers and granule proteins termed as neutrophil extracellular traps (NETs) that can trap and kill microbes extracellularly. NET formation is a part of active cell death; NETs are released when the activated neutrophils dies.

Neutrophils can also present antigens via MHC-II, thereby stimulating T cell activation and proliferation (Sandilands, 2005). Primed neutrophils actively synthesize and secrete cytokines, chemokines, leukotrienes and prostaglandins. In particular, neutrophils synthesize and secrete IL-8, IL-1, IL-1RA, IL-6, IL-12, TGF-β, and TNF-α (Cassatella, 1999; Fujishima, 1993). These cytokines can subsequently stimulate both neutrophils and other cells of the immune system. Neutrophils are significant source of leukotrienes and prostaglandins, especially leukotriene B4 (LTB4) and prostaglandin E2 (PGE2). PGE2 is an anti-inflammatory molecule, and has been reported to delay neutrophil apoptosis (Ottonello, 1998).

3.1 Neutrophils and AASV

The presence of activated neutrophils has been demonstrated at sites of injury in vasculitis lesions, both in lung infiltrates and renal biopsies (Brouwer, 1994; Travis, 1991). The number of activated neutrophils in renal biopsies correlated with extent of tissue damage. In a mouse model of MPO-ANCA associated vasculitis, neutrophil depletion reduced the number of vasculitic lesions(Xiao, 2005). In another Brown-Norway rat model of systemic necrotizing leukocytoclastic vasculitis induced by mercuric chloride and characterized by development of MPO-ANCA, a monoclonal antibody that depletes neutrophils could ameliorate vasculitis lesions (Qasim, 1996). These observations stand testimony to the key role of neutrophils in the pathogenesis of AASV.

The classical pathophysiological model of neutrophil activation can be divided into the following steps: an initial event (antigenic stimulus) primes neutrophils via cytokines (TNFα/IL-18/LPS) which subsequently induces membrane expression of PR3 and MPO. Priming induces the clustering of FcγRIIa and β2-integrins, formation of NADPH oxidase complex, increased expression of CD11b/CD18 and loose adherence of neutrophils to the endothelial cells. This is followed by binding of circulating ANCA to MPO and PR3 expressed on the neutrophil membrane. In the activation process, F(ab)´2 fragments of ANCA bind to their autoantigens, while Fc fragments bind to neutrophil Fcγ-receptors (FcγRIIa and FcγRIIIb) resulting in full activation of neutrophils (Falk, 1990).

There is substantial evidence for the activated state of neutrophils in AASV. In patients with active WG, neutrophils show increased expression of β1-(CD29), β2-(CD18) and α-(CD11b) integrin subunits (Haller, 1996). AASV neutrophils have been shown to have increased mPR3 expression and higher basal production of superoxide radicals. Alcorta et al have studied the leukocyte gene expression in ANCA positive vasculitis and showed >200 up-regulated genes, which correlated with disease activity (Alcorta, 2007). In normal situations, the short-lived neutrophils die by apoptosis and are subsequently phagocytosed by macrophages. Circulating apoptotic neutrophils are cleared from circulation by macrophages located in the liver (29%), spleen (31%) and the bone marrow (32%) (Saverymuttu, 1985). Tissue neutrophils, which migrate to tissues during infections, are removed by local macrophages that secrete anti-inflammatory cytokines TGF-β and IL-10 upon phagocytosis of these neutrophils. For normal homeostasis to take place and in order to keep normal counts of neutrophils in the circulation (2.5-7.5 ×109/l), neutrophil turn-over must be tightly balanced between granulopoiesis and neutrophil apoptosis/clearance. Delayed neutrophil apoptosis has been associated with several acute and chronic inflammatory diseases (Simon, 2003).

3.2 Neutrophil apoptosis

Apoptosis, or "programmed" cell death, is a physiological form of cell death characterized by cell shrinkage, nuclear and chromatin condensation, DNA fragmentation, membrane blebbing, externalization of phosphatidylserine (PS), and formation of membrane-bound apoptotic bodies (Edwards, 2003). Many players are known to regulate apoptosis, including caspases, cell death receptors (of the TNF family), adaptor proteins, inhibitor of apoptosis (IAP) proteins and the bcl-2 family.

Neutrophil apoptosis occurs via the intrinsic or the extrinsic pathways. The intrinsic pathway is regulated by various proteins and molecules, including Mcl-1 and Bcl-2-A1 (Bfl 1) gene product and SHIP-1 (Edwards, 2003). Mitochondria play an important role in the intrinsic pathway of apoptosis through three key mitochondrial proteins; cytochrome c (cyt c), Smac/DIABLO and apoptosis inducing factor (AIF). The release of cyt c from the mitochondria is recognized as an initiator of apoptosis via interaction with Apaf-1 (apoptotic protease activating factor-1), leading to activation of caspase 9, formation of the apoptosome, and triggering of the caspase cascade. The Bcl-2 family regulates mitochondrial membrane permeability and cyt c release, thus playing a central role in apoptosis (Fossati, 2003). Neutrophils possess very few mitochondria and express low amounts of cyt c and Smac/ DIABLO, which are nonetheless sufficient to induce apoptosis. The tendency of neutrophils towards spontaneous apoptosis is inversely correlated with Bcl-2 expression.

The extrinsic pathway is initiated by an extracellular death signal. Death receptors bind to extrinsic factors (FasL, TNF-α, TRAIL) and activate the caspase cascade, which in turn generates intracellular death signals culminating in apoptosis. Death receptors such as Fas and the TNF receptor are integral membrane proteins. Fas and Fas ligand (FasL) interaction initiates apoptosis in a caspase-dependent manner. Neutrophils undergo spontaneous apoptosis more than other leukocytes, probably because they express both Fas and FasL on their plasma membrane (Edwards, 2003; Liles, 1996). Apoptosis-inducing factor (AIF) is a flavoprotein that is normally located in the inter-membrane space of mitochondria. When cells receive a signal for apoptosis, AIF is released from the mitochondria and translocates into the nucleus and causes nuclear fragmentation and cell death. The DNA destruction mediated by AIF is not blocked by caspase inhibitors and is thus considered a caspase-independent pathway. In neutrophils, AIF does not leave the mitochondria and the caspase-independent pathway is mediated by mitochondria-derived reactive oxygen species (ROS) (Edwards, 2003).

The mechanisms regulating spontaneous neutrophil apoptosis are not fully understood. Disturbance in the normal apoptotic process can enhance survival time, leading to a persistent inflammatory response. Blood neutrophils express fairly high levels of a range of pro-apoptotic proteins like Bad, Bax and Bik, but do not express the anti-apoptotic Bcl-2 and Bcl-xL proteins. Several pro-inflammatory agents, including IL-1β, L-2, IL-4, IL-6, IL-15, IFN- γ, G-CSF, GM-CSF and LPS, can delay neutrophil apoptosis (Simon, 2003). G-CSF induces survival of PMNs via the MEK-ERK pathway, leading to phosphorylation of Bad (inactivation) (Chuang, 1998). GM-CSF induces survival via the tyrosine kinase LynK-PI3K and JAK-2. G-CSF up-regulates the expression of Bcl-2-A1 and down-regulates the expression of Bax. GM-CSF up-regulates the expression of Mcl-1 and down-regulates the expression of Bax (Moulding, 2001). G-CSF, but not GM-CSF, selectively up-regulates the expression of cIAP-2, at the protein as well as mRNA levels. IAPs regulate apoptosis by binding to TNF-receptor associated factor-1 (TRAF-1)/ TRAF-2 heterocomplex to suppress activation of caspase 8. IAPs suppressing activation of caspase 9 and are capable of inhibiting the activation of caspases 3 and 7 directly (Edwards, 2003). TNF-α has a dual action on neutrophil apoptosis, leading to accelerated apoptosis in a susceptible subpopulation and delayed apoptosis in the surviving cells. TNF-α differential effects are dependant on concentration and the time of exposure. Adhesion of neutrophils to activated endothelial cells, IL-8, as well as transmigration of neutrophils through endothelial cell layer inhibits apoptosis.

During an inflammatory response, neutrophils produce numerous cytokines and chemokines, via up-regulation of gene expression. Once phagocytosis is accomplished, these functions are down-regulated in tandem with induction of apoptosis, leading to a decrease in pro-inflammatory capacity. This process is tightly regulated to prevent tissue damage caused by lingering neutrophils. Walcheck et al. have shown that phagocytosis-induced neutrophil apoptosis is accompanied by increase in the surface expression of ADAM17, followed by ADAM17-mediated release of IL-6R from cells, which then recruits mononuclear phagocytes to the site of infection (Walcheck, 2006). Recruitment of macrophages to sites of inflammation is also promoted by resolvins and protectins including lipoxin A4 (LXA4).The removal of apoptotic neutrophils is a non-phlogistic process, largely due to release of anti-inflammatory mediators.

3.3 Neutrophil apoptosis and AASV

Pathological specimens from patients of WG show clear presence of apoptotic and necrotic neutrophils (Travis, 1991). Leucocytes, with degraded nuclear material, undergoing disintegration and apoptotic cells have been observed in tissue specimens from ANCA-positive renal vasculitis (Rastaldi, 2000). Histologically, AASV is characterized by leukocytoclasis, with infiltration and accumulation of unscavenged apoptotic and necrotic neutrophils in tissues around blood vessels. E/M studies of the leukocytoclastic lesions, have suggested that there may be a defect in the clearance of apoptotic neutrophils. The minority of neutrophils in this study showed typical apoptotic changes of the condensed and marginated nuclei, while the majority showed intact nuclei with disintegrated cytoplasmic organelles and plasma membranes (Yamamoto, 2000). We have demonstrated significantly higher rate of survival and lower rate of apoptosis in AASV neutrophils as compared to neutrophils from healthy blood donors (HBDs) (Un-published data). It can be presumed that reduced apoptosis in AASV might be secondary to chronic inflammation.

However, the rate of apoptosis did not correlate with clinical parameters such as disease activity, CRP concentration, BVAS score or reduced GFR.

Interestingly, when neutrophils from AASV patients and HBDs were incubated with plasma from AASV patients, neutrophil survival was enhanced, suggesting that specific factors in the plasma influenced the apoptosis mechanism or rate. Growth factors are known to prolong survival by up-regulating anti-apoptotic factors and down-regulating pro-apoptotic factors. G-CSF, GM-CSF and LPS up-regulate expression of anti-apoptotic Bcl-2A1 and promote neutrophil survival, while Mcl-1 is up-regulated by GM-CSF, IL-1β and LPS. G-CSF up-regulates c-IAP2 (Inhibitor of Apoptosis Protein, IAP) (Santos-Beneit, 2000). IAP-2 is strongly up-regulated in mature neutrophils from patients with chronic neutrophilic leukemia, which also show prolonged in vitro survival. Christensson et al. showed that AASV patients in remission had higher circulating levels of soluble Fas than HBD and other disease controls (Christensson, 2002). No data from functional tests was available, and the effect of soluble Fas on Fas-mediated neutrophil apoptosis is not known. G-CSF, GM-CSF and IL-3 are known to enhance neutrophil survival, and delay or prevent neutrophil apoptosis. In our study, G-CSF and IL-3 levels were normal in plasma from AASV; GM-CSF level was higher than normal in four of 44 AASV patients. It is still possible that GM-CSF and IL-3 could be related to delayed apoptosis; neutrophils may have increased sensitivity to these cytokines. We tested this hypothesis and observed increased sensitivity in only three patients, who were more sensitive to GM-CSF/IL-3 than HBD. The proapoptotic factor Bax is down-regulated in response to G-CSF, GM-CSF, IL-3 and IFN-γ. Our group did not observe any correlation between the reduced rate of apoptosis or necrosis in AASV patients with higher levels of mRNA encoding these factors. A statistically insignificant increase in expression of Bcl-2A1 (1.45), Mcl-1 (1.78) and Bax (1.56) was noted in AASV neutrophils, compared to HBD neutrophils. Another possible mechanism of reduced apoptosis is alteration in neutrophil growth factor signaling. Our group has shown that the level of mRNA encoding three transcription factors, involved in steady-state and emergency granulopoiesis (C/EBP-α, C/EBP-β and PU.1), is significantly higher in AASV than in HBD (Un-published data). The target genes of these transcription factors include important neutrophil proteins including G-CSF receptor, GM-CSF receptor, myeloperoxidase, PR3, elastase, lysozyme and lactoferrin. It is possible that elevated expression of C/EBP-α, C/EBP-β and PU.1 in AASV neutrophils could lead to enhanced sensitivity to cytokines; a defect/deficiency of inhibitory factors may lead to perpetuation and exaggeration of survival signals and increased transcription factors.

Gilligan et al. showed that aging neutrophils (unprimed) were capable of translocating PR3 and MPO to the membrane during apoptosis, as assessed by increased ANCA binding (Gilligan, 1996). Another study showed that a small sub-fraction of TNFα-accelerated apoptotic neutrophils expressed higher levels of PR3 and MPO than TNFα-primed live neutrophils (Kettritz, 2002). Also, Kantari et al have shown that scramblase-1 translocates PR3 to the plasma membrane in a flip-flop manner during apoptosis (Kantari, 2007). In contrast, Yang et al demonstrated that the level of mPR3 is similar between apoptotic and non-apoptotic primed neutrophils (Yang, 2000). Our group has shown that though there is an increased fraction of neutrophils double-positive for membrane PR3 and CD177 in AASV (69% for AASV, 58% for HBD; $p=0.004$) expression, the percentage of double positive neutrophils does not correlate with the rate of neutrophil apoptosis, suggesting that membrane PR3 is not a pre-apoptotic marker (un-published data). Thus, although evidence for increased membrane expression of auto-antigen in apoptotic neutrophils is inconclusive, it can be concluded that MPO and PR3 remain accessible for ANCA on the membrane of apoptotic neutrophils. Interestingly, Patry et al showed that injection of syngenic apoptotic neutrophils, but not freshly isolated neutrophils, into Brown Norway rats resulted in development of p-ANCA, with the majority being specific for elastase, again indicating that apoptotic neutrophils may boost an autoimmune response (Patry, 2001). Intraperitoneal infusion of live or apoptotic human neutrophils (but not formaline fixed or lysed neutrophils) into C57BL/6J mice resulted in development of ANCA specific for lactoferrin or myeloperoxidase. A second intravenous infusion of apoptotic neutrophils resulted in the development of PR3-specific ANCA. Again no vasculitic lesions were found in those mice developing ANCA.

ANCA themselves may dysregulate the process of neutrophil apoptosis. In an in vitro study conducted by Harper et al., ANCAs accelerated apoptosis of TNF-α-primed neutrophils by a mechanism dependent on NADPH oxidase and the generation of ROS (Harper, 2000). This was accompanied by uncoupling of the nuclear and cytoplasmic changes from the surface membrane changes. That is, while apoptosis progressed more rapidly, there was no corresponding change in the rate of externalization of PS (phosphatidyl serine) following activation of neutrophils by ANCAs. This dysregulation created a 'reduced window of opportunity' for phagocyte clearance by macrophages, leading to a more pro-inflammatory environment. It must be noted here that ANCAs were unable to accelerate apoptosis in unprimed neutrophils. Additionally, although there was increased expression of PR3 and MPO as apoptosis progressed, ANCAs were unable to activate these neutrophils. In fact, there was a time dependent decrease in ROS generation as these neutrophils aged. ANCA accelerates neutrophil apoptosis via generation of ROS, which act as amplifying factors for apoptosis. ROS are critical since neutrophils isolated from patients with chronic granulomatous disease (causing a defect in ROS production) do not show accelerated apoptosis after ANCA activation. The same authors, in a later study, as well as another independent group have shown that ANCA binding to apoptotic neutrophils enhanced phagocytosis by human monocyte-derived macrophages but also increased the secretion of pro-inflammatory cytokines like IL-1, IL-8 and TNF-α (Harper, 2000; Harper, 2001). IL-1 and IL-8 are capable of retarding apoptosis and are powerful chemoattractants. A pro-inflammatory neutrophil clearance will result in further cell recruitment and perpetuation of inflammation.

Apoptosis plays a crucial role in resolution of inflammation and maintaining self-tolerance. Defects in apoptotic pathways could potentially lead to the persistence of autoreactive T- or B-cells and contribute to development of autoimmune disease. Apoptotic neutrophils are a potential source of immunologically exposed neutrophil antigens that promote the production of ANCAs. From the available evidence, it may be inferred that there exists an altered neutrophil phenotype in AASV, which may be directly related to disease pathogenesis.

Enough evidence has accumulated for us to reasonably conclude that the neutrophils constitute two, molecularly well demarcated, sub-populations; one is positive for mPR3 and CD177 and the other subpopulation is negative for PR3 and CD177. The proportion of mPR3+/CD177+ cells is remarkably stable in a given individual, while a wide inter-individual variation can be observed. It is likely that these two subpopulations have distinct functions, which may have a direct bearing on pathophysiological processes. Membrane CD177 helps neutrophils adhere to the endothelium, while m-PR3 helps this positive subpopulation to migrate through the endothelium and interstitial tissues. It may be inferred that the mPR3+/CD177+ cells possess greater killing capabilities, including higher NET and ROS production, than the mPR3-/CD177- sub-population. In simplistic terms, the mPR3+/CD177+ neutrophils may be the designated "fighting" neutrophils, designed to migrate from blood into tissues and promote pro-inflammatory, microbicidal functions, while mPR3-negative neutrophils are destined to stay in the intra-vascular compartment, until they are filtered by bone marrow, liver or pancreas and undergo apoptosis. Functional defects that lead to change in the proportion of mPR3+/CD177+ cells would, by default, promote a pro-inflammatory state. The elevated/ up-regulated transcription factors in patients of AASV, may potentially explain the increased PR3-mRNA expression and the decreased neutrophil apoptosis; decreased apoptosis rate as well as the elevated transcription factors provide indirect evidence for an altered neutrophil phenotype in AASV. Alteration in apoptosis and membrane expression of PR3/CD177 are clearly linked to the pathophysiology of this disease. Future studies must be aimed at elucidating the mechanisms underlying the altered neutrophil phenotype. Possible directions include: measurement of Fas in the plasma as well as membrane expression of Fas and Fas Ligand on neutrophils, evaluation of G-CSF receptor, GM-CSF receptor and IL-3 receptor over-expression by neutrophils, measurement of JAK-2 inhibition by measurement of SHIP-1, SOCS-1 and SOCS-3 in neutrophils. It may also be worthwhile to search for, hitherto unknown, exogenous survival factors in the plasma or endogenous survival factors inside the neutrophils. The significance of an altered neutrophil phenotype in AASV is certainly intriguing and, will hopefully stimulate detailed and quality research into its mechanisms and pathophysiological role.

4. References

Abdgawad M, Gunnarson L, Bengtsson AA, et al. Elevated neutrophil membrane expression of proteinase 3 is dependent upon CD177 expression. Clin Exp Immunol 2010;161: 89–97

Abdgawad M, Hellmark T, Gunnarson L, Westman KWA, Segelmark M. Increased neutrophil membrane expression and plasma level of proteinase 3 in systemic vasculitis are not a consequence of the – 564 A/G promotor polymorphism. Clin Exp Immunol 2006;145: 63-70

Alcorta DA, Barnes DA, Dooley MA, et al. Leukocyte gene expression signatures in antineutrophil cytoplasmic autoantibody and lupus glomerulonephritis. Kidney Int 2007;72(7):853-64.

Baggiolini M, Bretz U, Dewald B, Feigenson ME. The polymorphonuclear leukocyte. Agents Actions 1978;8(1-2):3-10.

Ballieux BE, Zondervan KT, Kievit P, et al. Binding of proteinase 3 and myeloperoxidase to endothelial cells: ANCA-mediated endothelial damage through ADCC? Clin Exp Immunol 1994;97(1):52-60.

Bauer S, Abdgawad M, Gunnarson L, Segelmark M, Tapper H, Hellmark T. Proteinase 3 and CD177 are expressed on the plasma membrane of the same subset of neutrophils. J Leuk Biol 2007;81: 458-464

Beaudreuil S, Lasfargues G, Laueriere L, et al. Occupational exposure in ANCA positive patients: a case-control study. Kidney Int 2005;67(5):1961-6.

Booth AD, Almond MK, Burns A, et al. Outcome of ANCA-associated renal vasculitis: a 5-year retrospective study. Am J Kidney Dis 2003;41(4):776-84

Brinkmann V, Reichard U, Goosmann C, et al. Neutrophil extracellular traps kill bacteria. Science 2004;303(5663):1532-5.

Brouwer E, Huitema MG, Mulder AH, et al. Neutrophil activation in vitro and in vivo in Wegener's granulomatosis. Kidney Int 1994;45(4):1120-31.

Bux J GK, Wolff J, Kissel Karen, Doppl W, Schmidt KL, Fenchel K, Pralle H, Sibelius U. Expression of NB1 glycoprotein (HNA-2a, CD177) on neutrophils is upregulated in inflammatory diseases and during G-CSF expression. Blood 2002;100:462a.

Campbell EJ, Campbell MA, Owen CA. Bioactive proteinase 3 on the cell surface of human neutrophils: quantification, catalytic activity, and susceptibility to inhibition. J Immunol 2000;165(6):3366-74.

Campbell EJ, Campbell MA, Owen CA. Bioactive proteinase 3 on the cell surface of human neutrophils: quantification, catalytic activity, and susceptibility to inhibition. J Immunol 2000;165(6):3366-74.

Caruccio L, Bettinotti M, Director-Myska AE, Arthur DC, Stroncek D. The gene overexpressed in polycythemia rubra vera, PRV-1, and the gene encoding a neutrophil alloantigen, NB1, are alleles of a single gene, CD177, in chromosome band 19q13.31. Transfusion 2006;46(3):441-7.

Cassatella MA. Neutrophil-derived proteins: selling cytokines by the pound. Adv Immunol 1999;73:369-509.

Choi HK, Lamprecht P, Niles JL, Gross WL, Merkel PA. Subacute bacterial endocarditis with positive cytoplasmic antineutrophil cytoplasmic antibodies and antiproteinase 3 antibodies. Arthritis Rheum 2000;43(1):226-31

Christensson M, Pettersson E, Eneslatt K, et al. Serum sFAS levels are elevated in ANCA-positive vasculitis compared with other autoimmune diseases. J Clin Immunol 2002;22(4):220-7.

Chuang PI, Yee E, Karsan A, Winn RK, Harlan JM. A1 is a constitutive and inducible Bcl-2 homologue in mature human neutrophils. Biochem Biophys Res Commun 1998;249(2):361-5

Csernok E, Ai M, Gross WL, et al. Wegener autoantigen induces maturation of dendritic cells and licenses them for Th1 priming via the protease-activated receptor-2 pathway. Blood 2006;107(11):4440-8.

Csernok E, Ernst M, Schmitt W, Bainton DF, Gross WL. Activated neutrophils express proteinase 3 on their plasma membrane in vitro and in vivo. Clin Exp Immunol 1994;95(2):244-50.

Csernok E, Szymkowiak CH, Mistry N, Daha MR, Gross WL, Kekow J. Transforming growth factor-beta (TGF-beta) expression and interaction with proteinase 3 (PR3) in anti-neutrophil cytoplasmic antibody (ANCA)-associated vasculitis. Clin Exp Immunol 1996;105(1):104-11.

Edwards SW, Moulding DA, Derouet M, Moots RJ. Regulation of neutrophil apoptosis. Chem Immunol Allergy 2003;83:204-24.

Elzouki AN, Segelmark M, Wieslander J, Eriksson S. Strong link between the alpha 1-antitrypsin PiZ allele and Wegener's granulomatosis. J Intern Med 1994;236(5):543-8.

Falk RJ, Terrell RS, Charles LA, Jennette JC. Anti-neutrophil cytoplasmic autoantibodies induce neutrophils to degranulate and produce oxygen radicals in vitro. Proc Natl Acad Sci U S A 1990;87(11):4115-9.

Firestein GS BR, Harris Jr ED, McInnes IB, Ruddy S, Sergent JS. Vasculitis. The classification and epidemiology of systemic vasculitis. Kelley´s Tetbook of Rheumatology 8th edition 2008;Philadelphia, WB Saunders:Part 13, chapter 80.

Fossati G, Moulding DA, Spiller DG, Moots RJ, White MR, Edwards SW. The mitochondrial network of human neutrophils: role in chemotaxis, phagocytosis, respiratory burst activation, and commitment to apoptosis. J Immunol 2003;170(4): 1964-72.

Fridlich R, David A, Aviram I. Membrane proteinase 3 and its interactions within microdomains of neutrophil membranes. J Cell Biochem 2006;99(1):117-25.

Fujishima S, Hoffman AR, Vu T, et al. Regulation of neutrophil interleukin 8 gene expression and protein secretion by LPS, TNF-alpha, and IL-1 beta. J Cell Physiol 1993;154(3):478-85.

Gencik M, Meller S, Borgmann S, Fricke H. Proteinase 3 gene polymorphisms and Wegener's granulomatosis. Kidney Int 2000;58(6):2473-7.

Gilligan HM, Bredy B, Brady HR, et al. Antineutrophil cytoplasmic autoantibodies interact with primary granule constituents on the surface of apoptotic neutrophils in the absence of neutrophil priming. J Exp Med 1996;184(6):2231-41.

Gohring K, Wolff J, Doppl W, et al. Neutrophil CD177 (NB1 gp, HNA-2a) expression is increased in severe bacterial infections and polycythaemia vera. Br J Haematol 2004;126(2):252-4.

Goldschmeding R, van Dalen CM, Faber N, et al. Further characterization of the NB 1 antigen as a variably expressed 56-62 kD GPI-linked glycoprotein of plasma membranes and specific granules of neutrophils. Br J Haematol 1992;81(3):336-45.

Halbwachs-Mecarelli L, Bessou G, Lesavre P, Lopez S, Witko-Sarsat V. Bimodal distribution of proteinase 3 (PR3) surface expression reflects a constitutive heterogeneity in the polymorphonuclear neutrophil pool. FEBS Lett 1995;374(1): 29-33.

Haller H, Eichhorn J, Pieper K, Gobel U, Luft FC. Circulating leukocyte integrin expression in Wegener's granulomatosis. J Am Soc Nephrol 1996;7(1):40-8.

Harper L, Cockwell P, Adu D, Savage CO. Neutrophil priming and apoptosis in antineutrophil cytoplasmic autoantibody-associated vasculitis. Kidney Int 2001;59(5): 1729-38.

Harper L, Ren Y, Savill J, Adu D, Savage CO. Antineutrophil cytoplasmic antibodies induce reactive oxygen-dependent dysregulation of primed neutrophil apoptosis and clearance by macrophages. Am J Pathol 2000;157(1):211-20.

Hay EM, Beaman M, Ralston AJ, Ackrill P, Bernstein RM, Holt PJ. Wegener's granulomatosis occurring in siblings. Br J Rheumatol 1991;30(2):144-5.

Hellmich B, Csernok E, Trabandt A, Gross WL, Ernst M. Granulocyte-macrophage colony-stimulating factor (GM-CSF) but not granulocyte colony-stimulating factor (G-CSF) induces plasma membrane expression of proteinase 3 (PR3) on neutrophils in vitro. Clin Exp Immunol 2000;120(2):392-8.

Henshaw TJ, Malone CC, Gabay JE, Williams RC, Jr. Elevations of neutrophil proteinase 3 in serum of patients with Wegener's granulomatosis and polyarteritis nodosa. Arthritis Rheum 1994;37(1):104-12.

Kantari C, Pederzoli-Ribeil M, Amir-Moazami O, et al. Proteinase 3, the Wegener autoantigen, is externalized during neutrophil apoptosis: evidence for a functional association with phospholipid scramblase 1 and interference with macrophage phagocytosis. Blood 2007;110(12):4086-95

Kantari C, Pederzoli-Ribeil M, Amir-Moazami O, et al. Proteinase 3, the Wegener autoantigen, is externalized during neutrophil apoptosis: evidence for a functional association with phospholipid scramblase 1 and interference with macrophage phagocytosis. Blood 2007;110(12):4086-95.

Kettritz R, Scheumann J, Xu Y, Luft FC, Haller H. TNF-alpha--accelerated apoptosis abrogates ANCA-mediated neutrophil respiratory burst by a caspase-dependent mechanism. Kidney Int 2002;61(2):502-15.

Knight A, Ekbom A, Brandt L, Askling J. Increasing incidence of Wegener's granulomatosis in Sweden, 1975-2001. J Rheumatol 2006;33(10):2060-3.

Lalezari P, Murphy GB, Allen FH, Jr. NB1, a new neutrophil-specific antigen involved in the pathogenesis of neonatal neutropenia. J Clin Invest 1971;50(5): 1108-15

Lenny N, Westendorf JJ, Hiebert SW. Transcriptional regulation during myelopoiesis. Mol Biol Rep 1997;24(3):157-68.

Ley K, Laudanna C, Cybulsky MI, Nourshargh S. Getting to the site of inflammation: the leukocyte adhesion cascade updated. Nat Rev Immunol 2007;7(9):678-89.

Liles WC, Kiener PA, Ledbetter JA, Aruffo A, Klebanoff SJ. Differential expression of Fas (CD95) and Fas ligand on normal human phagocytes: implications for the regulation of apoptosis in neutrophils. J Exp Med 1996;184(2):429-40.

Lord BI, Gurney H, Chang J, Thatcher N, Crowther D, Dexter TM. Haemopoietic cell kinetics in humans treated with rGM-CSF. Int J Cancer 1992;50(1):26-31.

Mohammad AJ, Jacobsson LT, Mahr AD, Sturfelt G, Segelmark M. Prevalence of Wegener's granulomatosis, microscopic polyangiitis, polyarteritis nodosa and Churg- Strauss syndrome within a defined population in southern Sweden. Rheumatology (Oxford) 2007; 46(8):1329-37.

Mohammad AJ, Jacobsson LT, Westman KW, Sturfelt G, Segelmark M. Incidence and survival rates in Wegener's granulomatosis, microscopic polyangiitis, Churg-Strauss syndrome and polyarteritis nodosa. Rheumatology (Oxford) 2009;48(12):1560-5.

Moosig F, Csernok E, Kumanovics G, Gross WL. Opsonization of apoptotic neutrophils by anti-neutrophil cytoplasmic antibodies (ANCA) leads to enhanced uptake by macrophages and increased release of tumour necrosis factor-alpha (TNFalpha). Clin Exp Immunol 2000;122(3):499-503.

Moulding DA, Akgul C, Derouet M, White MR, Edwards SW. BCL-2 family expression in human neutrophils during delayed and accelerated apoptosis. J Leukoc Biol 2001;70(5):783-92.

Ohlsson K, Olsson I. The neutral proteases of human granulocytes. Isolation and partial characterization of two granulocyte collagenases. Eur J Biochem 1973;36(2):473-81.

Ohlsson S, Wieslander J, Segelmark M. Increased circulating levels of proteinase 3 in patients with anti-neutrophilic cytoplasmic autoantibodies-associated systemic vasculitis in remission. Clin Exp Immunol 2003;131(3):528-35.

Ottonello L, Gonella R, Dapino P, Sacchetti C, Dallegri F. Prostaglandin E2 inhibits apoptosis in human neutrophilic polymorphonuclear leukocytes: role of intracellular cyclic AMP levels. Exp Hematol 1998;26(9):895-902.
Patry YC, Trewick DC, Gregoire M, et al. Rats injected with syngenic rat apoptotic neutrophils develop antineutrophil cytoplasmic antibodies. J Am Soc Nephrol 2001;12(8):1764-8.
Pederzoli M, Kantari C, Gausson V, Moriceau S, Witko-Sarsat V. Proteinase-3 induces procaspase-3 activation in the absence of apoptosis: potential role of this compartmentalized activation of membrane associated procaspase-3 in neutrophils. J Immunol 2005;174(10):6381-90.
Pieters K, Pettersson A, Gullberg U, Hellmark T. The□564 A/G polymorphism in the promoter region of the proteinase 3 gene associated with Wegener's granulomatosis does not increase the promoter activity. Clin Exp Immunol 2004; 138:266–70.
Qasim FJ, Mathieson PW, Sendo F, Thiru S, Oliveira DB. Role of neutrophils in the pathogenesis of experimental vasculitis. Am J Pathol 1996;149(1):81-9.
Rao NV, Wehner NG, Marshall BC, Gray WR, Gray BH, Hoidal JR. Characterization of proteinase-3 (PR-3), a neutrophil serine proteinase. Structural and functional properties. J Biol Chem 1991;266(15):9540-8.
Rarok AA, Stegeman CA, Limburg PC, Kallenberg CG. Neutrophil membrane expression of proteinase 3 (PR3) is related to relapse in PR3-ANCA-associated vasculitis. J Am Soc Nephrol 2002;13(9):2232-8.
Rastaldi MP, Ferrario F, Crippa A, et al. Glomerular monocyte-macrophage features in ANCA-positive renal vasculitis and cryoglobulinemic nephritis. J Am Soc Nephrol 2000;11(11):2036-43.
Sachs UJ, Andrei-Selmer CL, Maniar A, et al. The neutrophil-specific antigen CD177 is a counter-receptor for platelet endothelial cell adhesion molecule-1 (CD31). J Biol Chem 2007;282(32):23603-12.
Sandilands GP, Ahmed Z, Perry N, Davison M, Lupton A, Young B. Cross-linking of neutrophil CD11b results in rapid cell surface expression of molecules required for antigen presentation and T-cell activation. Immunology 2005;114(3):354-68.
Santos-Beneit AM, Mollinedo F. Expression of genes involved in initiation, regulation, and execution of apoptosis in human neutrophils and during neutrophil differentiation of HL-60 cells. J Leukoc Biol 2000;67(5):712-24.
Saverymuttu SH, Peters AM, Keshavarzian A, Reavy HJ, Lavender JP. The kinetics of 111indium distribution following injection of 111indium labelled autologous granulocytes in man. Br J Haematol 1985;61(4):675-85
Schreiber A, Busjahn A, Luft FC, Kettritz R. Membrane expression of proteinase 3 is genetically determined. J Am Soc Nephrol 2003;14(1):68-75
Segelmark M, Baslund B, Wieslander J. Some patients with anti-myeloperoxidase autoantibodies have a C-ANCA pattern. Clin Exp Immunol 1994;96(3):458-65
Segelmark M, Elzouki AN, Wieslander J, Eriksson S. The PiZ gene of alpha 1- antitrypsin as a determinant of outcome in PR3-ANCA-positive vasculitis. Kidney Int 1995;48(3):844-50.
Simon HU. Neutrophil apoptosis pathways and their modifications in inflammation. Immunol Rev 2003;193:101-10.

Skold S, Rosberg B, Gullberg U, Olofsson T. A secreted proform of neutrophil proteinase 3 regulates the proliferation of granulopoietic progenitor cells. Blood 1999;93(3):849-56.

Skold S, Rosberg B, Gullberg U, Olofsson T. A secreted proform of neutrophil proteinase 3 regulates the proliferation of granulopoietic progenitor cells. Blood 1999;93(3):849-56.

Spitznagel JK. Antibiotic proteins of human neutrophils. J Clin Invest 1990;86(5): 1381-6.

Stroncek DF, Caruccio L, Bettinotti M. CD177: A member of the Ly-6 gene superfamily involved with neutrophil proliferation and polycythemia vera. J Transl Med 2004;2(1):8.

Sturrock A, Franklin KF, Hoidal JR. Human proteinase-3 expression is regulated by PU.1 in conjunction with a cytidine-rich element. J Biol Chem 1996;271(50): 32392-402.

Sturrock AB, Espinosa R, 3rd, Hoidal JR, Le Beau MM. Localization of the gene encoding proteinase-3 (the Wegener's granulomatosis autoantigen) to human chromosome band 19p13.3. Cytogenet Cell Genet 1993;64(1):33-4.

Travis WD, Hoffman GS, Leavitt RY, Pass HI, Fauci AS. Surgical pathology of the lung in Wegener's granulomatosis. Review of 87 open lung biopsies from 67 patients. Am J Surg Pathol 1991;15(4):315-33.

Travis WD, Hoffman GS, Leavitt RY, Pass HI, Fauci AS. Surgical pathology of the lung in Wegener's granulomatosis. Review of 87 open lung biopsies from 67 patients. Am J Surg Pathol 1991;15(4):315-33.

Vong L, D'Acquisto F, Pederzoli-Ribeil M, et al. Annexin 1 cleavage in activated neutrophils: a pivotal role for proteinase 3. J Biol Chem 2007;282(41):29998-30004

Walcheck B, Herrera AH, St Hill C, Mattila PE, Whitney AR, Deleo FR. ADAM17 activity during human neutrophil activation and apoptosis. Eur J Immunol 2006;36(4): 968-76

Ward AC, Loeb DM, Soede-Bobok AA, Touw IP, Friedman AD. Regulation of granulopoiesis by transcription factors and cytokine signals. Leukemia 2000;14(6): 973-90.

Watts R SD. Vasculitis. Baillière's clinical rheumatology 1995;9(3):529-54.

Witko-Sarsat V, Cramer EM, Hieblot C, et al. Presence of proteinase 3 in secretory vesicles: evidence of a novel, highly mobilizable intracellular pool distinct from azurophil granules. Blood 1999;94(7):2487-96

Witko-Sarsat V, Lesavre P, Lopez S, et al. A large subset of neutrophils expressing membrane proteinase 3 is a risk factor for vasculitis and rheumatoid arthritis. J Am Soc Nephrol 1999;10(6):1224-33

Witko-Sarsat V, Rieu P, Descamps-Latscha B, Lesavre P, Halbwachs-Mecarelli L. Neutrophils: molecules, functions and pathophysiological aspects. Lab Invest 2000;80(5):617-53.

Wolff J, Brendel C, Fink L, Bohle RM, Kissel K, Bux J. Lack of NB1 GP (CD177/ HNA-2a) gene transcription in NB1 GP- neutrophils from NB1 GP-expressing individuals and association of low expression with NB1 gene polymorphisms. Blood 2003;102(2):731-3.

Xiao H, Heeringa P, Liu Z, et al. The role of neutrophils in the induction of glomerulonephritis by anti-myeloperoxidase antibodies. Am J Pathol 2005;167(1): 39-45

Yamamoto T, Kaburagi Y, Izaki S, Tanaka T, Kitamura K. Leukocytoclasis: ultrastructural in situ nick end labeling study in anaphylactoid purpura. J Dermatol Sci 2000;24(3):158-65.

Yang JJ, Tuttle RH, Hogan SL, et al. Target antigens for anti-neutrophil cytoplasmic autoantibodies (ANCA) are on the surface of primed and apoptotic but not unstimulated neutrophils. Clin Exp Immunol 2000;121(1):165-72

Part 2

Pathogenesis and Pathology of Vasculitis

7

Pathology of the Cutaneous Vasculitides: A Comprehensive Review

Adrienne C. Jordan, Stephen E. Mercer, and Robert G. Phelps
The Mount Sinai Medical Center, New York, NY United States of America

1. Introduction

Vasculitis has historically been poorly defined and the histological and clinical manifestations are protean, further complicating the diagnostic process. The definitive diagnosis is made by evidence of histologic effacement of a vessel with associated transumural inflammatory infiltrate of that vessel. Vasculitis can be a primary process or secondary to disseminated intravascular coagulation, ulceration, arthropod assault, and/or suppurative infiltrates (for example pyoderma gangrenosum). Vasculitis must further be distinguished from vasculopathies, particularly livedoid vasculopathy and connective tissue diseases (namely scleroderma and systemic lupus erythematosus) in which the primary process is vascular fibrin thrombi of the upper dermal vessels. A necrotizing vasculitis resulting secondary to the thrombotic process can occur, blurring the lines between true vasculitis and vasculopathy. Very few vasculitic processes have pathognomonic histological findings. Often times the dermatopathologist and clinician must work in concert and combine clinical, histological, and laboratory data to determine what the primary process is. As previously stated, histological evidence of inflammatory infiltrate within the vessel wall must be seen in order to diagnose vasculitis. Associated findings include fibrinoid necrosis, endothelial swelling, and endothelial cell apoptosis (Carlson, et al., 2005). Other secondary changes including extravasation of red blood cells, necrosis, ulceration, and neovascularization suggest that there has been vascular damage (Carlson et al., 2005). Associated changes can also be seen in the sweat glands and include basal cell degeneration, necrosis, and basal cell hyperplasia (Akosa & Lampert, 1991). Changes in the adjacent tissue can aid the dermatopathologist in determining what the underlying etiology causing the vasculitis could be. Extravascular granulomas characterized by degenerating collagen bundles surrounded by eosinophils and flame figures ("red" granulomas) are seen in Churg Strauss Syndrome while extravascular granulomas characterized by degenerating collagen bundles surrounded by basophilic debris ("blue" granulomas) are seen in Wegener's granulomatosis and rheumatoid vasculitis (Carlson, 2010). Dermal lamellar fibrosis can be seen in erythema elevatum diutinum and granulomas faciale (Carlson et al., 2005). Direct immunofluorescence adds another important diagnostic piece of information. Absence of immune complex deposition (pauci-immune vasculitis) is seen in Wegener's granulomatosis, microscopic polyangiitis, and Churg Strauss syndrome (Carlson, 2010).

Peri-vascular deposition of IgG, IgM, and/or C3 is seen in cutaneous leukocytoclastic angiitis, urticarial vasculitis, and connective tissue disease vasculitis (Carlson et al., 2005). Vascular deposits of IgA are found in Henoch Schonlein purpura while deposition of IgM is seen in cryoglobulinemic vasculitis (Carlson, 2010). Basement membrane zone deposition of immunoglobulins can be seen in urticarial vasculitis and connective tissue disease vasculitis (Carlson et al., 2005).

The most common classification system of vasculitides is based on the size of the affected vessel. While biopsy is required for definitive diagnosis, the size of the affected vessel correlates with the cutaneous lesions seen. Large vessel involvement manifests as limb claudication, absent pulses, aortic dilation, bruits, and/or asymmetric blood pressure (Chen & Carlson, 2008). Giant cell (temporal) arteritis and Takayasu's arteritis are examples of this (Carlson, 2010). Vasculitis involving medium sized (muscular) vessels manifest as subcutaneous nodules, deep ulcers, livedo reticularis, palmar or digital scars, digital gangrene, mononeuritis, erythematous nodules, and aneurysms (Chen & Carlson, 2008). Examples of this include polyarteritis nodosa, Kawasaki disease, and nodular vasculitis (Carlson, 2010). Small vessel vasculitis can be further subdivided into two categories: immune complex mediated vasculitis arising in small post-capillary venules or non-immune complex mediated vasculitis arising in small muscular arteries and arterioles. Small vessel vasculitis appears as purpura, erythema, urticaria, vesiculobullous lesions, superficial ulcers, and splinter hemorrhages (Chen & Carlson, 2008). Examples of this include cutaneous leukocytoclastic vasculitis, Henoch Schonlein purpura, urticarial vasculitis, Churg Strauss vasculitis, Wegener's granulomatosis, and microscopic polyangiitis (Carlson, 2010).

Biopsy location, depth, and timing must be taken into consideration by the clinician to increase the diagnostic yield. Since small vessels reside in the upper dermis while medium sized, muscular vessels are found in the deep dermis and subcutis, a punch or excisional biopsy is required to ensure adequate sampling of all vessel sizes (Carlson et al., 2005). Biopsies performed within 48 hours after the onset of lesions can show a neutrophilic, eosinophilic, or lymphocytic infiltration, depending on the underlying process (Chen & Carlson, 2008). However, after 48 hours, lymphocytes replace the other inflammatory cells, regardless of the underlying etiology and will therefore be non-diagnostic (Chen & Carlson, 2008). Fibrosis, luminal obliteration, and lamination of the vessel wall is seen in healed lesions of vasculitis (Chen et al., 2005). Biopsy from a patient with livedo racemosa must be taken from the center white areas rather then the peripheral red areas since this is where the vascular stenosis can be seen (Carlson, 2010). Biopsy of superficial ulcers should be taken from non-ulcerated skin or from the edge of the ulcer whereas biopsy of deep ulcers should be taken central to the ulcer and include subcutaneous tissue to increase the diagnostic yield of medium sized vessel vasculitis (Chen & Carlson, 2008).

2. Small vessel vasculitis

2.1 Immune complex mediated vasculitis in post capillary venules

2.1.1 Cutaneous leukocytoclastic angiitis

Cutaneous leukocytoclastic angiitis (CLA) is also known as cutaneous leukocytoclastic vasculitis, hypersensitivity vasculitis/angiitis, allergic vasculitis, and necrotizing vasculitis (Carlson & Chen, 2006). The Chapel Hill Consensus Conference (CHCC) defines CLA as an isolated cutaneous leukocytoclastic vasculitis in the absence of systemic vasculitis (Carlson et al., 2005). Patients are typically middle aged adults with a recent history of exercise in hot weather (Chen & Carlson, 2008). Less than 10% of patients may present with renal or gastrointestinal involvement, however, this systemic vasculitis variant of CLA has yet to be formally recognized (Carlson, 2010). Etiology may be secondary to medications, viral upper respiratory infection, or collagen vascular diseases; however, in the majority of cases no etiology will be identified (Grunwald et al., 1997).

The cutaneous manifestations include crops of palpable purpura over the lower extremities associated with pruritus, stinging, tenderness, or burning (Chen & Carlson, 2008). Rarely patients may present with erythema and hemorrhagic bullae on the lower extremities (Carlson, 2010). Areas of ecchymoses and hyperpigmenation are seen as the lesions resolve over a period of 3-4 weeks (Chen & Carlson, 2008).

The general pathologic features of CLA on a skin biopsy include fibrin deposits, neutrophilic perivascular infiltration of small vessels, and nuclear debris (leukocytoclasia) (Carlson & Chen, 2006) (see Figures 1 and 2). Hemophagocytosis can also be seen (Draper & Morgan, 2007). The pathologic features of CLA change with temporal evolution. Early lesions are characterized by a neutrophil dominant vasculitis in the upper to mid dermis which then progresses to a mononuclear predominant vasculitis within 120 hours after the onset of the lesions (Zax et al., 1990) (see Figure 3). Epidermal involvement including vesicle formation and ulceration can also be identified (Grunwald et al., 1997). The healing lesions show regenerative endothelial cells, fibrin deposits within vessel walls, and a mild monocytic perivascular infiltrate (Grunwald et al., 1997) (see Figure 4). The other classic features of CLA including extravasation of erythrocytes, fibrinoid necrosis, and epidermal necrosis fade as the lesions age (Zax et al., 1990). Rarely a necrotizing venulitis can be seen extending through the mid and deep dermis (Carlson, 2010).

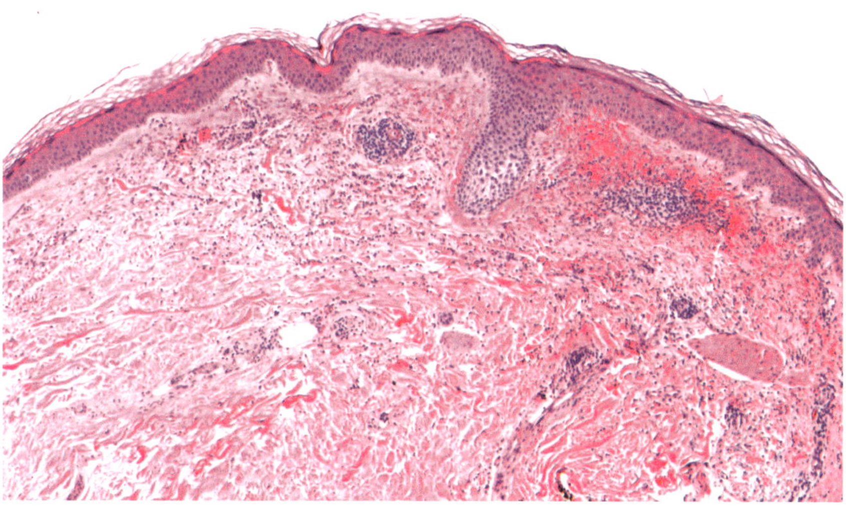

Fig. 1. Cutaneous Leukocytoclastic Angiitis. Small vessel vasculitides demonstrate many common features including fibrinoid necrosis, marked inflammation, leukocytoclasia and red cell extravasation (H&E, 40x).

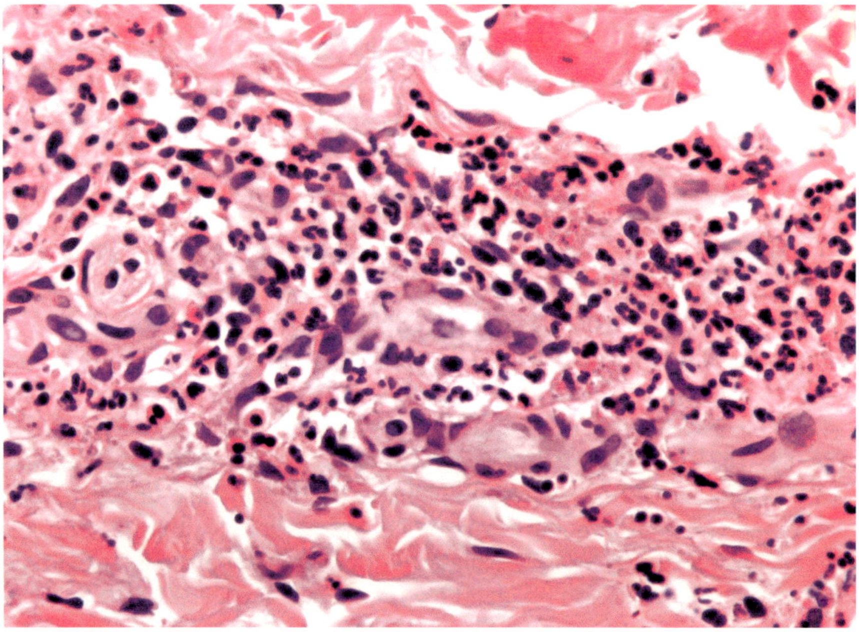

Fig. 2. Cutaneous Leukocytoclastic Angiitis. Neutrophilic perivascular infiltration of small vessels with accompanying leukocytoclasia consisting of karryorhectic nuclear debris (H&E, 400x).

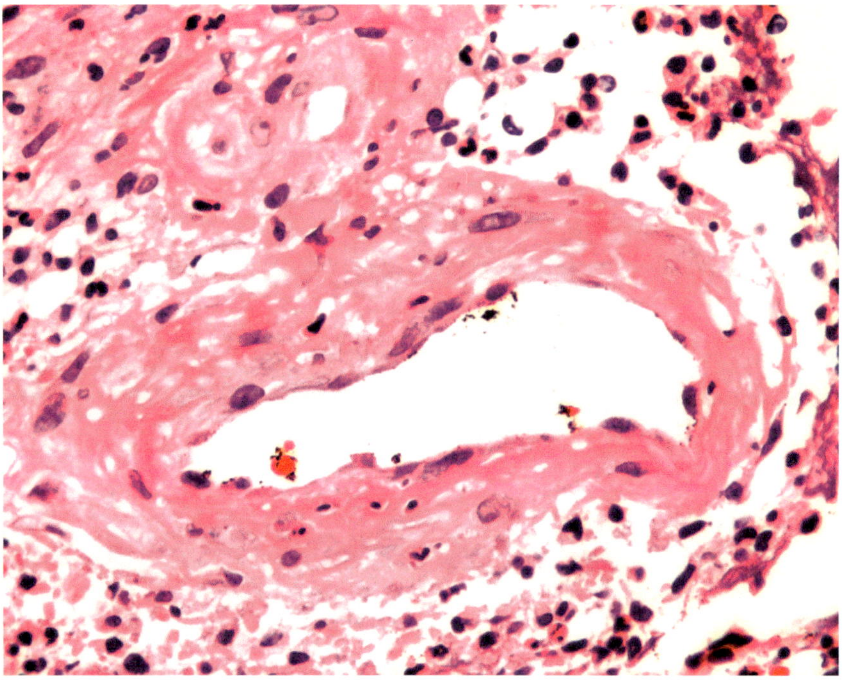

Fig. 3. Cutaneous Leukocytoclastic Angiitis. Fibrinoid necrosis of the vessel walls is characteristic (H&E, 400x).

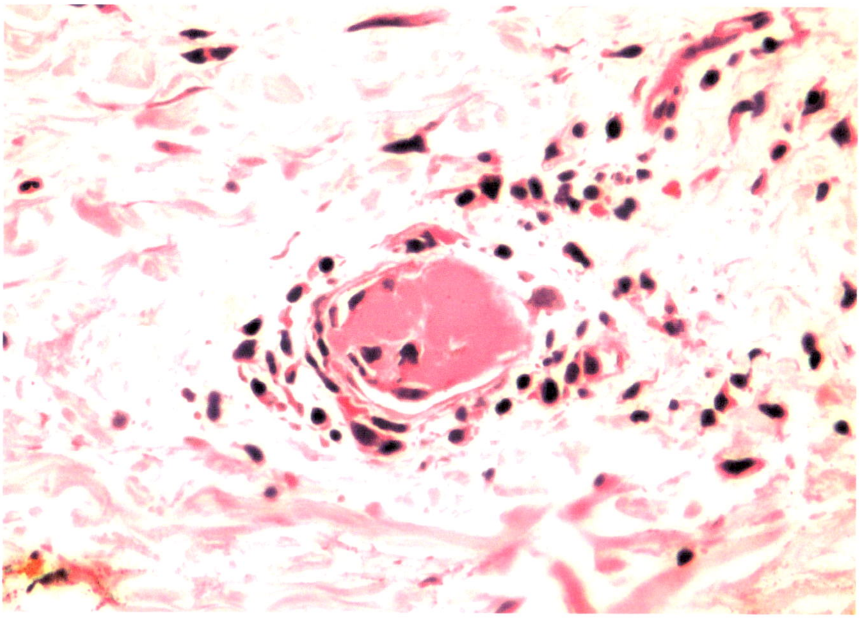

Fig. 4. Cutaneous Leukocytoclastic Angiitis. Intravascular fibrin thrombi are common and may be accompanied by epidermal infarction (H&E, 400x).

Nuclear dust was previously considered to be pathoneumonic for CLA, however, several reports have shown it is also present in linear IgA bullous dermatosis, inflammatory type of epidermolysis bullosa acquisita, septic vasculitis, and dermatitis herpetiformis (LeBoit, 2005). Further, not all nuclear dust is neutrophilic in origin. Lymphocytic inflammation can also result in nuclear dust in entities such as subcutaneous panniculitis like T-cell lymphoma, Kikuchi's disease, and irritated lichenoid keratosis (LeBoit, 2005).

Direct immunofluorescence is positive in 92% of cases and can be used during all stages of lesions (Grunwald et al., 1997). Detection of immunoreactants has the highest yield when taken from lesional rather than peri-lesional skin (Barnadas et al., 2004). Deposits of fibrinogen, C3 and IgM are most frequently present, but rarely IgG and C4 can also be seen (Grunwald et al., 1997). Deposition of IgA can also be seen in conjunction with IgM or IgG, distinguishing CLA from Henoch Schonlein Purpura in which IgA deposition is found in isolation (Sais & Vidaller, 2005).

2.1.2 Urticarial vasculitis

Urticarial vasculitis (UV) is a clinicopathologic entity characterized by urticarial lesions or faint purpura persisting longer than 24 hours which on histology show a leukocytoclastic vasculitis (Aboobaker & Greaves, 1986). Patients are typically female in their fourth to fifth decade of life (Chen & Carlson, 2008). Systemic symptoms such as fever, angioedema, arthralgias, and abdominal pain are usually present (Mehregan et al., 1992). Two clinical variants, hypocomplementemia UV (HUV) and normocomplementemia UV (NUV), exist. Patients with HUV are more likely to be female and present with more severe disease along with arthralgia, glomerulonephritis, uveitis, recurrent abdominal pain, and/or obstructive lung disease (Chen & Carlson, 2008). The cause of UV is mostly unknown;, however, it can be a manifestation of connective tissue diseases such as systemic lupus erythematosus or Sjögren's syndrome or be associated with viral infections, serum sickness, drug reactions, and exercise (Carlson & Chen, 2006).

Cutaneous findings which help to distinguish UV from chronic urticaria include burning, painful, or pruritic hive-like plaques persisting longer than 24 hours but which fade within 72 hours leaving residual areas of hypopigmentation (Carlson, 2010). Lesions tend to favor the trunk and proximal extremities (Fiorentino, 2003).

The minimal criteria required for diagnosis of UV are leukocytoclasia or fibrin deposits with or without extravasated red blood cells, features which can be subtle and overlap with the histologic findings seen in cutaneous leukocytoclastic angiitis (Black, 1999). There is a wide spectrum of histologic findings in UV, ranging from sparse neutrophilic infiltrate of small vessels to more severe lesions with a dense neutrophilic vasculitis, leukocytoclasia, extravasated red blood cells, endothelial cell swelling and fibrin deposits (Jones et al., 1983). The superficial and mid-dermal vessels are most commonly affected, however, vascular destruction can extend into the deep dermal and pannicular vessels (Davis et al., 1998; Mehregan et al., 1992). Neutrophilic vasculitis is more common in HUV whereas eosinophilic vasculitis predominates in NUV (see Figure 5) (Davis et al., 1998).

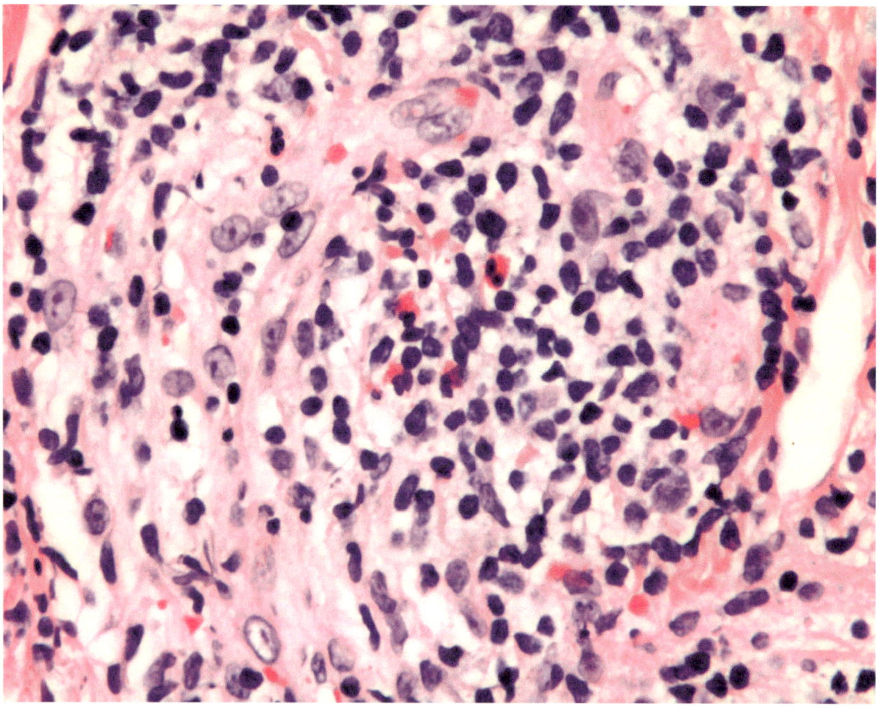

Fig. 5. Urticarial Vasculitis. A prominent eosinophilic infiltrate is present (H&E, 400x)

Direct immunofluorescence reveals peri-vascular deposits of C3 and immunoglobulins, mostly IgM, however, DIF is more frequently positive in HUV as opposed to NUV (87% versus 29%) (Mehregan et al., 1992). Likewise, basement membrane deposition of immunoglobulins and/or C3 is seen on DIF, but more commonly in HUV than NUV (70%

versus 18%) (Mehregan et al., 1992). 70% of patients with basement membrane deposition of immunoreactants will also have glomerulonephritis (Chen & Carlson, 2008).

2.1.3 Henoch schonlein purpura

Henoch Schonlein Purpura (HSP) represents approximately 10% of all cutaneous vasculitis cases and is the most common vasculitis in children, comprising about 90% of all cases (Carlson, 2010). HSP typically occurs in children aged four to eight years old with a history of upper respiratory tract infection one to two weeks prior to onset of symptoms (Fiorentino, 2003). The initial diagnosis of HSP required palpable purpura, gastrointestinal involvement, arthritis, and nephritis, however, it is now recognized that not all patients present with this tetrad of symptoms (Fiorentino, 2003). The only diagnostic criterion for HSP according to the Chapel Hill Consensus Conference (CHCC) guidelines is demonstration of IgA deposits affecting small vessels (Carlson et al., 2005). The CHCC definition is not specific for HSP, however, since IgA vascular deposits are also seen in erythema nodosum, venous stasis, cryoglobulinemia, coagulopathic vasculopathies, and livedoid vasculitis (Carlson & Chen, 2006). The diagnosis of HSP according to the American College of Rheumatology (ACR) requires two of the following: palpable purpura, age less than 20 years, abdominal pain, and/or neutrophilic vasculitis (Carlson et al., 2005). One could confuse HSP with mixed cryoglobulinemia, Wegener's granulomatosis, collagen vascular disease, hypocomplementemic vasculitis, and microscopic polyarteritis nodosa if only the more clinical ACR criteria are used for diagnosis, which does not require the demonstration of IgA deposits on direct immunofluorescence (DIF) (Magro & Crowson, 1999). Therefore, features more sensitive and specific for HSP include IgA vascular deposits and two or more of the following clinical features: age less than or equal to 20 years, abdominal pain or hematochezia, preceding upper respiratory tract infection, and/or hematuria or renal biopsy with mesangioproliferative glomerulonephritis with or without IgA deposits (Carlson, 2010).

Long term follow up of these patients is paramount as 20% of children who present with renal involvement or who have an abnormal urinalysis at the time of diagnosis will progress to chronic renal failure within 20 years (Chen & Carlson, 2008). The presence of nephrotic syndrome, hypertension, or renal failure at the outset are poor prognostic factors in children (Carlson & Chen, 2006). Adults who present with fever, rash above the waist, and an elevated erythrocyte sedimentation rate are more likely to have renal involvement (Chen & Carlson, 2008).

Cutaneous manifestations of HSP include symmetric macular erythema of the buttocks and lower extremities which progresses to palpable purpura that usually resolves within 10 to 14 days (Fiorentino, 2003).

The prototypic pathology of HSP shows a small vessel neutrophilic vasculitis indistinguishable from that seen in CLA (see Figure 6) (Carlson & Chen, 2006). At least three of the following features have been suggested as being specific for HSP: superficial plaques rather than palpable purpura, skin necrosis, retiform margins of lesions, or a livedoid pattern of hemorrhage (Piette & Stone, 1989). While the vasculitis is usually limited to the superficial and mid-dermal vessels, pandermal involvement can be seen (Magro & Crowson, 1999). A severe reaction which recapitulates a Sweet's like vascular reaction, neutrophilic interface dermatitis, dermatitis herpetiformis like abscesses, and adnexal infiltration by neutrophils can also be seen (Magro & Crowson, 1999).

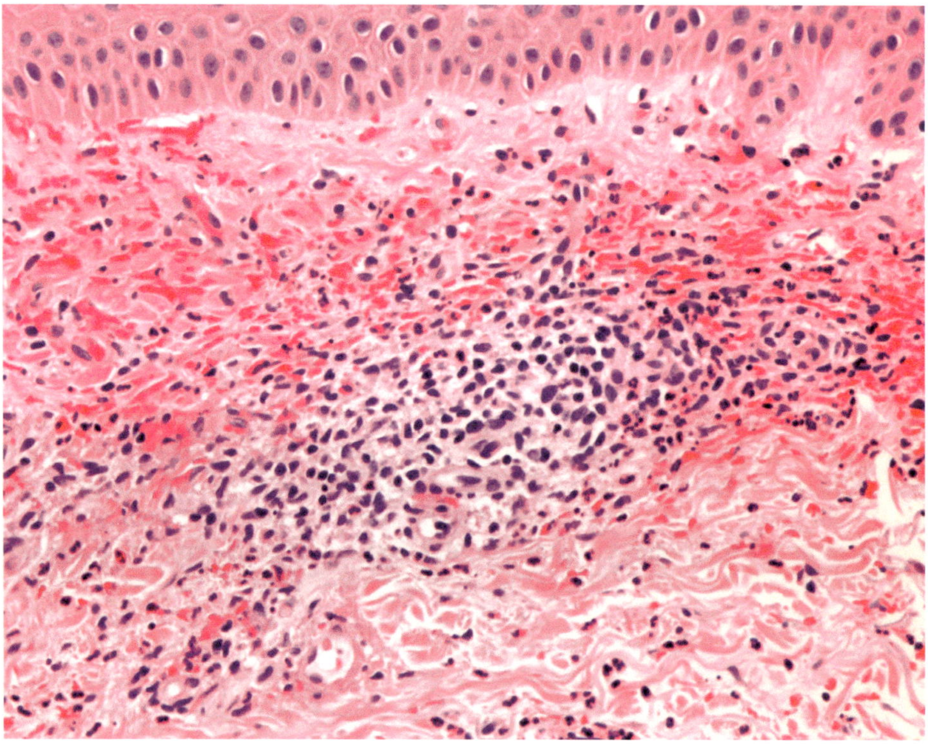

Fig. 6. Henoch Schonlein Purpura. Lesions of HSP are notable for marked red cell extravasation (H&E, 200x).

DIF reveals vascular deposits of IgA, predominately the IgA1 subclass (Egan et al., 1998). The sensitivity of DIF increases dramatically when performed on biopsies of lesions less than 48 hours in duration as compared to lesions of longer duration (85% versus 27%) (Murali et al., 2002).

Acute infantile hemorrhagic edema (AIHE) (also known as Finkelstein's Disease) is considered by some to be a variant of HSP characterized by fever, annular or targetoid skin lesions, and edema, (Carlson & Chen, 2006). Other authors consider AIHE a distinct entity from HSP owing to the fact that patients with AIHE are younger and have shorter disease courses than those patients with HSP (Karremann et al., 2009). Additionally, complications common to HSP, such as intestinal bleeding and renal involvement, are rare in AIHE (Karremann et al., 2009). Sudden onset of symptoms is seen after an upper respiratory infection, drug ingestion, or vaccination (Millard et al., 1999). The same small vessel neutrophilic vasculitis seen in HSP is also seen in AIHE, however, deposition of IgA is not a feature in AIHE (Legrain et al., 1991). Patients typically follow a benign clinical course with spontaneous resolution in 12-20 days (Millard et al., 1999).

2.1.4 Cryoglobulinemic vasculitis

Cryoglobulins are immunoglobulins which will precipitate when serum is cooled to temperatures less than 37° C (Cohen et al., 1991). Cryoglobulinemia is divided into three types: Type I is composed of monoclonal immunoglobulins, type II has mixed monoclonal and polyclonal immunoglobulins (monoclonal IgM and polyclonal IgG), and type III has only polyclonal immunoglobulins (polyclonal IgM and IgG) (Sansonno & Dammacco, 2005). Type I produces small vessel hyaline thrombi, not a true vasculitis, while types II and III result in cryoglobulinemic vasculitis (CV) (Carlson & Chen, 2006). Mixed cryoglobulinemia (types II and II) is associated with connective tissue diseases, lymphoproliferative disorders (although these are more frequently seen in association with type I), and infectious diseases (Cohen et al., 1991). Mixed cryoglobulinemia is frequently a manifestation of hepatitis C infection, although these patients less frequently present with vasculitis (Kapur et al., 2002).

The clinical triad of CV (mixed cryoglobulinemia with vasculitis) includes purpura induced by exposure to cold or prolonged standing, arthralgia, and weakness (Chen & Carlson, 2008). Non-pruritic, intermittent purpura invariably involving the lower extremities with facial and trunk sparring is always seen, however, petechiae, livedo reticularis, skin necrosis, ulcerations, and urticaria can rarely be present (Fiorentino, 2003). Other rare cutaneous presentations include polyarteritis nodosa like lesions, splinter hemorrhages, and palmar erythema (Chen & Carlson, 2008). Systemic manifestations include renal disease (presenting as hematuria, edema, or hypertension), liver disease (presenting from elevated liver enzymes and hepatomegaly to frank cirrhosis), gastrointestinal involvement (presenting as abdominal pain or gastrointestinal bleeding), lymphadenopathy, polyneuropathy, and pericarditis (Gorevic et al., 1980).

Skin biopsy of CV will demonstrate a neutrophilic vasculitis equally affecting small vessels in the papillary dermis and subcutaneous tissue (Cohen et al., 1991). Other histologic findings include endothelial swelling, extravasation of red blood cells, hyaline thrombi, and fibrinoid necrosis (Cohen et al., 1991; Gorevic et al., 1980). Rarely a lymphocytic small vessel vasculitis can be seen (Cohen et al., 1991). Direct immunofluorescence frequently reveals the presence of immunoreactants in vessel walls (typically IgG, IgM and/or C3) (Cohen et al., 1991; Gorevic et al., 1980). Deposition of immunoreactants along the basement membrane zone is not commonly seen (Gorevic et al., 1980). Hepatitis C proteins can be detected within vessel walls, even in the absence of vasculitis, and also within keratinocytes in patients with Hepatitis C virus and concurrent acute vasculitis (Sansonno & Dammacco, 2005).

2.1.5 Drug induced vasculitis

Approximately 20% of all cutaneous vasculitis eruptions result from an adverse drug reaction (Carlson, 2010). The interval between ingestion of the drug and onset of the vasculitis varies from hours to years and can commence with dosage increases or re-challenge with the agent (Carlson & Chen, 2006). The most common offenders in drug induced vasculitis include propylthiouracil, hydralazine, granulocyte-colony stimulating factor, cefaclor, minocycline, allopurinol, penicillamine, phenytoin, isotretinoin, and methotrexate (ten Holder et al., 2002).

While specific cutaneous and systemic findings vary with the offending drug (see Table 1), patients who present with limited cutaneous vasculitis in the absence of systemic involvement usually present with a maculopapular or vesicular rash over the extremities while patients with systemic vasculitis typically present with a maculopapular, vesicular, or purpuric rash which is not limited to the extremities (Mullick et al., 1979).

	Systemic Organs Involved	Cutaneous Findings	Duration of Therapy before Onset of Symptoms
Propylthiouracil	Renal (focal segmental glomerulosclerosis, mesangial proliferation), Pulmonary (hemoptysis, wheezing, congestion, cough, dyspnea), Musculoskeletal (myositis, cramping, elevated creatine kinase), Ear (decreased hearing, bilateral deafness, tinnitus)	Purpuric lesions progressing to necrotic ulcers	3 days-7 years
Hydralazine	Renal (pauci-immune glomerulonephritis), Pulmonary, Musculoskeletal (arthralgias, myalgias)	Palpable purpura, maculopapular eruptions on the lower extremities and hemorrhagic blisters on the legs, arms, trunk, nasal septum, and uvula	6 months-13 years
Granulocyte Colony Stimulating Factor	Systemic symptoms less common; Renal (vasculitis), Musculoskeletal (arthralgias)	Subcutaneous nodules, purpura, hemorrhagic bullae, erythematous macules	Days to Weeks
Allopurinol	Always presents with systemic symptoms; Renal (glomerulonephritis), Hepatic (elevated liver enzymes, granulomatous infiltration), Musculoskeletal (myalgias), Other (lymphadenopathy, seizures)	Macular rash more prominent on the back and abdomen, non-follicular macular exanthem on trunk and proximal extremities, erythema multiforme	2 hours-9 years
Cefaclor	Renal and Musculoskeletal	Serum sickness like reaction limited to the face and extremities	1-2 weeks
Minocycline	Renal (elevated creatinine), Hepatic (elevated liver enzymes), Ocular (conjunctivitis, swelling of the eye), Musculoskeletal (arthralgias, polyarthritis)	Urticarial eruption, erythema nodosum, non-palpable purpura, livedo reticularis, erythematous macular eruptions	9 days-9 months
Penicillamine	Renal (glomerulonephritis), Pulmonary (coughing, hemoptysis, lung infiltrates)	Cutaneous ulcers on hands and ears, purpuric rash	2 months-18 years
Phenytoin	High mortality rate; vasculitis involving the kidney, liver, spleen, and lung	Pruritic maculopapular rash	1 week-17 years
Isotretinoin	Renal (glomerulonephritis), Pulmonary (Wegener's granulomatosis), Musculoskeletal (myalgias, arthralgias)	Pruritic papules	6-16 weeks
Methotrexate	Fever	Erythematous palpable purpura	1-5 days

Adapted from ten Holder et al., 2002

Table 1. Drugs Most Frequently Associated with Vasculitis

Numerous cases report positive ANCA following ingestion of certain drugs. The drugs most commonly associated with ANCA positive vasculitis are propylthiouracil and hydralazine. Methimazole, phenytoin, thiazide, minocycline, allopurinol, penicillamine, sulfasalazine, cephotaxime, and retinoids have also been implicated (Cuellar, 2002). Cutaneous findings in patients with drug induced ANCA associated vasculitis include acral purpuric plaques and nodules, most commonly found on the extremities, face, breast, and ears (Fiorentino, 2003). Systemic involvement is more common in the ANCA associated drug induced vasculitides (Chen & Carlson, 2008).

Other drugs can cause a vasculitis which clinically and histologically resembles urticarial vasculitis (appetite suppressants, methotrexate, procainamide, fluoxetine), Churg Strauss syndrome (leukotriene inhibitors, macrolides), Henoch-Schonlein purpura (propylthiouracil, levodopa, carbidopa), and Wegener's granulomatosis (propylthiouracil) (Cuellar, 2002).

Skin biopsy usually reveals a leukocytoclastic vasculitis (LCV) similar to that seen in other small vessel vasculitis syndromes characterized by vascular and interstitial neutrophilic infiltration, leukocytoclasis, endothelial cell swelling, fibrinoid necrosis, and extravasation of red blood cells (Bahrami et al., 2006). Determining a drug induced versus non-drug induced etiology is a diagnostic dilemma for clinicians and pathologists. Tissue eosinophilia can be present in drug induced LCV, however, its existence does not exclude other non-drug induced etiologies such as arthropod assault, which will also show prominent interstitial eosinophils (Bahrami et al., 2006). One study suggested the presence of vascular fibrin deposition should exclude a drug related LCV, however, later studies have failed to replicate this findings (Bahrami et al., 2006; Mullick et al., 1979). Intravascular fibrin thrombi and epidermal changes including vesicle formation can occasionally be seen (Bahrami et al., 2006).

Recent attention has been given to vasculitis secondary to cocaine adulterated with levamisole. Patients present clinically with retiform purpura and skin biopsy shows a leukocytoclastic vasculitis with thrombosis (Walsh et al., 2010). Mural fibrin, extravasated red blood cells, nuclear dust, and luminal thrombosis can also be seen (see Figure 7) (Waller et al., 2010). A diagnostic pit fall for clinicians and dermatopathologists is "cocaine-induced pseudovasculitis" in which the clinical and serologic findings are suggestive of vasculitis, but the histopathologic findings of vasculitis are absent (Friedman & Wolfsthal, 2005). These patients can also present with retiform purpura and skin biopsy shows fibrin thrombi occluding small superficial and deep dermal vessels without evidence of vasculitis (Waller et al., 2010).

Recent attention has been given to vasculitis secondary to cocaine adulterated with levamisole. Patients present clinically with retiform purpura and skin biopsy shows a leukocytoclastic vasculitis with thrombosis (Walsh et al., 2010). Mural fibrin, extravasated red blood cells, nuclear dust, and luminal thrombosis can also be seen (see Figure 7) (Waller et al., 2010). A diagnostic pit fall for clinicians and dermatopathologists is "cocaine-induced pseudovasculitis" in which the clinical and serologic findings are suggestive of vasculitis, but the histopathologic findings of vasculitis are absent (Friedman & Wolfsthal, 2005). These patients can also present with retiform purpura and skin biopsy shows fibrin thrombi occluding small superficial and deep dermal vessels without evidence of vasculitis (Waller et al., 2010).

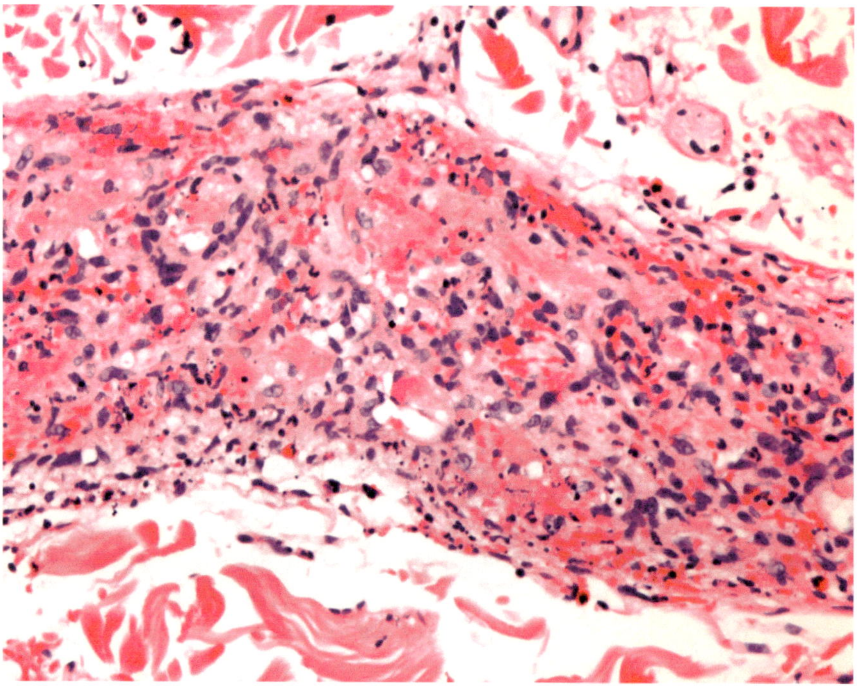

Fig. 7. Levamisole-Induced Vasculitis. Complete effacement of the vessel wall with extensive fibrin thrombosis and neutrophilic infiltrates reminiscent of an infectious etiology (H&E, 200x).

2.1.6 Connective tissue disease associated vasculitis

Connective tissue disease (CTD) vasculitis is an uncommon complication most frequently seen in patients with systemic erythematosus (SLE), rheumatoid arthritis (RA), and Sjögren's syndrome (SS) but can also rarely be seen in dermatomyositis, scleroderma, and polychondritis (Carlson & Chen, 2006). The usual presentation is arterial and capillary involvement represented clinically by purpura, vesiculobullous lesions, urticaria, and splinter hemorrhages (Carlson, 2010). Ulcers, subcutaneous nodules, gangrene, livedo racemosa, and pyoderma gangrenosum can also be seen and represent arterial involvement (Carlson, 2010).

Skin biopsy typically reveals a vasculitis of small vessels, although medium sized vessel involvement can occasionally be seen (see Figure 8) (Carlson, 2010). The findings of both small and medium sized vessel vasculitis in the same biopsy are characteristic of CTD vasculitis (Chen & Carlson, 2008). Patients with CTD vasculitis can show p-ANCA or, more rarely, c-ANCA on indirect immunofluorescence (Carlson & Chen, 2006). Serology for anti-proteinase 3 and anti-myeloperoxidase is typically negative in these patients, ruling out Wegener's granulomatosis and Churg Strauss syndrome, respectively (Merkel et al., 1997). While the histologic features of CTD vasculitis are similar despite the etiology, certain extravascular findings may help aid in distinguishing which specific CTD is present. Interface dermatitis with increased dermal mucin is seen in SLE and dermatomyositis; dermal sclerosis is seen in scleroderma; granulomatous dermatitis is seen in RA and SLE; and interstitial neutrophilia is seen in SLE and SS (Chen & Carlson, 2008). Chronic lymphocytic vasculitis is the suspected etiology for endarteritis obliterans, a vasculopathy characterized by progressive blood vessel occlusion with subsequent internal organ ischemia seen in patients with CTD vasculitis (Carlson & Chen, 2006).

2.1.7 Rheumatoid vasculitis

Rheumatoid vasculitis (RV) is an uncommon complication of rheumatoid arthritis (RA) with significant mortality (Chen et al., 2002). RV is associated with high rheumatoid factor titer, joint erosions, extra-articular symptoms, rheumatoid nodules, male gender, increasing number of treatment with disease modifying agents, and prior treatment with D-penicillamine or azathioprine (Sayah & English, 2005). Onset is typically 10-14 years after the onset of RA (Sayah & English, 2005). Diagnosis of RV requires RA plus one or more of the following: mononeuritis multiplex, acute peripheral neuropathy, peripheral gangrene, acute necrotizing vasculitis seen on biopsy plus systemic symptoms, or deep cutaneous ulcers or extra-articular disease if associated with infarcts or vasculitis (Sayah & English, 2005). Cutaneous findings are the most common extra-articular manifestation in RV and can be seen in 80-89% of all patients and are frequently the presenting symptom (Chen et al., 2002). Patients with cutaneous RV generally have a good prognosis while those with RV involving nerves or bowel typically have a fatal outcome (Carlson & Chen, 2006).

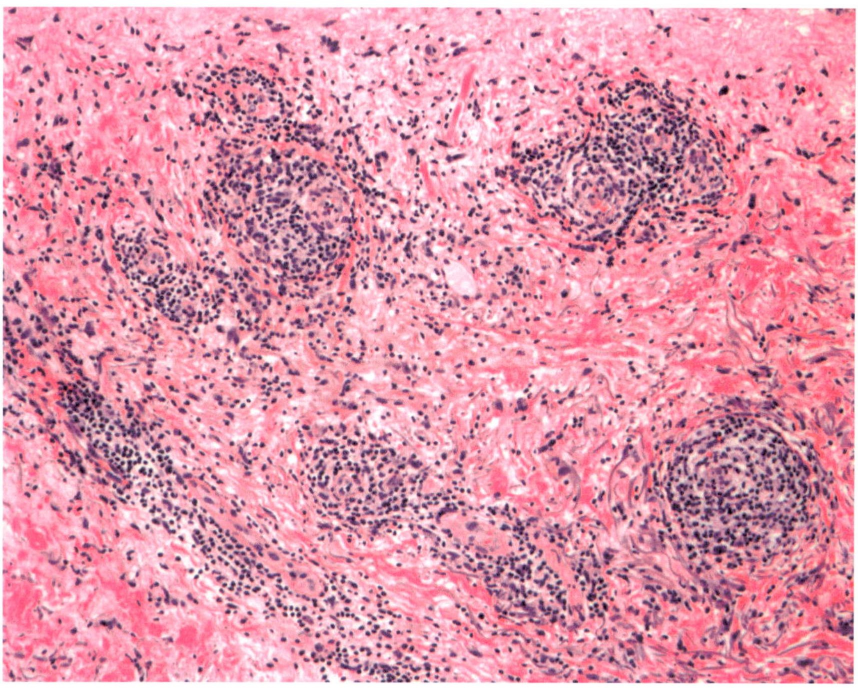

Fig. 8. Lymphocytic Vasculitis. Connective tissue disease may present with a predominately lymphocytic infiltrate (H&E, 100x).

Palpable purpura on the lower extremities is the most common cutaneous presentation (Genta et al., 2006). Other manifestations include ulcers, maculopapular erythema, hemorrhagic blisters, erythema elevatum diutinum, livedo reticularis, subcutaneous nodules, and atrophie blanche (Chen et al., 2002). Ulcers tend to be found on the dorsum of the foot or upper calf, locations which are different from ulcerations due to atherosclerosis and diabetes, a finding which may help clinically distinguish these entities (Genta et al., 2006). Small, brown, painless infarcts of the nail fold or edge, also known as Bywaters lesions, are characteristic of RV (Sayah & English, 2005).

Histologic diagnosis of RV is complicated by the fact that vessels ranging from subcutaneous muscular arteries to venules can be involved and vessels in all stages of acute and healing vasculitis can be identified in the same specimen (Chen et al., 2002). Three histologic patterns of vasculitis may be seen. A necrotizing leukocytoclastic vasculitis of dermal venules is seen in patients with palpable purpura, hemorrhagic bullae, maculopapular erythema, and erythema elevatum diutinum (Chen et al., 2002). An acute or healing arteritis of the dermal-subcutaneous vessels similar to that seen in polyarteritis nodosa is seen in patients with subcutaneous nodules, livedo reticularis, and ulcers (Carlson & Chen, 2006). The last pattern is a mixed venulitis and arteritis and is seen in patients with subcutaneous nodules, atrophie blanche, and palpable purpura (Chen et al., 2002). Other histologic patterns that can be seen include folliculocentric neutrophilic vasculitis, pustular vasculitis with epidermal microabscess formation resembling dermatitis herpetiformis, and granulomatous vasculitis composed namely of lymphocytes and histiocytes (Magro & Crowson, 2003). Small vessel occlusive arteritis is seen in Bywaters lesions (Sayah & English, 2005). Vascular deposition of immunoglobulin, typically IgM, can frequently be seen on direct immunofluorescence and is associated with the presence of extra-articular manifestations (Rapoport et al., 1980).

2.1.8 Lupus vasculitis

Lupus vasculitis (LV) can be seen in 19-36% of patients with systemic lupus erythematosus (SLE) and 7-12% of patients with subacute cutaneous lupus erythematous (SCLE) (Carlson & Chen, 2006). Patients with LV are more frequently younger, male patients when compared to SLE patients without vasculitis (Carlson & Chen, 2006). Laboratory abnormalities include anemia, an elevated erythrocyte sedimentation rate and anti-La/SS-B antibodies, which are more common in patients with LV than those with non-vasculitis SLE (Chen & Carlson, 2008). Systemic LV, with or without cutaneous LV, is associated with a higher rate of mortality (Carlson & Chen, 2006).

The most common cutaneous findings are small painful macules or depressed punctuate scars over the palmar surfaces and finger tips which represent palmar and digital infarcts (Carlson & Chen, 2006). Other manifestations include palpable purpura, urticaria, and livedo reticularis of the lower extremities (Fiorentino, 2003).

Neutrophilic vasculitis of small vessels is the most frequent histological findings on skin biopsy (Drenkard et al., 1997). Neutrophilic or lymphocytic vasculitis involving medium sized muscular vessels can also be seen (Carlson & Chen, 2006). Biopsies of punctuate palmar lesions or areas of livedo reticularis show typical findings of livedoid vasculitis such as thickening and hyalinization of dermal and subcutaneous small and muscular vessels, inconspicuous lymphocytic perivascular infiltration, endothelial swelling, occlusion of the vessel lumen by fibrin, and endothelial necrosis can also be seen (Yasue, 1986). Livedoid vasculitis is associated with an increased risk of developing SLE involving the central nervous system (Yasue, 1986). Concomitant findings of cutaneous lupus erythematosus and LV can be seen within the same biopsy (Carlson & Chen, 2006). Direct immunofluorescence will reveal vascular deposition of IgG, IgM, or complement in approximately 55% of cases and co-existing basement membrane zone deposition of immunoglobulins (mostly IgM but rarely IgG) and complement in 60% of cases (Yasue, 1986).

2.1.9 Sjögren's syndrome

Sjögren's syndrome (SS) is an autoimmune disease primarily affecting exocrine glands leading to dry mouth and dry eyes (Ramos-Casals et al., 2004). Patients with SS vasculitis are more likely to have systemic involvement of their disease such as arthritis, peripheral neuropathy, central nervous system vasculitis, Raynaud's phenomenon, and renal disease (Carlson & Chen, 2006). Presence of antinuclear antibodies, anti-Ro/SS-A antibodies, rheumatoid factor, and cryoglobulins are frequent laboratory findings (Carlson & Chen, 2006).

The most common cutaneous findings are urticaria, palpable purpura, and ecchymoses (Fiorentino, 2003). Erythema multiforme, erythema perstans, and erythema nodosum can also be seen (Alexander & Provost, 1987).

Two distinct histologic patterns are seen. A neutrophilic vasculitis with extravasation of red blood cells, fibrin deposition, and nuclear dust is seen in patients with antinuclear antibodies, high titers of anti-Ro/SS-A and anti-La/SS-B antibodies, hypergammaglobulinemia, hypocomplementemia, and positive rheumatoid factor (Alexander & Provost, 1987). A lymphocytic vasculitis with fibrinoid necrosis is associated with negative antinuclear antibodies, low titers of anti-RO/SS-A and anti-La/SS-B antibodies, normocomplementemia, and normal globulin levels (Alexander & Provost, 1987). Necrotizing vasculitis of medium sized vessels can occasionally be seen (Ramos-Casals et al., 2004).

2.1.10 Erythema elevatum diutinum

Erythema elevatum diutinum (EED) is a chronic relapsing and remitting cutaneous vasculitis occurring in middle aged patients (Wahl et al., 2005). While the etiology is largely unknown, there is an association between EED and connective tissue disease, infectious agents (hepatitis, syphilis, HIV, and Streptococcus), and hematological abnormalities (myelodysplasia, multiple myeloma, and lymphoma) (Wahl et al., 2005). ANCA can occasionally be detected in patients with EED (Carlson & Chen, 2006). Lesions are typically symmetric, tender, red or brown papules, plaques, or nodules on the extensor surfaces of the extremities (Yiannias et al., 1992).

Skin biopsy of early lesions reveals a leukocytoclastic vasculitis of small vessels in which neutrophils are the predominant inflammatory cell (see Figure 9) (Yiannias et al., 1992). The dermis is relatively cellular with fibroblasts, histiocytes, and neutrophils predominating with relatively sparring of the epidermis and papillary dermis (Wahl et al., 2005). Older lesions show predominately fibrosis and granulation tissue with some lesions showing xanthomatization of the mid-dermis (Yiannias et al., 1992). Dense areas of laminated fibrosis contributes to the nodular appearance seen clinically (LeBoit & Cockerell, 1993). Direct immunofluorescence is generally non-diagnostic, but vascular deposition of IgG, IgM, complement (C3), and fibrinogen can be seen (Yiannias et al., 1992).

2.1.11 Granuloma faciale

Granuloma faciale (GF) usually presents in middle aged adults as red-brown plaques, nodules, or papules which usually arise on the face (Ortonne et al., 2005). Clinically, these lesions can be mistaken for sarcoidosis, lymphoma, discoid lupus erythematosus, and basal cell carcinoma (Carlson & Chen, 2006).

Skin biopsy shows a leukocytoclastic vasculitis within in the upper and reticular dermis and rarely involves the hypodermis (Marcoval et al., 2004). The dermis densely infiltrated by inflammatory cells, predominately eosinophils and plasma cells, distinguishing this entity from erythema elevatum diutinum, where neutrophils predominate (see Figure 10) (LeBoit, 2002). The cellular dermis is separated from the unremarkable epidermis by a grenz zone (see Figure 11) (Ortonne et al., 2005). Fibrinoid necrosis, extravasated red blood cells, and hemosiderin deposition can also be seen (Marcoval et al., 2004). Concentric perivascular fibrosis can be seen in older lesions (LeBoit, 2002). Perivascular and basement membrane deposition of immunoglobulins (mostly IgG but also IgA and IgM), complement (C3), and fibrinogen can be seen on direct immunofluorescence (Barnadas et al., 2005).

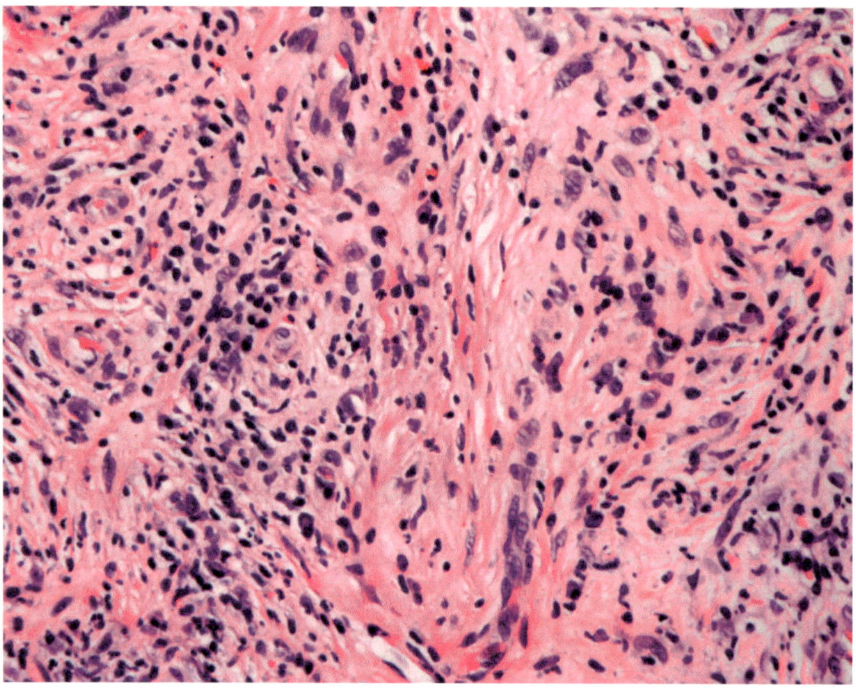

Fig. 9. Erythema Elevatum Diutinum. Older lesions are characterized by dermal sclerosis and scarring (H&E, 100x).

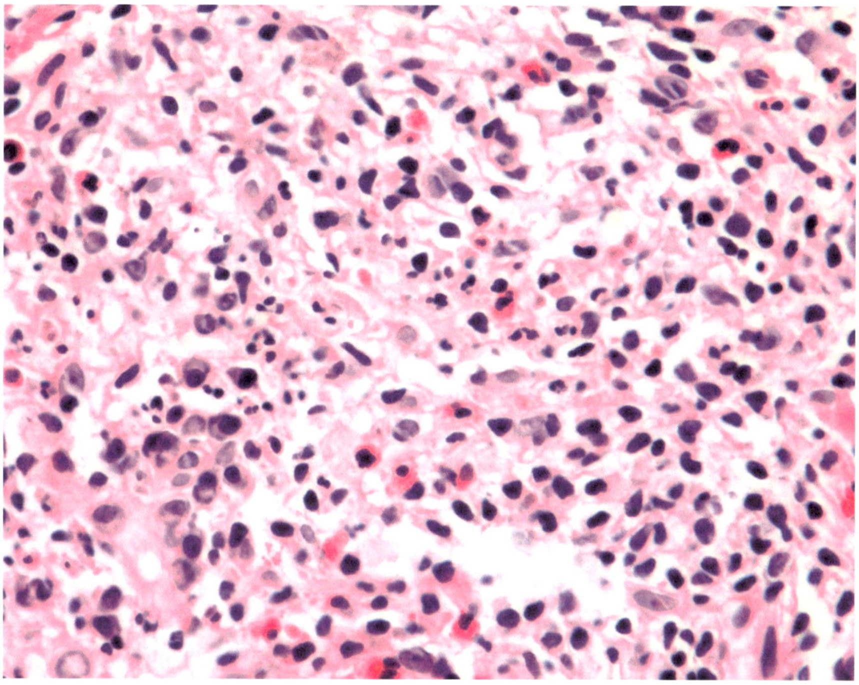

Fig. 10. Granuloma Faciale. Numerous eosinophils are present in the mixed dermal infiltrate (H&E, 400x)

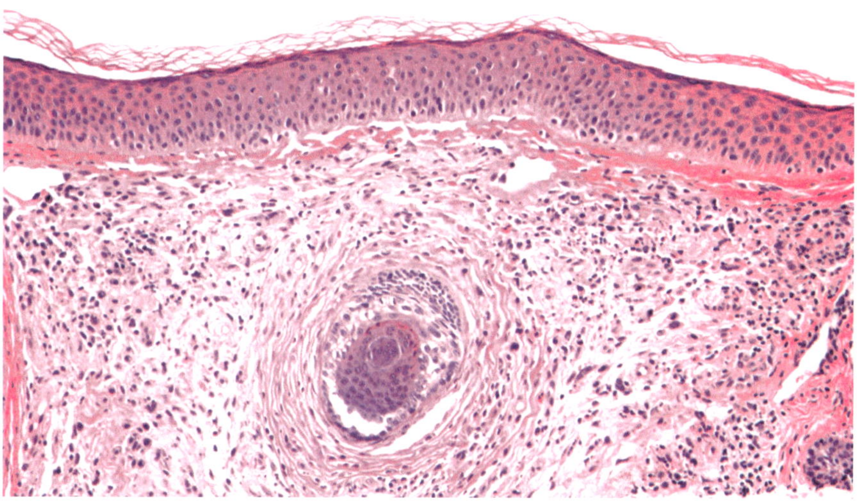

Fig. 11. Granuloma Faciale. A dense inflammatory infiltrate fills the dermis underneath a prominent Grenz zone (H&E, 100x).

2.2 Non-immune complex mediated vasculitis in small muscular arteries and arterioles

2.2.1 Churg strauss syndrome

Churg Strauss Syndrome (CSS) is a clinically distinct entity characterized by asthma (usually adult onset), allergic symptoms (ex. allergic rhinitis), peripheral and tissue eosinophilia, and systemic vasculitis affecting small to medium sized vessels (Chen & Carlson, 2008). The classic presentation follows three phases, the prodromal phase which consists of atopic disease, namely asthma or allergic rhinitis followed by the second phase consisting of peripheral and tissue eosinophilia and finally the third phase which is heralded by a life threatening systemic vasculitis (Lanham et al., 1984). Cutaneous lesions accompanied by peripheral neuropathy are the most common clinical symptoms (Chen et al., 2007). Other clinical findings include pulmonary infiltrates, abdominal pain, intestinal obstruction leading to perforation (secondary to obstructive submucosal eosinophilic infiltrates), pericarditis, congestive heart failure, neuropathy, joint pain, and myalgia (Lanham et al., 1984). Renal involvement in the form of focal segmental glomerulonephritis is rarely seen (Lanham et al., 1984). The renal findings in CSS and Wegener's granulomatosis are indistinguishable; however, renal involvement in CSS is extraordinarily rare and follows a benign course whereas renal disease is common in Wegener's granulomatosis and frequently leads to renal failure (Lanham et al., 1984).

Laboratory findings typically include eosinophilia and elevated IgE; approximately two thirds of patients will have a positive ANCA, usually p-ANCA (Frankel et al., 2002). Patients with a positive p-ANCA are more likely to have vasculitis and renal and central nervous system involvement (Choi et al., 2008). Vaccination, leukotriene inhibitors, and withdraw of corticosteroids have all been implicated as possible factors precipitating the onset of symptoms (Fiorentino, 2003).

Three main types of cutaneous lesions are seen: erythematous maculopapules, hemorrhagic lesions (ranging from petechiae to ecchymosis) associated with necrosis and ulceration, and tender, deep seated nodules on the scalp and temple (Choi et al., 2008). Other cutaneous manifestations include livedo reticularis, wheals, vesicles, and bullae (Chen et al., 2007).

Skin biopsy reveals three major histologic features: eosinophilic and neutrophilic vasculitis of small to medium sized vessels in the superficial and mid-dermal vessels ranging from a mild perivascular cuffing of inflammatory cells to a necrotizing arteritis which can recapitulate polyarteritis nodosa (PAN); interstitial dermal infiltration with eosinophils; or granulomas (see Figure 12) (Carlson & Chen, 2006; Lanham et al., 1984). All three histologic patterns may be seen in the same biopsy (Lanham et al., 1984). While the vasculitis typically involves small vessels, medium sized vasculitis can also occasionally be seen (Lanham et al., 1984). Lesions in the healing stages will show fibrosis with calcified nodules and a sparse or complete absence of inflammatory cells (Carlson & Chen, 2006; Chen et al., 2007). This is in contrast to PAN where the acute stage is marked by neutrophils and the healing stage by lymphocytes and histiocytes (Chen et al., 2007).

Two types of extravascular granulomas exist. The "blue" granulomas show palisading histiocytes surrounding basophilic degenerated collagen bundles (Chen et al., 2007). "Red" granulomas are also characterized by palisading histiocytes which surround a central zone of eosinophilic debris and collagen bundles (Carlson, 2010). While granulomatous arteritis may be found within internal organs of patients with CSS, the initial series report by Churg and Strauss only demonstrated perivascular or extravascular granulomas within skin

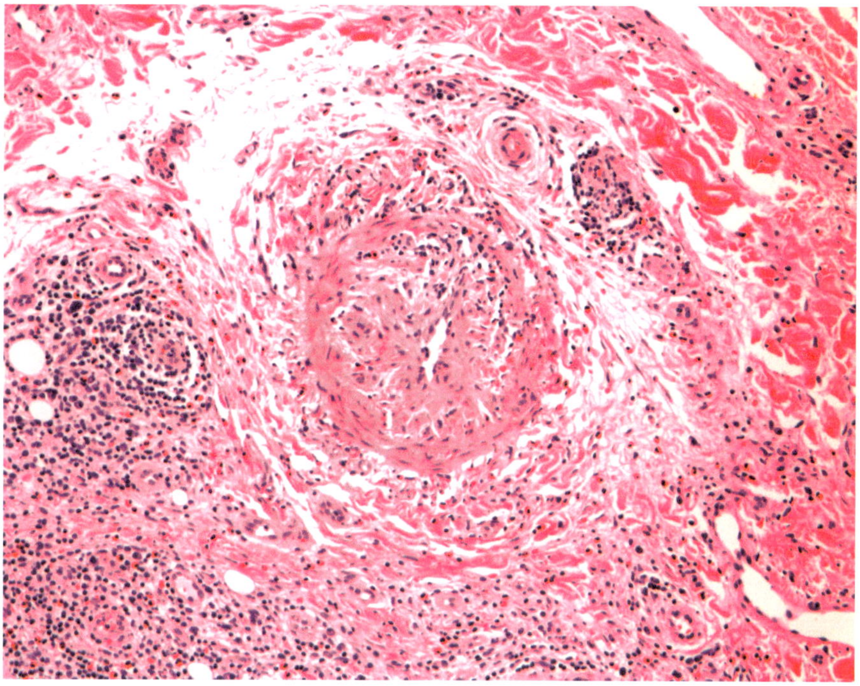

Fig. 12. Churg-Strauss Syndrome. Medium-sized vessel vasculitis with a prominent eosinophilic infiltrate (H&E. 100x).

lesions (Churg & Strauss, 1951). Granulomatous arteritis is a relatively rare findings in CSS. Chen et al recently suggested five scenarios which may contribute to the infrequency of this finding: biopsy was not performed over areas of livedo reticularis; biopsy did not extend into the subcutis; serial sections on the specimen were not performed; biopsy was taken after the start of treatment; or biopsy was not taken during the granulomatous stage (Chen et al., 2007). Direct immunofluorescence is typically negative giving rise to the name "pauci-immune" vasculitis (Carlson, 2010).

2.2.2 Wegener's granulomatosis

The initial description of Wegener's granulomatosis (WG) included three clinical findings: necrotizing granulomas with a predilection for the upper and lower airways, systemic small vessel vasculitis, and pauci-immune glomerulonephritis (Fiorentino, 2003). The most common initial presentation involves the upper and lower airways, with renal development occurring later (Frankel et al., 2002). Since all three clinical features are only concurrently present in 16% of patients, other criteria are used to establish the diagnosis (Carlson & Chen, 2006). The Chapel Hill Consensus Conference (CHCC) defined WG as necrotizing vasculitis of the small to medium size vessels and granulomatous inflammation of the respiratory tract (Jennette et al., 1994). The documentation of granulomas does not necessarily require histology, but can rather be made using non-invasive techniques such as radiology (Jennette et al., 1994). The CHCC recognized, however, that the broad definition they used to classify WG left significant overlap between WG and microscopic polyangiitis (Jennette et al., 1994). The American College of Rheumatology (ACR) criteria for diagnosis requires two or more of the following: nasal or oral inflammation, chest x-ray showing nodules, infiltrates, or cavities, microscopic hematuria, and/or granulomatous inflammation on biopsy (Carlson et al., 2005). The positive predictive value of the ACR criteria for diagnosing WG ranges from 25-40% (Rae et al., 1998). Typical laboratory findings include a positive C-ANCA in 75-80% of patients (Fiorentino, 2003). WG is highly fatal, with a one year mortality rate of greater than 80% in untreated patients (Chen & Carlson, 2008). Relapse within 5 years occurs in 50% of patients (Carlson & Chen, 2006).

A limited form of WG which typically involves younger patients is characterized by no or minimal renal dysfunction, limited pulmonary involvement, and no critical organ involvement (i.e., gastrointestinal, ocular, or central nervous system) exists (Carlson & Chen, 2006). The cutaneous presentation is usually limited to purpura or ulcers (Carlson & Chen, 2006).

Cutaneous lesions are found in 50% of patients but may be the presenting symptoms in up to 10% of cases (Chen & Carlson, 2008). Cutaneous manifestations fall into three categories: palpable or non-palpable purpura which reflects a small vessel vasculitis; ulcers or digital infarcts secondary to small to medium sized vessel vasculitis; or polymorphic lesions including rheumatoid like nodules over the extensor surfaces, urticaria, vesiculobullous lesions, gingival hyperplasia, or ulcers like those seen in pyoderma gangrenosum, resulting from extravascular granulomas (Carlson, 2010). Other dermatological manifestations include petechiae, bullae, and erythema (Daoud et al., 1994). Mucosal ulcerations, xanthomas, and livedo reticularis can also be seen (Francès et al., 1994). A larger, suppurative ulceration involving the entire orbit and zygoma has been reported in a patient with limited WG (Bull et al., 1993). Hemorrhagic bullous plaques and erythematous pustules reminiscent of Sweet's syndrome have been described (Gürses et al., 2000).

Four histological patterns can be seen on skin biopsies: (1) Leukocytoclastic vasculitis (LCV) characterized by necrotizing, neutrophilic vasculitis of small to medium sized dermal blood vessels; (2) Palisading granulomas with a central core of basophilic collagen surrounded by histiocytes and neutrophils reminiscent of granulomas seen in Churg-Strauss syndrome; (3) Granulomatous vasculitis with perivascular and periadnexal lymphohistiocytic granulomatous infiltrate and giant cells within the walls of muscular vessels of the subcutis; and (4) Perivascular and periadnexal infiltration of granulomas composed of large, atypical lymphocytes (see Figure 13) (Hu et al., 1977). Other non-specific histological findings include fibrin deposition within the lumen of and surrounding blood vessels, extravasation of red blood cells, endothelial cell swelling, and nuclear debris (Barksdale et al., 1995). Histological findings in patients with WG but without cutaneous vasculitis include foreign body giant cell reaction, fibrosis, hemorrhage, pseudoepitheliomatous hyperplasia, and interstitial eosinophilia (Carlson & Chen, 2006). Epidermal changes are rarely seen and include bulla formation and epidermal necrosis (Daoud et al., 1994). Biopsies of cutaneous lesions from patients with limited WG will often show granulomatous dermatitis but will seldom show vasculitis (Carlson & Chen, 2006).

Patients presenting with necrotizing vasculitis or granulomas composed of lymphocytes have a higher mortality rate than those presenting with palisading granulomas or granulomatous vasculitis (Hu et al., 1977). The cutaneous pathology correlates with the presence of systemic disease, specifically with respect to articular and renal involvement (Francès et al., 1994). Patients presenting with LCV are more likely to have concurrent musculoskeletal and renal involvement and a more rapidly progressive disease course when compared to patients without cutaneous manifestations and are more likely to, over time, develop renal, musculoskeletal, and ocular manifestations when compared to patients with granulomatous dermatitis (Barksdale et al., 1995).

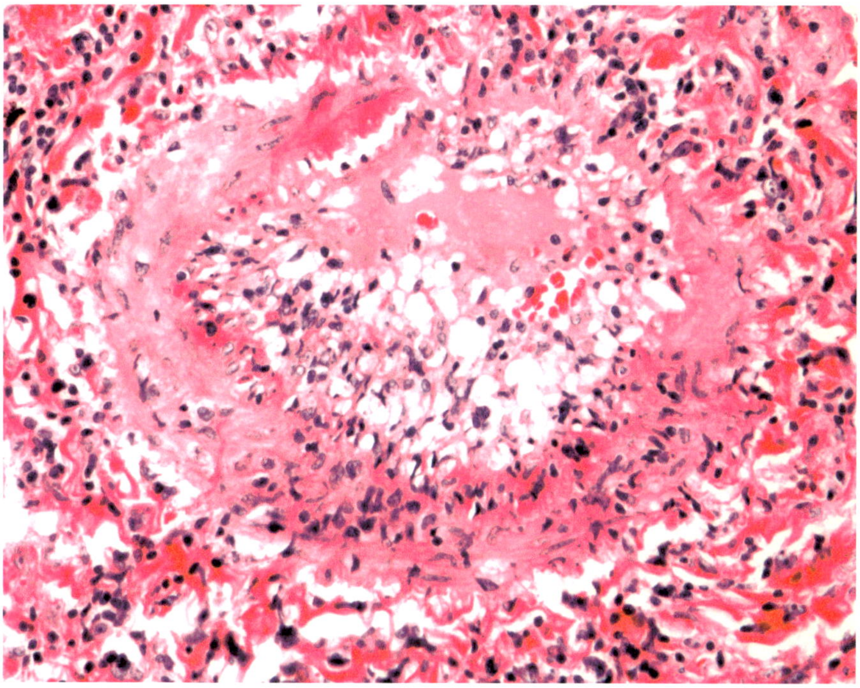

Fig. 13. Wegener's Granulomatosis. Granulomatous and necrotizing vasculitis can be seen in this section of pulmonary artery (H&E, 200x).

While direct immunofluorescence typically fails to demonstrate immunoglobulin or complement deposition on renal biopsies, skin biopsies frequently show perivascular deposits of IgG, IgM, IgA, and C3 in subepidermal and dermal vessels (Brons et al., 2001). In patients who have had a relapse of WG, immunoglobulin deposits can be seen along the basement membrane and within the dermis (Brons et al., 2001).

2.2.3 Microscopic polyangiitis (microscopic polyarteritis)

Microscopic polyangiitis (MPA) is a systemic neutrophilic vasculitis of small vessels (Carlson, 2010). Men are slightly more affected then women and the average age of onset is 50 years (Guillevin et al., 1999). The major systemic finding includes rapidly progressive focal segmental necrotizing glomerulonephritis; pulmonary hemorrhage, skin involvement, and antibodies to p-ANCA are also frequently present (Frankel et al., 2002). A prodromal phase consisting of weight loss, fatigue, fevers, arthralgias, and myalgias is often present months to years before the acute onset of the disease (Fiorentino, 2003). Drugs (specifically antibiotics), hepatitis B, streptococcal infection, and neoplasia have all been implicated as inciting factors in MPA (Savage et al., 1985). The overall mortality rate for MPA is 32%, similar to polyarteritis nodosa (PAN), Wegener's granulomatosis (WG), and Churg-Strauss syndrome (CSS), however, relapses are more frequent in MPA than seen in the other vasculitis syndromes (Guillevin et al., 1999). Since the histologic features of MPA are similar and in some instances indistinguishable from WG and CSS, the following criteria have been suggested for diagnosis: 1) no evidence of granulomatous inflammation (either by histology or radiology), 2) neutrophilic vasculitis of small vessels and/or glomerulonephritis without immune complex deposition, and 3) involvement of two or more organ systems as documented by biopsy or other laboratory or radiological markers (i.e., proteinuria, hematuria) (Chen & Carlson, 2008).

Up to 15% of patients with MPA will present with skin disease and 65% or less will develop skin disease throughout the course of their illness (Carlson & Chen, 2006). The most common cutaneous presentation is palpable purpura and petechiae (Seishima et al., 2004). Other manifestations include splinter hemorrhages, nodules, palmar erythema, livedo, urticaria, hemorrhagic bullae, infarcts, facial edema, annular purpura, ulcers, and telangiectases (Carlson & Chen, 2006). One case of MPA reported in a patient with palpable purpura, myalgias, anorexia, and synovitis but no evidence of pulmonary or renal involvement suggests that a cutaneous limited variant of MPA may exist (Irvine et al., 1997).

While a wide spectrum of pathologic changes can be seen, the classic histologic features of MPA on skin biopsy include a neutrophilic vasculitis of small vessels in the upper to mid-dermis and subcutis (Carlson & Chen, 2006). Rarely medium sized vessels can be involved (Lhote et al., 1998). Other findings on the histologic continuum of MPA include lymphocytic perivascular infiltration in the upper dermis, mixed lymphocytic and neutrophilic perivascular infiltration in the mid to deep dermis, and mixed lymphocytic and histiocytic perivascular infiltration in the mid dermis (Seishima et al., 2004). Other non-specific findings of leukocytoclastic vasculitis similar to those seen in cutaneous leukocytoclastic angiitis (CLA) include fibrinoid necrosis and leukocytoclasis (Homas et al., 1992). The clinical appearance of livedo racemosa presents histologically as a vasculitis affecting deep dermal and subcutaneous vessels and a deep incisional biopsy is indicated in these patients to ensure that the subcutis is sampled (Nagai et al., 2009). Rarely patients can present with oral ulcerations which will also reveal a small vessel vasculitis on histologic examination (Savage et al., 1985). A unique histologic finding in MPA is the presence of active vasculitis, healed vessels, and unaffected vessels in the same tissue biopsy (Lhote et al., 1998).

Small vessel vasculitis is diagnostic of MPA and excludes the diagnosis of PAN, even if medium sized vessels are involved (Lhote et al., 1998). Further, vascular nephropathy is the common renal finding in PAN whereas MPA is characterized by rapidly progressive focal segmental necrotizing glomerulonephritis (Lhote et al., 1998). WG is another small vessel vasculitis similar to MPA, however, granulomatous inflammation characteristic of WG is absent in MPA (Lhote et al., 1998). Absence of immunoglobulin deposition on direct immunofluorescence distinguishes MPA from CLA (Carlson & Chen, 2006).

2.2.4 Septic vasculitis

Approximately 22% of all cases of cutaneous vasculitis are associated with an infectious etiology (viruses, bacteria, fungi, protozoa, and helminthes) (Chen & Carlson, 2008). Organisms that have been implicated include *Neisseria meningitides, Neisseria gonnorhoeae, Pseudomonas, Staphylococcus aureus, Hemophilus influenzae, Streptococcus, and Rickettsia* (Carlson & Chen, 2006).

Cutaneous findings include hemorrhagic petechiae, pustular purpura, vesicles, bullae, erythematous macules, and nodules surrounded by pustules (Carlson & Chen, 2006). Patients with chronic gonococcemia and chronic meningococcemia typically present with petechiae surrounded by a rim of erythematous vesicles and pustules with a necrotic surface on the extremities, particularly acral surfaces (Chen & Carlson, 2008).

Biopsy reveals a mixed small and medium sized vessel neutrophilic vasculitis of deep dermal and subcutaneous vessels (see Figure 14) (Chen & Carlson, 2008). Vessel occlusion with thrombi composed of platelets and red blood cells is also seen (Sotto et al., 1976). As compared to conventional small vessel neutrophilic vasculitis, septic vasculitis has scant perivascular fibrin and fibrin thrombi and little to no nuclear debris (Carlson, 2010). Arteriolar involvement, hemorrhage, and subepidermal and intraepidermal pustules help distinguish septic vasculitis from cutaneous leukocytoclastic angiitis (Shapiro et al., 1973). Epidermal changes include edema, intra-epidermal or subcorneal pustules, and epidermal necrosis (Shapiro et al., 1973). Gram stain is typically negative in septic vasculitis, however, gram negative rods can be seen within the cytoplasm of neutrophils, within endothelial cells, and admixed with extravasated red blood cells in acute meningococcemia (Sotto et al., 1976). Gram negative diplococci can be isolated in gonococcemia if there is a high bacterial load and if lesions are biopsied early (Ackerman et al., 1965). Deposition of IgG, IgM, IgA, complement, and fibrinogen can be seen on direct immunofluorescence in acute meningococcemia (Sotto et al., 1976).

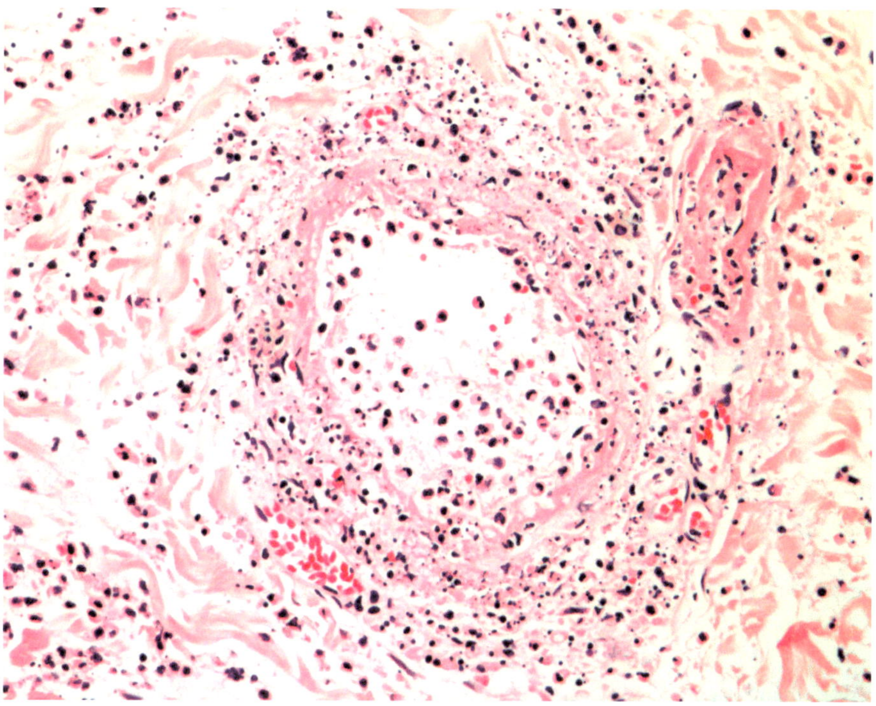

Fig. 14. Septic Vasculitis. Note the distinct neutrophilia and abundant karyorrhectic debris and near complete destruction of the vessel wall (H&E, 200x).

2.2.5 Behçet's disease

Behçet's disease (BD) is a chronic inflammatory disease characterized by oral and genital ulcers, arthralgias, gastrointestinal symptoms, and central nervous system involvement (Chen et al., 1997). Cutaneous manifestations include erythema nodosum like nodules, follicular lesions, or papulopustular lesions or rarely can include palpable purpura, hemorrhagic bullae, erythema multiforme like lesions, or pyoderma gangrenosum like lesions (Chen et al., 1997).

While BD is typically classified as a neutrophilic dermatosis, recent evidence has suggested that it should rather be categorized as a cutaneous vasculitis (Chen et al., 1997). BD is unique in that it involves the entire spectrum of blood vessels, ranging from capillaries to the aorta (Carlson & Chen, 2006). Biopsy reveals a neutrophilic, and rarely a lymphocytic, vasculitis of medium sized vessels in the subcutis and venules throughout the dermis and subcutis (Chen et al., 1997). Biopsy of erythema nodosum like lesions show a subcutaneous thrombophlebitis with a lymphocytic vasculitis in the overlying dermis (Carlson & Chen, 2006). Fibrinoid necrosis, nuclear dust, panniculitis, venulitis in the dermis and subcutis, and necrotizing venulitis can also be seen (Chen et al., 1997). Direct immunofluorescence rarely shows deposition of IgA, IgM, and/or complement (C3 or C1q) (Chen et al., 1997).

3. Medium sized vessel vasculitis

3.1 Polyarteritis nodosa

Polyarteritis nodosa (PAN) is a relatively rare vasculitis of medium sized vessels which presents equally in men and women between the ages of 40 to 60 years (Carlson & Chen, 2007). While the etiology in most cases of PAN is unknown, there is a strong association with hepatitis B virus (Frankel et al., 2002). Patients may present with a wide range of constitutional symptoms including fever, weight loss, arthralgias, muscle wasting, abdominal pain (usually as a result of bowel infarction and perforation), mononeuritis multiplex, hypertension, orchitis, and congestive heart failure (Colmegna & Maldonado-Cocco, 2005). Renal manifestations in PAN typically include a primary vascular nephropathy presenting as multiple aneurysms in branches of the renal artery which leads to hypertension and rare pulmonary involvement, in contrast to Wegener's granulomatosis and microscopic polyangiitis which presents with glomerulonephritis and frequent pulmonary manifestations (Frankel et al., 2002; Colmegna & Maldonado-Cocco, 2005).

Cutaneous manifestations occur in 20-50% of patients with classic PAN and include palpable purpura, while this is a manifestation of small vessel vasculitis, it does not exclude the diagnosis of PAN (Fiorentino, 2003). Other cutaneous findings indicative of medium sized vessel vasculitis include livedo reticularis, ulcers, and subcutaneous nodules (Fiorentino, 2003). Rare findings include ecchymosis, gangrene, and urticaria (Colmegna & Maldonado-Cocco, 2005).

The classic histologic description of PAN requires the presence of a necrotizing vasculitis in medium sized vessels (see Figure 15) (Colmegna & Maldonado-Cocco, 2005). Four stages of histologic findings in PAN have been identified: degenerative, acute inflammatory, granulation tissue, and healed end-stage (Arkin, 1930). The degenerative stage shows destructive coagulative necrosis of the media, fibrinous exudates surroundings the internal elastic lamina, neutrophilic infiltration, and partial destruction of the internal and external elastic lamina (Arkin, 1930). The acute inflammatory stage is characterized by infiltration of neutrophils, lymphocytes, and eosinophils, complete destruction of the internal elastic lamina, fibrinous exudates extending from the intima to the adventitia with complete destruction of the media, fibroblastic proliferation and edematous changes of the surrounding connective tissue, and total obliteration of the vessel lumen with fibrin thrombi (Arkin, 1930). In the granulation tissue stage, neutrophils are replaced by increasing numbers of lymphocytes, marked granulation tissue that replaces the media and extends into the adventitia and can invade through defects in the internal elastic lamina into the vessel lumen, and prolific intimal thickening (Arkin, 1930). The final stage, healed granulation tissue stage, is characterized by acellular scar tissue replacing the arterial wall and perivascular fibroblastic proliferation (Arkin, 1930).

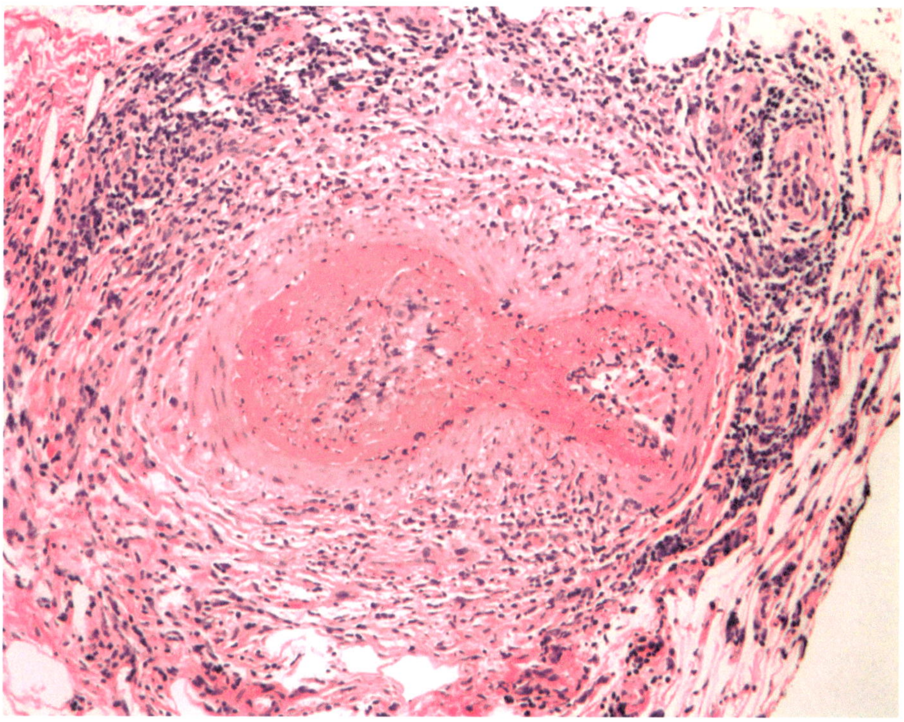

Fig. 15. Polyarteritis Nodosa. Necrotizing vasculitis in a medium sized vessel (H&E, 100x).

When an ulcerated lesion is present, a biopsy including adequate subcutis central to the ulcer border is essential to optimize the diagnostic yield (Ricotti et al., 2007). Biopsy of ulcerated lesions will demonstrate a vasculitis of medium sized vessels at the dermal subcutaneous junction with associated neutrophilic infiltration, leukocytoclasia, and endothelial swelling with overlying dermal fibrosis and necrosis and epidermal ulceration

(Ricotti et al., 2007). Lesions which present as subcutaneous nodules show a neutrophilic vasculitis of medium sized muscular vessels with a predilection for areas where arteries bifurcate (Carlson & Chen, 2007).

3.1.1 Cutaneous polyarteritis nodosa

Cutaneous polyarteritis nodosa (CPAN) is a limited form of PAN which presents with cutaneous findings, fever, myalgias, arthralgias, and peripheral neuropathy, but no other systemic symptoms (Fiorentino, 2003). It typically affects women more then men between the ages of 20 to 40 years (Chen & Carlson, 2008). Classic cutaneous manifestations include tender subcutaneous nodules which are usually limited to the lower extremities and buttocks (Carlson & Chen, 2007). Ulcerations with surrounding irregular livedo reticularis in a "burst" pattern are common in CPAN (Morgan & Schwartz, 2010). Other cutaneous findings include petechiae, purpura, necrosis, and gangrene (Morgan & Schwartz, 2010). Ulcerated lesions are more frequently found in patients with associated neuropathy and rare reports exist of these patients eventually progressing to classic PAN (Chen & Carlson, 2008). Patients with mononeuritis multiplex may also present with atrophie blanche without evidence of venous insufficiency and/or thrombophilia (Carlson & Chen, 2007). While patients with classic PAN can present with similar cutaneous findings, the lack of systemic multi-organ involvement in CPAN is an essential distinction between the two diseases (Morgan & Schwartz, 2010).

The clinical severity of CPAN can be graded into three classes: class I or mild disease presents with subcutaneous nodules, livedo reticularis, and/or mild polyneuropathy; class II or severe disease presents with livedo, painful ulcerations, sensory neuropathy, fever, malaise, and arthralgia; and class III or progressive systemic disease presents with fever, malaise, arthralgia, deep ulcerations, necrotizing livedo, acral gangrene, foot drop mononeuropathy multiplex, worsening musculoskeletal symptoms, positive autoimmune serology, and eventual systemic involvement (Chen & Carlson, 2008).

Similar to classic PAN, the etiology of CPAN is usually unknown although there is an association between CPAN and Group A β hemolytic Streptococcus, hepatitis B (although this association is not as well documented in CPAN as it is in classic PAN), hepatitis C, parvovirus B-19, tuberculosis, and minocycline (Morgan & Schwartz, 2010).

The traditional description of CPAN on deep skin biopsy is a neutrophilic, necrotizing vasculitis of small to medium sized muscular arteries at the dermal-subcutaneous junction (Morgan & Schwartz, 2010). Similar to classic PAN, four stages of histologic findings in CPAN have been described;, however, the progression of arterial destruction is different in CPAN than classic PAN. The acute stage is characterized by a neutrophilic vasculitis of small to medium sized blood vessels and the dermal subcutaneous junction, damage to endothelial cells, fibrin thrombi within the vascular lumen, and no disruption of the internal elastic lamina (Ishibashi & Chen, 2008). The subacute stage shows focal disruption of the internal elastic lamina with fibrinoid necrosis of the media adjacent to the disruption, a targetoid appearance of vessels caused by subendothelial fibrinoid necrosis lined by an inner layer of intact endothelial cells and surrounded by the internal elastic lamina, and infiltration of the vessel wall by neutrophils, lymphocytes, and histiocytes (Ishibashi & Chen, 2008). The reparative stage shows a shift in the inflammatory cells to mostly lymphocytes and histiocytes, complete occlusion of the vascular lumen by fibrin thrombi, and fibroblastic proliferation (Morgan & Schwartz, 2010). The healed stage shows discernible thickening of the intima with a scant inflammatory infiltrate surrounding the artery and perivascular neovascularization (Ishibashi & Chen, 2008). Direct immunofluorescence frequently reveals IgM and C3 deposition in and around deep dermal vessels, however, interestingly, IgG and IgA are almost universally negative in all cases of CPAN (Diaz-Perez et al., 1980). Since the histologic features diagnostic of CPAN, including neutrophilic vasculitis of medium sized vessels and the dermal subcutaneous junction, are segmental and focal, repeated and deeper biopsies followed by serial sectioning may be required for diagnosis (Chen & Carlson, 2008).

The main diagnostic challenge for clinicians and dermatopathologists is the distinction between CPAN and thrombophlebitis. Thrombophlebitis is a vasculitis involving veins and venules while CPAN affects arteries (Chen, 2010). The distinction between veins and arteries is an important one in differentiating these two conditions. Features that histologically define an artery include a round vessel with a concentric, continuous wreath of smooth muscle fibers and a band of wavy elastic fibers between the intimal and medial layers of the vessel wall known as the internal elastic lamina while features of a vein include oval vessels with collagen admixed with smooth muscle and elastic fibers, but lacks an internal elastic lamina (Carlson, 2010). The presence or absence of an internal elastic lamina has long been cited by pathology textbooks as the distinction between arteries and veins, however, this distinction is blurred by increased hydrostatic pressure in the lower extremities which causes hypertrophy of the muscular layer and proliferation of elastic fibers in veins which can resemble the muscular layer and internal elastic lamina of arteries (Dalton et al., 2006). In fact, up to 44% of veins demonstrate an internal elastic lamina-like layer (Dalton et al., 2006). Three possible solutions have been suggested to avoid this diagnostic pitfall. The muscular pattern in arteries demonstrates a continuous wreath of smooth muscle while veins show bundles of smooth muscle admixed with collagen (Dalton et al., 2006). Next, the internal elastic lamina of an artery has an even thickness while the internal elastic lamina-like layer seen in veins is thinner and uneven in thickness (Chen, 2010). It is important to note, however, that the internal elastic lamina seen in arteries can lose its regular wavy appearance and thickness during the healing stages of arteritis (Ishiguro & Kawashima, 2010). Perhaps the most helpful tool in the histological distinction of a vein and artery is the use of an elastic stain which will demonstrate numerous elastic fibers in the muscular layers of a vein, but only scant fibers in the muscular layers of an artery (Chen, 2010).

3.2 Kawasaki disease (also known as mucocutaneous lymph node syndrome)

Kawasaki disease typically occurs in children less than four years of age and is defined clinically as a fever of 1-2 weeks duration which is unresponsive to antibiotics in conjunction with a constellation of symptoms including non-exudative conjunctivitis, oral manifestations (dry lips, strawberry tongue, etc.), erythematous and edematous palms and soles, polymorphous rash, and cervical lymphadenopathy (Hirose & Hamashima, 1978; Weston & Huff, 1981). Presence of at least five of the previously mentioned symptoms or four of the symptoms plus evidence of coronary artery aneurysm should be identified to diagnose Kawasaki disease (Kimura et al., 1988). The most feared complication of Kawasaki disease is a coronary artery aneurysm which develops in 20-25% of untreated patients and is the leading cause of acquired heart disease in children (Gedalia & Cuchacovich, 2009).

Cutaneous changes include edema and redness of the palms and soles which evolves into a macular eruption beginning on the extremities and spreading to the trunk (Kawasaki et al., 1974). The eruption then progresses into a morbilliform, scarlatiniform, or multiform eruption (Kawasaki et al., 1974). The morbilliform lesions consist of generalized macular and papular lesions which are clinically indistinguishable from a viral exanthem (Weston & Huff, 1981). The scarlantiniform eruption mimics the rash seen in scarlet fever or a drug eruption (Weston & Huff, 1981). The multiform lesions are typically targetoid lesions which do not progress to form blisters and can resemble erythema multiforme (Weston & Huff, 1981). Rarely patients can present with pustules superimposed on erythema (Kimura et al., 1988). Regardless of the initial presentation of the eruption, all patients advance to desquamation beginning in the periungual regions and progressing centrally to the trunk, a finding characteristic of but not unique to Kawasaki disease (Kawasaki et al., 1974).

Skin biopsies reveal a superficial perivascular dermatitis characterized by dermal edema and mild perivascular lymphocytic inflammation (Weston & Huff, 1981). Papillary edema and minimal extravasation of red blood cells can be seen if the exanthem is biopsied within six days of onset (Hirose & Hamashima, 1978). Deposition of fibrinoid material and focal endothelial cell necrosis has been reported (Hirose & Hamashima, 1978). Vessel changes are most prominent in the medium sized vessel of the subcutis (Carlson & Chen, 2007). The pustular lesions show intraepidermal neutrophilic pustules, epidermal hyperplasia, superficial perivascular infiltrate with lymphocytes, neutrophils, and histiocytes, and neutrophilic inflammation around intraepidermal eccrine ducts (Kimura et al., 1988). Other diseases which present histologically with intraepidermal pustules such as pustular psoriasis, subcorneal pustular dermatosis, staphylococcal scalded skin syndrome, and milia should also be considered in the differential diagnosis (Kimura et al., 1988). Rare cases of psoriasiform-like hyperkeratosis have been reported (Passeron et al., 2002).

3.3 Nodular vasculitis (also known as erythema induratum or erythema induratum of bazin)

Nodular vasculitis (NV) is characterized by tender, indurated plaques on the calves of young to middle aged women and is associated with *Mycobacterium tuberculosis* (Schneider JW, 1997). The prodromal phase of NV occurs 1-3 weeks prior to the onset of lesions and consists of fever, malaise, arthritis, and arthralgias (Gilchrist & Patterson, 2010). NV presents as reoccurring crops of lesions lasting 2 weeks which heal with residual scarring and hyperpigmentation (Segura et al., 2008).

Histologically, lobular panniculitis with necrotizing vasculitis that can be neutrophilic, lymphocytic, or granulomatous, is seen (see Figure 16) (Carlson & Chen, 2007). Early lesions show neutrophilic infiltration between fat lobules while established lesions show granulomatous infiltration of lobules (Segura et al., 2008). Two types of lesions can be seen. Type I is characterized by focal panniculitis and neutrophilic vasculitis of muscular vessels (Schneider & Jordaan, 1997). Type II lesions are characterized by diffuse septolobular panniculitis with numerous foci of neutrophilic small and medium sized vessel vasculitis (Schneider & Jordaan, 1997). Neutrophilic septal venulitis and arteritis is also common (Segura et al., 2008). Caseous necrosis can also be seen extending to the epidermal surface (Segura et al., 2008).

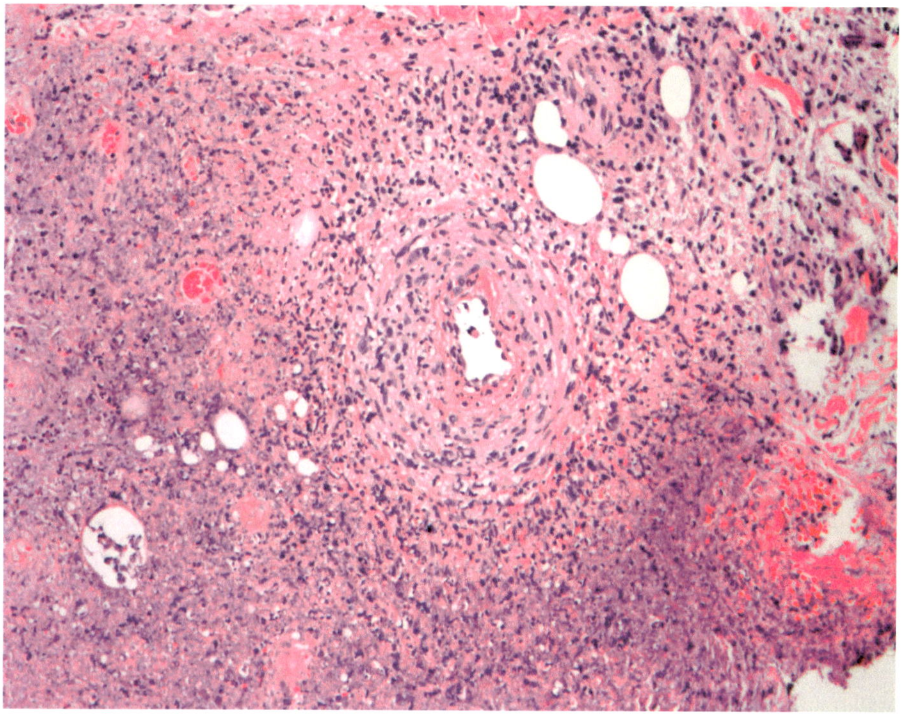

Fig. 16. Nodular Vasculitis. Suppurative necrosis of the subcutaneous fat surrounds this deep, inflamed vessel (H&E, 100x).

4. Large vessel vasculitis

4.1 Takayasu arteritis

Takayasu arteritis (TA) is a large vessel granulomatous arteritis which typically involves the aorta and its main branches (Carlson & Chen, 2007). Patients are more commonly female in their second to third decade of life (Gedalia & Cuchacovich, 2009). The initial symptoms are nonspecific and usually consist of fever, fatigue, myalgias, arthralgias, and weight loss (Frankel et al., 2002). The most common clinical presentation is arterial hypertension, however, patients can also present with cardiac failure, bruits, and pulselessness (Gedalia & Cuchacovich, 2009). Other symptoms resulting from vessel occlusion and ischemia include claudication, syncope, headache, and visual disturbances (Frankel et al., 2002). Stenosis or aneurysm of the aorta or its major branches seen on angiography is the gold standard for the diagnosis of TA (Gedalia & Cuchacovich, 2009).

Cutaneous involvement is rare in TA, occurring in 8-28% of patients (Carlson & Chen, 2007). Clinical findings include erythematous nodules, pyoderma gangrenosum-like ulcer, erythema nodosum, erythema induratum, and purpura (Perniciaro et al., 1987).

During the acute phase of TA, the characteristic findings of granulomatous arteritis with transmural inflammation can be seen in the aorta or its branches (Lie, 1990). The morphologic findings on skin biopsy are generally non-specific and include granulomatous vasculitis, necrotizing vasculitis of the deep dermal medium sized vessels, and septal and lobular panniculitis with or without vasculitis (Pascual-Lòpez et al., 2004).

4.2 Giant cell arteritis (also known as temporal arteritis)

Giant cell arteritis (GCA) is a granulomatous vasculitis of large arteries, particularly affecting the branches of the external carotid artery (Tsianakas et al., 2009). The prevalence is higher in women, the elderly, Caucasians, and patients with polymyalgia rheumatica (Chen & Carlson, 2008). Clinical symptoms are usually due to ischemia secondary to endarteritis obliterans and include headache, jaw cladication, and visual and neurological problems (Carlson & Chen, 2007). Timely diagnosis is imperative since significant morbidity, including visual loss, and even death may occur if treatment is delayed (Goldberg et al., 1987).

Cutaneous findings in GCA are rare, presenting in less than 1% of cases, and include scalp tenderness, loss or decrease in temporal pulse, scalp necrosis, and scalp blanching (Chen & Carlson, 2008). Erythema, ecchymoses, purpura, ulceration, gangrene, urticaria, erythema nodosum, and hyperpigmentation on the lower extremities have also been reported (Goldberg et al., 1987). Scalp necrosis is associated with increased risk of vision loss and carries a higher mortality rate (Tsianakas et al., 2009).

The diagnostic features of GCA on temporal artery biopsy are segmental inflammation of the artery and infiltration of the media, adventitia, and internal elastic lamina by lymphocytes, neutrophils, and multinucleated giant cells (see Figures 17 and 18) (Goldberg et al., 1987). The segmental arterial involvement makes histologic diagnosis a challenge.

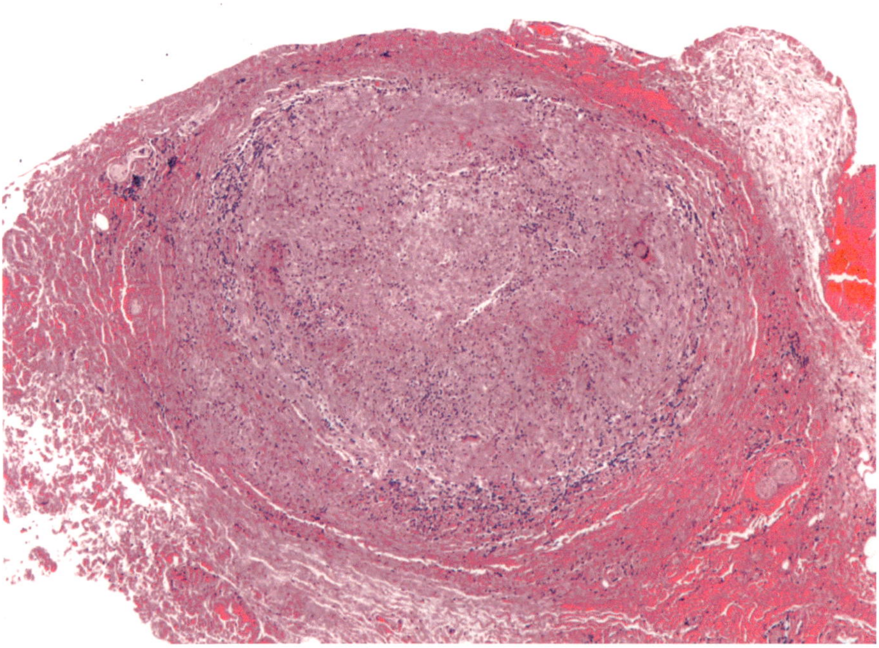

Fig. 17. Giant Cell (Temporal) Arteritis. A dense granulomatous infiltrate effaces the elastic artery. The intima and media are particularly affected and giant cells may be conspicuous (H&E, 40x).

Lack of histologic evidence of GCA on temporal artery biopsy should not delay treatment in a patient clinically suspected of having GCA (Lie, 1990). Elastophagocytosis is a common finding (Carlson & Chen, 2007). Granulomatous infiltration of medium sized muscular vessels in the deep dermis or subcutaneous tissue is typically seen on skin biopsy (Chen & Carlson, 2008). Healing lesions are characterized by segmental stenosis and loss of the elastic lamina as well as myxomatous stromal replacement of the vessel wall (Carlson & Chen, 2007). The lack of inflammation seen in completely healed lesions makes the distinction between GCA and atherosclerosis impossible (Carlson & Chen, 2007).

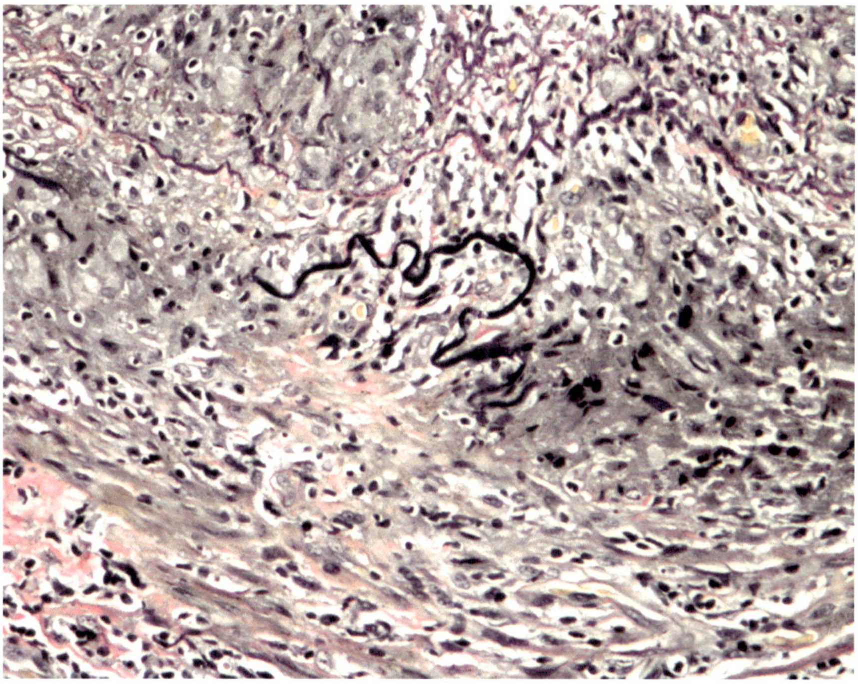

Fig. 18. Giant cell arteritis. Staining for elastin fibers demonstrates fragmentation of the internal elastic lamina (elastic von Giesen stain, 200x).

5. Conclusion

Vasculitis is a broad, poorly defined category of diseases. The clinical presentation, progression of disease, and treatment vary as widely as the diseases themselves. Often times it is the compilation of clinical, laboratory, and pathologic findings which aid in formulating the diagnosis.

6. References

Aboobaker J. & Greaves M. (1986). Urticarial vasculitis. *Clin Exp Dermatol*, Vol. 11, No. 5, (September 1986), pp. 436-444

Ackerman A., Miller R., & Shapiro L. (1965). Gonococcemia and its cutaneous manifestations. *Arch Dermat*, Vol. 91, (March 1965), pp. 227-232

Akosa A. & Lampert I. (1991). The sweat gland in cutaneous vasculitis. *Histopathology*, Vol. 18, No. 6, (June 1991), pp. 553-558.

Alexander E. & Provost T. (1987). Sjögren's syndrome. Association of cutaneous vasculitis with central nervous system disease. *Arch Dermatol*, Vol. 123, No. 6, (June 1987), pp. 801-810

Arkin A. (1930). A clinical and pathological study of periarteritis nodosa: a report of five cases, one histologically healed. *Am J Pathol*, Vol. 6, No. 4, (July 1930), pp. 401-426

Bahrami S., Malone J., Webb K., & Callen J. (2006). Tissue eosinophilia as an indicator of drug-induced cutaneous small-vessel vasculitis. *Arch Dermatol*, Vol. 142, No. 2, (February 2006), pp. 155-161

Barksdale S., Hallahan C., Kerr G., Fauci A., Stern J., & Travis W. (1995). Cutaneous pathology in Wegener's granulomatosis. A clinicopathologic study of 75 biopsies in 46 patients. *Am J Surg Pathol*, Vol. 19, No. 2, (February 1995), pp. 161-172

Barnadas M., Pérez E., Gich I., Llovet J., Ballarín J., Calero F., Facundo C., & Alomar A. (2004). Diagnostic, prognostic and pathogenic value of the direct immunofluorescence test in cutaneous leukocytoclastic vasculitis. *Int J Dermatol*, Vol. 43, No. 1, (January 2004), pp. 19-26

Barnadas M., Curell R., & Alomar A. (2006). Direct immunofluorescence in granuloma faciale: a case report and review of the literature. *J Cutan Pathol*, Vol. 33, No. 7, (July 2006), pp. 508-511

Black A. (1999). Urticarial vasculitis. *Clinics in Dermatol*, Vol. 17, No. 5, (September-October 1999), pp. 565-569

Brons R., de Jong M., de Boer N., Stegeman C., Kallenberg C., & Cohen Tervaert J. (2001). Detection of immune deposits in skin lesions of patients with Wegener's granulomatosis. *Ann Rheum Dis*, Vol. 60, No. 12, (December 2001), pp. 1097-1102

Bull R., Marsden R., Cook M., & Ryan J. (1993). Fatal facial ulceration. *Clin Exp Dermatol*, Vol. 18, No. 4, (July 1993), pp. 356-359

Carlson J. (2010). The histological assessment of cutaneous vasculitis. *Histopathology*, Vol. 56, No. 1, (January 2010), pp 3-23

Carlson J. & Chen K. (2006). Cutaneous vasculitis update: small vessel neutrophilic vasculitis syndromes. *Am J Dermatopathol*, Vol. 28, No. 6, (December 2006), pp. 486-506

Carlson J., Ng B., & Chen K. (2005). Cutaneous vasculitis update: diagnostic criteria, classification, epidemiology, etiology, pathogenesis, evaluation and prognosis. *Am J Dermatopathol*, Vol. 27, No. 6, (December 2005), pp. 504-528

Carlson J. & Chen K. (2007). Cutaneous vasculitis update: neutrophilic muscular vessel and eosinophilic, granulomatous, and lymphocytic vasculitis syndromes. *Am J Dermatopathol*, Vol. 29, No. 1, (February 2007), pp. 32-43

Chen K., Kawahara Y., Miyakawa S., & Nishikawa T. (1997). Cutaneous vasculitis in Behçet's disease: a clinical and histopathologic study of 20 patients. *J Am Acad Dermatol*, Vol. 36 No. 5, (May 1997), pp. 689-696

Chen K., Toyohara A., Suzuki A., & Miyakawa S. (2002). Clinical and histopathological spectrum of cutaneous vasculitis in rheumatoid arthritis. *Br J Dermatol*, Vol. 147, No. 5, (November 2002), pp. 905-913

Chen K., Sakamoto M., Ikemoto K., Abe R., & Shimizu H. (2007). Granulomatous arteritis in cutaneous lesions of Churg-Strauss syndrome. *J Cutan Pathol*, Vol. 34, No. 4, (April 2007), pp. 330-337

Chen K. & Carlson J. (2008). Clinical approach to cutaneous vasculitis. *Am J Clin Dermatol*, Vol. 9, No. 2, pp. 71-92

Chen K. (2010). The misdiagnosis of superficial thrombophlebitis as cutaneous polyarteritis nodosa: features of the internal elastic lamina and the compact concentric muscular layer as diagnostic pitfalls. *Am J Dermatopathol*, Vol. 32, No. 7, (October 2010), pp. 688-693

Choi J., Ahn I., Lee H., Park C., Lee C., & Ahn H. (2009). A case of Churg-Strauss syndrome. *Ann Dermatol*, Vol. 21, No. 2, (May 2009), pp. 213-216

Churg J. & Strauss L. (1951). Allergic granulomatosis, allergic angiitis, and periarteritis nodosa. *Am J Pathol*, Vol. 27, No. 2, (March-April 1951), pp. 277-301

Cohen S., Pittelkow M., & Su W. (1991). Cutaneous manifestations of cryoglobulinemia: clinical and histopathologic study of seventy-two patients. *J Am Acad Dermatol*, Vol. 25, No. 1, (July 1991), pp. 21-27

Colmegna I. & Maldonado-Cocco J. (2005). Polyarteritis nodosa revisited. *Curr Rheumatol Rep*, Vol. 7, No. 4, (August 2005), pp. 288-296

Cuellar M. (2002). Drug induced vasculitis. *Curr Rheumatol Rep*, Vol. 4, No. 1, (February 2002), pp. 55-59

Dalton S., Fillman E., Ferringer T., Tyler W., & Elston D. (2006). Smooth muscle pattern is more reliable than the presence or absence of an internal elastic lamina in distinguishing an artery from a vein. *J Cutan Pathol*, Vol. 33, No. 3, (March 2006), pp. 216-219

Daoud M., Gibson L., DeRemee R., Specks U., el-Azhary R., & Daniel Su W. (1994). Cutaneous Wegener's granulomatosis: clinical, histopathologic, and immunopathologic features of thirty patients. *J Am Acad Dermatol*, Vol. 31, No. 4, (October 1994), pp. 605-612

Davis M., Daoud M., Kirby B., Gibson L., & Rogers R. (1998). Clinicopathologic correlation of hypocomplementemic and normocomplementemic urticarial vasculitis. *J Am Acad Dermatol*, Vol. 38, No. 6, (June 1998), pp. 899-905

Diaz-Perez J., Schroeter A., & Winkelmann R. (1980). Cutaneous periarteritis nodosa: immunofluorescence studies. *Arch Dermatol*, Vol. 116, No. 1, (January 1980), pp. 56-58

Draper N. & Morgan M. (2007). Dermatologic perivascular hemophagocytosis: a report of two cases. *Am J Dermatopathol*, Vol. 29, No. 5, (October 2007), pp. 467-469

Drenkard C., Villa A., Reyes E., Abello M., & Alarcón-Segovia D. (1997). Vasculitis in systemic lupus erythematosus. *Lupus*, Vol. 6, No. 3, (1997), pp. 235-242

Egan C., Taylor T., Meyer L., Petersen M., & Zone J. (1999). IgA1 is the major IgA subclass in cutaneous blood vessels in Henoch-Schonlein purpura. *Br J Dermatol*, Vol. 141, No. 5, (November 1999), pp. 859-862

Fiorentino D. (2003). Cutaneous vasculitis. *J Am Acad Dermatol*, Vol. 48, No. 3, (March 2003), pp. 311-340

Francès C., Huong L., Piette J., Saada V., Boisnic S., Wechsler B., Blétry O., & Godeau P. (1994). Wegener's granulomatosis: dermatological manifestations in 75 cases with clinicopathologic correlation. *Arch Dermatol*, Vol. 130, No. 7, (July 1994), pp. 861-867

Frankel S., Sullivan E., & Brown K. (2002). Vasculitis: Wegener granulomatosis, Churg-Strauss syndrome, microscopic polyangiitis, polyarteritis nodosa, and Takayasu arteritis. *Crit Care Clin*, Vol. 18, No. 4, (October 2002), pp. 855-879

Friedman D. & Wolfsthal S. (2005). Cocaine-induced pseudovasculitis. *Mayo Clin Proc*, Vol. 80, No. 5, (May 2005), pp. 671-673

Gedalia A. & Cuchacovich R. (2009). Systemic vasculitis in childhood. *Curr Rheumatol Rep*, Vol. 11, No. 6, (December 2009), pp. 402-409

Genta M., Genta R., & Cabay C. (2006). Systemic rheumatoid vasculitis: a review. Sem Arthritis Rheum, Vol. 36, No. 2, (October 2006), pp. 88-98

Gilchrist H. & Patterson J. (2010). Erythema nodosum and erythema induratum (nodular vasculitis): diagnosis and management. *Dermatologic Therapy*, Vol. 23, No. 4, (July-August 2010), pp. 320-327

Goldberg J., Lee M., & Sajjad S. (1987). Giant cell arteritis of the skin simulating erythema nodosum. *Ann Rheum Dis*, Vol. 46, No. 9, (September 1987), pp. 706-708

Gorevic P., Kassab H., Levo Y., Kohn R., Meltzer M., Prose P., & Franklin E. (1980). Mixed cryoglobulinemia: clinical aspects and long-term follow-up of 40 patients. *Am J Med*, Vol. 69, No. 2, (August 1980), pp. 287-308

Grunwald M., Avinoach I., Amichai B., & Halevy S. (1997). Leukocytoclastic vasculitis-correlation between different histologic stages and direct immunofluorescence results. *Int J Dermatol*, Vol. 36, No. 5, (May 1997), pp. 349-352

Guillevin L., Durand-Gasselin B., Cevallos R., Gayraud M., Lhote F., Callard P., Amouroux J., Casassus P., & Jarrousse B. (1999). Microscopic polyangiitis: clinical and laboratory findings in eighty-five patients. *Arthritis Rheum*, Vol. 42, No. 3, (March 1999), pp. 421-30

Gürses L., Yücelten D., Cõmert A., Ergun T., & Gürbüz O. (2000). Wegener's granulomatosis presenting as neutrophilic dermatosis: a case report. *Br J Dermatol*, Vol. 143, No. 1, (July 2000), pp. 198-233

Hirose S. & Hamashima Y. (1978). Morphological observations on the vasculitis in the mucocutaneous lymph node syndrome. *Eur J Pediatr*, Vol. 129, No. 1, (August 1978), pp. 17-27

Homas P., David-Bajar K., Fitzpatrick J., West S., & Tribelhorn D. (1992). Microscopic polyarteritis. Report of a case with cutaneous involvement and antimyeloperoxidase antibodies. *Arch Dermatol*, Vol. 128, No. 9, (September 1992), pp. 1223-1228

Hu C., O'Loughlin S., & Winkelmann R. (1977). Cutaneous manifestations of Wegener granulomatosis. *Arch Dermatol*, Vol. 113, No. 2, (February 1977), pp. 175-182

Irvine A., Bruce I., Walsh M., & Bingham E. (1997). Microscopic polyangiitis. Delineation of a cutaneous-limited variant associated with antimyeloperoxidase autoantibody. *Arch Dermatol*, Vol. 133, No. 4, (April 1997), pp. 474-477

Ishibashi M. & Chen K. (2008). A morphological study of evolution of cutaneous polyarteritis nodosa. *Am J Dermatopathol*, Vol. 30, No. 4, (August 2008), pp. 319-326

Ishiguro N. & Kawashima M. (2010). Cutaneous polyarteritis nodosa: a report of 16 cases with clinical and histopathological analysis and a review of the published work. *J Dermatol*, Vol. 37, No. 1, (January 2010), pp. 85-93

Jennette J., Falk R., Andrassy K., Bacon P., Churg J., Gross W., et al. (1994). Nomenclature of systemic vasculitides. Proposal of an international consensus conference. *Arthritis Rheum*, Vol. 37, No. 2, (February 1994), pp. 187-192

Jones R., Bhogal B., Dash A., & Schifferli J. (1983). Urticaria and vasculitis: a continuum of histological and immunopathological changes. *Br J Dermatol*, Vol. 108, No. 6, (June 1983), pp. 695-703

Kapur N., Tympanidis P., Colville C., & Yu R. (2002). Long-term follow-up of a patient with cutaneous vasculitis secondary to mixed cryoglobulinaemia and Hepatitis C virus. *Clin Exp Dermatol*, Vol. 27, No. 2, (March 2002), pp. 37-39

Karremann M., Jordan A., Bell N., Witsch M. & Dürken M. (2009). Acute hemorrhagic edema of infancy: report of 4 cases and review of the current literature. *Clin Pediatr (Phila)*, Vol. 48, No. 3, (Apirl 2009), pp. 2009

Kawasaki T., Kosaki F., Okawa S., Shigematsu I., & Yanagawa H. (1974). A new infantile acute febrile mucocutaneous lymph node syndrome (MLNS) prevailing in Japan. *Pediatrics*, Vol. 54, No. 3, (September 1974), pp. 271-276

Kimuyra W., Miyazawa H., Watanabe K., & Moriya T. (1988). Small pustules in Kawasaki disease: a clinicopathological study of four patients. *Am J Dermatopathol*, Vol. 10, No. 3, (June 1988), pp. 218-223

Lanham J., Elkon K., Pusey C., & Hughes G. (1984). Systemic vasculitis with asthma and eosinophilia: a clinical approach to the Churg-Strauss syndrome. *Medicine (Baltimore)*, Vol. 63, No. 2, (March 1984), pp. 65-81

LeBoit P. & Cockerell C. (1993). Nodular lesions of erythema elevatum diutinum in patients infected with the human immunodeficiency virus. *J Am Acad Dermatol*, Vol. 28, No. 6, (June 1993), pp. 919-922

LeBoit P. (2002). Granuloma faciale. A diagnosis deserving of dignity. *Am J Dermatopathol*, Vol. 24, No. 5, (October 2002), pp. 440-443

LeBoit P. (2005). Dust to dust. *Am J Dermatopathol*, Vol. 27, No. 3, (June, 2005), pp. 277-278

Legrain V., Lejean S., Taieb A., Guillard J., Battin J., & Maleville J. (1991). Infantile acute hemorrhagic edema of the skin: a study of ten cases. *J Am Acad Dermatol*, Vol. 24, No. 1, (January 1991), pp. 17-22

Lhote F., Cohen P., & Guillevin L. (1998). Polyarteritis nodosa, microscopic polyangiitis and Churg-Strauss syndrome. *Lupus*, Vol. 7, No. 4, (1998), pp. 238-258

Lie J. (1990). Illustrated histopathologic classification criteria for selected vasculitis syndromes. American College of Rheumatology Subcommittee on Classification of Vasculitis. *Arthritis Rheum*, Vol. 33, No. 8, (August 1990), pp. 1074-1087

Magro C. & Crowson N. (1999). A clinical and histologic study of 37 cases of immunoglobulin A-associated vasculitis. *Am J Dermatopathol*, Vol. 21, No. 3, (June 1999), pp. 234-240

Magro C. & Crowson A. (2003). The spectrum of cutaneous lesions in rheumatoid arthritis: a clinical and pathological study of 43 patients. *J Cutan Pathol*, Vol. 30, No. 1, (January 2003), pp. 1-10

Marcoval J., Moreno A., & Peyrí J. (2004). Granuloma faciale: a clinicopathological study of 11 cases. *J Am Acad Dermatol*, Vol. 51, No. 2, (August 2004), pp. 269-273

Mehregan D., Hall M., & Gibson L. (1992). Urticarial vasculitis: a histopathologic and clinical review of 72 cases. *J Am Acad Dermatol*, Vol. 26, No. 3, (March 1992), pp. 441-448

Merkel P., Polisson R., Chang Y., Skates S., & Niles J. Prevalence of antineutrophil cytoplasmic antibodies in a large inception cohort of patients with connective tissue disease. *Ann Intern Med*, Vol. 126, No. 11, (June 1997), pp. 866-873

Millard T., Harris A., & MacDonald D. (1999). Acute infantile hemorrhagic oedema. *J Am Acad Dermatol*, Vol. 41, No. 5, (November 1999), pp. 837-839

Morgan A. & Schwartz R. (2010). Cutaneous polyarteritis nodosa: a comprehensive review. *Int J Dermatol*, Vol. 49, No. 7, (July 2010), pp. 750-756

Mullick F., McAllister H., Wagner B., & Fenoglio J. (1979). Drug related vasculitis. Clinicopathologic correlations in 30 patients. *Hum Pathol*, Vol. 10, No. 3, (May 1979), pp. 313-325

Murali N., George R., John G., Chandi S., Jacob M., Jeyaseelan L., Thomas P., & Jacob C. (2002). Problems of classification of Henoch Schonlein purpura: an Indian perspective. *Clin Exp Dermatol*, Vol. 27, No. 4, (June 2002), pp. 260-263

Nagai Y., Hasegawa M., Igarashi N., Tanaka S., Yamanaka M., & Ishikawa O. (2009). Cutaneous manifestations and histological features of microscopic polyangiitis. *Eur J Dermatol*, Vol. 19, No. 1, (January-February 2009), pp. 57-60

Ortonne N., Wechsler J., Bagot M., Grosshans E., & Cribier B. (2005). Granuloma faciale: a clinicopathologic study of 66 patients. *J Am Acad Dermatol*, Vol. 53, No. 6, (December 2005), pp. 1002-1009

Pascual-López M., Hernández-Núñez A., Aragüés-Montañes M., Daudén E., Fraga J., & Garcia-Diez A. (2004). Takayasu's disease with cutaneous involvement. *Dermatology*, Vol. 208, No. 1 (2004), pp. 10-15

Passeron T., Olivier V., Sirvent N., Khalfi A., Boutté P., & Lacour J. (2002). Kawasaki disease with exceptional cutaneous manifestations. *Eur J Pediatr*, Vol 161, No. 4, (April 2002), pp. 228-230

Perniciaro C., Winkelmann R., & Hunder G. (1987). Cutaneous manifestations of Takayasu's arteritis. *J Am Acad Dermatol*, Vol. 17, No. 6, (December 1987), pp. 998-1005

Piette W. & Stone M. (1989). A cutaneous sign of IgA associated small dermal vessel leukocytoclastic vasculitis in adults (Henoch-Schonlein purpura). *Arch Dermatol*, Vol. 125, No. 1, (January 1989), pp. 53-56

Ramos-Casals M., Anaya J., Garcia-Carrasco M., Rosas J., Bove A., Claver G., Diaz L., Herrero C., & Font J. (2004). Cutaneous vasculitis in primary Sjogren syndrome: classification and clinical significance of 52 patients. *Medicine (Baltimore)*, Vol. 83, No. 2, (March 2004), pp. 96-106

Rae J., Allen N., & Pincus T. (1998). Limitations of the 1990 American College of Rheumatology classification criteria in the diagnosis of vasculitis. *Ann Intern Med*, Vol. 129, No. 5, (September 1998), pp. 345-352

Rapoport R., Kozin F., Mackel S., & Jordon R. (1980). Cutaneous vascular immunofluorescence in rheumatoid arthritis. Correlation with circulating immune complexes and vasculitis. Am J Med, Vol. 68, No. 3, (March 1980), pp. 325-331

Ricotti C., Kowalczyk J., Ghersi M., & Nousari C. (2007). The diagnostic yield of histopathologic sampling techniques in PAN-associated cutaneous ulcers. *Arch Dermatol*, Vol. 143, No. 10, (October 2007), pp. 1334-1336

Sais G. & Vidaller A. (2005). Role of direct immunofluorescence test in cutaneous leukocytoclastic vasculitis. *Int J Dermatol*, Vol. 44, No. 11, (November 2005), pp. 970-971.

Sansonno D. & Dammacco F. (2005). Hepatitis C virus, cryoglobulinaemia, and vasculitis: immune complex relations. *Lancet Infect Dis*, Vol. 5, No. 4, (April 2005), pp. 227-236

Savage C., Winearls C., Evans D., Rees A., & Lockwood C. (1985). Microscopic polyarteritis: presentation, pathology and prognosis. *Q J Med*, Vol. 56, No. 220, (August 1985), pp. 467-483

Sayah A. & English J. (2005). Rheumatoid arthritis: a review of the cutaneous manifestations. *J Am Acad Dermatol*, Vol. 53, No. 2, (August 2005), pp. 191-205

Schneider J. & Jordaan F. (1997). The histopathologic spectrum of erythema induratum of Bazin. *Am J Dermatopathol*, Vol. 19, No. 4, (August 1997), pp. 323-333

Segura S., Pujol R., Trindade F., & Requena L. (2008). Vasculitis in erythema induratum of Bazin: a histopathologic study of 101 biopsy specimens from 86 patients. *J Am Acad Dermatol*, Vol. 59, No. 5, (November 2008), pp. 839-851

Seishima M., Oyama Z., & Oda M. (2004). Skin eruptions associated with microscopic polyangiitis. *Eur J Dermatol*, Vol. 14, No. 4, (July-August 2004), pp. 255-258

Shapiro L., Teisch J., & Brownstain M. (1973). Dermatohistopathology of chronic gonococcal sepsis. *Arch Dermatol*, Vol. 107, No. 3, (March 1973), pp. 403-406

Sotto M., Langer B., Hoshino-Shimizu S., & de Brito T. (1976). Pathogenesis of cutaneous lesions in acute meningococcemia in humans: light, immunofluorescent, and electron microscopic studies of skin biopsy specimens. *J Infect Dis*, Vol. 133, No. 5, (May 1976), pp. 506-514

ten Holder S., Joy M., & Falk R. (2002). Cutaneous and systemic manifestations of drug-induced vasculitis. *Ann Pharmacother*, Vol. 36, No. 1, (January 2002), pp. 130-147

Tsianakas A., Ehrchen J., Presser D., Fischer T., Kruse-Loesler B., Luger T., & Sunderkoetter C. (2009). Scalp necrosis in giant cell arteritis: case report and review of the relevance of this cutaneous sign of large-vessel vasculitis. *J Am Acad Dermatol*, Vol. 61, No. 4, (October 2009), pp. 701-706

Wahl C., Bouldin M., & Gibson L. (2005). Erythema elevatum diutinum. Clinical, histopathologic, and immunohistochemical characteristics of six patients. *Am J Dermatopathol*, Vol. 27, No. 5, (October 2005), pp. 397-400

Waller J., Feramisco J., Alberta-Wszolek L., McCalmont T., & Fox L. (2010). Cocaine-associated retiform purpura and neutropenia: is levamisole the culprit? *J Am Acad Dermatol*, Vol. 63, No. 3, (September 2010), pp. 530-535

Walsh N., Green P., Burlingame R., Pasternak S., & Hanly J. (2010). Cocaine-related retiform purpura: evidence to incriminate the adulterant, levamisole. *J Cutan Pathol*, Vol. 37, No. 12, (December 2010), pp. 1212-1219

Weston W. & Huff J. (1981). The mucocutaneous lymph node syndrome: a critical re-examination. *Clin Exp Dermatol*, Vol. 6, No. 2, (March 1981), pp. 167-178

Yasue T. (1986). Livedoid vasculitis and central nervous system involvement in systemic lupus erythematosus. *Arch Dermatol*, Vol. 122, No. 1, (January 1986), pp. 66-70

Yiannias J., El-Azhary R., & Gibson L. (1992). Erythema elevatum diutinum: a clinical and histopathologic study of 13 patients. *J Am Acad Dermatol*, Vol. 26, No. 1, (January 1992), pp. 38-41

Zax R., Hodge S., & Callen J. (1990). Cutaneous leukocytoclastic vasculitis. Serial histopathologic evaluation demonstrates the dynamic nature of the infiltrate. *Arch Dermatol*, Vol. 126, No. 1, (January 1990), pp. 69-72

8

Endothelial Cells and Vasculitis

Vidosava B. Djordjević, Vladan Ćosić , Lilika Zvezdanović-Čelebić,
Vladimir V. Djordjević and Predrag Vlahović
University of Niš, School of Medicine/Clinical Centre Niš
Serbia

1. Introduction

The vascular endothelium is a specific organ consisting of the endothelial cell (EC) monolayer, weighting about 1 kg which makes a unique border between the circulating blood and the underlying tissues. Because of its strategic location, the endothelium interacts with cellular and neurohumoral mediators, thus controlling the vascular contractile state and cellular composition. Endothelial cells (ECs) used to be considered a layer of "nucleated cellophane", an inert lining to blood vessels, endowed with negative properties, and the most important of which is its ability to act as a non-thrombogenic substrate for blood. Further, the endothelium was thought to participate in tissue reactions as target for injurious agents. Now the endothelium is recognized as a semipermeable barrier that regulates the transfer of small and large molecules, a highly specialized, metabolically active organ having vital metabolic, secretory, synthetic and immunologic functions. It performs significant autocrine, paracrine and endocrine actions and exerts influences on smooth muscle cells, platelets and peripheral leucocytes. Therefore, haemostasis, inflammatory reactions and immunity involve close interactions between immunocompetent cells and vascular endothelium.

ECs arise from hemangioblasts, blast-like bipotential cells (Choi et al., 1998). They can also transdifferentiate into mesenchymal cells and intimal smooth muscle cells. It is known that there is a marked phenotypic variation between ECs in different parts of the vascular system. The cells from different location in the same person not only express different surface antigens and receptors, but can generate different responses to the same stimulus. Further, cells from the same part of the vasculature can have varied responses (Galley & Webster, 2004).

The vascular endothelium senses mechanical stimuli, such as pressure and shear stress, and hormonal stimuli, such as vasoactive substances. In respons, it releases agents that regulate vasomotor function, trigger inflammatory processes and affect hemostasis. Among the vasodilatory substances the endothelium produces are nitric oxide (NO), prostacyclin, different endothelium derived hyperpolarizing factors and C-type natriuretic peptide. Vasoconstricting molecules include endothelin-1 (ET-1), angiotensin II (Ang II), thromboxane A_2 and reactive oxygen species (ROS) (Endemann & Schiffrin, 2004). Inflammatory modulators include NO, intercellular adhesion molecule-1 (ICAM-1), vascular adhesion molecule-1 (VCAM-1), E-selectin, and NF-κB. The endothelium realizes the modulation of hemostasis by releasing: plasminogen activator, tissue factor inhibitor, von

Willebrand factor, NO, prostacyclin, thromboxane A_2, plasminogen/activator, inhibitor/1 and fibrinogen. The endothelium also contributes to mitogenesis, angiogenesis, vascular permeability and fluid balance. The endothelium is indispensable for body homeostasis. An controlled endothelium cell response is involved in many disease processes including atherosclerosis, hypertension, pulmonary hypertension, sepsis and inflammatory syndromes including vasculitis. These diseases are related to endothelial injury, dysfunction and activation.

2. Physiological functions of endothelial cell

In order for ECs to perform their physiological functions, they should exist in the so-called resting or quiescent state. It seems that, under normal resting conditions, ECs constitutively express certain "protective" genes, such as that encoding Bcl-x_L, the purpose of which is to maintain ECs in their quiescent phenotype by inhibiting nuclear factor κB (NFκB) activation and exerting anti-apoptotic functions (Bach et al., 1997). In this state ECs can perform their normal barrier and anticoagulant functions even in the presence of low levels of stimulans, such as shear stress, circulating endotoxins or reactive oxygen species. In the quiescent state, the antithrombotic, anti-inflammatory and antiproliferative properties of the endothelium are maintained by the dominance of nitric oxide (NO) signaling and the formation of S-NO modifications of proteins, shear stress signaling through the surface glycocalyx and signaling between pericytes and the endothelium.

2.1 Transport functions

ECs makes an important barrier to the free passage of molecules and cells from the blood to the underlying interstitium and cells. Transport functions are realized by protein transporters, caveolae and tight junctions. Specific transport mechanisms transport essential circulating macromolecules across ECs to the subendothelial space to enable the metabolic needs of the surrounding tissue cells. ECs express glucose transporters GLUT-1 and GLUT-4. GLUT-1 is the most abundant endothelial isoform. The blood-brain barrier is the major endothelial tissue expressing GLUT transporters, although these transporters have been also detected in other ECs including the umbilical vein, adrenal capillaries, aorta, retina, heart, placenta, the eye and testis (Mann et al., 2003).
Aminoacids are transported by multiple transport systems in ECs, but the system y^+ catonic amino acid transporter is perhaps most relevant, since this system transports L-arginine, the substrate for nitric oxide. Cytokines such as TNFα can stimulate L-arginine transport in ECs resulting in increased NO production (Bogle et al., 1995).
Transcellular transport in ECs occurs via caveolae which represent invaginations in the cell membrane and which are primary important in albumin transport across the endothelium. Albumin binding proteins (albumin binding glycoprotein, gp60) initiate the endocytosis of albumin by associating with the scaffolding protein caveolin-1 and activating the kinase Src. The Src enzyme phosphorylates caveolin-1 and a second protein dynamin (Galley & Webster, 2004). This results in the fission of caveolae and internalization of albumin. In the endothelium, caveolin-1 regulates nitric oxide signaling by binding to and maintaining endothelial nitric oxide synthase (NOS) in an inactive state (Bucci et al., 2000). Caveolin-1 is also an important determinant of calcium signaling in ECs because calcium influx channels and pumps are localized in caveolae (Fujimoto, 1993).

Paracellular transport is realized through tight junctions. Within multicellular organisms, several organs are relatively independent of whole body homeostasis and are wrapped by EC sheets. For example, the blood brain barrier is made of highly specialized ECs whose tight junctions protect the central nervous system. Tight junctions can function as either a „gate" (selected passage of molecules) or a „fence" (no passage) (Sawada et al., 2003). The gate function regulates the passage of ions, water and various macromolecules, even of cancer cells, through paracellular spaces. This type of function is important in oedema, jaundice, diarrhoea and blood-borne metastasis. The fence function maintains cell polarity by preventing the mixing of molecules in the apical EC membrane with those in the lateral membrane. Some pathogenic bacteria and viruses target and affect the tight junction function, leading to diseases affecting the vascular system (oedema), the gastrointestinal tract (bacterial enteritides) and respiratory tract (acute respiratory distress syndrome) (Galley & Webster, 2004).

2.2 Vascular tone regulation

The endothelium produces a number of vasodilator and vasoconstrictor substances which regulate vasomotor tone, but the most important is NO.

2.2.1 Nitric oxide

Nitric oxide is the most powerful vasodilator. Resting ECs constitutively express an endothelial specific isoform of nitric oxide synthase (eNOS, NOS3) which synthesizes NO from L-arginine (Palmer et al., 1988) maintaing the vasculature in a state of vasodilatation. The most important stimuli are physical factors such as shear stress and pulsatil stretching of the vessel wall as well as circulating and locally released vasoactive substances. The endothelium can be taken as a biosensor reacting to a large variety of stimuli and therefore maintaing an adequate NO release. ECs can express both, Ca-dependent constitutive NOS and Ca^{2+}-independent inducible NOS (iNOS, NOS2). In unstimulated ECs, eNOS is targeted to specific microdomains in the plasma membrane called caveolae, where eNOS is associated with a scaffold protein caveolin, resulting in the tonic inhibition of the enzyme activity (Garcia-Cardena et al., 1997; Michel et al., 1997). The elevation of Ca^{2+} induced by Ca^{2+}-elevating agonists stimulates the binding of calmodulin to eNOS challenging the dissociation of the enzyme from caveolin and thereby its activation (Michel et al., 1997). Some stimuli such as shear stress and ceramide can induce the Ca^{2+}-independent activation of eNOS (Igarashi et al., 1999). Shear stress and receptor agonists (such as bradykinin and vascular endothelial growth factor) can induce the phosphorylation of eNOS by Akt and its translocation to the cytosol where it interacts with calmodulin and the chaperone Hsp90. There is evidence that the some situations are associated with an increased activity and the amount of constitutive eNOS indicating that this isoform can also be induced. Although caveolae play an integral part in regulating the activity of eNOS, proinflammatory cytokines also increase the activity of GTP-cyclohydrolase, the rate-limiting enzyme for tetra-hydrobiopterin production, which is a cofactor for NOS (Harrison, 1997). The y+ amino acid transporter channels are co-located with NOS on caveolae, and the recirculation of L-arginine from L-citruline mediated by cytokines occurring in vascular ECs (Lee & Yu, 2002) makes substrate for NO production available . NO is subsequently produced by the enzyme only when the substrate L-arginine and the cofactor tetrahydrobiopterine are available. NO can then react with the cysteine motifs in proteins throughout ECs to make S-NO modifications to these proteins (S-nitrosylation), thereby silencing multiple metabolic processes, including apoptotic cell death regulation (Mannick, 2007) and the inhibition of mitochondrial oxidative phosphorylation during hypoxia or a protection against hypoxia by increasing the binding activity of hypoxia-inducible factor 1α. S-nitrosylation of NF-κB can suppress inflammation (Rabelink & Luscher, 2006). L-arginine depletion occurs when it is diverted into alternative metabolic pathways through the redox induction of enzymes such as arginase and protein methyltransferases.

Under prolonged redox signaling, eNOS itself may switch from being an enzyme that produces NO into the one that produces reactive oxygen species. This event is known as NOS "uncoupling", and it is dependent on the lack of availability of the cofactor tetrahydrobiopterine, which is essential for the eNOS-dependent production of NO. The amount of tetrahydrobipterin can be reduced as a result of direct oxidation by ROS derived from another source followed by the amplification of oxidative stress or when hydrogen peroxide induces the inactivation of the enzymes GTP-cyclohydrolase and dihydrofolate reductase, which generate and regenerate tetrahydrobiopterine. When its levels are low the heme group in eNOS will directly yield superoxide and hydrogen peroxide (Crabtree et al., 2009). The enzyme may reduce molecular oxygen rather than transfer electrons to L-arginine, thereby generating superoxide. Superoxide is believed to originate from the oxygenase domain of the enzyme through the dissociation of a ferrous-dioxygen complex that is normally stabilized by tetrahydrobiopterine (Xia et al., 1998). This uncoupling converts eNOS into an accelerator of redox signaling followed by the production of large amounts of ROS inducing a proinflammatory state (Rabelink & Luscher, 2006). Several enzymes such as the hemoxygenase system (Ryter et al., 2006), antioxidant enzymes, thioredoxin reductase and glutathione reductase (Hojo et al., 2002) can scavenge ROS and "fine-tune" this activation cascade, to the extent that ROS exceed the antioxidative capacity of cellular antioxidants (Cai & Harrison, 2000). This process explains how the chronic activation of the endothelium or impaired activity of eNOS can lead to the endothelial dysfunction.

Endothelial iNOS may be induced in both physiological and pathological conditions. Known physiological settings include pregnancy, treatment with oestradiol (Weiner et al 1994), shear stress, chronic exercise or receptor agonists (such as bradykinine and vascular endothelial growth factor). In activated ECs iNOS can be induced producing much higher levels of NO then those present under physiological conditions and that is implicated in the pathogenesis of a wide variety of diseases involving endothelium (Djordjević et al., 2004; Djordjević et al., 2008). iNOS is highly regulated by cytokines, some of which promote while others inhibit the enzyme induction. Although there are indices suggesting that a cocktail of three cytokines (TNF-α, IL-1β and IFN-γ) (Steiner et al., 1997), is neccesery for NOS induction, most data showed that NOS induction can be triggered by a mixture of two cytokines especially IL-1 and TNF (Mantovani et al., 1997). Transforming growth factor -β (TGF-β) reduces cytokine-induced iNOS activity by inhibiting iNOS mRNA translation and increasing iNOS protein degradation, while IL-4 interferes with iNOS transcription (Bogdan et al., 1991). The disruption of genes encoding IFN-γ, part of its receptor or an IFN regulatory factor results in a phenotypic deficiency in iNOS expression. EC produced NO may exert an autocrine function. It inhibits the cytokine-induced expression of adhesion molecules and cytokine production by ECs through inducing and stabilizing of NF-κB inhibitor (Peng et al., 1995), thus attenuating proinflammatory responses.

2.2.2 NADPH oxidase

An emerging paradigm in vascular homeostasis involves the balance between ROS-mediated and NO-mediated signals. ROS contribute to cellular signaling, affecting almost all aspects of cellular function including gene expression, proliferation, migration and cell death. It is now clear that ROS play an important role in regulating the normal function of the endothelium. However, the generation of ROS both within ECs and in adjacent cells such as vascular smooth muscle cells, adventitial fibroblasts and inflammatory cells has a major role in the genesis of endothelial activation and dysfunction. The potential sources of superoxide in ECs include the mitochondrial electron transport chain, xanthine oxidase, cytochrome p450 enzymes, uncoupled NOS and NADPH oxidases. Mitochondria are both a source and a target for ROS. Because they are susceptible to oxidative damage it can result in enhanced mitochondrial ROS production (Cai & Harrison, 2000). Xanthine oxidase is expressed on the luminal surface of the endothelium and catalyses the conversion of hypoxanthine into urate in the process that generates superoxide. An increased xanthine-oxidase-derived superoxide production is involved in endothelial dysfunction in several diseases.

NADPH oxidase is considered as a rather special source of ROS generation since its the primary function is the regulation of ROS production, primarily identified and characterized in phagocytes where it plays an essential role in host defense against microbial organisms. Furthermore it has become apparent that ROS production by NADPH oxidase homologues in non-phagocytic cells also plays an important role in the regulation of signal transduction via the modulation of kinase and phosphatase activities or through gene transcription (Finkel, 2003; Groemping & Rittinger, 2005). The phagocytic enzyme is normally quiescent, but becomes activated during the neutrophil oxidative burst when it generates large amounts of superoxide (Brandes & Kreuzer, 2005). The classical phagocytic NADPH oxidase is composed of two subunits, a catalytic subunit $gp91^{phox}$ (91 kDa glycosylated protein; where phox is phagocyte oxidase), and $p22^{phox}$ subunit forming a membrane-bound heterodimeric flavo-cytochrome b_{558}. For fully enzyme activation a number of cytosolic regulatory subunits are required namely $p67^{phox}$, $p47^{phox}$, $p40^{phox}$ and the small GTPase Rac2 which are translocated to and assembled with the membrane cytochrome in a highly regulated process (DeLeo & Quinn, 1996) that involves the post-translational modification of several cytosolic subunits and specific protein-protein binding through tandem SH3 (Src homology) domains. The tight regulation of enzymatic activity is achieved by two mechanisms: the separation of the oxidase subunits into different subcellular locations during the resting state and the modulation of reversible protein-protein and protein-lipid interactions. In the activated enzyme complex, the flavin-containing catalytic subunit functions as an electron transport system which uses NADPH as a donor of electrons that are transferred to molecular oxygen, resulting in the generation of superoxide.

Initially, several homologues of the $gp91^{phox}$ catalytic subunit have been identified, each encoded by separate genes and designated Noxs. These are now seven members: Nox1, Nox2, Nox3, Nox4, Nox5, Duox1 and Duox2. Nox2 contains $gp91^{phox}$. It seems that all the Nox homologues may bind to $p22^{phox}$ in a similar manner to the $gp91^{phox}$/ $p22^{phox}$ complex. In the case of Nox1, homologues of $p47^{phox}$ and $p67^{phox}$ (NOXO1 and NOXA1) have been found to be important for its activation. On the other side, Nox4 activation does not require either $p47^{phox}$ and $p67^{phox}$ (Ray & Shah, 2005).

ECs express all the classical NADPH oxidase subunits. However, there are a few significant differences between phagocytic oxidase and the enzyme in ECs. Firstly, endothelial oxidase continuously generates small amounts of superoxide even in unstimulated cells, but its activity can be augmented by specific agonists. Secondly, a large proportion of the superoxide generated in ECs is intracellular, whereas neutrophil superoxide generation is mainly in the extracellular compartment. The Nox2 oxidase is predominantly located in a perinuclear distribution in association with the cytoskeleton. There are also many fully preassembled ROS generating oxidase complexes which can explain both the continuous low-level superoxide generation in unstimulated endothelium and the intracellular site of ROS production. The Nox4 isoform is expressed in greater amounts in ECs and seems to contribute to the basal constitutive superoxide generation.. Additionally, ECs express the Nox1 enzyme in smaller amounts than the Nox2 isoform. Endothelial NADPH oxidase may be stimulated by a variety of (patho)physiological stimuli: 1. Agonists of G-protein coupled receptors such as angiotensin II and endothelin, 2. Growth factors such as thrombin and vascular endothelial growth factor, 3. Cytokines such as TNF-α, 4. Metabolic factors such as increased glucose, insulin, non-esterified fatty acids, advanced glycation end products, 5. Oxidized lipids, 6. Oscillatory shear stress , and 7. Hypoxia/reoxygenation and nutrient deprivation.

A major mechanism involved in NADPH oxidase activation is the PKC (protein kinase C)-dependent phosphorylation of the $p47^{phox}$ regulatory subunit and its translocation to the membrane heterodimer. TNF-α induced endothelial oxidase activation downstream phosphorylation of extracellular signal-regulated kinase, involves not only the phosphorylation of $p47^{phox}$, but also its binding to TRAF4 (TNF-receptor associated factor 4) (Li et al., 2005). The other mechanism, occurs via the action of Src, EGF receptor transactivation and the subsequend activation of PI3- kinase which leads to the robust activation of Rac and an enhanced and prolonged oxidase dependent ROS production. The activation of the oxidase by Rac 1 is therapeutically relevant because Rac 1 activation requires its post-translational modification by isoprenylation, a process that is inhibited by β-hydroxy-3-methylglutaryl-CoA reductase inhibitors (statins).

3. Endothelial cell activation

Generally, ECs are constantly a target for a wide variety of stimuli which can induce an EC response in three different ways: 1) stimulation - a rapid response of resting ECs initiated by agonists such as histamine, 2) activation - a slower protein synthesis-dependent response mostly initiated by inflammatory cytokines, (these two responses are normal EC functions), 3) injury - a process occurring by strong stimuli which can induce either endothelial necrosis or endothelial dysfunction.

A large number of distinct pathogens including viruses, bacteria and their products, protozoa, anti-EC antibodies, reactive oxygen species, rickettsiae and toxins can be directly or indirectly involved in EC activation (Figure 1). ECs can be also a target for angiogenic signals in neoplasia, and a major target for an immune reaction directed against alloantigens or xenoantigens. Some of them (like viruses) infect ECs, others (viruses, bacteria and their products, anti-EC antibodies) interact with ECs and induce or modify cytokine production.

EC activation triggered by inflammatory cytokines (e.g. TNF-α, IFN-γ, IL-1) or growth factors (e.g. angiotensin II) can induce the expression of a functional program related to thrombosis and inflammation. Thus, under stronger insults ECs initially acquire a proinflammatory and procoagulant phenotype. Since the ultimate goal of the activated EC is to survive, it leads the cell to add to the constitutively- expressed protective machinery by initiating the upregulation of a new set of protective genes, including those for A1 and A20 (Bach et al., 1997).

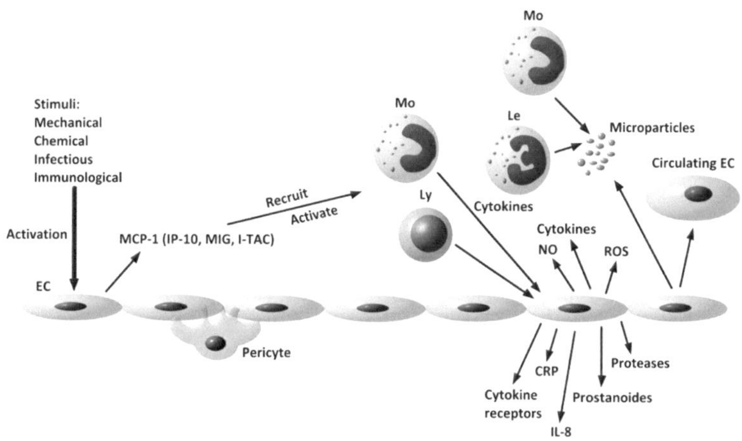

Fig. 1. Endothelial cell activation

During activation ECs not only develop a characteristic morphology but also synthesize a new surface protein and soluble mediators not present in the resting vascular endothelium. Many of these morphologic and functional changes can be induced in cultured ECs by purified immune mediators, such as monokines, lymphokines and bacterial LPS. Numerous inducible genes involved in endothelial activation, including cell adhesion molecule 1, E-selectin, tissue factor, interleukin-1 (IL-1), interleukin-6 (IL-6), G-CSF, interleukin-8 (IL-8) and c-myc contain elements in their promoter regions that could be recognized by the NF-κB 1/Rel family of transcription factors. ECs also express an inhibitor of NF-κB, IκB-α, and can dramaticaly modulate the level of this inhibitor in parallel with the activation process.

One of the earliest changes in the endothelium activation is an alteration in the glycocalyx composition. Glycocalyx contains anchoring proteoglycans (CD44, the syndecan protein family) and conecting glycosaminoglycans. The major class of negatively charged polysaccharides that contribute to the glycocalyx include heparan sulfate, chondroitin sulfate and the nonsulfated hyaluronan. The various combinations of possible sulfation modifications within a heparan sulfate chain can give rise to many structurally distinct binding sites for a wide rage of different ligands, including chemokines, growth factors, lipoproteins, lipases, serine protease inhibitors, thrombomodulin, extracellular SOD and complement factors (Weinbaum et al., 2007). The endothelial glycocalyx (Tarbell & Ebong, 2008) markedly changes its properties under inflammatory conditions which facilitates rolling adhesion and tight adhesion of leucocytes. Cytokines activate proteases either located in glycocalyx or secreted by activated ECs and leucocytes which partially degrade the glycocalyx layer and thereby provide a mechanism for leucocyte recruitment (Mulivor & Lipowsky, 2004). Also, the release of glycocalyx components into the circulation can be considered as a very early sign of endothelial activation. So, syndecan 1 and heparan sulfates have been shown to be released from the endothelium following stimulation by thrombin or endotoxin (Fitzgerald et al., 2000), and circulating glycocalyx components have been explored as a measure of endothelial activation in patients with type 2 diabetes and the coronary artery disease

(Bruegger et al., 2009; Wang et al., 2009). During sustained endothelial activation platelets and leucocytes bind to the endothelial surface leading to the formation of proinflammatory factors such as thrombin and the membrane attached complex which can cause further activation of the endothelium and promote the formation of membrane particules so called microparticles. Microparticles from ECs, platelets and leucocytes are released into the circulation. The interaction between ECs and pericytes is disrapted and pericytes begins to produce proteases that damage the endothelial basement membrane. These processes may lead to the apoptosis or necrosis of ECs or ECs can be detached and detected in the circulation (Haubitz & Woywodt, 2004).

3.1 Nuclear factor-κB

NF-κB is a redox sensitive transcription factor associated with rapid-response activation mechanisms. It consists of homo- or heterodimeric complexes of members of the Rel family of proteins: p50/p105 (NF-κB1, derived from its p105 precursor), p52/100 (NF-κB2 and its p100 precursor), p65/RelA, c-Rel and Rel-B. The best characterized form is the heterodimer p50/p65. These proteins share a 300 amino acid region known as the Rel homology domain, which mediates DNA binding and dimerization. In resting cells, NF-κB binding proteins are in an inactive cytosolic form and are complexed to members of a family of inhibitory proteins referred to as IκB (IκB-α, IκB-β, IκB-γ, IκB-σ and IκB-ε). IκB-α is the best characterized inhibitor, which binds to the p65 subunit of NF-κB (Baldwin, 1996). All IκB forms contain multiple ankyrin repeats which are involved in interactions with NF-κB. NF-κB can be activated by a number of divers agents such as the citokines, IL-1β, and TNF-α, LPS, oxidative stress, oxidatively modified LDL particles, viral products, advanced glycosylation end products and physical forces. These stimuli may activate the NF-κB kinase complex through distinct signaling pathways that culminate in the activation of the IκB kinase. In this way they induce IκB-α release from the p65 subunit after its phosphorilation. After phosphorilation IκB is ubiquitinated and targeted for degradation via the nonlysosomal ATP-dependent proteosome pathway followed by a rapid loss of this protein. Alterations in IκB-α at the levels Ser^{32} and Ser^{36}, which prevent its phosphorilation and degradation, lead to blocking IκB-α ubiquitination and subsequent degradation (Brown et al., 1995). A removal of IκB-α exposes a nuclear localisation sequence in NF-κB which is then able to translocate to the nucleus, bind to a specific DNA sequence (5'-GGGRNNYYCC-3') and activate NF-κB dependent genes.

IκB-α is rapidly resinthesized after the loss, suggesting an autoregulatory mechanism for NF-κB regulation in the endothelium (Thurberg & Collins, 1998). When the IκB-α pool is replenished, IκB-α translocates to the nucleus and displaces the transactivating form of NF-κB from promotor elements. The NF-κB/IκB-α complex is then transported back to the cytoplasm in the inactive form. Further, the genes that code for p65, p105 and IκB-α are highly inducible in ECs in response to the stimuli that activate NF-κB. The promoter of the IκB-α-gene contains κB binding sites. p65 stimulates IκB-α gene expression (Baldwin, 1996) and p65 stabilises IκB-α protein indicating that p65 and IκB-α have been directly linked in an autoregulatory loop. The NF-κB/IκB-α autoregulatory system may ensure that the induction of NF-κB is transient, and that the activated cell returns to a quiescent state. It allows a continuous maintenance of the cytoplasmatic reservoirs of NF-κB complexes for stimulation in an acute response, and also prepares the EC to return NF-κB to its uninduced condition.

The rapid cytokine-induced activation of NF-κB in ECs is probably similar to that seen in other cell types. However, the recovery kinetics of the NF-κB/IκB-α response in the endothelium may be different. The NF-κB remains activated and IκB-α levels remain below basal levels for long periods of time than seen in cells programmed for rapid responses, such as macrophages (Read et al., 1994). It is possible that cytokines released by activated ECs result in an autocrine activation of NF-κB and continued degradation of IκB-α. Such prolonged endothelial activation may play a role in recruiting circulating cells to the sites of ongoing inflammatory (artherosclerosis) (Ahn et al., 2006; Brand et al., 1997) or immune processes (autoimmune diseases). The NF-κB activation can be blocked by sodium salicylate and aspirin (Kopp & Ghosh, 1994).

However, in addition to the proinflammatory genes, activated NF-κB may induce a set of protective genes, including antiapoptotic genes that may limit the activation process and thereby regulate the respons to injury. The protective genes include IκB-α and hemoxygenase, as well as the antiapoptotic genes A20, Bcl-2, and Bcl-XL. Besides the antiapoptotic activity, the antiapoptotic genes also inhibit the activation of NF-κB in ECs and thus block the induction of the proinflammatory genes (Bach et al., 1997). Some stimuli, such as laminar shear stress, upregulate genes for manganese superoxide dismutase, cyclooxygenase-2 and endothelial specific nitric oxide synthase. Since this set of genes has antioxidant, antithrombotic and antiadhesive properties, they can be also recognised as "protective". When the protective effect is not adequate, ECs undergo apoptosis.

To maintain an antiinflammatory and anticoagulant state the endothelium also requires environmental cues. Laminar shear stress is a key contributor to the integrity of ECs through the inhibition of apoptosis. Shear stress also activates specific transcription factors, such as kruppel-like factor 2 and nuclear factor erythroid 2-related factor 2 (Dekker et al., 2002; Chen et al., 2003). These transcription factors regulate about 70% of the genes responsive to shear stress, including those that encode typical protective endothelial factors such as eNOS, thrombomodulin and antioxidant enzymes, but at the same time they down regulate genes that encode procoagulant factors such as plasminogen activator inhibitor 1, IL-8 and the tissue factor (Fledderus et al., 2008). It seems that kruppel-like factor 2 can be directly regulated by shear stress, while the nuclear factor erythroid 2-related factor 2 is released from its inhibitor, kelch-like ECH associated protein 1, through the generation of ROS, which suggests that it functions as a defense mechanism against antioxidants (Kraft et al., 2004).

However, in the stabilisation of the endothelial phenotype a key role belongs to the reciprocal interaction of stromal or epithelial cells with the endothelium. ECs have direct physical contact with pericytes and vascular smooth muscle cells through myoendothelial junctions. Pericytes send signals to the endothelium through number of factors including hydrogen sulfide, all isoforms of VEGF (vascular endothelial growth factor), sphingosine-1-phosphate, platelet-derived growth factor, basic fibroblast growth factor and angiopoietin I (Gaengel et al., 2009; Diaz-Flores et al., 2009). Angiopoietin I is best known to stabilize the endothelium and to maintain its quiescent state. If the signaling between angiopoietin I and the ECs is interrupted ECs sprout and migrate; this results in neoangiogenesis (Chen & Stinnett, 2008).

3.1.1 Regulation of NF-κB dependent gene expression

The activation of the pleiotropic mediator NF-κB in ECs could coordinate the expression of numerous endothelial products which are important in endothelial activation including some cell surface adhesion proteins, cytokines, growth factors, NADPH oxidase, NOS, prostanoides, acute phase reactants and components of the coagulation system. They may be multiple phosphorylation events which play a key role in NF-κB activation. Some of the cytosolic NF-κB/IκB-α is associated with the catalitic subunit of the cAMP-dependent protein kinase, PKAc, in an inactive state. The signal-induced degradation of IκB-α leads to the activation of PKAc which phosphorilates the p65 subunit of NF-κB on Ser^{276}. This causes a conformational change which unmasks the CREB binding protein (cAMP-responsive binding protein) interacting domain on p65. Once CREB interacting domain on p65 is unmasked, NF-κB interaction with a coactivator is enhanced and NF-κB can enter the nucleus (Zhong et al., 1997). Lysophosphatidylcholine, one of the active molecules present in oxLDL, has been shown to activate NF-κB in primary cultured ECs via a PKC dependent pathway. ECs can also be shown to be responsive to oxLDL *in vivo*. When unmodified human LDL particles are injected into a rat model, they are localized in the arterial wall were they undergo oxidative modification which is accompanied by an increase in endothelial NF-κB activation and expression of NF-κB dependent genes (Calara et al., 1998). In the nucleus, the p65 subunit can be phosphoregulated by the components of the p38 and ERK MAP kinase signal patways (Berghe et al., 1998).

4. Endothelial cells and inflammation

ECs actively participate in the inflammatory process acting as both a target and a responder to a variety of stimuli. Whatever the initial stimuli (mechanical, chemical, infectious or immunological) they activate ECs. There are two stages of EC activation; the first-EC activation type I which does not require *de novo* protein synthesis or gene upregulation, occurs rapidly and it is followed by the retraction of ECs, expression of P selectin and release of von Willebrand factor. The second response, EC activation type II, requires time for the stimulating agent to cause an effect via gene transcription and protein synthesis. A stimulating agent acting on the EC surface causes the expression of many genes via the activation of NF-κB (Baldwin, 1996). EC activation is a graded rather than an all response. For example, changes in EC integrity range from simple increases in local permeability to major EC contraction, exposing large areas of subendothelium. Activation may proceed as an acute response or as a chronic EC activation such as in atherosclerosis and in vascular diabetic complications. Ligands of RAGE (the receptor for advanced glycation end products) mediate continuous NF-κB activation which results in persistent endothelial tissue factor induction. The activation may occur locally, as in transplant rejection, or systematically, as in septicaemia and the systemic inflammatory response.

Generaly, EC activation is associated with five core changes including the loss of vascular integrity, expression of leucocyte adhesion molecules, change in phenotype from antithrombotic to prothrombotic, cytokine production and upregulation of HLA molecules. The loss of vascular integrity can expose subendothelium and cause the efflux of fluids from the intravascular space.

The first step in EC activation, independently on the initial stimuli, involves inflammatory cytokines mostly TNF-α, IL-1 and IFN-γ (Steiner et al., 1997). They stimulate ECs to produce monocyte chemotactic protein-1 (MCP-1). Vascular cells produce three more chemokines including IP-10, MIG, I-TAC, when exposed to the inflammatory mediator IFN-γ, a molecule produced by activated T cells and perheps macrophages. MCP-1 recruits and activates immune and inflammatory cells which produce inflammatory cytokines and induce the expression of adhesion molecules. The upregulation of surface glycoproteins such as endothelial leucocyte adhesion molecule-1 (ELAM-1, also known as E-selectin), intercellular adhesion molecule-1 (ICAM-1), vascular cell adhesion molecule-1 (VCAM-1) and MHC molecules allows leucocytes to adhere to the endothelium and then move into tissues.

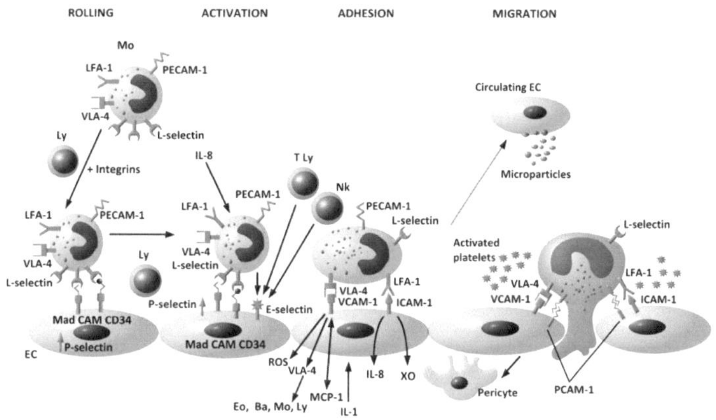

Fig. 2. Endothelial cells and inflammation

Tissue infiltration by circulating leucocytes is a four-step process involving low affinity attachment, roling on the endothelium, high affinity attachment to the endothelium, followed by transmigration across the ECs lining blood vessel walls. These processes are mediated by adhesion molecules. Four distinct families of adhesion molecules including cadherins, immunoglobulin superfamily members, selectins and integrins are involved in vascular cell-cell adhesion. These molecules are requred four: 1. The formation of the junctional complexes that enable the assembly of ECs into functional vascular networks; 2. They mediate the leucocyte-endothelial adhesive interactions involved in the trafficking of leucocytes out of the circulation but the set of adhesion molecules expressed by ECs depends on the stimuli (Cook-Mills & Deem, 2005) while the specificity of the adhesion molecules regulates the specificity of leucocyte homing to tissues; and 3. They contribute to contacts between pericytes and the endothelium that are important to the regulation of EC proliferation, addressin interaction, rolling which can also be mediated by the interaction of leucocyte $\alpha 4\beta 1$-integrin and VCAM-1/CD106. A transitory contact of leucocytes with the endothelium or their rolling are mediated by low-affinity receptors, selectins and addressins.

The binding of selectins on leucocytes stimulates "outside-in" signals in leucocytes, increasing the affinity of the integrin family of receptors, which then bind to EC adhesion molecules such as ICAM-1/CD54 and VCAM-1. The regulation of the expression of the adhesion molecules occurs by negative control as well as at the level of gene transcription. For example, NO can reduce leucocyte adhesion to arteries and can counteract the induction of VCAM-1 expression by ECs stimulated by inflammatory cytokines such as IL-1 or TNF-α. At the transcriptional level, NO inhibits VCAM-1 gene expression in ECs by interfering with the NF-κB signaling pathway via a non-cyclic GMP-mediated mechanism (Peng et al., 1995). Instead, NO inhibits NF-κB by inducing its inhibitor IκB-α. Thus, NO acts as an anti-inflammatory mediator. Leucocyte integrin affinity is also rapidly increased by "inside-out" signals from leucocyte chemokine receptors triggered by chemokines expressed on the surface of ECs. When leucocyte integrin affinity is increased, leucocyte roling is arrested.

More sustained sticking of leucocyte to the endothelium is mediated by VCAM-1 which binds to the cognate ligand VLA-4 (very late adhesion molecule-4) that is expressed by the very types of leucocytes recruited to the intima: monocytes and lymphocytes, respectively. Once adherent, the leucocytes enter the vascular wall. Leucocyte migration from the blood into tissues is vital for immune surveillance and inflammation. Leucocytes can stimulate "outside-in" signal transduction in ECs and some of these signals can cause localized alterations in EC junctions.

At the sites of inflammation, activated antigen specific lymphocytes are the first to migrate across activated endothelium expressing adhesiom molecules. During the leucocyte-EC interaction, the EC promotes the migration of leucocytes or removes leucocytes that are in the early stages of apoptosis. Leucocytes can be found within the vacuolar structures of ECs only when ECs phagocytose apoptotic leucocytes. This function of ECs may be a mechanism by which the endothelium is protected from the localised vascular damage which would occur if apoptotic leucocytes were to undergo necrosis. Thus, we can say that ECs modulate leucocyte migration by promoting leucocyte migration or removing leucocytes undergoing apoptosis.

While lymphocytes migrate acros activated endothelium neutrophils and monocytes migrate between ECs (Mamdouh et al., 2003). It has been shown that neutrophils roll across the luminal surface of human umbilical vein ECs to bicellular and tricellular EC junctions. In response to peptid N-formyl-methionyl-leucyl-phenylalanine neutrophils migrate through a pore in nonactivated cutaneous ECs. Adhesion molecule signals result in alterations in the function of cell junction proteins and/or contractile forces in the EC, thereby opening an EC junction and permitting leucocyte migration into the tissue. During neutrophil and monocyte migration, localized EC retraction of lateral junctions occurs at the site of leucocyte migration showing that contractile forces in ECs have an active role in leucocyte migration.

4.1 Selectins

Three selectins have been characterized and named according to their cell of original discovery: P-selectin (platelet selectin), E-selectin (EC selectin) and L-selectin (leucocyte selectin). These are glycosylated proteins, which share several structural features and support leukocyte-EC and leukocyte-platelet adhesion. L-selectin is constitutively expressed by most leucocytes, but not by other cell-types. The ECs of high endothelial venules of lymph nodes constitutively express ligand for L-selectin (lymphocyte homing receptors) and L-selectin plays a central role in the normal recirculation of lymphocytes. ECs from other vascular beds also support L-selectin-mediated adhesion after the exposure to cytokines. P-selectin, which is expressed by ECs and platelets, is stored in intracellular granules and mobilized to the surface upon cell activation where it supports the adhesion of granulocytes, monocytes and some lymphocyte subsets. E-selectin is expressed by cytokine-activated ECs and supports adhesion of granulocytes, monocytes, some memory T-lymphocytes and natural killer cells (Bevilacqua & Nelson, 1993; Brady, 1994).

4.2 Integrins

Selectin - mediated adhesion facilitates the immobilization of phagocytes by the interaction of phagocyte integrins with immunoglobulin-like molecules on the endothelium. Integrins are heterodimeric glycoproteins composed of non-covalently associated α and β subunits. Integrins mediate diverse cell-cell and cell-matrix interactions. The most important integrins in leukocyte-endothelial adhesion include the very late activation antigen-4 β1 integrin (VLA-4) and the CD11/CD18 β-2 integrins. VLA-4 is constitutively expressed by lymphocytes, monocytes, basophiles and eosinophils, but not neutrophils. This protein is a ligand for the inducible vascular cell adhesion molecule-1 (VCAM-1) and also mediates cell attachment to fibronectin and possibly other matrix components. β-2 integrins include three well characterized members: CD11a/CD18 (LFA-1, Lymphocyte function-associated antigen-1), CD11b/CD18 (Mac-1) and CD11c/CD18 where CD11 and CD18 are the α and β subunits, respectively. LFA-1 is found on all T- cells and also on B-cells, macrophages and neutrophils. CD11 subunits are encoded by distinct genes in a cluster on chromosome 16, while CD18 is encoded by a single gene on chromosome 21. CD18 contains a short cytoplasmic tail which has several potential phosphoregulation sites, a highly conserved transmembrane domain and a long extracellular region which contains a conserved cystein-rich region that is necessary for surface expression (Brady, 1994). The major ligands for CD11a/CD18 are the intercellular adhesion molecules-1 and 2 (ICAM-1 and ICAM-2). ICAM-1 is also a ligand for CD11b/CD18 which supports phagocyte adhesion to cellular and acellular substrates by ICAM-1 independent mechanisms. Other ligands for CD11b/CD18 include fibrinogen, clotting factors and complement fragments (C3bi).

4.3 Immunoglobulin-like molecules

4.3.1 Platelet-EC adhesion molecule-1 (PECAM-1)

PECAM-1 adhesion at the lateral borders of nonactivated ECs participates in the formation of EC junctions and my be a critical regulator of phagocyte diapedesis between ECs. PECAM-1 also mediates the binding with PECAM-1 on leucocytes. Although there is PECAM-1 independent models of lymphocyte, neutrophil and monocyte migration anti-PECAM-1 antibodies can block monocyte diapedesis across TNF-α or IL-1β-activated ECs (Schenkel et al., 2002). PECAM-1 can activate signals that increase leukocyte adhesion (Chiba et al., 1999). Also, PECAM-1 has been shown to recycle between the cell membrane and a cytoplasmic compartment juxtaposed to the membrane. PECAM-1 is recruited to the EC surface at the sites of monocyte transmigration (Mamdouh et al., 2003). A treatment of nonactivated cells with an inducer of oxidative stress increases PECAM-1 phosphorylation followed by an increase in leukocyte migration. PECAM-1 phosphorylation is regulated by ser/thr phosphatases which can be blocked with anti-PECAM-1 antibodies, antioxidants or inhibitors of PKC, Ras and glutathione synthesis (Rattan et al., 1997). The homophilic adhesion of PECAM-1 stimulates its binding to several intracellular proteins involved in signaling including Src homology containing phosphatase, phospholipase C-γ and Pi-3k (Jackson et al., 1997; Pellegatta et al., 1998; Pumphrey et al., 1999). Phosphorylated PECAM-1 can be linked to the cytoskeletal catenins thereby limiting their translocation to the nucleus thus modulating gene expression.

PECAM-1 localization in ECs is modulated by cytokines. The simultaneous treatment with TNF-α and IFN-γ moves PECAM-1 out of lateral junctions without inhibiting the ability of monocytes to migrate across these ECs under laminar flow conditions suggesting that sufficient PECAM-1 is still available for migration (Shaw et al., 2001).

4.3.2 Intercellular adhesion molecule-1 (ICAM-1)

ICAM-1 is a glycoprotein which contains five tandem immunoglobulin domains. It is constituvely expressed on many cell types but can be increased on endothelium by inflammatory mediators (Roebuck & Finnegan, 1999). The first and third immunoglobulin-like domain of ICAM-1 bind to the counter-receptors of LFA-1 and membrane-activated complex-1 (CD11b/CD18) respectively, on leucocytes, but it can also bind to fibrinogen on lymphocytes (Dupperay et al., 1997). A chelation of intracellular calcium or the inhibition of PKC in IFN-γ treated brain EC lines blocks ICAM-1 dependent lymphocyte migration without affecting lymphocyte adhesion (Etienne-Manneville et al., 2000). ICAM-1 stimulates ECs to produce chemokines through the activation of ERK1 and ERK2 (Sano et al., 1998) suggesting that ICAM-1 induces EC signals that are required for lymphocyte migration.

ICAM-1 signals can also regulate the EC actin cytoskeletion. The antibody cross-linking of ICAM-1 on TNF-α-activated pulmonary microvascular ECs activates xanthine oxidase and p38 MAPK (Wang & Doerschuk, 2001), resulting in actin rearrangement, and can also induce phosphorylation of another cytoskeleton protein ezrin. ICAM-1 associates with the cytoskeletal protein ezrin through phosphatidylinositol 4,5-biphosphate (Heiska et al., 1998).

Homotypic and heterotypic lymphocyte adhesion mediated by the interaction of ICAM-1 and CD11a/CD18 facilitates other important lymphocyte functions including antigen recognition, lymphocyte co-stimulation and cytotoxicity.

4.3.3 Vascular cell adhesion molecule-1 (VCAM-1)

VCAM-1 is a glycoprotein containing seven immunoglobulin-like domains which predominates in ECs. A second form of VCAM-1, consisting of six immunoglobulin-like domains, is produced in some tissues by alternate splicing. VCAM-1 is constitutively expressed at low levels by ECs and can be induced on these and other cell-types by cytokines. VCAM-1 supports the adhesion of eosinophils, basophils, monocytes and lymphocytes but not neutrophils, through the interaction with VLA-4. The binding of lymphocytes to VCAM-1 stimulates localized EC-shape changes and the "opening of a narrow passage way" through which leucocytes can migrate (Cook-Mills & Deem, 2005; Matheny et al., 2000). Lymphocyte binding to VCAM-1 activates ECs NADPH oxidase for the generation of ROS in ECs which constitutively express VCAM-1 and the MCP-1. The VCAM-1-mediated activation of NADPH oxidase is dependent on calcium flux and the small molecular weight G protein Rac1. Rac1 is involved in the assembly of the active NAPH oxidase complex in ECs such as in neutrophils (Dorseuil et al., 1995).

ICAM-1 and PECAM-1 do not activate EC NADPH oxidase. The VCAM-1-stimulated EC NADPH oxidase activity is required for VCAM-1-dependent lymphocyte migration because the inhibition of EC NADPH oxidase blocks MCP-1 stimulated, VCAM-1 dependent lymphocyte migration without altering lymphocyte adhesion. ROS scavengers inhibit VCAM-1 dependent lymphocyte migration while VCAM-1 dependent lymphocyte migration is not blocked by the inhibition of ROS-generating enzymes NOS, xanthine oxidase or cytochrome p450 on ECs (Matheny et al., 2000).

Lymphocyte binding to VCAM-1 induces a low concentration of hydrogen peroxide (1μmol) production in ECs (Tudor et al., 2001) much lower than those (50-200 μmol) produced by neutrophils and macrophages for the destruction of pathogens (DeLeo & Quinn, 1996) or released in some diseases (Thannickal & Fanburg, 2000). Low levels of ROS induce rapid, transient and reversible signals. This is important, since once a leucocytes reach an EC junction, the process of transmigration occurs within a couple of minutes. Another function of the ROS produced during VCAM-1-dependent lymphocyte migration is the activation (within minutes) of matrix metalloproteinases (MMPs) associated with ECs or IL-4 activated ones. The EC-derived hydrogen peroxide also activates lymphocyte-associated MMPs but 2-5 hours later. These results show that the ECs-associated rather than the lymphocyte-associated MMPs are required for VCAM-1-dependent lymphocyte migration across VCAM-1-expressing ECs (Deem & Cook-Mills, 2004).

Hydrogen peroxide produced by VCAM-1 stimulation has a direct, rapid effect on EC-associated MMPs. ROS activate purified MMPs by oxidizing the cysteine in the propeptide arm opening the arm and exposing the MMP active site (Murphy et al., 1994) which stimulate the autocatalytic removal of the arm, forming an active MMP (Van Wart & Birkedal-Hansen, 1990). Contrary to EC-associated MMPs, hydrogen peroxide indirectly activates lymphocyte-associated MMPs through the down-regulation of the expression of the high levels of tissue inhibitors of MMPs (TIMPs) on lymphocytes (Deem & Cook-Mills, 2004) which takes several hours indicating that lymphocyte MMPs are likely involved in the leukocyte migration through the extravascular tissue (Cook-Mills & Deem, 2005).

MMPs associated with ECs are more important than secreted MMPs during lymphocyte migration. Among MMPs the EC-associated MMP-2 and MMP-9 are likely to degrade matrix and EC junction molecules at the site of transmigration (Herren et al., 1998).

5. Endothelial cells and vasculitis

5.1 Vasculitis triggered by infectious agents

Vasculitis can be a primary disease, that is not associated with another cause. Or, it may be a complication of some other diseases such as infections, malignancy, reactions to certain medications (Zhang et al., 2010), a complication after an organ transplant, a connective tissue disease or other causes.

The participation of ECs in the pathogenesis of vascular inflammation is complex. On one hand, the vascular endothelium may be the target for injury. On the other hand, ECs may actively participate in amplifying and maintaining the inflammatory process. The role of ECs seems to be more prominent in small vessel vasculitis, such as hypersensitivity vasculitis and vasculitis associated with antineutrophil cytoplasmic antibodies (ANCA). In larger vessel vasculitis, ECs are the crucial protagonist of the vascular response to inflammation which leads to the amplification of the inflammatory response, vessel remodeling and repair, and eventually, vessel occlusion, which is the source of some of the most severe complications in patients with systemic vasculitis.

Although most of the infection related vasculitides are immune-complex-mediated (hepatitis B virus-related polyarteritis nodosa, and hepatitis C virus associated cryoglobulinemia) some pathogens are able to directly infect the ECs. Primary vasculitis can be induced by several pathogenic mechanisms. The direct infection of ECs include: bacterial vasculitis (naisserial), spirochetal vasculitis (syphilitic), mycobacterial vasculitis (tuberculous), rickettsial vasculitis (Rocky Mountain spotted fever), fungal vasculitis (aspergillosis) and viral vasculitis (herpes virus, herpes zoster) (Heeringa et al., 2004). Rickettsiae and herpes virus family members, particularly cytomegalovirus are the best documented (Mandell & Calabrese, 1998). Serious infections by these agents frequently include vasculitis lesions. The proliferation of the rickettsial organism in small-vessel walls elicits an inflammatory response that results in focal vascular inflammation, often with necrosis and hemorrhage. However most forms of vasculitis do not appear to be caused by the direct infection of vessel walls by pathogens.

5.2 Immune complex-mediated vasculitis

Noninfection immunologic mechanisms that cause vasculitis include cell-mediated inflammation, immune complex-mediated inflammation and inflammation induced by ANCA. Immune complex-mediated vasculitis include: cryoglobulinemic vasculitis, Henoch-Schonlein purpura, serum sickness vasculitis, lupus vasculitis, infection-induced immune complex vasculitis (hepatitis virus), some drug-induced vasculitis (sulfonamide-induced vasculitis), some paraneoplastic vasculitis, and Goodpasture's syndrome (mediated by anti GMB antibodies) (Heeringa at al., 2004).

In immune complex-mediated vasculitis, EC morphology is altered and the luminal endothelium may be destroyed. Complement-mediated lysis as well as neutrophil-mediated EC damage are the main mechanisms of endothelium cell injury in these processes (Cid, 2002). The membrane attack complex C5b-9, final product of the complement activation cascade, has been detected in the necrotizing vasculitis of the polyarteritis nodose type (Kissel et al., 1989).

5.3 ANCA-mediated vasculitis

Wegener's granulomatosis, microscopic polyangitis, and Churg-Strauss syndrome are the major forms of small-vessel vasculitis that are strongly associated with ANCA (Heeringa et al., 2004). ANCA vasculitis may be induced by some drugs, such as thiouracil. There are two clinically important forms: cytoplasmatic ANCA (cANCA) and perinuclear ANCA (pANCA). ANCA are autoantibodies that are directed against constituents of the primary granules of neutrophils and the peroxidase positive lysosomes of monocytes. The primary antigenic targets for ANCA are proteinase-3 (PR3), a 29kD neutral serin protease, and myeloperoxidase (MPO), a 140kD enzyme involved in the generation of ROS (Falk & Jennette, 1988; Jennette et al., 1990). ANCA recognizes MPO or PR3 translocated to the neutrophil membrane on TNF-α or interleukin-8 (IL-8) primed neutrophils (Flint et al., 2010) or may bind to Fc receptors through their Fc portion. Both interactions, specific and Fc-mediated appear to be functionally relevant (Falk et al., 1990; Porges et al., 1994). ANCA immunoglobulin G can activate neutrophils and monocytes. ANCA binding to neutrophils may stimulate or amplify many neutrophil functions including respiratory bursts which generate ROS, degranulation and protease release (Falk et al., 1990), NO production (Tse et al., 2001), and chemotactic activity. ANCA binding also stimulates integrin expression and integrin-mediated homotypic adhesion and adhesion to ECs (Radford et al., 2000). Homotypic interactions mediated by neutrophil integrins are required for enhanced TNF-α induced neutrophil activation by ANCA. ANCA-stimulated neutrophil function results in an augmentation of neutrophil-mediated EC injury by inducing EC detachment and lyse of ECs previously damaged by other mediators. Further, in an inflammatory microenvironment, enzymes released by activated neutrophils, including MPO and PR3, may induce EC apoptosis (Yang et al., 2001).

ANCA-mediated monocyte and neutrophil activation has also been shown to induce the expression and secretion of proinflammatory cytokines (IL-1, IL-6, IL-8, TNF- α), chemokines (MCP-1) and prostanoids (Cid, 2002; Cid et al., 2004). Such mediators may contribute to the amplification and propagation of the inflammatory process.

The detection of ANCA is an important diagnostic and prognostic marker. Testing of ANCA is indicated in patients with evidence for the ANCA disease such as severe pulmonary hemorrhage, especially if accompanied by evidence for glomerulonephritis, peripheral

neuropathy, purpura, hemorrhagic sinusitis or other manifestations of small-vessel vasculitis.
However, the use of ANCA as a marker of the disease and its activity show a number of limitations such as the occurrence of high ANCA titers with no disease activity, or ANCA presence in non-vasculitis disorders, such as endocarditis (Choi et al., 2000) or tuberculosis (Flores-Suarez et al., 2003). In addition, circulating ECs have been used as markers in a variety of vascular disorders (Dignat-George & Sampol, 2000) and also their use is demonstrated in ANCA-associated small-vessel vasculitis (Haubitz and Woywodt, 2004). Recently it has been documented that an increase risk for relapse appears to be related to the presence of anti-PR3 antibody seropositivity.

5.4 Anti endothelial cell antibodies

Circulating anti-EC antibodies have been detected in several vasculitides including Wegener's granulomatosis, microscopic polyangitis, Kawasaki diseases, thromboangiitis obliterans, Bechet's disease and Takayasu's arthritis (Praprotnik et al., 2001). It seems that a large, highly heterogeneous group of antigens can be recognized by anti-EC antibodies. Some anti-endothelial antibodies, such as those detected in Kawasaki disease, recognize cytokine-inducible molecules, while others, such as those detected in Wagener's granulomatosis and microscopic polyangitis, recognize constitutive EC antigens (Del Papa et al., 1996).
Studies *in vitro* have shown that some anti-EC antibodies may trigger complement activation or anti-body-dependent cellular cytotoxicity. These mechanisms might contribute to EC damage in systemic vasculitis. That alloantigens can activate ECs is well recognized within transplantation where HLA-specific antibodies can activate EC NF-κB (Savage & Williams, 2007; Smith et al., 2000). EC antibodies arise most probably as a secondary event to endothelial injury. Initial endothelial injury may result from pathogenic processes that may be unleashed during the development of the vasculitis process itself (for example, by proteolytic enzymes released from neutrophils after their inappropriate activation by ANCA). It is also likely that sequestered viral infections, such as cytomegalo-virus that can replicate within ECs, may become relatively more activated during the development of an autoimmune response and particularly after the introduction of immnosuppression. That cytomegalovirus can induce anti-EC antibodies is recognized (Toyoda et al., 1999). The binding of anti-EC antibodies to EC *in vitro* elicits a calcium-flux, the secretion of the chemokines MCP-1 and GCP-2 (but not IL-8 or GRO-α), and the upregulation of the ligands MHC-class I related antigen A (MICA) and vascular adhesion protein-1 (VAP-1). Signal transduction via the SAPK/JNK pathway appears to be important in the increased expression of MCP-1, GCP-2 and MICA. In addition, anti-EC antibodies also activate NF-κB. However, it has been demonstrated that anti-EC antibodies have an ability to induce EC apoptosis via the recognition of Hsp60 (Jamin et al., 2005). Once present, anti EC antibodies have the potential to inhibit potent antiinflammatory mechanisms (Nara et al., 2006).

5.5 The endothelial cell as an inflammation amplifier

ECs are able to amplify the inflammatory response by three main mechanisms: adhesion molecule expression, cytokine production and angiogenesis. Most of the primary immunopathogenic mechanisms playing a role in the pathogenesis of blood vessel inflammation in vasculitis include adhesion molecule expression and function (Cid et al., 2002). The studies *in vitro* show that complement activation products induce adhesion molecule expression by cultured ECs. C1q induces E-selectin, ICAM-1 and VCAM-1 (Del Papa et al., 1996) and C5a can upregulate P-selectin expression (Foreman et al., 1994). Immune complex and complement-mediated vessel damage *in vivo* require adhesion molecule expression and function. Also, ANCA binding to EC membrane-associated PR3 or related epitopes may induce E-selectin and VCAM-1 expression by ECs. PR3 released by neutrophils in the vicinity of ECs may induce EC ICAM-1 expression. Anti-EC antibody binding to ECs also induces endothelial adhesion molecule expression (Cid, 2002). The main inducers of endothelial adhesion molecules are the cytokines IL-1, TNF-α and IFN-γ which are produced by activated lymphocytes and macrophages in an vasculitis area (Raines & Ferri, 2005).

The expression of inducible adhesion molecules E-selectin and VCAM-1 by ECs as well as the upregulated constitutive expression of ICAM-1 were detected in patients with cutaneous leucocytoclastic vasculitis, Kawasaki disease, classical polyarteritis nodosa and gian-cell arteritis (Cid et al., 2000). In Wegener's granulomatosis, microscopic polyangitis and ANCA associated glomerulonephritis VCAM-1 and ICAM-1 expression were observed at the glomerular tuft as well as in tubular epithelial cells and peritubular capillaries (Rastaldi et al., 1996).

In small vessel vasculitis, endothelial adhesion molecule expression occurs in luminal endothelium (Sais et al., 1997). In medium-sized vasculitis, the luminal endothelium only expresses constitutive or inducible adhesion molecules at early stages. As the inflammatory process proceeds, the luminal endothelium is damaged and the vascular lumen is occluded. Then, endothelial adhesion molecules are expressed by adventitial neovessels (Coll-Vinent et al., 1998). In sclerotic glomeruli of kidney ANCA-associated vasculitis glomerular expression of ICAM-1 and VCAM-1 declines (Patey et al., 1996). In large-vessel vasculitis, adhesion molecule expression occurs in neovessels at the adventitia and at the intima/media junction. These observations suggest that infiltrating leucocytes penetrate the vessel wall through the adventitial vasa vasorum and neovessels in large- and medium-sized vessels.

In an inflammatory setting ECs have the potential to produce a variety of cytokines, chemokines and growth factors. In vasculitides a stimulation of ECs arises by ANCA binding, some anti-EC antibodies and cytokines released by infiltrating cells. By IL-1α and IL-6 production ECs contribute to the systemic acute phase in many systemic vasculitides. Colony-stimulating factors produced by ECs prolong the half-life of infiltrating leucocytes, while chemokines (IL-8, RANTES, Groα and SLC) selectively attract leucocyte subpopulations which bear specific receptors contributing to tissue targeting and amplifying vessel inflammation.

6. Conclusion

The endothelium has long been considered a passive physical barrier that only separates blood from tissues. Currently, it is clear that the endothelium is one of the most active organs which regulates many physiological functions and helps to coordinate functions of differentiated tissues in a way that meets the requirements of the organism as a whole. It has also emerged that ECs are the key immuno-reactive cells involved in host defence and inflammation. These cells both produce and react to a wide variety of mediators including cytokines, growth factors, adhesion molecules, vasoactive substances and chemokines, with effects on various cells. Prolonged or exaggerated endothelial activation leads to dysfunction (an early predclinical event of vascular disease) that is regulated by stromal cells and that can drive the vasculitis process with leucocyte recruitment, thrombosis and platelet plugging. Such local vascular inflammation has distant effects on the vascular endothelium leading to systemic endothelial dysfunction. Besides a whole panel of inflammatory markers used to monitor disease activity in systemic vasculitis circulating endothelial cells seem to be a promising new marker of this systemic disorder.

7. References

Ahn, Y.; Kim, Y.S. & Jeong, M.H. (2006). The role of nuclear factor kappa B activation in atherosclerosis and ischemic cardiac injury. *Korean Circulation J*, Vol.36, pp. 245-251, ISSN 1738-5520

Bach, F.H.; Hancock W.W. & Ferran, C. (1997). Protective genes expressed in endothelial cells: a regulatory response to injury. *Immunology today*, Vol.18, No.10, pp. 483-486, ISSN 0167 -5699

Baldwin, A. S. (1996). The NF-[kappa]B-[alpha] proteins: new discoveries and insights, *Ann Rev Immunol*, Vol.14, pp. 649-681, ISSN 0732-0582

Berghe, W. V.; Plaisance, S.; Boone, E.; De Bosscher, K.; Schmitz, M. L.; Fiers, W. & Haegeman, G. (1998). p38 and extracellular signal-regulated kinase mitogen-activated protein kinase pathways are required for nuclear factor-[kappa]B p65 transactivation mediated by tumor necrosis factor. *J Biol Chem*, Vol.273, pp. 3285-3290, ISSN 0021-9258

Bevilacqua, M.P. & Nelson, R.M. (1993). Selectins. *J Clin Invest*, Vol.91, pp. 379-387, ISSN 0021-9738

Bogdan, C.; Vodovotz, Y.; Paik, J.; Xie, Q.W. & Nathan, C. (1991). Mechanism of suppression of nitric oxide synthase expression by interleukin-4 in primary mouse macrophages. *J Leuk Biol*, Vol.55, pp. 227- 233, ISSN 0741-5400

Bogle, R.G.; Macallister, R.J.; Whitley, G.S.J. & Vallance, P. (1995). Induction of NG-monomethyl-L-arginine uptake: a mechanism for differential inhibition of NO synthases? *Am J Physiol Cell Physiol*, Vol.269, pp. C750–756, ISSN 0363-6143

Brady, R.H. (1994). Leukocyte adhesion molecules and kidney diseases. *Kidney Int*, Vol.45, pp. 1285-1300, ISSN 0085-2538

Brand, K.; Page, S.; Walli, A.K.; Neumerier, D. & Baeuerle, P.A. (1997). Impared endothelial function and smooth muscle cell function in oxidative stress: role of nuclear factor-[kappa]B in atherogenesis. *Exp Physiol*, Vol.82, pp. 297-304, ISSN 0958-0670

Brandes, R.P. & Kreuzer, J. (2005). Vascular NADPH oxidases: molecular mechanisms of activation. *Cardiovasc Res*, Vol.65, pp. 16-27, ISSN 0008-6363

Brown, K.; Gerstberger, S.; Carlson, L.; Franzoso, G. & Siebenlist, U. (1995). Control of [kappa]B-[alpha] proteolysis by sitespecific, signal-induced phosphorylation. *Science*, Vol.267, pp. 1485-1488, ISSN 0036-8075

Bruegger, D.; Rehm, M.; Abicht, J.; Paul, J.O.; Stoeckelhuber, M.; Pfirrmann, M.; Reichart, B.; Becker, B.F. & Christ, F. (2009). Shedding of the endothelial glycocalyx during cardiac surgery: on-pump versus off-pump coronary artery bypass graft surgery. *J Thorac Cardiovasc Surg*, Vol.138, pp. 1445–1447, ISSN 0022-5223

Bucci, M.; Gratton, J.P. & Rudic, R.D. (2000). In vivo delivery of the caveolin-1 scaffolding domain inhibits nitric oxide synthesis and reduces inflammation. *Nature Med*, Vol.6, pp. 1362–1367, ISSN 1078-8956

Cai, H. & Harrison, D. G. (2000). Endothelial dysfunction in cardiovascular diseases: the role of oxidant stress. *Circ Res,* Vol.87, pp. 840–844, ISSN 0009-7330

Calara, F.; Dimayuga, P.; Neimann, A.; Thyberg, J.; Diczfalusy, U. & Witztum J.L. (1998). Regnstrom: an animal model to study local oxidation of LDL and its biological effects in the arterial wall. *Arterioscler Thromb Vasc Biol,* Vol.18, pp. 884-893, ISSN 1079-5642

Chen, J.X. & Stinnett, A. (2008). Disruption of Ang-1/Tie-2 signaling contributes to the impaired myocardial vascular maturation and angiogenesis in type II diabetic mice. *Arterioscler Thromb Vasc Biol,* Vol.28, pp. 1606–1613, ISSN 1079-5642

Chen, X.L.; Varner, S.E.; Rao, A.S.; Grey, J.Y.; Thomas, S.; Cook, C.K.; Wasserman, M.A.; Medford, R.M.; Jaiswal, A.K. & Kunsch, C. (2003). Laminar flow induction of antioxidant response element-mediated genes in endothelial cells. A novel anti-inflammatory mechanism. *J Biol Chem,* Vol.278, pp. 703–711, ISSN 0021-9258

Chiba, R.; Nakagawa, N.; Kurasawa, K.; Tanaka, Y.; Saito, Y. & Iwamoto, I. (1999). Ligation of CD31 (PECAM-1) on endothelial cells increases adhesive function of αvß3 integrin and enhances ß1 integrin-mediated adhesion of eosinophils to endothelial cells. *Blood,* Vol.94, pp. 1319-1329, ISSN 0006-4971

Choi, H.K.; Lamprecht, P.; Niles, J.L.; Gross, W.L. & Merkel, P.A. (2000). Subacute bacterial endocarditis with positive cytoplasmic antineutrophil cytoplasmic antibodies and anti-proteinase 3 antibodies. *Arthritis Rheum,* Vol.43, pp. 226-231, ISSN 1529-0131

Choi, K.; Kennedy, M.; Kazarov, A.; Papadimitriou, J.C.; Keller, G.A. (1998). A common precursor for hematopoietic and endothelial cells. *Development,* Vol.125, pp. 725–732, ISSN 1011-6370

Cid, M.C. (2002). Endothelial cell biology, perivascular inflammation, and vasculitis. *Clev Clin J Med,* Vol.69, Suppl 2, pp. S1145-1149, ISSN 0891-1150

Cid, M.C.; Cebrián, M.; Font, C.; Coll-Vinent, B.; Hernández-Rodríguez, J.; Esparza, J.; Urbano-Márquez, A. & Grau, J. M . (2000). Cell adhesion molecules in the development of inflammatory infiltrates in giant-cell arteritis.Inflammation-induced angiogenesis as the preferential site of leukocyte-endothelial cell interactions. *Arthritis Rheum,* Vol.43, pp. 184-194, ISSN 1529-0131

Cid, M.C.; Coll-Vinent, B. & Bielsa, I. (2002). Endothelial cell adhesion molecules. In: *Inflammatory Diseases of Blood Vessels,* G.S. Hoffman, & C.M. Weyand, (Ed.), 13-28, Marcel Dekker, ISBN 978-082-4702-69-4

Cid, M.C.; Segarra, M.; García-Martínez, A. & Hernández-Rodríguez, J. (2004). Endothelial cells, antineutrophil cytoplasmic antibodies, and cytokines in the pathogenesis of systemic vasculitis. *Curr Rheumatol Rep,* Vol.6, No.3, pp. 184-194, ISSN 1523-3774

Coll-Vinent, B.; Cebrián, M.; Cid, M.C.; Font, C.; Esparza, J. & Juan, M. (1998). Dynamic pattern of endothelial cell adhesion molecule expression in muscle and perineural vessels from patients with classical polyarteritis nodosa. *Arthritis Rheum,* Vol.41, pp. 435-444, ISSN 1529-0131

Cook-Mills, J.M. & Deem, T.L. (2005). Active participation of endothelial cells in inflammation. *J Leukocyte Biol,* Vol.77, pp. 487-495, ISSN 0741-5400

Crabtree, M.J.; Tatham, A.L.; Hale, A.B.; Alp, N.J. & Channon, K.M. (2009). Critical role for tetrahydrofolate reductase in regulation of endothelial nitric-oxide synthase coupling: relative importance of the *de novo* biopterin synthesis versus salvage pathways. *J Biol Chem,* Vol.284, pp. 28128-28136, ISSN 0021-9258

Deem, T.L. & Cook-Mills, J.M. (2004). Vascular cell adhesion molecule-1 (VCAM-1) activation of endothelial cell matrix metalloproteinases: role of reactive oxygen species. *Blood,* Vol.104, pp. 2385-2393, ISSN 0006-4971

Dekker, R.J.; Soest, S.; Fontijn, R.D.; Salamanca, S.; Groot, P.; VanBavel, E.; Pannekoek, H. & Horrevoets, A. (2002). Prolonged fluid shear stress induces a distinct set of endothelial cell genes, most specifically lung Krüppel-like factor (KLF2). *Blood,* Vol.100, pp. 1689–1698, ISSN 0006-4971

Del Papa, N.; Guidalhi, L.; Sironi, M.; Shoenfeld, Y.; Mantovani, A. & Tincani, A. (1996). Anti-endothelial cell IgG antibodies from patients with Wegener's granulomatosis bind to human endothelial cells in vitro and induce adhesion molecule expression and cytokine secretion. *Arthritis Rheum,* Vol.39, pp. 758-766, ISSN 1529-0131

DeLeo, F.R. & Quinn, M.T. (1996). Assembly of the phagocyte NADPH oxidase: molecular interaction of oxidase proteins. *J Leukoc Biol,* Vol.60, pp. 677-691, ISSN 0741-5400

Díaz-Flores, L.; Gutiérrez, R.; Madrid, J.F.; Varela, H.; Valladares, F.; Acosta, E.; Martín-Vasallo, P.; Díaz-Flores, L. (2009). Pericytes. Morphofunction, interactions and pathology in a quiescent and activated mesenchymal cell niche. *Histol Histopathol,* Vol.24, pp. 909–969, ISSN 0213-3911

Dignat-George, F. & Sampol J. (2000). Circulating endothelial cells in vascular disorders: new insights into an old concept. *Eur J Haematol,* Vol.65, pp. 215-220, ISSN 0902-4441

Djordjević, B.V.; Stanković, T.; Ćosić, V.; Zvezdanović, L.; Kamenov, B.; Tasić-Dimov, D. & Stojanović, I. (2004). Immune system-mediated endothelial damage is associated with NO and antioxidant system disorders. *Clin Chem Lab Med,* Vol.42, No.10, pp. 1117 - 1121, ISSN 1434-6621

Djordjević, B.V.; Stojanović, I.; Ćosić, V.; Zvezdanović, L.; Deljanin-Ilić, M.; Dimić, S.; Kundalić, B.; Cvetković, T. & Jevtović-Stoimenov T. (2008). Serum neopterin, nitric oxide, inducible nitric oxide synthase and tumor necrosis factor-α levels in patients with ischemic heart disease. *Clin Chem Lab Med,* Vol.46, No.8, pp. 1149–1155, ISSN 1434-6621

Dorseuil, O.; Quinn, M.T. & Bokoch, G.M. (1995). Dissociation of Rac translocation from p47phox/p67phox movements in human neutrophils by tyrosine kinase inhibitors *J Leukoc Biol,* Vol.58, pp. 108-113, ISSN 0741-5400

Duperray, A.; Languino, L.R.; Plescia, J.; McDowall, A.; Hogg, N.; Craig, A.G.; Berendt, A.R. & Altieri, D.C. (1997). Molecular identification of a novel fibrinogen binding site on the first domain of ICAM-1 regulating leukocyte-endothelium bridging. *J Biol Chem,* Vol.272, pp. 435-441, ISSN 0021-9258

Endemann, D. & Schiffrin E. (2004). Endothelial dysfunction. *J Am Soc Nephrol,* Vol.15, pp. 1983-1992, ISSN 1046-6673

Etienne-Manneville, S.; Manneville, J.B.; Adamson, P.; Wilbourn, B.; Greenwood, J. & Couraud, P.O. (2000). ICAM-1-coupled cytoskeletal rearrangements and transendothelial lymphocyte migration involve intracellular calcium signaling in brain endothelial cell lines. *J Immunol,* Vol. 165, pp. 3375-3383, ISSN 0022-1767

Falk, R.J. & Jennette J.C. (1988). Anti-neutrophil cytoplasmatic autoantibodies with specificity for myeloperoxidase in patients with systemic vasculitis and idiopathic necrotizing and crescentic glomerulonephritis. *N Engl J Med,* Vol. 318, pp. 1651-1657, ISSN 0028-4793

Falk, R.J.; Terell, R.S.; Charles, R.A. & Jennette J.C. (1990). Anti-neutrophil cytoplasmic autoantibodies induce neutrophils to degranulate and produce oxygen radicals in vitro. *Proc Natl Acad Sci USA,* Vol.87, pp. 4115-4119, ISSN 0027-8424

Finkel T. (2003). Oxidant signals and oxidative stress. *Curr Opin Cell Biol,* Vol. 15, pp. 247-254, ISSN 1369-5266

Fitzgerald, M.L.; Wang, Z.; Park, P.W.; Murphy, G. & Bernfield, M. (2000). Shedding of syndecan-1 and -4 ectodomains is regulated by multiple signaling pathways and mediated by a TIMP-3-sensitive metalloproteinase. *J Cell Biol,* Vol.148, pp. 811–824, ISSN 1540-8140

Fledderus, J.O.; Boon, R.A.; Volger, O.L.; Hurttila, H.; Ylä-Herttuala, S.; Pannekoek, H.; Levonen, A.L. & Horrevoets, A.J. (2008). KLF2 primes the antioxidant transcription factor Nrf2 for activation in endothelial cells. *Arterioscler Thromb Vasc Biol,* Vol.28, pp. 1339–1346, ISSN 1079-5642

Flint, J.; Morgan, M.D. & Savage, C.O.S. ((2010). Pathogenesis of ANCA-associated vasculitis. *Rheum Dis Clin North Am,* Vol.36, No.3, pp. 463-477, ISSN 1558-3163

Flores-Suarez, L.F.; Cabiedes, J.; Villa, A.R.; van der Woude, F.J. & Alcocer-Varela, J. (2003). Prevalence of antineutrophil cytoplasmic autoantibodies in patients with tuberculosis. *Rheumatology (Oxford),* Vol.42, pp. 223-229, ISSN 1462-0324

Foreman, K.E.; Vaporciyan, A.A.; Bonish, B.K.; Jones, M.L.; Johnson, K.J.; Glovsky, M.M.; Eddy, S.M. & Ward P.A. (1994). C5a-induced expression of P-selectin in endothelial cells. *J Clin Invest,* Vol.94, pp. 1147-1155, ISSN 0021-9738

Fujimoto T. (1993). Calcium pump of the plasma membrane is localized in caveolae. *J Cell Biol,* Vol.120, pp. 1147–1157, ISSN 1540-8140

Gaengel, K.; Genové, G.; Armulik, A. & Betsholtz, C. (2009). Endothelial-mural cell signaling in vascular development and angiogenesis. *Arterioscler Thromb Vasc Biol,* Vol.29, pp. 630–638, ISSN 1079-5642

Galley, H. & Webster, N. (2004). Physiology of the endothelium. *Brit J Anaesth,* Vol.93, pp. 105-113, ISSN 0007-0912

Garcia-Cardena, G.; Martasek, P.; Masters, B.S.S.; Skidd, P.M.; Couet, J.; Li, S; Lisanti, M.P. & Sessa, W. (1997). Dissecting the interaction between nitric oxide synthase (NOS) and caveolin. Functional significance of the NOS caveolin binding domain *in vivo. J Biol Chem,* Vol.272, pp. 25437- 25440, ISSN 0021-9258

Groemping, Y. & Rittinger, K. (2005). Activation and assembly of the NADPH oxidase: a structural perspective. *Biochem J,* Vol.386, pp. 401-416, ISSN 0264-6021

Harrison, D.G. (1997). Cellular and molecular mechanisms of endothelial cell dysfunction. *J Clin Invest,* Vol.100, pp. 2153–2157, ISSN 0021-9738

Haubitz, M. & Woywodt A. (2004). Circulating endothelial cells and vasculitis. *Intern Med,* Vol.43, No.8, pp. 660-667, ISSN 0918-2918

Heeringa, P.; Schreiber, A.; Falk, R.J. & Jennette, J.C. (2004). Pathogenesis of pulmonary vasculitis. *Semin Respir Crit Care Med,* Vol.25, No.5, pp. 465-474, ISSN 1069-3424

Heiska, L.; Alfthan, K.; Gronholm, M.; Vilja, P.; Vaheri, A. & Carpen, O. (1998). Association of ezrin with intercellular adhesion molecule-1 and -2 (ICAM-1 and ICAM-2). Regulation by phosphatidylinositol 4, 5-bisphosphate. *J Biol Chem,* Vol.273, pp. 21893-21900, ISSN 0021-9258

Herren, B.; Levkau, B.; Raines, E.W. & Ross, R. (1998). Cleavage of ß-catenin and plakoglobin and shedding of VE-cadherin during endothelial apoptosis: evidence for a role for caspases and metalloproteinases. *Mol Biol Cell,* Vol.9, pp. 1589-1601, ISSN 1059-1524

Hojo, Y.; Saito, Y.; Tanimoto, T.; Hoefen, R.; Baines, C.; Yamamoto, K.; Haendeler, J.; Asmis, R. & Berk, B. (2002). Fluid shear stress attenuates hydrogen peroxide-induced c-Jun NH2-terminal kinase activation via a glutathione reductase-mediated mechanism. *Circ Res,* Vol.91, pp. 712–718, ISSN 0009-7330

Igarashi, J.; Thatte, H.S.; Prabhakar, P.; Golan, D.E. & Michel T. (1999). Calcium-independent activation of endothelial nitric oxide synthase by ceramide. *Proc Natl Acad Sci USA,* Vol.96, pp. 12583–12588, ISSN 0027-8424

Jackson, D.E.; Ward, C.M.; Wang, R. & Newman, P.J. (1997). The protein-tyrosine phosphatase SHP-2 binds platelet/endothelial cell adhesion molecule-1 (PECAM-1) and forms a distinct signaling complex during platelet aggregation. Evidence for a mechanistic link between PECAM-1- and integrin-mediated cellular signaling. *J Biol Chem,* Vol.272, pp. 6986-6993, ISSN 0021-9258

Jamin, C.; Dugue, C.; Alard, J.E.; Jousse, S.; Saraux, A.; Guillevin, L.; Piette, J.C. & Youinou P. (2005). Induction of endothelial cell apoptosis by the binding of anti-endothelial cell antibodies to Hsp60 in vasculitis-associated systemic autoimmune diseases. *Arthritis Rheum,* Vol.52, pp. 4028 -4038, ISSN 1529-0131

Jennette, J.C.; Hoidai, J.R. & Falk R.J. (1990). Specificity of anti-neutrophil cytoplasmatic autoantibodies for proteinase 3. *Blood,* Vol.75, pp. 2263-2264, ISSN 0006-4971

Kissel, J.T.; Riethman, J.L.; Omerza, J.; Rammohan, K.W. & Mendell J.R. (1989). Peripheral nerve vasculitis: immune characterization of the vascular lesions. *Ann Neurol,* Vol.25, pp. 291-297, ISSN 0364-5134

Kopp, E. & Ghosh S. (1994). Inhibition of NF-[kappa]B by sodium salicylate and aspirin. *Science,* Vol.265, pp. 956-959, ISSN 0036-8075

Kraft, A.D.; Johnson, D.A. & Johnson, J.A. (2004). Nuclear factor E2-related factor 2-dependent antioxidant response element activation by tert-butylhydroquinone and sulforaphane occurring preferentially in astrocytes conditions neurons against oxidative insult. *J Neurosci,* Vol.24, pp. 1101–1112, ISSN 0270-6474

Lee, T.J. & Yu, J.G. (2002). L-Citrulline recycle for synthesis of NO in cerebral perivascular nerves and endothelial cells. *Ann NY Acad Sci,* Vol.962, pp. 73–80, ISSN 0077-8923

Li, J.M.; Fan, L.M.; Christie, M.R. & Shah, A.M. (2005). Acute tumor necrosis factor alpha signaling via NADPH oxidase in microvascular endothelial cells: role of $p47^{phox}$ phosphorylation and binding to TRAF4. *Mol Cell Biol,* Vol.25, pp. 2320-2330, ISSN 1471-0072

Mamdouh, Z.; Chen, X.; Pierini, LM.; Maxfield, F.R. & Muller, W.A. (2003). Targeted recycling of PECAM from endothelial surface-connected compartments during diapedesis. *Nature,* Vol.421, pp. 748-753, ISSN 1078-8956

Mandell, B.F. & Calabrese L.H. (1998). Infections and systemic vasculitis. *Curr Opin Rheumatol,* Vol.10, pp. 51-57, ISSN 1040-8711

Mann, G.E.; Yudilevich, D.L. & Sobrevia, L. (2003). Regulation of amino acid and glucose transporters in endothelial and smooth muscle cells. *Physiol Rev,* Vol.83, pp. 183–252, ISSN 0031-9333

Mannick J.B. (2007). Regulation og apoptosis by protein S-nitrosylation. *Amino Acids,* Vol.32, pp. 523-526, ISSN 0939-4451

Mantovani, A.; Bussolino, F. & Introna M. (1997). Cytokine regulation of endothelial cell function: from molecular level to the bedside. *Immunol Today,* Vol.18, pp. 231- 240, ISSN 0167 -5699

Matheny, H.E.; Deem, T.L. & Cook-Mills, J.M. (2000). Lymphocyte migration through monolayers of endothelial cell lines involves VCAM-1 signaling via endothelial cell NADPH oxidase *J Immunol,* Vol.164, pp. 6550-6559, ISSN 0022-1767

Michel, J.B.; Feron, O.; Sacks, D. & Michel T. (1997). Reciprocal regulation of endothelial nitric-oxide synthase by Ca2+-calmodulin and caveolin. *J Biol Chem,* Vol.272, pp. 15583- 15586, ISSN 0021-9258

Mulivor, A.W. & Lipowsky, H.H. (2004). Inflammation- and ischemia-induced shedding of venular glycocalyx. *Am J Physiol Heart Circ Physiol,* Vol.286, pp. H1672–H1680, ISSN 0363-6135

Murphy, G.; Willenbrock, F.; Crabbe, T.; O'Shea, M.; Ward, R.; Atkinson, S.; O'Connell, J. & Docherty, A. (1994). Regulation of matrix metalloproteinase activity. *Ann N Y Acad Sci,* Vol.732, pp. 31-41, ISSN 0077-8923

Nara, H.; Okamoto, H.; Minota, S. & Yoshio, T. (2006). Mouse monoclonal anti-human thrombomodulin antibodies bind to and activate endothelial cells through NF-kappaB activation in vitro. *Arthritis Rheum,* Vol.54, pp. 1629 -1637, ISSN 1529-0131

Palmer, R.M.J.; Ashton, D.S. & Moncada, S. (1988). Vascular endothelial cells synthesize nitric oxide from L-arginine. *Nature,* Vol.333, pp. 664 - 666, ISSN 1078-8956

Patey, N.; Lesavre, P; Halbwachs-Mecarelli, L. & Noel L.H. (1996). Adhesion molecules in human crescentic glomerulonephritis. *J Pathol,* Vol.179, pp. 414-420, ISSN 0022-3417

Pellegatta, F.; Chierchia, S.L. & Zocchi, M.R. (1998). Functional association of platelet endothelial cell adhesion molecule-1 and phosphoinositide 3-kinase in human neutrophils *J Biol Chem,* Vol.273, pp. 27768-27771, ISSN 0021-9258

Peng, H.B.; Libby, P. & Liao, J.K. (1995). Induction and stabilization of I kappa B alpha by nitric oxide mediates inhibition of NF-kappa B. *J Biol Chem,* Vol.270, pp. 14214–14219, ISSN 0021-9258

Porges, A.J.; Redecha, P.B. & Kimberly, W.T. (1994). Anti-neutrophil cytoplasmic antibodies engage and activate human neutrophils via Fc-RIIa. *J Immunol,* Vol.153, pp. 1271-1280, ISSN 0022-1767

Praprotnik, S.; Blank, M.; Meroni, P.L.; Rozman, B.; Eldor, A. & Shoenfeld Y. (2001). Classification of anti-endothelial cell antibodies into antibodies against microvascular and macrovascular endothelial cells: the pathogenic and diagnostic implications. *Arthritis Rheum,* Vol.44, pp. 1484-1494, ISSN 1529-0131

Pumphrey, N.J.; Taylor, V.; Freeman, S.; Douglas, M.R.; Bradfield, P.F.; Young, S.P.; Lord, J.M.; Wakelam, M.J.; Bird, I.N.; Salmon, M. & Buckley, CD. (1999). Differential association of cytoplasmic signalling molecules SHP-1, SHP-2, SHIP and phospholipase C-γ1 with PECAM-1/CD31. *FEBS Lett,* Vol.450, pp. 77-83, ISSN 0014-5793

Rabelink, T.J. & Luscher, T.F. (2006). Endothelial nitric oxide synthase: host defense enzyme of the endothelium? *Arterioscler Thromb Vasc Biol,* Vol.26, pp. 267–271, ISSN 1079-5642

Radford, D.J.; Savage, C.O. & Nash G.B. (2000). Treatment of rolling neutrophils with antineutrophil cytoplasmic antibodies causes conversion to firm integrin-mediated adhesion. *Arthritis Rheum,* Vol.43, pp. 1337-1345, ISSN 1529-0131

Raines, E. & Ferri N. (2005). Cytokines affecting endothelial and smooth cells in vascular disease. *J Lipid Res,* Vol.46, pp. 1081-1092, ISSN 0022-2275

Rastaldi, M.P.; Ferrario, F.; Tunesi, S.; Yang, L. & d'Amico G. (1996). Intraglomerular and interstitial leukocyte infiltration, adhesion molecules, and interleukin-1 alpha expression in 15 cases of anti–neutrophil cytoplasmic autoantibody–associated renal vasculitis. *Am J Kidney Dis,* Vol.27, pp. 48-57, ISSN 0272-6386

Rattan, V.; Sultana, C.; Shen, Y. & Kalra, V.K. (1997). Oxidant stress-induced transendothelial migration of monocytes is linked to phosphorylation of PECAM-1. *Am J Physiol,* Vol.273, pp. E453-E461, ISSN 0885-8276

Ray, R. & Shah, A.M. (2005). NADPH oxidase and endothelial cell function. *Clin Sci,* Vol.109, pp. 217-226, ISSN 0143-5221

Read, M.A.; Whitley, M.Z.; Williams, A.J. & Collins T. (1994). NF-κB and IκBα: An inducible regulatory system in endothelial activation. *J Exp Med,* Vol.179, pp. 503-512, ISSN 1540-9538

Roebuck, K.A. & Finnegan, A. (1999). Regulation of intercellular adhesion molecule-1 (CD54) gene expression *J Leukoc Biol,* Vol.66, pp. 876-888, ISSN 0741-5400

Ryter, S.W.; Alam, J. & Choi, A.M. (2006). Heme oxygenase-1/carbon monoxide: from basic science to therapeutic applications. *Physiol Rev,* Vol.86, pp. 583–650, ISSN 0031-9333

Sais, G.; Vidaller, A.; Jugcla, A.; Condom, E. & Peyri J. (1997). Adhesion molecule expression and endothelial cell activation in cutaneous leukocytoclastic vasculitis: an immunohistologic and clinical study in 42 patients. *Arch Dermatol,* Vol. 133, pp. 443-450, ISSN 0003-987X

Sano, H.; Nakagawa, N.; Chiba, R.; Kurasawa, K.; Saito, Y. & Iwamoto, I. (1998). Cross-linking of intercellular adhesion molecule-1 induces interleukin-8 and RANTES production through the activation of MAP kinases in human vascular endothelial cells. *Biochem Biophys Res Commun,* Vol.250, pp. 694-698, ISSN 0006-291X

Savage, C.; & Williams, J. (2007). Anti–Endothelial Cell Antibodies in Vasculitis. *J Am Soc Nephrol,* Vol.18, pp. 2424-2426, ISSN 1046-6673

Sawada, N.; Murata, M. & Kikuchi K. (2003). Tight junctions and human diseases. *Med Electron Microsc,* Vol.36, pp. 147–156, ISSN 1437-773X

Schenkel, A.R.; Mamdouh, Z.; Chen, X.; Liebman, R.M. & Muller, W.A. (2002). CD99 plays a major role in the migration of monocytes through endothelial junctions. *Nat Immunol,* Vol.3, pp. 143-150, ISSN : 1529-2908

Shaw, S.K.; Perkins, B.N.; Lim, Y.C.; Liu, Y.; Nusrat, A.; Schnell, F.J.; Parkos, C.A. & Luscinskas, F.W. (2001). Reduced expression of junctional adhesion molecule and platelet/endothelial cell adhesion molecule-1 (CD31) at human vascular endothelial junctions by cytokines tumor necrosis factor-α plus interferon-γ does not reduce leukocyte transmigration under flow. *Am J Pathol,* Vol.159, pp. 2281-2291, ISSN 0887-8005

Smith, J.D.; Lawson, C.; Yacoub, M.H. & Rose, M.L. (2000). Activation of NF-kappa B in human endothelial cells induced by monoclonal and allospecific HLA antibodies. *Int Immunol,* Vol.12, pp. 563 –571, ISSN 0953-8178

Steiner, L.; Kroncke, K.; Fehsel, K. & Kolb-Bachofen V. (1997). Endothelial cells as cytotoxic effector cells: cytokine-activated rat islet endothelial cells lyse syngeneic islet cells via nitric oxide. *Diabetologia,* Vol.40, pp. 2150–2155, ISSN 0012-186X

Tarbell, J.M. & Ebong, E.E. (2008). The endothelial glycocalyx: a mechano-sensor and -transducer. *Sci Signal* 1, pt8, ISSN 1945-0877

Thannickal, V.J. & Fanburg, BL. (2000). Reactive oxygen species in cell signaling. *Am J Physiol Lung Cell Mol Physiol,* Vol.279, pp. L1005-L1028, ISSN 1040-0605

Thurberg, B.L. & Collins, T. (1998). The nuclear factor-kappa B/inhibitor of kappa B autoregulatory system and atherosclerosis. *Curr Opin Lipidol,* Vol.9, pp. 387–396, ISSN 0957-9672.

Toyoda, M.; Petrosian, A. & Jordan S.C. (1999). Immunological characterisation of anti-endothelial cell antibodies induced by cytomegalovirus infection. *Transplantation,* Vol.68, pp. 1311 -1318, ISSN 0931-0509

Tse, W.Y.; Williams, J.; Pall, A.; Wilkes, M.; Savage, C.O. & Adu, D. (2001). Antineutrophil cytoplasmic antibody-induced neutrophil nitric oxide production is nitric oxide synthase independent. *Kidney Int,* Vol.9, pp. 593-600, ISSN 0085-2538

Tudor, S.; Hess, K.L. & Cook-Mills, J.M. (2001). Cytokines modulate endothelial cell intracellular signal transduction required for VCAM-1-dependent lymphocyte transendothelial migration *Cytokine,* Vol.15, pp. 196-211, ISSN 1043-4666

Van Wart, H.E. & Birkedal-Hansen, H. (1990). The cysteine switch: a principle of regulation of metalloproteinase activity with potential applicability to the entire matrix metalloproteinase gene family. *Proc Natl Acad Sci, USA,* Vol.87, pp. 5578-5582, ISSN 0027-8424

Wang, J.B.; Guan, J.; Shen, J.; Zhou, L.; Zhang, Y.J.; Si, Y.F.; Yang, L.; Jian, X.H. & Sheng Y. (2009). Insulin increases shedding of syndecan-1 in the serum of patients with type 2 diabetes mellitus. *Diabetes Res Clin Pract,* Vol.86, pp. 83–88, ISSN 0168-8227

Wang, Q. & Doerschuk, C.M. (2001). The p38 mitogen-activated protein kinase mediates cytoskeletal remodeling in pulmonary microvascular endothelial cells upon intracellular adhesion molecule-1 ligation *J Immunol,* Vol.166, pp. 6877-6884, ISSN 0022-1767

Weinbaum, S.; Tarbell, J.M. & Damiano, E.R. (2007). The structure and function of the endothelial glycocalyx layer. *Annu Rev Biomed Eng,* Vol.9, pp. 121–167, ISSN 1523-9829

Weiner, C.P.; Lizasoain, I.; Baylis, S.A.; Knowles, R.C.; Charles, I.C. & Moncada S. (1994). Induction of calcium-dependent nitric oxide synthase by sex hormones. *Proc Natl Acad Sci USA,* Vol.91: pp. 5212– 5216, ISSN 0027-8424

Xia, Y; Tsai, A; Berka, V. & Zweier J.L. (1998). Superoxide generation from endothelial nitric oxide synthase. A Ca2+ /calmodulin-dependent and tetrahydrobiopterin regulatory process. *J Biol Chem,* Vol.273, pp. 25804-25808, ISSN 0021-9258

Yang, J.J; Preston, G. & Pendergraft W. (2001). Internalization of proteinase 3 is concomitant with endothelial cell apoptosis and internalization of myeloperoxidase with generation of intracellular oxidants. *Am J Pathol,* Vol. 158, pp. 581-592, ISSN 0887-8005

Zhang, J.; DeFelice, A.F.; Hanig, J.P. & Colatsky, T. (2010). Biomarkers of endothelial cell activation serve as potential surrogate markers for drug-induced vascular injury. *Toxicol Pathol,* Vol.38, No.6, (October 2010), pp. 856-871, ISSN 0192-6233

Zhong, H.; SuYang, H; Erdjument-Bromage, H; Tempst, P. & Ghosh S. (1997). The transcriptional activity of NF-[kappa]B is regulated by the I[kappa]B-associated PKAc subunit through a cyclic AMP-independent mechanism. *Cell,* Vol.89, pp. 413-424, ISSN 0092-8674

9

Markers of Vascular Damage and Repair

Uta Erdbruegger[1], Ajay Dhaygude[2] and Alexander Woywodt[2]
[1]*Division of Nephrology, University of Virginia at Charlottesville, Charlottesville,*
[2]*Renal Unit, Lancashire Teaching Hospitals NHS Foundation Trust, Preston, Lancashire,*
[1]*USA*
[2]*United Kingdom*

1. Introduction

Damage to endothelial cells is a crucial event during the pathogenesis of vasculitis. The vasculitides cause different clinical manifestations, depending on the extent and acuity of endothelial damage as well as their preponderance to affect some organ-specific endothelial cells and spare others. About 40 years ago circulating endothelial cells (CEC) were first observed in peripheral blood. Since then CEC have been established as a reliable indicator of vascular injury and damage and more sophisticated detection techniques, such as immunomagnetic isolation and fluorescence-activated cell sorting (FACS), have become available to detect and enumerate them. Based on current concepts of pathogenesis, detached endothelial cells, and/or their soluble and cellular debris, must be detectable in peripheral blood of vasculitis patients. In hindsight, it is therefore surprising that for many years few, if any, attempts were made to evaluate their use as clinically relevant markers of endothelial damage. Endothelial Microparticles (eMP) have been described as another potential marker of endothelial damage. eMP are markers of activation, cell injury or apoptosis. They are the product of exocytic budding and consist of cytoplasmic components and phospholipids. Fluorescence-activated cell sorting (FACS) is the preferred technology for isolating MP and different surface markers of the parent cells have been used. eMP can reflect endothelial activation and damage, although differences between eMP and CEC remain ill-defined. Another approach to measuring endothelial damage is to assay soluble markers, such as thrombomodulin or von Willebrand factor. However, these markers also have their limitations. It is also worthwhile to remember that all approaches struggle with the fact that many endothelial markers are also expressed on non-endothelial cells (Table 1). More recently, interest has focused on endothelial repair and damage and endothelial progenitor cells have been studied, again with different methodologies. Recent evidence has also revealed interesting interactions between CEC and healthy endothelium in vitro although the relevance of these findings for human vascular disease in vivo remains unclear. Here, we review markers of endothelial damage and repair in vasculitis. We discuss the implications of these findings for the pathogenesis, their potential clinical utility, and also review the limitations of each approach. Finally, we review the phenotype of CEC, mechanisms of detachment and interactions with other cell subsets.

2. Soluble endothelial markers

Endothelial cells express a broad variety of proteins [1] but only few of these have been studied in serum or plasma in vascular disease. Currently, von Willebrand factor (vWF), thrombomodulin [2], soluble E-Selectin and circulating angiopoietin [3] are best described [4-7]. It must be noted that several factors may influence the levels of these circulating proteins. For example, thrombomodulin undergoes renal excretion. Hence, serum levels are influenced by renal function. Other confounding factors, such as liver function, clotting or fibrinolysis may also influence these proteins. In addition, these soluble markers do not distinguish between endothelial activation and damage. Some investigators compared levels of these markers with numbers of CECs. A recent study found a correlation between CECs, von Willebrand factor ($p=0.002$) and plasma tissue factor ($p=0.02$) [8]. It is also clear that necrotic endothelial cells will release, either in situ or after their detachment from the basement membrane, a variety of other, nonspecific, soluble factors. In this regard, Bruchfeld and colleagues recently reported elevated levels of High-mobility group box-1 protein (HMGB1), a nuclear and cytosolic protein that is released from necrotic cells [9]. However HMGB1 is also actively secreted from monocytes and macrophages. Angiopoietin-2 (Ang-2) is another new soluble marker investigated in small vessel vasculitis. Ang-2 is bound to the endothelial specific angiopoietin Tie Ligand–receptor, which is a regulator of endothelial cell detachment. Circulating Ang-2 is elevated in small vessel vasculitis and closely correlates with vasculitis activity score [3]. Ang-2 therefore reflects a potential new mediator of endothelial cell detachment in vasculitis although theses findings need to be validated by analyzing a larger cohort.

CD/antigen name	Other names	Expression by non-endothelial cells
CD31	PECAM-1	Platelets, monocytes, neutrophils, T cell subsets
CD62e	E-selectin	Activated endothelial cells
CD54	ICAM-1	Endothelial cells, activated B and T lymphocytes, monocytes
CD105	Endoglin	Endothelial cells, activated monocytes, tissue macrophages, erythroid marrow precursors
CD106	VCAM-1	Activated endothelial cells, stromal cells
CD141	Thrombomoduli n	Endothelial cells, keratinocytes, platelets, monocytes, neutrophils
CD146	P1H12, S-endo-1	Endothelial cells, activated T-Lymphocytes, melanoma cells, trophoblast
Tissue factor		Endothelial cells, monocytes/macrophages

Table 1. Antigens of endothelial cells, which are also present on non-endothelial cells

3. Circulating endothelial cells in vasculitis

Circulating endothelial cells (CEC) are detectable in peripheral blood after they have been detached from the damaged endothelial monolayer, probably leaving behind a denuded basement membrane. Those cells were first described almost 40 years ago [10] although methods of their identification were rather primitive. ANCA-associated small-vessel vasculitis serves as a paradigm of an endothelial disorder. Therefore it is not surprising that high numbers of CEC are detected in ANCA vasculitis and correlate with disease activity [11]. Phenotypic analysis, however, proved more difficult than anticipated. It is quite clear from the concept of small vessel vasculitis that CEC cannot be specific to ANCA vasculitis. Dang and colleagues reported elevated CEC numbers in aortoarteritis [12] while Nakatani et al. demonstrated CECs in patients with Kawasaki disease [13]. CEC are also elevated in systemic lupus erythematosus [14] and Behcet's [15]. In a broader sense, CEC are also markedly elevated in other, non-vasculitic, forms of widespread acute vasculopathy, such as thrombotic microangiopathy [16]. In addition, CEC can be useful to monitor treatment and to distinguish between relapse and infection in difficult cases [17]. Patients with relapse of vasculitis had markedly elevated numbers of circulating endothelial cells and indeed similar cell numbers when compared to patients at their initial vasculitic presentation[18]. Patients with limited disease due to granulomatous ANCA-associated vasculitis had only slightly elevated cell numbers, which were similar to those seen in remission. Patients with infection had no elevated CEC numbers [18]. These findings gave us confidence in the clinical use of CEC in vasculitis [17, 19] although prospective data on the clinical use of CEC are lacking.

	CEC	EPC
Cell type	Mature endothelium	Endothelial progenitor cell
Origin	Vessel wall	Bone marrow
Morphology	Cells, a-nuclear carcasses or sheets of multiple cells 10-100μm	Diameter less than 20μm
Characteristic properties	VWF CD 31 Thrombomodulin CD 146 UEA-1	CD 133 CD 34 TIE-2 KDR Uptake of acetylated LDL UEA-1 (unclear)
Colony-forming potential	None (controversial)	Yes
Laboratory methods	Immunomagnetic isolation, FACS	FACS, culture assays

Table 2. Characteristic properties of CEC and EPC

3.1 CEC and vasculitis: Immunomagnetic isolation and FACS in competition

The mainstay of immunomagnetic isolation is the use of paramagnetic particles (Dynabeads™), which have been coated with anti-endothelial antibodies as reviewed in great detail elsewhere [10]. Briefly, whole blood is incubated with antibody-labeled magnetic Dynabeads™. Next, target cells with bound anti-endothelial antibody and Dynabeads™ are recovered with a magnet. CEC can then be enumerated after acridine staining. Immunomagnetic capturing is mostly performed using the cell surface marker CD 146 [20].

A variety of factors has been considered to influence CEC counts [21]. To avoid false positive results caused by traumatic venepuncture (resulting in dislodgement of endothelial cells from the vessel wall) it is recommended to discard the first tube of blood [20]. Adding albumin or EDTA and Fc-blocking agents is employed to reduce non-specific binding of anti-CD 146-coupled beads to leukocytes although this remains a concern even in experienced hands [22]. Moreover, activated T-lymphocytes and other cell subsets may under some circumstances also harbor CD 146 and lead to artifacts [23]. We therefore developed a secondary stain with Ulex Europaeus lectin 1 (UEA-1). [24] Even so and despite the proposal of a consensus for definition of CEC the approach remains time consuming and require considerable experience. Automated systems have been described but these are costly [25].

Flow cytometry is an alternative technique to isolate and enumerate CEC [26-31]. The technique holds considerable promise, as several surface markers can be used concurrently. For example, CD 146 expression on activated T cells can be distinguished from CD 146 on endothelial cells by co-staining with CD45 or CD3 (or both). CD 133 may help to identify EPC because it is not present on CEC or any mature endothelial cells. The addition of viability stains, such as propidium iodide or 7-AAD, may also help to identify EPC. Markers of endothelial activation can be studied as well. Most groups define CEC using flow cytometry as CD146+, CD34+ and CD45- [32]. Others have defined CEC as CD31bright, CD34+CD45-, CD133- [33 34]. However, CD31 bright could also include platelets, resulting in falsely elevated numbers of CEC [35].

Unlike immunomagnetic isolation, FACS does not permit visualization of the cell. Furthermore the cell numbers obtained with FACS differ markedly from those obtained with immunomagnetic isolation, whereby higher numbers are usually observed with FACS. In addition, there is considerable discrepancy in these numbers between different groups that employ FACS. It is remarkable that most if not all investigators using immunomagnetic isolation enumerate in the range of 10 CEC/ml blood in healthy individuals while those using FACS report cell numbers in the thousands per ml with a fairly broad range [10]: Holmen and colleagues measured a mean of 50 CEC/ml in healthy controls [26], Mancuso et al. counted 1,200 CEC/ml of rested cells [36] and Jacques N et al. 6.5 CEC/ml [37]. Two groups compared CEC counts measured with both methods in the same populations. Goon et al. measured 8 CEC/ml in healthy controls comparable to CEC detection by IB (4.5CEC/ml) [32]. In contrast, Clarke et al. detected lower numbers of CEC by FC compared to IB [38] suggesting limited sensitivity for the detection of CECs. Further validation studies are required to determine the influence of gating, CEC phenotype, and "lysing", which could reduce recovery of CEC.

In comparison to immuno-magnetic isolation, FACS holds considerable promise and technical advantages. In addition, FACS is less time consuming and easily amenable to standardization. Cost is difficult to compare with immunomagnetic isolation, given the expenditure for the FACS counter and the fact that the cost of experienced staff is difficult to gauge. Very recently alternative approaches have combined the two techniques [39]. This novel tool has to be validated in other clinical settings and populations.

3.2 Phenotype and mechanisms of detachment of CEC in vasculitis

Endothelial cells can be activated by various stimuli, such as pro-inflammatory cytokines, growth factors, infectious agents, lipoproteins, or oxidative stress. Loss of integrity of the endothelial layer eventually leads to cell detachment of cells [40]. Such detachment can be caused by defective adhesive properties of the endothelial cells, by action of proteases and/or cytokines or, by mechanical injury. Endothelial adhesive molecules of the integrin and cadherin family, such as vitronectin and fibronectin and VE cadherin, respectively, promote adhesion of endothelial cells to matrix [40-41]. Loss of these survival signals triggers detachment and apoptosis of endothelial cells [42]. Protective factors have been described as well: In sickle cell disease endothelial apoptosis is impaired by VEGF. This has also been shown in vitro, where VEGF inhibits apoptosis of unanchored culture cells [43]. Release of proteases by granulocytes is another well-documented cause of endothelial cell detachment [44-45 46 47]. Finally, mechanical force can detach endothelial cells from the basement membrane as shown in patients undergoing percutaneous catheter interventions [48].

Not much is known regarding the phenotype of CEC. This is caused mainly by the paucity of CEC even in active disease and in the difficulty of characterizing these cells further. Moreover, it is difficult to say with certainty whether or not phenotypic changes were induced by the isolation procedure itself. The viability of CEC remains particularly controversial. Our own data suggest that CEC in ANCA-associated small-vessel vasculitis are mainly necrotic [11] and we were unable to culture these cells. Others, however, describe culture of CEC that were isolated by FACS. In contrast, two-thirds of CEC in normal subjects are believed to be apoptotic [49]. Lin et al could also demonstrate that vessel-wall derived CD146+ CEC can be viable, although they have limited growth capability [50]. Another group was recently able to grow CEC for about 10 days, but no significant proliferative capacity was observed [26].

3.3 Circulating endothelial cells as potential mediators of disease

It has been speculated that CEC themselves could be pro-inflammatory [40]. In general, damaged eukaryotic cells have been shown to release a variety of pro-inflammatory factors, to initiate pro-inflammatory pathways in other cell subsets, such as a Toll-like-receptor-2/NFκB-dependent reaction in monocytes [51]. In highly active vasculitis, the healthy endothelium must surely encounter a vast array of apoptotic and/or necrotic endothelial cells and their debris. Disturbed clearance of apoptotic cells may play a role in systemic lupus erythematosus [52]. Interestingly, apoptotic and necrotic endothelial cells and their fragments are rapidly internalized by healthy endothelium [53]. Support for these findings came from other studies demonstrating the phagocytic capability of endothelial cells [54]. We could also show that endothelial cells exposed to apoptotic and necrotic cells exhibit enhanced adhesion properties for leukocytes and that isolated CEC from patients with vasculitis aggravated these effects further [53]. These effects on binding properties could be explained in part by release of IL-8 and MCP1, which serve as chemo-attractants. Interestingly, apoptotic and necrotic cells induced different patterns of effects in healthy endothelium. Enhanced IL-8 and MCP1 levels in serum have been detected in patients with active vasculitis and ANCA induce the synthesis of these chemokines in various cell subsets [55]. Endothelial synthesis of these mediators triggered by ANCA [56] and circulating endothelial cells [53] may contribute to the pro-inflammatory state associated with vasculitis.

We have investigated this topic further and became interested in thrombospondin (TSP-1) as a possible mediator. This multi-functional glycoprotein is a known endogenous inhibitor of angiogenesis [57] and modulates cell adhesion and proliferation [58]. We were able to show that apoptotic cells induce expression of TSP-1 in endothelial cells [59] and that TSP-1 facilitates engulfment of apoptotic cells by phagocytes [59]. We speculate that under pathological conditions with high numbers of un-cleared dying cells in the circulation endothelial-derived elevated TSP-1 level may serve as an attraction signal for phagocytes promoting enhanced recognition and clearance of apoptotic cells.

It is probably fair to say that at present we do not understand the interactions between CEC and healthy endothelium and other cell subsets. Further studies, for example in animal models, are surely warranted. Figure 1 summarizes proven and proposed interactions of circulating endothelial cells with healthy endothelium.

4. Microparticles in vasculitis: Just smaller than CEC or different, too?

Microparticles (MP) are sub-micrometric fragments derived from plasma membranes in response to a variety of events, such as activation, injury, or apoptosis. Loss of phospholipid asymmetry and increased surface expression of phosphatidylserine are crucial events in this process [60-61]. On their surface these particles express antigens that reflect their cellular origin, which permits their enumeration and characterisation by flow cytometry. In addition eMP have a functional role as mediators of inflammation or coagulation. In general, microparticles have attracted considerable interest in vascular disease although a consensus definition of these particles and a uniformly accepted protocol for their enumeration is still lacking [62]. To make matters even more complicated, endothelial microparticles represent a small subgroup of all MP found in plasma[63]. Specific endothelial microparticles were first described in 1990 by Hamilton and colleagues [64]. On balance, it is probably fair to say that the field of microparticles is fraught with similar technical issues as that of CEC and that further standardisation is eagerly awaited.

We studied endothelial microparticles (EMP) by FACS analysis and found elevated EMP in active vasculitis [65]. Similar results had previously been obtained in a paediatric cohort of vasculitis patients [60 66]. Particle counts also correlated with disease activity [65]. The difficult bit is that CECs and microparticles may not reflect the same disease process. Incidentally, the same holds true for soluble endothelial markers, such as soluble von Willebrand factor or thrombomodulin: CEC, EMP and soluble markers may represent different mechanisms of endothelial activation and damage. For example, soluble markers and EMP may already be elevated in endothelial activation whereas presence of CEC probably reflects true damage. Interestingly CEC and eMP also follow different kinetics in ANCA-associated vasculitis: CEC decline slowly during successful immunosuppressive therapy while activated eMP probably represent an early marker that normalises quickly [65]. To make matters even more complicated, each of these markers may underlie different confounding factors: eMP are elevated in patients with renal diseases including those on hemodialysis [67] and could reflect vascular damage in these patients whereas CEC are not increased in renal failure [11]. Nevertheless, ESRD patients with and without a history of cardiovascular disease causing possible endothelial damage had similar levels of EMP [68]. This illustrates that phenotyping of microparticles and characterization of subgroups of microparticles for each different disease process will be crucial as each disease process will release different microparticles.

Finally, EMP may also have pathogenetic importance in vasculitis. Microparticles are now regarded as crucial players at the interface of atherosclerosis and inflammation [69]. MP are generally capable of inducing cytokine release [70] and leukocyte MP induce endothelial IL-6 and MCP-1 production [71]. It has been demonstrated that endothelial microparticles convert plasminogen into plasmin [72] and are tissue-factor positive [73] . Burkhart et al. demonstrated recently that microparticle tissue factor activity is increased in PR3-ANCA vasculitis patients with active disease [74].

Evidence has also emerged to suggest that endothelial release of microparticles from adherent cells is actually protective and that inhibition of microparticle release leads to endothelial detachment [75]. Moreover, pre-treatment of endothelial cells and monocytes with platelet derived MP modulates monocyte-endothelial cell interactions by increasing the expression of adhesion molecules on both cell types [76]. EMP have been shown to decrease nitric-oxide-dependent vasodilation and to be both pro-inflammatory and pro-coagulant [61]. MP have also been found to stimulate angiogenesis and differentiation of progenitor cells [77]. Finally, elegant studies in flow chambers have demonstrated that MP enhance leukocyte rolling [78]. Taken together, current data suggest that EMP may not only be a surrogate marker of vasculitis but that they may contribute to the pro-inflammatory and pro-coagulant status of the endothelium. It must be remembered, however, that findings in generic microparticles may not be applicable to EMP and vice versa.

5. CEC and EPC – an ongoing controversy

The role of endothelial progenitor cells (EPC) [79] in vascular disease and their potential role for therapy [80] have been reviewed recently [81]. Of note, the field of EPC is particularly hampered by lack of standardisation [82 83]. Our knowledge about the kinetics of CEC detachment and EPC mobilisation as well as their interaction is equally limited. Very recently, the margins between endothelial progenitor cells and haematopoietic stem cells became somewhat blurred after proof that endothelial cells can be haematopoietic in mice [84]. We have previously studied numbers of circulating CD34+ progenitor cells and EPCs in vasculitis and demonstrated that these cells increased significantly after the institution of immunosuppressive therapy and with disease remission [85]. Others have previously described an increase in EPCs in inflammatory vascular diseases: Avouac and colleagues, for instance, described increased EPC numbers in scleroderma [86]. In contrast to de Groot and co-workers [85], other studies postulate an imbalance between CECs and EPCs in patients with vasculitis [26 87]. Another study by Zavada and colleagues reports reduced EPC numbers as a risk factor for relapse in vasculitis [88]. Of note, the pattern of EPC in vasculitis may be different in children and one group reports increased numbers in active vasculitis [66]. EPCs were also measured in other subgroups of vasculitis. In Behcet's vasculitis EPC were decreased [89], in children with Kawasaki disease EPC were increased [90].

What make these studies so difficult to compare is, again, the lack of standardisation and the use of different assays and surface markers. Of note, the field of EPC is particularly hampered by lack of standardisation [82 83]. The population of EPC may include a group of cells existing in a variety of stages ranging from immature hematopoietic stem cells to completely differentiated endothelial cells. Endothelial markers, such as CD-146 and UEA-1 are also present on EPC. However, the severely damaged morphology of cells obtained by CD-146-driven immunomagnetic isolation and our inability to growth these cells in culture [11] was regarded as indication that these cells are not EPC. Our own experience shows that CD 146 positive cells were CD 133 negative [91]. Very recently, however, Delorme and co-workers clearly demonstrated EPC among a population of cells isolated by CD-146-driven immunomagnetic isolation [92]. Although their findings need corroboration, new protocols of immunomagnetic isolation may be needed to exclude EPC. Table 2 summarizes characteristic properties of CEC and EPC.

Therefore, the studies mentioned above provide interesting food for thought but require independent confirmation. What stimulates EPCs in reaction to ischemia or other forms of insult? There is conclusive evidence that EPC are not stimulated by the non-specific acute phase response [93] but by microvascular injury [94]. A variety of specific factors have been implicated in this mechanism: First, it is worthwhile to remember that erythropoietin (EPO) regulates EPCs [95]. Hence EPO treatment must always be corrected for when EPCs are measured in renal patients. Statins also influence EPC numbers [96]. Other factors that have been implicated as regulators of EPCs include vascular endothelial growth factor (VEGF), the angiopoetins, and platelet-derived growth factor CC (PDGF-CC). Haeme oxygenase 1 (HO1) has been implicated as well [97]. It is clear that EPCs are capable of homing in to sites of vascular damage. Mechanisms include CD18/ICAM-1 and sdf-1/CXCR4. Endothelial commitment requires histone deacylase (HDAC) activity and depends on the expression of the homoeobox transcription factor HoxA9 [98]. It is probably fair to say that EPCs will receive further scientific attention in vasculitis while a standard as to their definition and enumeration is eagerly awaited.

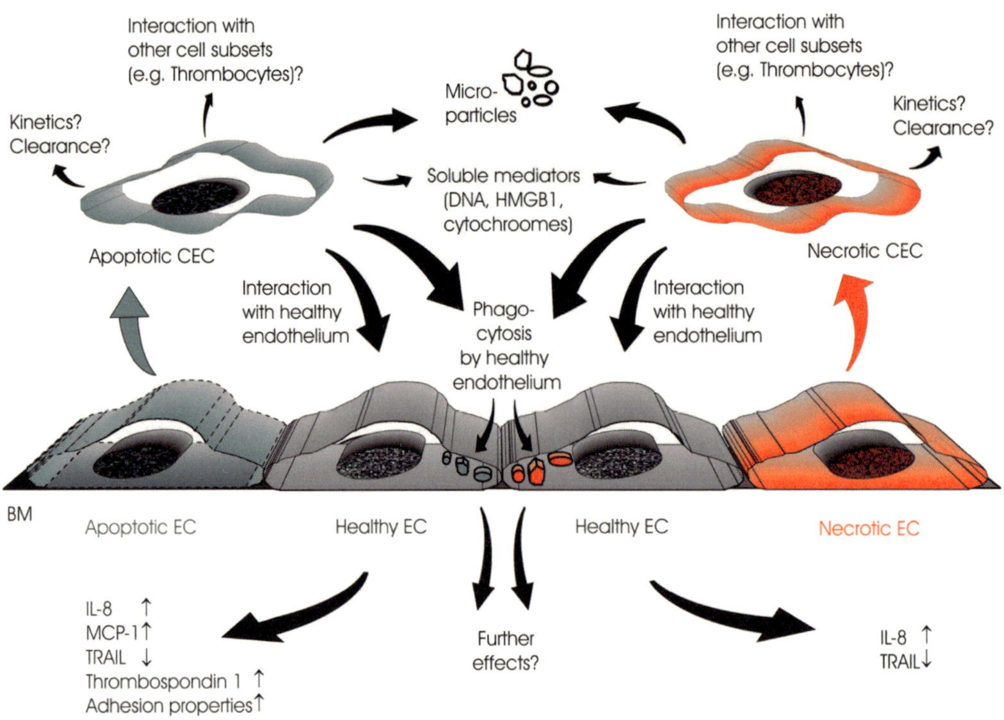

Fig. 1. Interactions of apoptotic and necrotic circulating endothelial cells with healthy endothelium; from [100], with permission

6. Conclusion

Endothelial activation and damage is a crucial event during the pathogenesis of vasculitis. Not surprisingly, markers of such damage are detectable in peripheral blood. Several markers have been studied. Circulating endothelial cells are an established and reliable marker of vascular damage. Cell numbers do correlate with the activity of vascular disease and their use in a clinical setting is on the horizon. In comparison, endothelial microparticles are smaller and their presence may reflect a different stage of the inflammatory process. For both approaches, the lack of standardization remains a matter of particular concern and further multi-centre efforts should be encouraged. Interactions of CEC with the healthy endothelium and other cells deserve further attention, as does the phenotype of CEC. Endothelial repair is another facet of the inflammatory process although, again, progress is hampered by lack of standardization. Taken together, all of these markers may be useful to assess vascular inflammation and repair in a clinical setting.

7. References

[1] Garlanda C, Dejana E. (1997) Heterogeneity of endothelial cells. Specific markers. *ArterioscIerThromb VascBiol*; Vol. 17: pp. 1193-202. ISSN

[2] Zycinska K, Wardyn KA, Zielonka TM, Krupa R, Lukas W. (2009) Clinical implications of serum thrombomodulin in PR3-ANCA-associated vasculitis. *Eur J Med Res*; Vol. 14 Suppl 4: pp. 268-70. ISSN 0949-2321 (Print) 0949-2321 (Linking)

[3] Kumpers P, Hellpap J, David S, et al. (2009) Circulating angiopoietin-2 is a marker and potential mediator of endothelial cell detachment in ANCA-associated vasculitis with renal involvement. *Nephrol Dial Transplant*; Vol. 24: pp. 1845-50. ISSN 1460-2385 (Electronic) 0931-0509 (Linking)

[4] Federici AB, Fox RI, Espinoza LR, Zimmerman TS. (1984) Elevation of von Willebrand factor is independent of erythrocyte sedimentation rate and persists after glucocorticoid treatment in giant cell arteritis. *Arthritis Rheum*; Vol. 27: pp. 1046-9. ISSN

[5] Hergesell O, Andrassy K, Nawroth P. (1996) Elevated levels of markers of endothelial cell damage and markers of activated coagulation in patients with systemic necrotizing vasculitis. *ThrombHaemost*; Vol. 75: pp. 892-8. ISSN

[6] Gabat S, Keller C, Kempe HP, et al. (1996) Plasma thrombomodulin: a marker for microvascular complications in diabetes mellitus. *Vasa*; Vol. 25: pp. 233-41. ISSN

[7] Kozuka K, Kohriyama T, Nomura E, Ikeda J, Kajikawa H, Nakamura S. (2002) Endothelial markers and adhesion molecules in acute ischemic stroke--sequential change and differences in stroke subtype. *Atherosclerosis*; Vol. 161: pp. 161-8. ISSN

[8] Makin AJ, Blann AD, Chung NA, Silverman SH, Lip GY. (2004) Assessment of endothelial damage in atherosclerotic vascular disease by quantification of circulating endothelial cells. Relationship with von Willebrand factor and tissue factor. *Eur Heart J*; Vol. 25: pp. 371-6. ISSN

[9] Bruchfeld A, Wendt M, Bratt J, et al. (2011) High-mobility group box-1 protein (HMGB1) is increased in antineutrophilic cytoplasmatic antibody (ANCA)-associated vasculitis with renal manifestations. *Mol Med*; Vol. 17: pp. 29-35. ISSN 1528-3658 (Electronic)1076-1551 (Linking)

[10] Blann AD, Woywodt A, Bertolini F, et al. (2005) Circulating endothelial cells. Biomarker of vascular disease. *Thromb Haemost*; Vol. 93: pp. 228-35. ISSN

[11] Woywodt A, Streiber F, de Groot K, Regelsberger H, Haller H, Haubitz M. (2003) Circulating endothelial cells as markers for ANCA-associated small-vessel vasculitis. *Lancet*; Vol. 361: pp. 206-10. ISSN

[12] Dang A, Wang B, Li W, et al. (2000) Plasma endothelin-1 levels and circulating endothelial cells in patients with aortoarteritis. *Hypertens Res*; Vol. 23: pp. 541-4. ISSN

[13] Nakatani K, Takeshita S, Tsujimoto H, Kawamura Y, Tokutomi T, Sekine I. (2003) Circulating endothelial cells in Kawasaki disease. *Clin Exp Immunol;* Vol. 131: pp. 536-40. ISSN

[14] Clancy RM. (2000) Circulating endothelial cells and vascular injury in systemic lupus erythematosus. *Curr Rheumatol Rep;* Vol. 2: pp. 39-43. ISSN

[15] Kutlay S, Calayoglu R, Boyvat A, et al. (2008) Circulating endothelial cells: a disease activity marker in Behcet's vasculitis? *Rheumatol Int;* Vol. 29: pp. 159-62. ISSN 0172-8172 (Print) 0172-8172 (Linking)

[16] Erdbruegger U, Woywodt A, Kirsch T, Haller H, Haubitz M. (2006) Circulating endothelial cells as a prognostic marker in thrombotic microangiopathy. *Am J Kidney Dis;* Vol. 48: pp. 564-70. ISSN 1523-6838 (Electronic)

[17] Haubitz M, Woywodt A. (2004) Circulating endothelial cells and vasculitis. *Intern Med;* Vol. 43: pp. 660-7. ISSN

[18] Woywodt A, Goldberg C, Kirsch T, et al. (2005) Circulating endothelial cells in relapse and limited granulomatous disease due to ANCA-associated vasculitis. *Ann Rheum Dis;* Vol. 65: pp. 164-8. ISSN

[19] Erdbruegger U, Haubitz M, Woywodt A. (2006) Circulating endothelial cells: A novel marker of endothelial damage. *Clin Chim Acta;* Vol. 373: pp. 17-26. ISSN

[20] George F, Brisson C, Poncelet P, et al. (1992) Rapid isolation of human endothelial cells from whole blood using S-Endo1 monoclonal antibody coupled to immuno-magnetic beads: demonstration of endothelial injury after angioplasty. *Thromb Haemost;* Vol. 67: pp. 147-53. ISSN

[21] Woywodt A, Blann AD, Kirsch T, et al. (2006) Isolation and enumeration of circulating endothelial cells by immunomagnetic isolation: proposal of a definition and a consensus protocol. *J Thromb Haemost;* Vol. 4: pp. 671-7. ISSN

[22] Woywodt A, Goldberg C, Scheer J, Regelsberger H, Haller H, Haubitz M. (2004) An improved assay for enumeration of circulating endothelial cells. *Ann Hematol;* Vol. 83: pp. 491-4. ISSN

[23] CD146. Protein reviews on the web, 2003. (Accessed Jam 24, 2006, 2003, at http://mpr.nci.nih.gov/prow/.)

[24] Woywodt A, Blann A, Kirsch T, Erdbruegger U, Haubitz M, Dignat-George F. (2006) Isolation and enumeration of circulating endothelial cells by immunomagnetic isolation: proposal of a definition and a consensus protocol. *J Thromb Haemost;* Vol. 4: pp. 671-7. ISSN

[25] Rowand JL, Martin G, Doyle GV, et al. (2007) Endothelial cells in peripheral blood of healthy subjects and patients with metastatic carcinomas. *Cytometry A;* Vol. 71: pp. 105-13. ISSN 1552-4922 (Print)

[26] Holmen C, Elsheikh E, Stenvinkel P, et al. (2005) Circulating inflammatory endothelial cells contribute to endothelial progenitor cell dysfunction in patients with vasculitis and kidney involvement. *J Am Soc Nephrol;* Vol. 16: pp. 3110-20. ISSN

[27] Moroni G, Del Papa N, Moronetti LM, et al. (2005) Increased levels of circulating endothelial cells in chronic periaortitis as a marker of active disease. *Kidney Int;* Vol. 68: pp. 562-8. ISSN

[28] Del Papa N, Colombo G, Fracchiolla N, et al. (2004) Circulating endothelial cells as a marker of ongoing vascular disease in systemic sclerosis. *Arthritis Rheum*; Vol. 50: pp. 1296-304. ISSN
[29] Mancuso P, Rabascio C, Bertolini F. (2003) Strategies to investigate circulating endothelial cells in cancer. *Pathophysiol Haemost Thromb*; Vol. 33: pp. 503-6. ISSN
[30] Mancuso P, Burlini A, Pruneri G, Goldhirsch A, Martinelli G, Bertolini F. (2001) Resting and activated endothelial cells are increased in the peripheral blood of cancer patients. *Blood*; Vol. 97: pp. 3658-61. ISSN
[31] Khan SS, Solomon MA, McCoy JP, Jr. (2005) Detection of circulating endothelial cells and endothelial progenitor cells by flow cytometry. *Cytometry B Clin Cytom*; Vol. 64: pp. 1-8. ISSN 1552-4949 (Print) 1552-4949 (Linking)
[32] Goon PK, Boos CJ, Stonelake PS, Blann AD, Lip GY. (2006) Detection and quantification of mature circulating endothelial cells using flow cytometry and immunomagnetic beads: a methodological comparison. *Thromb Haemost*; Vol. 96: pp. 45-52. ISSN 0340-6245 (Print) 0340-6245 (Linking)
[33] Mancuso P, Antoniotti P, Quarna J, et al. (2009) Validation of a standardized method for enumerating circulating endothelial cells and progenitors: flow cytometry and molecular and ultrastructural analyses. *Clin Cancer Res*; Vol. 15: pp. 267-73. ISSN 1078-0432 (Print) 1078-0432 (Linking)
[34] Duda DG, Cohen KS, Scadden DT, Jain RK. (2007) A protocol for phenotypic detection and enumeration of circulating endothelial cells and circulating progenitor cells in human blood. *Nat Protoc*; Vol. 2: pp. 805-10. ISSN 1750-2799 (Electronic)
[35] Strijbos MH, Gratama JW, Kraan J, Lamers C, Bakker Md, Sleijfer S. (0000) Circulating endothelial cells in oncology: pitfalls and promises. *Br J Cancer*; Vol. 98: pp. 1731-5. ISSN 0007-0920
[36] Mancuso P, Calleri A, Cassi C, et al. (2003) Circulating endothelial cells as a novel marker of angiogenesis. *Adv Exp Med Biol*; Vol. 522: pp. 83-97. ISSN
[37] Jacques N, Vimond N, Conforti R, et al. (2008) Quantification of circulating mature endothelial cells using a whole blood four-color flow cytometric assay. *J Immunol Methods*; Vol. 337: pp. 132-43. ISSN 0022-1759 (Print) 0022-1759 (Linking)
[38] Clarke LA, Shah V, Arrigoni F, et al. (2008) Quantitative detection of circulating endothelial cells in vasculitis: comparison of flow cytometry and immunomagnetic bead extraction. *J Thromb Haemost*; Vol. 6: pp. 1025-32. ISSN 1538-7836 (Electronic) 1538-7836 (Linking)
[39] Widemann A, Sabatier F, Arnaud L, et al. (2008) CD146-based immunomagnetic enrichment followed by multiparameter flow cytometry: a new approach to counting circulating endothelial cells. *J Thromb Haemost*; Vol. 6: pp. 869-76. ISSN 1538-7836 (Electronic) 1538-7836 (Linking)
[40] Woywodt A, Bahlmann FH, de Groot K, Haller H, Haubitz M. (2002) Circulating endothelial cells: Life, death and detachment of the endothelial cell layer. *Nephrol Dial Transplant*; Vol. 17: pp. 1728-30. ISSN
[41] Ingber D. (1991) Extracellular matrix and cell shape: potential control points for inhibition of angiogenesis. *J Cell Biochem*; Vol. 47: pp. 236-41. ISSN

[42] Oguey D, George PW, Ruegg C. (2000) Disruption of integrin-dependent adhesion and survival of endothelial cells by recombinant adenovirus expressing isolated beta integrin cytoplasmic domains. *Gene Ther*; Vol. 7: pp. 1292-303. ISSN

[43] Grosjean J, Kiriakidis S, Reilly K, Feldmann M, Paleolog E. (2006) Vascular endothelial growth factor signalling in endothelial cell survival: A role for NFkappaB. *Biochem Biophys Res Commun*; Vol. 340: pp. 984-94. ISSN

[44] Ballieux BE, Hiemstra PS, Klar-Mohamad N, et al. (1994) Detachment and cytolysis of human endothelial cells by proteinase 3. *Eur J Immunol*; Vol. 24: pp. 3211-5. ISSN

[45] Boehme MW, Galle P, Stremmel W. (2002) Kinetics of thrombomodulin release and endothelial cell injury by neutrophil-derived proteases and oxygen radicals. *Immunology*; Vol. 107: pp. 340-9. ISSN

[46] Harlan JM, Killen PD, Harker LA, Striker GE, Wright DG. (1981) Neutrophil-mediated endothelial injury in vitro mechanisms of cell detachment. *J Clin Invest*; Vol. 68: pp. 1394-403. ISSN

[47] Ruegg C, Dormond O, Foletti A. (2002) Suppression of tumor angiogenesis through the inhibition of integrin function and signaling in endothelial cells: which side to target? *Endothelium*; Vol. 9: pp. 151-60. ISSN

[48] Mutin M, Canavy I, Blann A, Bory M, Sampol J, Dignat-George F. (1999) Direct evidence of endothelial injury in acute myocardial infarction and unstable angina by demonstration of circulating endothelial cells. *Blood*; Vol. 93: pp. 2951-8. ISSN

[49] Bull TM, Golpon H, Hebbel RP, et al. (2003) Circulating endothelial cells in pulmonary hypertension. *Thromb Haemost*; Vol. 90: pp. 698-703. ISSN

[50] Lin Y, Weisdorf DJ, Solovey A, Hebbel RP. (2000) Origins of circulating endothelial cells and endothelial outgrowth from blood. *JClinInvest*; Vol. 105: pp. 71-7. ISSN

[51] Li M, Carpio DF, Zheng Y, et al. (2001) An essential role of the NF-kappa B/Toll-like receptor pathway in induction of inflammatory and tissue-repair gene expression by necrotic cells. *J Immunol*; Vol. 166: pp. 7128-35. ISSN

[52] Botto M, Dell'Agnola C, Bygrave AE, et al. (1998) Homozygous C1q deficiency causes glomerulonephritis associated with multiple apoptotic bodies. *Nat Genet*; Vol. 19: pp. 56-9. ISSN

[53] Kirsch T, Woywodt A, Beese M, et al. (2007) Engulfment of apoptotic cells by microvascular endothelial cells induces proinflammatory responses. *Blood*; Vol. 109: pp. 2854-62. ISSN 0006-4971 (Print)

[54] Chen Q, Stone PR, McCowan LM, Chamley LW. (2006) Phagocytosis of necrotic but not apoptotic trophoblasts induces endothelial cell activation. *Hypertension*; Vol. 47: pp. 116-21. ISSN

[55] Yang JJ, Preston GA, Alcorta DA, et al. (2002) Expression profile of leukocyte genes activated by anti-neutrophil cytoplasmic autoantibodies (ANCA). *Kidney Int*; Vol. 62: pp. 1638-49. ISSN

[56] Mayet W, Schwarting A, Barreiros AP, Schlaak J, Neurath M. (1999) Anti-PR-3 antibodies induce endothelial IL-8 release. *Eur J Clin Invest*; Vol. 29: pp. 973-9. ISSN

[57] Isenberg JS, Martin-Manso G, Maxhimer JB, Roberts DD. (2009) Regulation of nitric oxide signalling by thrombospondin 1: implications for anti-angiogenic therapies. *Nat Rev Cancer*; Vol. 9: pp. 182-94. ISSN
[58] Bonnefoy A, Moura R, Hoylaerts MF. (2008) The evolving role of thrombospondin-1 in hemostasis and vascular biology. *Cell Mol Life Sci*; Vol. 65: pp. 713-27. ISSN
[59] Kirsch T, Woywodt A, Klose J, et al. (2009) Endothelial-derived thrombospondin-1 promotes macrophage recruitment and apoptotic cell clearance. *J Cell Mol Med*; Vol. Jun 5. [Epub ahead of print]: pp. ISSN
[60] Brogan PA, Shah V, Brachet C, et al. (2004) Endothelial and platelet microparticles in vasculitis of the young. *Arthritis Rheum*; Vol. 50: pp. 927-36. ISSN
[61] Chironi GN, Boulanger CM, Simon A, Dignat-George F, Freyssinet JM, Tedgui A. (2009) Endothelial microparticles in diseases. *Cell Tissue Res*; Vol. 335: pp. 143-51. ISSN 1432-0878 (Electronic)
[62] Burnier L, Fontana P, Kwak BR, Angelillo-Scherrer A. (2009) Cell-derived microparticles in haemostasis and vascular medicine. *Thromb Haemost*; Vol. 101: pp. 439-51. ISSN 0340-6245 (Print)
[63] Jy W, Horstman LL, Jimenez JJ, et al. (2004) Measuring circulating cell-derived microparticles. *J Thromb Haemost*; Vol. 2: pp. 1842-51. ISSN
[64] Hamilton KK, Hattori R, Esmon CT, Sims PJ. (1990) Complement proteins C5b-9 induce vesiculation of the endothelial plasma membrane and expose catalytic surface for assembly of the prothrombinase enzyme complex. *J Biol Chem*; Vol. 265: pp. 3809-14. ISSN 0021-9258 (Print)
[65] Erdbruegger U, Grossheim M, Hertel B, et al. (2008) Diagnostic role of endothelial microparticles in vasculitis. *Rheumatology (Oxford)*; Vol. 47: pp. 1820-5. ISSN 1462-0332 (Electronic)
[66] Clarke LA, Hong Y, Eleftheriou D, et al. (2010) Endothelial injury and repair in systemic vasculitis of the young. *Arthritis Rheum*; Vol. 62: pp. 1770-80. ISSN 1529-0131 (Electronic) 0004-3591 (Linking)
[67] Daniel L, Fakhouri F, Joly D, et al. (2006) Increase of circulating neutrophil and platelet microparticles during acute vasculitis and hemodialysis. *Kidney Int*; Vol. 69: pp. 1416-23. ISSN 0085-2538 (Print) 0085-2538 (Linking)
[68] Faure V, Dou L, Sabatier F, et al. (2006) Elevation of circulating endothelial microparticles in patients with chronic renal failure. *J Thromb Haemost*; Vol. 4: pp. 566-73. ISSN
[69] Ardoin SP, Shanahan JC, Pisetsky DS. (2007) The role of microparticles in inflammation and thrombosis. *Scand J Immunol*; Vol. 66: pp. 159-65. ISSN
[70] Mesri M, Altieri DC. (1998) Endothelial cell activation by leukocyte microparticles. *J Immunol*; Vol. 161: pp. 4382-7. ISSN
[71] Mesri M, Altieri DC. (1999) Leukocyte microparticles stimulate endothelial cell cytokine release and tissue factor induction in a JNK1 signaling pathway. *J Biol Chem*; Vol. 274: pp. 23111-8. ISSN
[72] Lacroix R, Sabatier F, Mialhe A, et al. (2007) Activation of plasminogen into plasmin at the surface of endothelial microparticles: a mechanism that

modulates angiogenic properties of endothelial progenitor cells in vitro. *Blood;* Vol.: pp. ISSN

[73] Sabatier F, Roux V, Anfosso F, Camoin L, Sampol J, Dignat-George F. (2002) Interaction of endothelial microparticles with monocytic cells in vitro induces tissue factor-dependent procoagulant activity. *Blood;* Vol. 99: pp. 3962-70. ISSN

[74] Burkart M, Glover S, McGregor JAG, et al. Microparticle Tissue Factor Activity Is Increased in PR3-ANCA Vasculitis Patients with Active Disease.

[75] Abid Hussein MN, Boing AN, Sturk A, Hau CM, Nieuwland R. (2007) Inhibition of microparticle release triggers endothelial cell apoptosis and detachment. *Thromb Haemost;* Vol. 98: pp. 1096-107. ISSN 0340-6245 (Print)

[76] Barry OP, Pratico D, Savani RC, FitzGerald GA. (1998) Modulation of monocyte-endothelial cell interactions by platelet microparticles. *J Clin Invest;* Vol. 102: pp. 136-44. ISSN

[77] Hristov M, Erl W, Linder S, Weber PC. (2004) Apoptotic bodies from endothelial cells enhance the number and initiate the differentiation of human endothelial progenitor cells in vitro. *Blood;* Vol. 104: pp. 2761-6. ISSN 0006-4971 (Print) 0006-4971 (Linking)

[78] Forlow SB, McEver RP, Nollert MU. (2000) Leukocyte-leukocyte interactions mediated by platelet microparticles under flow. *Blood;* Vol. 95: pp. 1317-23. ISSN

[79] Woywodt A, Erdbruegger U, Haubitz M. (2006) Circulating endothelial cells and endothelial progenitor cells after angioplasty: news from the endothelial rescue squad. *J Thromb Haemost;* Vol. 4: pp. 976-8. ISSN

[80] Dzau VJ, Gnecchi M, Pachori AS, Morello F, Melo LG. (2005) Therapeutic potential of endothelial progenitor cells in cardiovascular diseases. *Hypertension;* Vol. 46: pp. 7-18. ISSN

[81] Mobius-Winkler S, Hollriegel R, Schuler G, Adams V. (2009) Endothelial progenitor cells: implications for cardiovascular disease. *Cytometry A;* Vol. 75: pp. 25-37. ISSN 1552-4930 (Electronic)

[82] Fadini GP, Baesso I, Albiero M, Sartore S, Agostini C, Avogaro A. (2008) Technical notes on endothelial progenitor cells: ways to escape from the knowledge plateau. *Atherosclerosis;* Vol. 197: pp. 496-503. ISSN

[83] Hirschi KK, Ingram DA, Yoder MC. (2008) Assessing identity, phenotype, and fate of endothelial progenitor cells. *Arterioscler Thromb Vasc Biol;* Vol. 28: pp. 1584-95. ISSN 1524-4636 (Electronic)

[84] Eilken HM, Nishikawa S, Schroeder T. (2009) Continuous single-cell imaging of blood generation from haemogenic endothelium. *Nature;* Vol. 457: pp. 896-900. ISSN 1476-4687 (Electronic)

[85] de Groot K, Goldberg C, Bahlmann FH, et al. (2007) Vascular endothelial damage and repair in antineutrophil cytoplasmic antibody-associated vasculitis. *Arthritis Rheum;* Vol. 56: pp. 3847-53. ISSN 0004-3591 (Print)

[86] Avouac J, Juin F, Wipff J, et al. (2008) Circulating endothelial progenitor cells in systemic sclerosis: association with disease severity. *Ann Rheum Dis*; Vol. 67: pp. 1455-60. ISSN

[87] Zavada J, Kideryova L, Pytlik R, Vankova Z, Tesar V. (2008) Circulating endothelial progenitor cells in patients with ANCA-associated vasculitis. *Kidney Blood Press Res*; Vol. 31: pp. 247-54. ISSN

[88] Zavada J, Kideryova L, Pytlik R, Hruskova Z, Tesar V. (2009) Reduced number of endothelial progenitor cells is predictive of early relapse in anti-neutrophil cytoplasmic antibody-associated vasculitis. *Rheumatology (Oxford)*; Vol. 48: pp. 1197-201. ISSN 1462-0332 (Electronic) 1462-0324 (Linking)

[89] Fadini GP, Tognon S, Rodriguez L, et al. (2009) Low levels of endothelial progenitor cells correlate with disease duration and activity in patients with Behcet's disease. *Clin Exp Rheumatol*; Vol. 27: pp. 814-21. ISSN 0392-856X (Print) 0392-856X (Linking)

[90] Xu MG, Men LN, Zhao CY, et al. (2010) The number and function of circulating endothelial progenitor cells in patients with Kawasaki disease. *Eur J Pediatr*; Vol. 169: pp. 289-96. ISSN 1432-1076 (Electronic) 0340-6199 (Linking)

[91] Woywodt A, Scheer J, Hambach L, et al. (2004) Circulating endothelial cells as a marker of endothelial damage in allogeneic hematopoietic stem cell transplantation. *Blood*; Vol. 103: pp. 3603-5. ISSN

[92] Delorme B, Basire A, Gentile C, et al. (2005) Presence of endothelial progenitor cells, distinct from mature endothelial cells, within human CD146+ blood cells. *Thromb Haemost*; Vol. 94: pp. 1270-9. ISSN

[93] Padfield GJ, Tura O, Haeck ML, et al. (2010) Circulating endothelial progenitor cells are not affected by acute systemic inflammation. *Am J Physiol Heart Circ Physiol*; Vol. 298: pp. H2054-61. ISSN 1522-1539 (Electronic) 0363-6135 (Linking)

[94] Hohenstein B, Kuo MC, Addabbo F, et al. (2010) Enhanced progenitor cell recruitment and endothelial repair after selective endothelial injury of the mouse kidney. *Am J Physiol Renal Physiol*; Vol. 298: pp. F1504-14. ISSN 1522-1466 (Electronic)0363-6127 (Linking)

[95] Bahlmann FH, De Groot K, Spandau JM, et al. (2004) Erythropoietin regulates endothelial progenitor cells. *Blood*; Vol. 103: pp. 921-6. ISSN 0006-4971 (Print)

[96] Matsumura M, Fukuda N, Kobayashi N, et al. (2009) Effects of atorvastatin on angiogenesis in hindlimb ischemia and endothelial progenitor cell formation in rats. *J Atheroscler Thromb*; Vol. 16: pp. 319-26. ISSN 1880-3873 (Electronic)

[97] Smadja DM, d'Audigier C, Bieche I, et al. (2011) Thrombospondin-1 is a plasmatic marker of peripheral arterial disease that modulates endothelial progenitor cell angiogenic properties. *Arterioscler Thromb Vasc Biol*; Vol. 31: pp. 551-9. ISSN 1524-4636 (Electronic) 1079-5642 (Linking)

[98] Rossig L, Urbich C, Bruhl T, et al. (2005) Histone deacetylase activity is essential for the expression of HoxA9 and for endothelial commitment of progenitor cells. *J Exp Med*; Vol. 201: pp. 1825-35. ISSN 0022-1007 (Print)

[99] Woywodt A, Kirsch T, Haubitz M. (2008) Circulating endothelial cells in renal disease: markers and mediators of vascular damage. *Nephrol Dial Transplant*; Vol. 23: pp. 7-10. ISSN

[100] Haubitz M, Dhaygude A, Woywodt A. (2009) Mechanisms and markers of vascular damage in ANCA-associated vasculitis. *Autoimmunity*; Vol. 42: pp. 605-14. ISSN 1607-842X (Electronic)

10

Clinical Relevance of Cytokines, Chemokines and Adhesion Molecules in Systemic Vasculitis

Tsuyoshi Kasama, Ryo Takahashi,
Kuninobu Wakabayashi and Yusuke Miwa
Division of Rheumatology, Department of Medicine
Showa University School of Medicine, Tokyo
Japan

1. Introduction

Although the causes of most vasculitis syndromes remain unclear, advances in molecular and cellular immunology have enabled the definition of many effector mechanisms that mediate inflammatory vascular damage. Vascular endothelial dysfunction is observed in a variety of immune-mediated inflammatory diseases. Therefore, endothelial cells (ECs) play a pivotal role in the pathogenesis of systemic vasculitis (Buckley et al. 2005; Kaneider et al. 2006), in large part by amplifying and perpetuating the inflammatory process through the expression and secretion of various cytokines, chemokines, cell adhesion molecules, and other inflammatory molecules. In addition, specific cell-cell interactions, especially between ECs and invading mononuclear cells, including macrophages and lymphocytes, also contribute to the progression of systemic vasculitis and other autoimmune diseases, including rheumatoid arthritis (RA) and systemic lupus erythematosus (SLE). In addition, recent studies of the pathogenesis of atherosclerosis have shown that a key feature of atherosclerotic disease is the alternating interaction and amplification of thrombosis and inflammation, which is considered an unusual form of chronic inflammation of the artery wall that is triggered by chemical (e.g., smoking and hyperlipidemia), biological (e.g., Chlamydia pneumoniae) and/or mechanical (e.g., shear stress in hypertension) insults to ECs (Libby 2002).
Among the various mediators secreted by activated inflammatory cells are cytokines and chemokines, which appear to be involved in both systemic vasculitis and atherosclerosis. The purpose of this review is to provide an overview of the expression and function of the cytokines and chemokines during the pathogenesis of vasculitic diseases, including systemic vasculitis and related conditions.

2. Endothelial cells are an important cellular component of vascular inflammation

The endothelium is the first obstacle to leukocyte transmigration, and both the properties of the chemokines expressed and the functionality of the cells support the idea that ECs serve as a gateway, controlling leukocyte extravasation at sites of inflammation. In this role, the ECs engage in significant proinflammatory activities, including amplifying and perpetuating inflammatory processes. Among these processes is the proinflammatory facilitation of the expression and secretion of various cytokines, chemokines, cell adhesion molecules and other inflammatory mediators (Mantovani & Dejana 1989) that are critically involved in the pathogenesis of systemic vasculitis (Sneller & Fauci 1997; Cid et al. 2004; Bacon 2005; Buckley, Rainger et al. 2005; Kaneider, Leger et al. 2006). For example, the dysregulation of cytokine/chemokine expression and secretion is crucially involved in the pathogenesis of vasculitis (Cid & Vilardell 2001; Charo & Taubman 2004). Specific cell-cell interactions, especially between ECs and invading mononuclear cells, are also key contributors to the evolution of vascular inflammation and the progression of vasculitis and autoimmune diseases such as RA and SLE, as summarized briefly in Figure 1.

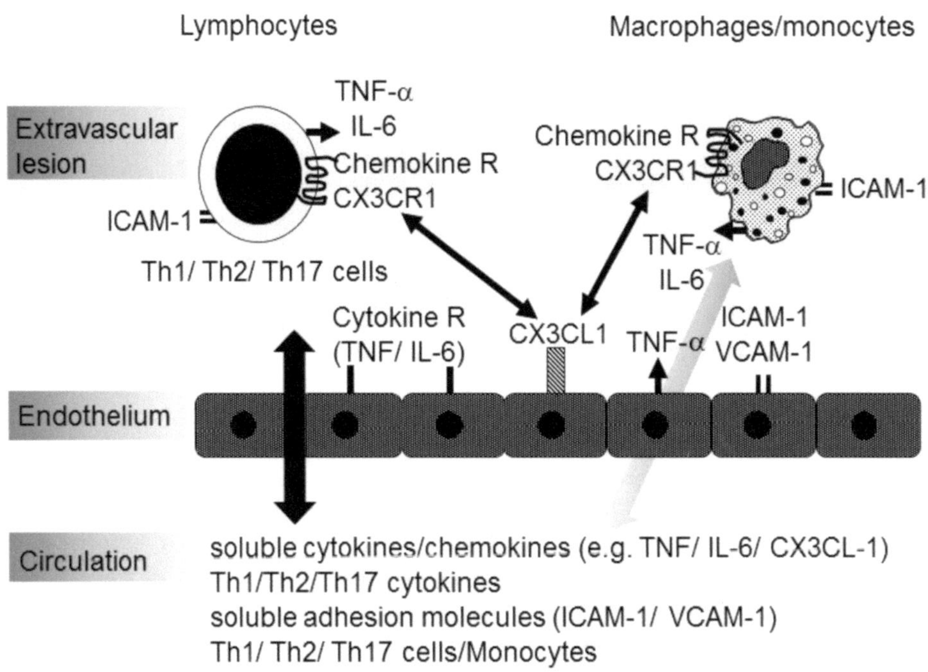

Fig. 1. Cytokines/chemokines and cell adhesion molecules involved in the interaction between endothelial cells and inflammatory/immune cells

The dysregulation of cytokine/chemokine expression, corresponding receptors (R) and adhesion molecules on inflammatory cells/endothelial cells is crucially involved in the pathogenesis of inflammatory vascular diseases.

3. Cytokines involved in systemic vasculitis and anti-neutrophil cytoplasmic antibody-associated vasculitis

Although little data are available regarding the participation of proinflammatory cytokines in the pathogenesis of systemic vasculitis, many cytokines are known to play a role in the pathogenesis of vasculitis syndrome (Sundy & Haynes 2000; Cid, Segarra et al. 2004; Muller-Ladner et al. 2005). The cross-talk between ECs, leucocytes, and cytokines fulfills a homeostatic function and acts as a rapid response in situations of the vascular injury seen in systemic vasculitis.

Anti-neutrophil cytoplasmic antibody (ANCA)-associated vasculitis (AAV) is the most common cause of rapidly progressive glomerulonephritis and immune-mediated pulmonary renal syndrome. Small-vessel vasculitis (SVV) is associated with the development of ANCA, which is directed against neutrophil intracellular enzymes, myeloperoxidase (MPO-ANCA), and proteinase-3 (PR3-ANCA). Now that the acute manifestations of the disease can generally be controlled using immunosuppressive drugs, ANCA-associated vasculitis has become a chronic and relapsing inflammatory disorder.

A number of cytokines are capable of cooperating with ANCA to mediate inflammatory events. A recent report by Nolan et al. indicates that circulating anti-MPO IgG acts synergistically with inflammatory stimuli to potentiate cytokine-induced leukocyte firm adhesion and transmigration within murine cremasteric venules and also promotes changes within leukocytes that drive injury at susceptible distant sites (Nolan et al. 2008). Taken together, these findings suggest that neutrophils primed by cytokines in the presence of anti-MPO IgG may exert systemic effects and target specific vascular beds.

Cytokines play a key role in the pathogenesis of systemic inflammation, both in systemic inflammatory processes, such as the upregulation of acute-phase protein synthesis, and as a focal point for the interplay of cytokines in the vascular endothelium (Kunkel et al. 1996; Firestein 2003; Middleton et al. 2004; McInnes & Schett 2007). This endothelial layer is the primary target of circulating mediators and thus, this layer controls the trafficking of cells and molecules from the bloodstream into the underlying tissue.

3.1 TNF

TNF has a wide range of biological effects, such as the cellular activation of cells that play a role in host defense, including monocytes/macrophages, B and T lymphocytes and neutrophils, and is considered a primary cytokine in chronic inflammation.

Recently, increasing evidence has indicated that TNF-α plays important roles in vasculitis inflammation. Turesson et al. showed that higher levels of TNF are observed in patients with clinical signs of systemic vasculitis compared with those without any evidence of systemic involvement (Turesson et al. 2001). In addition, Lamprecht et al. showed that intracytoplasmic TNF-α and IL-12 expression is significantly increased in Wegener's granulomatosis (WG) compared with healthy controls. The elevated TNF-α and IL-12 expression in monocytes normalized after clinical remission through treatment with cyclophosphamide and corticosteroid (CYC + GC) (Lamprecht et al. 2002).

In another study, serum levels of TNF-α and soluble CD4 (sCD4), sCD8, IL-6, and sIL-6 receptor (sIL-6R) were examined in RA patients to evaluate the relationship between extra-articular manifestations (EAMs) and immunological alterations (Kuryliszyn-Moskal 1998). Serum concentrations of TNF-α, IL-6, sIL-6R, and sCD4 are significantly increased in RA patients compared with those in healthy individuals. Furthermore, RA patients with clinical signs of systemic vasculitis show significantly higher levels of TNF-α (Kuryliszyn-Moskal 1998).

Recent clinical findings support that TNF-α plays important pathological roles. Indeed, TNF-target therapy such as infliximab in ANCA-associated vasculitis was recently reported to be beneficial in several open-label studies (Booth et al. 2004; Huugen et al. 2006). Taken together, the results of these studies demonstrate that TNF-α exerts crucial effects on the pathogenesis of vasculitis, and the results further suggest an important role for cellular immune activation in the pathogenesis of microvascular damage.

3.2 IL-6

Numerous investigations have demonstrated that IL-6 plays a central role in the regulation of inflammatory and immune responses and hematopoiesis, including B-cell maturation, immunoglobulin production, induction of acute-phase proteins in the liver, and T-cell maturation and activation (Akira et al. 1993). In response to diverse stimuli, IL-6 is expressed in a wide variety of cell types, including monocytes/macrophages, T cells, fibroblasts, and ECs (Akira, Taga et al. 1993; Naka et al. 2002). IL-6 potentially contributes to immune responses, especially B-cell maturation, stimulation and immunoglobulin production, and IL-6 may also play a role in the development of autoimmune disorders such as SLE, which is characterized by the dysregulated production of autoantibodies and polyclonal B-cell activation (Cross & Benton 1999).

Both anti-PR3 and anti-MPO positive IgG fractions from patients with AAV activate ECs in vitro. Interestingly, IL-6 is secreted by human umbilical vein endothelial cells (HUVEC) that are activated by the ANCA-positive IgG fraction isolated from patients with WG and/or microscopic polyangiitis (MPA) (Muller Kobold et al. 1999).

Increased serum levels of IL-6 can be detected in patients with giant cell arteritis (GCA) and polymyalgia rheumatica (PMR), and IL-6 concentrations are significantly correlated with the parameters of disease activity, such as C-reactive protein (CRP) levels and the erythrocyte sedimentation rate (ESR) (Roche et al. 1993; Emilie et al. 1994; Weyand et al. 2000). In addition, Emilie et al. showed that both IL-6 protein and mRNA are detectable in the biopsied temporal artery, and most of the IL-6-producing cells were macrophages and, to a lesser extent, fibroblasts in the intima (Emilie, Liozon et al. 1994).

As mentioned previously, Kuryliszyn-Moskal also observed increased IL-6 levels in RA patients with vasculitis (rheumatoid vasculitis; RV) (Kuryliszyn-Moskal 1998). Statistical analyses encompassing all RA patients, with and without vasculitis, demonstrated a significant correlation among the levels of IL-6, sCD4 and sCD8 and ESR. In turn, although IL-6 and sIL-6R levels were significantly higher in RA patients than in healthy controls, there were no significant differences between the RA groups with and without vasculitis. Furthermore, there was no association between the severity of microvascular damages and the levels of IL-6 and sIL-6R (Kuryliszyn-Moskal 1998). The lack of correlation between IL-6 or sIL-6R and vasculitis complications in RA patients suggests that the IL-6/IL-6R systems might be regulated during the development of vasculitis by different mechanisms or RV disease stage.

3.3 Th1 and Th2 cytokines

Churg-Strauss syndrome (CSS) is a type of AAV and is further characterized by severe eosinophilia and, often, granulomatous inflammation. Activated T cells from CSS patients are predominantly T-helper type 2 (Th2) cells, which exhibit an increased production of IL-4 and IL-13. In addition, the PBMCs isolated from patients with CSS and cultured with T-cell-specific stimuli secrete significantly increased amounts of IL-5 compared with PBMCs from healthy controls (Hellmich et al. 2005). The Th2-mediated immune response in CSS may result from an abnormal eosinophil response causing T cell activation and Th2 cytokine production. Similarly, in a majority of patients with CSS, there is a marked increase in Th1 cytokines, including IL-2 and interferon (IFN)-α, in the serum (Grau et al. 1989). IL-25, which is produced by epithelial cells and other innate cells such as eosinophils, basophils, and mast cells, links innate and adaptive immunity by enhancing Th2 cytokine production (Angkasekwinai et al. 2007). Increased levels of IL-25, which are correlated with disease activity and eosinophil levels, have been observed in the serum of active patients with CSS (Terrier et al. 2010). Furthermore, IL-25 has been found within the vasculitic lesions of patients with CSS. This suggests that eosinophils, through the production of IL-25, may play a critical role in promoting Th2 responses in the peripheral blood and target tissues in CSS.

WG is characterized by a predominance of the Th1 response. As described above, Lamprecht et al. showed that intracytoplasmic IL-12 and TNF-α expression is significantly increased in WG patients compared with healthy controls. Monocytic cytokines, especially IL-12, may play a role in the early determination and skewing of the immunoregulatory response toward a Th1 profile. The normalization of the skewed cytokine pattern by CYC + GC treatment may be a prerequisite and an indicator of inducing remission of WG (Lamprecht, Kumanovics et al. 2002). Furthermore, Lamprecht et al. clearly indicated the important role of the Th1-dominant axis in the pathogenesis of WG (Lamprecht et al. 2003).

Based on recent evidence, the Th1 phenotype expresses certain chemokine receptors, including CCR5 ligands for CCL3 and CCL5 (Sallusto et al. 1998; Rossi & Zlotnik 2000), while the Th2 phenotype expresses CCR4, ligands for CCL17 (TARC) and CCL22 (MDC). It now appears that chemokines not only have the ability to recruit specific subsets of lymphocytes but also aid in determining the type of immune response that is elicited. These and other aspects of chemokine function may have a significant effect on the development of autoimmune disorders.

Higher expression levels of CCR5, the functional receptor of CCL3-5 (MIP-1), in $CD4^{+}CD28^{-}$ T cells in localized WG may favor stronger CCR5-mediated recruitment of this T-cell subset into the granulomatous lesions in localized WG, and Th1 cells that lack CD28 expand independent of age and immunosuppressive therapy. The expansion of Th1-type $CD4^{+}CD28^{-}CCR5^{+}$ effector memory T cells might contribute to disease progression and autoreactivity, either directly by maintaining the inflammatory response or as a result of bystander activation (Lamprecht, Bruhl et al. 2003).

3.4 Th17 cytokines

The recently characterized IL-17-producing T helper cell lineage (Th17), rather than the Th1 lineage, is involved in several autoimmune diseases (Lyakh et al. 2008; Takatori et al. 2008). In addition, IL-23 is associated with the generation of the Th17 response and IL-17 production (Lyakh, Trinchieri et al. 2008). However, little is known about the role of IL-23 in AAV (Hruskova et al. 2008). Recently, Nogueira et al. showed that serum levels of IL-17A and IL-23 are significantly elevated in acute AAV patients compared with those in healthy controls. In contrast, no significant differences in IFN-γ levels were detected between the patient group and the control group. The patients with elevated levels of IL-23 compared with those with low levels of IL-23 had more active disease as measured by the Birmingham Vasculitis Activity Score (BVAS) and had higher ANCA titers. Critically, immunosuppressive therapy did not always effectively suppress the IL-23 or IL-17 production. Additionally, autoantigen-specific IL-17-producing, but not IFN-g-producing, cells were significantly elevated in patients during disease convalescence compared with healthy controls. Taken together, these findings indicate that the Th17 axis and specifically IL-23 may serve as important mediators in the severity of AAV (Nogueira et al. 2010).

The possible role of Th17 cells in WG has not yet been elucidated. Patients with WG who are in remission have a significantly decreased percentage of $CD69^{+}CD4^{+}$ T cells in response to PR3. These patients also tend to have a lower percentage of $CD69^{+}CD4^{+}$ T cells in response to other stimuli compared with healthy controls. WG patients who are in remission have significantly increased percentages of Th17 cells ($IL\text{-}4^{-}$, $IL\text{-}17^{+}$, $IFN\text{-}\gamma^{-}$) and Th2 cells ($IL\text{-}4^{+}$, $IL\text{-}17^{-}$, $IFN\text{-}\gamma^{-}$) within the activated $CD69^{+}CD4^{+}$ T cell population. Consistent with the results from Lamprecht, WG patients in remission and healthy controls have similar percentages of Th1 cells ($IL\text{-}4^{-}$, $IL\text{-}17^{-}$, $IFN\text{-}\gamma^{+}$). Furthermore, in Kawasaki disease (KD), Th17 proportions and the expression levels of relevant cytokines (IL-17, IL-6 and IL-23) are upregulated (Sohn et al. 2003; Jia et al. 2010). The skewed Th17 response found in ANCA-positive WG patients following stimulation with the autoantigen PR3 and also in KD patients suggests that IL-17 is involved in disease pathogenesis and may constitute a new therapeutic target (Abdulahad et al. 2008).

3.5 MIF

Macrophage migration inhibitory factor (MIF) was originally identified as a soluble factor in the culture medium of activated T lymphocytes that inhibited the migration of macrophages (Bloom & Bennett 1966; Bloom & Shevach 1975) and is recognized as a multipotential cytokine in the regulation of immune and inflammatory responses (Calandra & Roger 2003). Several cell populations, including T cells (Bacher et al. 1996), macrophages/monocytes (Calandra et al. 1994), synovial fibroblasts (Leech et al. 1999) and endothelial cells (Nishihira et al. 1998) express and secrete MIF. Furthermore, MIF is implicated in various inflammatory and immune-mediated diseases, including RA (Leech, Metz et al. 1999; Ayoub et al. 2008), SLE (Hoi et al. 2003; Foote et al. 2004), scleroderma (Selvi et al. 2003) and inflammatory bowel diseases (de Jong et al. 2001). Serum MIF levels are also increased in systemic vasculitis, including WG and AAV (Ohwatari et al. 2001; Becker et al. 2006).

We recently showed that patients with systemic vasculitis have increased serum MIF levels compared with normal controls. Interestingly, patients with MPA have significantly increased levels of serum MIF compared with patients with medium-vessel vasculitis (MVV) and large-vessel vasculitis (LVV). The elevated MIF levels seen in MPA patients are positively correlated with BVAS, CRP levels, ESR, and serum MPO-ANCA titers. Notably, MPA patients in clinical remission after treatment have significantly diminished levels of MIF. Similarly, Becker et al. showed that AAV patients have elevated serum MIF levels (Becker, Maaser et al. 2006). Patients with vasculitis have increased serum levels of endothelial-related molecules, such as adhesion molecules and EC-derived cytokines (Bradley et al. 1994; Johnson et al. 1997; Sundy & Haynes 2000). Indeed, vasculitis-affected small vessels, such as those found in MPA, may have dysregulated EC function (Filer et al. 2003). In patients with MPA, the increased serum MIF may originate from endothelial cells and/or inflammatory cells, including monocytes and neutrophils because these cells are capable of secreting MIF (Calandra, Bernhagen et al. 1994; Nishihira, Koyama et al. 1998; Riedemann et al. 2004) and secreted MIF participates in regulating the proliferation of ECs (Yang et al. 2000). However, there have been no data demonstrating the stimulating capacity of MPO-ANCA to secrete any cytokines including MIF. The lack of evidence may be related to the disease activity and MIF levels because there is a positive relationship between the MPO-ANCA titers and the disease activity of vasculitis (Sinico et al. 2005). Furthermore, MIF upregulates the expression of intercellular adhesion molecule-1 (ICAM-1) on endothelial cells (Lin et al. 2000). In addition, MIF stimulates the expression and secretion of other inflammatory cytokines, including TNF-α and IL-8 (Leech, Metz et al. 1999; Onodera et al. 2004). The recruitment of leukocytes to the sites of inflammation involves adhesion molecule-dependent interactions with ECs. Collectively, the dysregulated orchestration of MIF from ECs and/or leukocytes and adhesion molecules and the cytokines induced by MIF may play crucial roles in the development of SVV, including MPA.

Taken together, these results suggest that increased MIF appears to be involved in the pathogenesis of systemic vasculitis, especially the small vessel vasculopathy seen in MPA, and may serve as a useful serologic marker of disease activity in vasculitis.

3.6 IL-18

IL-18, originally called an IFN-γ-inducing factor, has recently been identified as a cytokine synthesized by Kupffer cells and activated macrophages. In combination with IL-12, IL-18 induces IFN-γ production by Th1 and NK cells in Th1 cells, B cells, and natural killer cells, promoting Th1-type immune responses (Okamura et al. 1998).

AAV patients have an increased deposition of IL-18 in their renal biopsies, as assessed by immunoperoxidase staining (Hewins et al. 2006). Immunofluorescence microscopy demonstrated that podocytes are the predominant glomerular IL-18-positive cell type, whereas in the interstitium, the myofibroblasts, distal tubular epithelium, and infiltrating macrophages stained positive for IL-18. In vitro, IL-18 primed the superoxide production by ANCA-activated neutrophils at similar levels as TNF-α. Hewins et al. concluded that IL-18 is likely to be important for neutrophil recruitment and priming in AAV (Hewins, Morgan et al. 2006).

The inflammatory activity of vascular lesions in GCA is mediated by adaptive immune responses, with $CD4^+$ T cells undergoing clonal expansion in the vessel wall and releasing IFN-γ (Weyand et al. 2005). Additionally, several polymorphisms within the IL-18 promoter gene are associated with different inflammatory and autoimmune diseases (Sivalingam et al. 2003). Therefore, IL-18 may be implicated in the pathogenesis of GCA. Indeed, a recent study showed that the IL18 -607 allele A is significantly increased in GCA patients compared with controls. In addition, an additive effect between the associated IL-18 and Toll-like receptor 4 genetic variants was observed (Palomino-Morales et al. 2010). In addition, serum IL-18 as well as IL-6 levels were elevated in patients with TA, especially in those with active disease (Park et al. 2006). Serum IL-18 levels correlated well with disease activity of TA. These results suggest that IL-6 and IL-18 might contribute to the pathogenesis of TA and that IL-18 could be a useful marker for monitoring the disease activity of TA.

3.7 AIF

The allograft inflammatory factor-1 (AIF-1) is an IFN-γ-inducible $Ca2^+$-binding cytokine originally cloned from activated macrophages in human and rat atherosclerotic allogenic heart grafts undergoing chronic transplant rejection (Utans et al. 1995). AIF-1 appears to play a role in the survival and proinflammatory activity of macrophages (Yang et al. 2005). Broglio et al. showed that the biopsied arterial walls of vasculitic neuropathies have increased AIF-1 compared with the nerves of chronic inflammatory demyelinating polyneuropathies and that vascular smooth muscle cells (VSMCs) in vasculitic nerves have increased expression of AIF-1 protein (Broglio et al. 2008). AIF-1 is involved in the proliferation and migration of VSMCs and is rapidly expressed in response to injury and inflammatory cytokines, but AIF-1 is not expressed in unstimulated VSMCs (Autieri et al. 2000). These studies suggest that AIF-1 plays an important role in inflammatory nerve disease, with either autocrine- or paracrine-induced vasculitis and VSMC proliferation in the damaged vascular tissues.

4. Chemokines involved in systemic vasculitis

Chemokines are a family of over 40 small secreted proteins that induce chemotaxis and other functional changes in subsets of leukocytes in vitro, and they are known to belong to two major superfamilies that share substantial homology via four conserved cysteine residues (Kunkel, Lukacs et al. 1996; Baggiolini 1998; Moser et al. 2004; Szekanecz et al. 2006). They are produced by a wide variety of cell types of both hematopoietic and nonhematopoietic origin (Kasama et al. 2005), and they play a key role in the migration and activation of leukocytes in vivo as well as in several autoimmune diseases (Arimilli et al. 2000; Haringman et al. 2004). The CXC chemokine family [e.g., CXCL1 (growth-related oncogene alpha; GRO-α), CXCL5 (expression of neutrophil-activating protein-78; ENA-78), CXCL8 (IL-8), CXCL9 (monokine induced by interferon-gamma; MIG), CXCL10 (interferon-inducible protein 10; IP-10), CXCL11 (interferon-inducible T cell A chemoattractant; I-TAC) and CXCL16 (CXC chemokine ligand 16)] induces chemotaxis mainly in neutrophils and T lymphocytes. The CC chemokine family [e.g., CCL2 (macrophage chemoattractant protein 1; MCP-1), CCL3 (macrophage inflammatory protein 1 alpha; MIP-1α), CCL4 (MIP-1β) and CCL5 (regulated on activation normal T cells expressed and secreted; RANTES)] induces chemotaxis in monocytes and subpopulations of T lymphocytes. There are two other minor groups, the C and CX3C chemokines, which include CX3CL1 (fractalkine). The members of these families show considerable structural homology and often possess overlapping chemoattractant specificities. In addition to their roles in chemoattraction, the chemokines have been implicated in rheumatic disorders, including RA and SLE (Kunkel, Lukacs et al. 1996; Gerard & Rollins 2001; Bodolay et al. 2002). Few studies have documented the localization of various chemokines in pathological conditions such as systemic vasculitis (Cid & Vilardell 2001; Charo & Taubman 2004; Eardley et al. 2009).

4.1 CC chemokines

4.1.1 CCL2

In contrast with CXCL8, CCL2 (MCP-1) plays an important role in chronic inflammation, particularly in activating the migration of macrophages and specific T cells (Daly & Rollins 2003). CCL2 is expressed in mesangial glomerulonephritis, including the vasculitic lesions of the WG kidney, in association with mononuclear cell infiltration (Rovin et al. 1994). Both the protein and the mRNA of CCL2 are detectable in the kidney with cryoglobulinemic vasculitis, which correlates with the infiltration of macrophages (Gesualdo et al. 1997). Furthermore, CCR5, a functional receptor for CCL2, also plays an important role in the tissue inflammation seen in WG. A recent report by Ohlsson et al. showed that elevated CCL2 levels are found in the urine of patients with AAV, even those in remission, and the CCL2 levels are associated with poor prognosis and possibly also with risk of relapse, suggesting that urinary CCL2 is a promising potential prognostic marker in SVV (Ohlsson et al. 2009).

CCL2 and CCL5 appear to be involved in LVV in similar ways as in SSV, including WG, cryoglobulinemic vasculitis, and Takayasu's arteritis (TA). TA is a chronic obliterative inflammatory disease involving the aorta and its main branches. Patients with TA have increased serum concentrations of both CCL2 and CCL5 compared with normal healthy controls; these concentrations closely correlate with disease activity (Noris et al. 1999; Dhawan et al. 2006). These findings suggest that CCL2 and CCL5 can be used as reliable markers in determining the activity of TA. In addition, patients with KD or MVV disease have elevated serum levels of CCL2 and CXCL10 (Shikishima et al. 2003).

4.1.2 CCL26 and CCL17

Recently, a chemokine family that specifically mediates the trafficking of eosinophils to inflammatory and allergic sites has been characterized. CCL11, CCL24 and CCL26 are grouped together as eotaxins (Bisset & Schmid-Grendelmeier 2005). Although these chemokines share only ~40% homology and their genes are located on different chromosomes, they all bind to a common receptor: CCR3. Interestingly, CCL26 (eotaxin-3), rather than the other eotaxins, has also been implicated in the pathogenesis of eosinophilic esophagitis (Blanchard et al. 2006). Eosinophilic infiltration into inflamed tissues is the histologic hallmark of CSS (Zwerina et al. 2009). Recently, studies showed that patients with CSS have increased CCL26, but not CCL11 or CCL24, in serum, and the elevated levels of CCL26 significantly diminished following successful treatment and clinical improvement. The serum CCL26 levels in CSS patients are significantly correlated with the levels of CRP and serum IgE (Polzer et al. 2008).

Recently, studies showed that CSS patients with active disease have significantly elevated serum CCL17 levels compared with controls and patients with inactive disease, and the serum CCL17 levels are correlated with the clinical disease course of CSS and with the absolute eosinophil counts as well as IgE levels (Dallos et al. 2010). CCL17 is a chemokine that is secreted from monocyte-derived dendritic cells (DCs) and ECs and is responsible for the selective recruitment and migration of activated Th2 lymphocytes to affected tissues. Regarding the polarization of Th responses, CSS is a Th2-mediated systemic vasculitis characterized by eosinophilic infiltration, blood eosinophilia, and high IgE levels (Zwerina, Axmann et al. 2009). CCL17 may serve as a biomarker for eosinophilic tissue damage. Taken together, CCL26 and CCL17 seem to be crucial pathogenic mediators that facilitate the development of a targeted pharmacotherapy for CSS.

4.1.3 Other CC and XC chemokines

CCL3, CCL4 and CCL5 may contribute to the pathophysiology of immune disorders including RA and SLE. Zhou et al. demonstrated that the lung tissues from patients with WG are infiltrated by CCR5-positive mononuclear cells and have increased protein concentrations for the ligands of CCR5, including CCL3, CCL4 and CCL5 (Zhou et al. 2003). Moreover, CCR5 and CXCR3 are highly expressed by infiltrating leucocytes that are in the tissue sections from patients with GCA, and the adventitia has a predominant clustering of CCR5- and CXCR3-positive leucocytes, which are co-localized with the expression of CCL5/RANTES mRNA (Bruhl et al. 2005). In addition, XCL1, also known as lymphotactin, is the sole member of the C subgroup of chemokines, and its primary chemotactic activity is controlling the movement of $CD4^+$ and $CD8^+$ T cells. XCL1 is mainly expressed by $CD4^+CD28^-$ T cells in WG patients (Blaschke et al. 2009). In renal biopsies, the presence of XCL1 is only detected within interstitial $CD4^+$ and $CD8^+$ T cells. Meanwhile, there are no significant differences in XCL1 serum concentrations between WG patients and controls. In functional studies, PMN stimulated with XCL1 demonstrated a significant enhancement of CXCL8 production. Considering its function as a lymphocyte-specific chemoattractant, XCL1 might be a key modulator of T cell recruitment in WG and may support vascular inflammation by the induction of CXCL8 secretion by the PMN. These chemokines and related T cell populations may contribute to the granuloma formation and disease progression in WG.

4.2 CXC chemokines

4.2.1 CXCL8

The main function of CXCL8 (IL-8) is its role in acute inflammation stimulating the migration of polymorphonuclear neutrophils. However, CXCL8 may be involved in the immune response that induces the migration of specific T cell populations (Moser & Loetscher 2001; Rot & von Andrian 2004). Indeed, CXCL8 has been implicated in lupus nephritis (Holcombe et al. 1994; Rovin et al. 2002).

CXCL8 has been implicated in MVV, including Kawasaki disease (KD) (Asano & Ogawa 2000). In the acute phase of KD, the expression of CXCL8 mRNA in mononuclear cells and polymorphonuclear neutrophils, the level of CXCL8 protein, and the neutrophil chemoattractant activity within the plasma were all increased. Patients with TA, particularly those with LVV, have increased serum levels of CXCL8 (Tripathy et al. 2004).

4.2.2 CXCL10

CXCL10 (IP-10) is expressed and secreted by monocytes, fibroblasts, and ECs after stimulation with IFN-γ (Neville et al. 1997; Luster 1998; Hanaoka et al. 2003) and plays important roles in the migration of some subsets of T cells into inflamed sites. In contrast to CXCL8, CXCL10 also promotes the regression of angiogenesis (Angiolillo et al. 1995; Strieter et al. 1995). Despite these findings, few studies have been conducted in the field of vasculitis. Mixed cryoglobulinemia (MC) + HCV patients have increased CXCL10 levels that are significantly associated with the presence of active vasculitis (Antonelli et al. 2008).

Recently, Panzer et al. showed that the damage of endothelial cells in different renal compartments induced in rats by selective renal artery perfusion with an anti-endothelial antibody leads to different chemokine expression patterns (Panzer et al. 2006). CXCL10 is expressed in the tubulointerstitium by peritubular capillaries, whereas glomerular endothelial cells do not express CXCL10. The CXCL10 expression pattern overlaps with the pattern of T cell influx. Massive tubulointerstitial T cell infiltration was observed, whereas no T cells were found inside the glomeruli. In this regard, we previously demonstrated that the interaction of monocytes with HUVECs resulted in synergistic increases in CXCL10 expression and secretion, which consequently inhibited endothelial tube formation *in vitro* (Kasama et al. 2002). This induction of CXCL10 was mediated via specific cell surface molecules such as CD40 molecules. This finding suggests the contribution of CXCL10 to the regulation of angiogenesis and the initiation of inflammatory vascular diseases. Taken together, the expression and regulation of CXCL10 play an important, but limited, functional role in microvascular damage.

4.2.3 CXCL13

CXCL13, also known as B cell-attracting chemokine 1 or B-lymphocyte chemoattractant, is a member of the CXC subtype of the chemokine superfamily. Similar to the increased levels of

CXCL10, significantly increased levels of CXCL13 were observed in HCV-related MC patients; these levels correlated with vasculitis disease activity (Sansonno et al. 2008). In this report, the mRNA expression of CXCL13 was detected in the portal tract of biopsied liver tissues and also in the skin tissues from MC patients with active cutaneous vasculitis. CXCL13 is mainly associated with extracellular fibrils and, to a much lower extent, with cells displaying a follicular dendritic cell phenotype. Extravasated monocytes, which are potent inducible producers of this chemokine, in inflammatory lesions such as cutaneous vasculitis of patients with cryoglobulinemia may give rise to cells capable of producing CXCL13. In these patients, CXCL13 production may be involved in the exacerbation of cryoglobulinemic vasculitis, particularly through the aberrant dissemination of antigen-priming information from the liver to extrahepatic sites.

4.3 CX3C chemokine

4.3.1 CX3CL1

The chemokine CX3CL1, also known as fractalkine, is synthesized as a type I transmembrane protein by ECs (Bazan et al. 1997). The unique CX3C chemokine domain of CX3CL1 is attached to a 241-amino acid mucin stalk, a 19-amino acid transmembrane domain, and a 37-amino acid intracellular domain of unknown function (Bazan, Bacon et al. 1997; Pan et al. 1997). The soluble form of CX3CL1 reportedly exerts a chemotactic effect on monocytes, natural killer (NK) cells, and T lymphocytes. CX3CL1 acts via its receptor CX3CR1 as an adhesion molecule that promotes the firm adhesion of a subset of leukocytes to the ECs under conditions of physiologic flow (Imai et al. 1997; Umehara et al. 2001). Thus, CX3CL1 appears to possess immunoregulatory properties that affect inflammatory and immune cell-EC interactions and the inflammatory responses at inflamed sites. Indeed, numerous studies have implicated CX3CL1 in a variety of inflammatory disorders, including glomerulonephritis, RA, systemic sclerosis, and SLE (Chen et al. 1998; Ruth et al. 2001; Blaschke et al. 2003; Hasegawa et al. 2005; Yajima et al. 2005).

We recently found that serum CX3CL1 levels were significantly higher in all vasculitis patients than in healthy controls (Matsunawa et al. 2009; Kasama et al. 2010). Among the vasculitis patients, CX3CL1 levels were highest in the SVV group, whereas patients with MPA had the strongest expression overall. The elevated CX3CL1 levels observed in MPA patients, as well as in all systemic vasculitis patients, were positively correlated with BVAS, CRP levels and ESR. Similarly, an increased expression of cell-surface CX3CR1 was observed on the peripheral blood $CD4^+$ and $CD8^+$ T cells from patients with MPA. Notably, MPA patients in clinical remission after treatment had significantly diminished levels of both CX3CL1 and CX3CR1. Recently, Bjerkeli et al. showed that serum CX3CL1 levels were significantly higher in patients with WG than in healthy controls (Bjerkeli et al. 2007), although no data were presented for the other types of SVV (MPA or CSS). The disease activity in patients with either WG or MPA is closely correlated with the markers of EC damage (Hergesell et al. 1996). Moreover, we found that higher serum CX3CL1 levels are observed in patients with RV than in those with RA without vasculitis or in healthy controls (Matsunawa et al. 2006). The elevated CX3CL1 levels in the RV patients are positively correlated with BVAS, VAI and serum parameters, including rheumatoid factor titers, immune complex (IC-C1q) levels, and ICAM-1 levels. CX3CL1 levels are negatively correlated with complement C4 levels. CX3CL1 levels are diminished in RV patients successfully treated with glucocorticoids and other immunosuppressive drugs. The correlation between CX3CL1 levels and ICAM-1 expression in RV patients suggests

endothelial damage and/or vascular inflammation (Blann et al. 1995; Boehme et al. 1996; Kuryliszyn-Moskal et al. 1996). The higher CX3CL1 levels observed in RV patients compared with RA or extraarticular manifestation (EAM)-RA patients may be an indicator of undiagnosed vasculitis in RA patients. The difference in CX3CL1 levels may also support the hypothesis that vasculopathy underlies EAMs in RA. The accumulation of activated cells and the upregulated expression of inflammatory molecules, including ICAM-1 and CX3CL1, reflect the pathophysiological events leading to vasculitis, suggesting the magnitude of activation and inflammation of ECs. In this regard, increasing evidence suggests that by mediating vascular endothelial activation, TNF-α, which is known to be a potent inducer of CX3CL1 in ECs (Fong et al. 1998; Ahn et al. 2004), plays a key role in the pathophysiology of systemic vasculitis (Kuryliszyn-Moskal 1998; Bacon 2005; Feldmann & Pusey 2006).
Thus, CX3CL1 and CX3CR1 appear to possess immunoregulatory properties that affect inflammatory and immune cell-EC interactions and inflammatory responses at inflamed sites. Moreover, their coordinated regulation appears to be involved in the pathogenesis of systemic vasculitis, especially the small vessel vasculopathy seen in MPA, WG and RV, and may serve as a useful serologic marker of vasculitis disease activity.

4.4 Adhesion molecules involved in systemic vasculitis

Intercellular adhesion is mediated through a variety of receptors that have unique physical and kinetic characteristics, regulatory patterns, and tissue and cell localization that is well suited to their diverse functions. Adhesion molecules, such as ICAM-1, vascular cell adhesion molecule-1 (VCAM-1), and other related molecules, are thought to mediate intercellular adhesion (Gearing et al. 1992). The adhesion molecules ICAM-1, VCAM-1, and E-selectin are regulated by proinflammatory cytokines and play an important role in the binding and activation of leukocytes in inflammatory diseases (Kaneider, Leger et al. 2006).

4.4.1 ICAM-1

ICAM-1, also known as CD54, is a cell surface glycoprotein that contributes to the interactions between leukocytes and several other cell types, including ECs, fibroblasts, and keratinocytes (Springer 1990; Mackay & Imhof 1993). Although ICAM-1 is constitutively expressed by numerous cell types, including monocytes/macrophages, lymphocytes, and ECs, the stimulation of cells with cytokines or microbial infections can induce a marked increase in ICAM-1 expression. ICAM-1 and endothelial selectin are expressed on the activated endothelium to facilitate the localization of leukocytes to the site of vascular injury.
The presence of adhesion molecules, such as ICAM-1, may reflect the presence of inflammation and damage to the vascular endothelium (Bradley, Lockwood et al. 1994) and suggests that ICAM-1 plays a crucial role in autoimmune rheumatic diseases, including vasculitis and RA (Sfikakis & Tsokos 1997).
Circulating ICAM-1 was detected in the serum of patients with systemic vasculitis and RA (Aoki et al. 1993; Blann, Herrick et al. 1995; Johnson, Alexander et al. 1997; Ara et al. 2001). Patients with active WG have significantly elevated serum levels of ICAM-1, which are correlated with disease activity. These findings suggest that ICAM-1 plays an important role in the pathogenesis of WG and may be used as an additional parameter of disease activity (Ohta et al. 2001). Di Lorenzo et al. showed that in MPO-ANCA-positive MPA patients, higher ICAM-1 and ELAM-1 levels during the active phase and their slower decline during

the treatment period could be a prognostic risk factor for chronic renal factor development (Di Lorenzo et al. 2004).
The ICAM-1 protein, TNF-α, and E-selectin are expressed in ECs and perivascular mononuclear cells in areas of microvascular damage in the salivary glands of RV patients (Flipo et al. 1997). Furthermore, RV patients have elevated levels of sICAM-1 (Voskuyl et al. 1995; Kuryliszyn-Moskal, Bernacka et al. 1996; Witkowska et al. 2003). In addition, Voskuyl et al. (Voskuyl, Martin et al. 1995) demonstrated the involvement of ICAM-3 and ICAM-1 in patients with RV. This involvement suggests that ICAM-1 and ICAM-3 in serum may be useful markers of vascular inflammation in patients with RV, and these proteins may play a crucial role in vasculitis development in RA.

4.4.2 VCAM-1

The immunoglobulin superfamily member VCAM-1 recognizes alpha 4 beta 1 integrin and is expressed on all leukocytes, but not neutrophils (Gearing, Hemingway et al. 1992; Zimmerman et al. 1996). The blockade or inhibition of VCAM-1/alpha 4 beta 1 interaction is expected to have therapeutic potential in treating various inflammatory disorders and autoimmune diseases because the VCAM-1/alpha 4 beta adhesion pathway has a major influence on eosinophil, lymphocyte, and monocyte trafficking (van Dinther-Janssen et al. 1991; Dean et al. 1993; Foster 1996; Matsuyama & Kitani 1996). Several investigators have shown that, in addition to the involvement with adhesion molecules such as ICAM-1, VCAM-1 is clinically involved in RA and systemic vasculitis.
Recently, the significance of VCAM-1 was shown in AAV (Ara, Mirapeix et al. 2001; Schneeweis et al. 2010). The levels of VCAM-1 were higher in all patient groups with vasculitis compared with healthy controls. Enhanced levels of VCAM-1 may be a marker for endothelial cell activation in AAV. The observed correlation between VCAM-1 and creatinine levels might indicate the influence of the vasculitic process on renal function (Schneeweis, Rafalowicz et al. 2010). Noguchi et al. clearly showed that patients with TA have significantly higher levels of VCAM-1 compared with those in healthy controls in Japanese populations and hypothesized that the increased levels of VCAM-1 may be related to disease activity (Noguchi et al. 1998).
In contrast to the role of ICAM-1, the role of VCAM-1 in RV and RA is contradictory. Immunohistological analysis revealed significantly greater expression of VCAM-1 and ICAM-1 in the muscle biopsies from RA patients with RV compared with those RA patients without vasculitis (Verschueren et al. 2000). In addition, Salih et al. (Salih et al. 1999) reported that RA patients with neuropathy had significantly higher serum levels of soluble VCAM-1 than patients without neuropathy and healthy controls. On the other hand, VCAM-1 was not immunohistochemically detected in the vasculitis lesions in the salivary glands of RV patients, despite the significant expression of ICAM-1 in ECs and perivascular cellular infiltrates (Flipo, Cardon et al. 1997). Taken together, these findings indicate that the role of VCAM-1 is limited in the pathogenesis of RV and RA compared with the role of ICAM-1.

4.4.3 E-selectin

The selectin family of adhesion molecules has been implicated in the initial steps of the interaction between lymphocytes and the endothelium during lymphocyte homing. E-selectin, also known as endothelial-leukocyte adhesion molecule-1, mediates the early phase of neutrophil binding, as well as the binding of eosinophils, basophils, monocytes, and certain subsets of T cells. E-selectin is also an inducible endothelial adhesion molecule, although its expression follows slower kinetics and reaches its maximum level after 4–6 hours of stimulation with inflammatory mediators. Antibodies against E-selectin strongly bind to the endothelium in the RA synovium, predominantly on the venules and capillaries. In osteoarthritic synovial sections, anti-E-selectin stained a substantially lower percentage of blood vessels and fewer endothelial cells.

Increased serum levels of E-selectin, ICAM-1 and VCAM-1 in active AAV and the normalization of E-selectin during the remission phase suggest that the concentration of soluble levels of these adhesion molecules reflects disease activity (Ara, Mirapeix et al. 2001). Importantly, Tripathy et al. showed the significant roles of these adhesion molecules in LVV, including TA. Patients with inactive TA have elevated levels of E-selectin, but not sVCAM-1 or sICAM-1, and the elevated levels of E-selectin may indicate persistent vasculopathy in clinically inactive disease (Tripathy et al. 2008). Because E-selectin is exclusively expressed on the activated endothelium, elevated levels of E-selectin in inactive TA indicate a persistence of subclinical vascular inflammation during remission of the disease.

Blann et al. (Blann, Herrick et al. 1995) observed a significant augmentation of soluble E-selectin in patients with RA, vasculitis, and scleroderma. Interestingly, the strongest correlations in RA patients were between ICAM-1 and VCAM-1, and a significant correlation between E-selectin and ICAM was observed in systemic vasculitis patients. Similar to other adhesion molecules and TNF-α, the E-selectin protein is expressed at significantly higher levels by ECs and perivascular cellular infiltrates according to immunohistochemistry in labial salivary glands of patients with RV compared with those of patients with inactive RV, RA, or Sjögren's syndrome (Flipo, Cardon et al. 1997). In contrast, Voskuyl et al. (Voskuyl, Martin et al. 1995.) reported no significant elevation of circulating E-selectin in patients with RV. Because the expression of E-selectin and other molecules in the salivary glands was especially high in active RV, the presence of microvascular damage in the salivary gland tissues of patients with RV may reflect the limited and specific dissemination of the vascular inflammatory process.

4.4.4 CD40 ligand

CD40 ligand (CD40L), a member of the tumor necrosis family of transmembrane glycoproteins, is expressed on the surface of recently activated $CD4^+$ T cells. The interactions between CD40L and CD40 help to activate B cells, induce immunoglobulin production and activate monocytes and dendritic cell differentiation (Grewal & Flavell 1998). Activated T lymphocytes that express CD40L engage CD40 on ECs to augment the expression of proinflammatory cytokines and adhesion molecules (Miller et al. 1998; Thienel et al. 1999). Kim et al. (Kim et al. 2005) described an eosinophilic vasculitis with an infiltration of CD40L-positive eosinophils and a marked increase in serum TNF-a levels. Furthermore, enhanced expression of CD40L on $CD4^+$ T cells and platelets and increased serum levels of sCD40L were observed in patients with Kawasaki disease, an acute febrile vasculitic syndrome in children (Wang et al. 2003). Although few studies have examined this, these findings suggest that sCD40L is a marker of pathogenic B-cell activation in RA, which often occurs in cases with vasculitis. CD40L and/or CD40 in B-cell-T-cell interactions or interactions of other cells may have important pathogenic roles in vasculitis.

4.4.5 CD44

CD44 is a broadly distributed transmembrane glycoprotein that plays a critical role in a variety of cellular behaviors, including adhesion, migration, invasion, and survival. CD44 mediates cell–cell and cell–matrix interactions primarily through its affinity for hyaluronan (HA), a glycosaminoglycan constituent of extracellular matrices, and potentially through its affinity for ligands, such as osteopontin, collagens, and matrix metalloproteinases (Lesley et al. 1993). Most primary cells express CD44 in a low-affinity state that does not confer sufficient binding to HA. Cellular activation can induce a CD44 transition to a high-affinity state, which then mediates HA binding. The transition from the "inactive" low-affinity state to the "active" high-affinity state of CD44 on leukocytes can be induced by the ligation of antigen receptors to leukocytes, ECs, and other mesenchymal cells by soluble factors, including cytokines (Levesque & Haynes 1997; Cichy & Pure 2000; Brown et al. 2001). In addition to its localization with adhesion molecules, a soluble form of CD44 has been detected in circulation. CD44 has been detected in the serum, lymph nodes, and arthritic synovial tissues (Haynes et al. 1991; Takahashi et al. 1992; Johnson et al. 1993; Katoh et al. 1994). Malignant disease, immune activation and inflammation are often associated with increased plasma levels of sCD44. These findings indicate that the release of CD44 correlates with enhanced local proteolytic activity and matrix remodeling, and CD44 may be a potential biomarker for immune activation and inflammation.

Seiter et al. (Seiter et al. 1998) observed some isoforms of CD44 (e.g., CD44v10) in the vasculitis of patients with either skin-associated vasculitis or autoimmune disease. However, as was the case with VCAM-1, CD44 protein is only weakly expressed in the vasculitis of the salivary glands of RV patients (Flipo, Cardon et al. 1997). These findings indicate that CD44 has a limited role in the development of vasculitis.

4.4.6 Fibronectin

Fibronectin (FN) is a large adhesive glycoprotein found in the extracellular matrix of many tissues. It is also present in body fluids such as synovial fluid (SF) and plasma. FN regulates cellular adhesion and spreading, cell motility, cell growth, differentiation and opsonization via heparin-binding domains (Ruoslahti 1988; Schwarzbauer 1991). Some splice variants of FN are expressed in the synovial endothelium in RA, and the expression of FN is upregulated by the proinflammatory cytokine IL-1 (Boyle et al. 2000). Circulating FN is increased in experimental vascular injury and in the serum of patients with active vasculitis syndromes (Peters et al. 1986; Peters et al. 1989). These observations indicate that the presence of FN reflects the inflammation and injury of the blood endothelium (Jennette et al. 1991).

FN and von Willebrand factor antigen (vWfAg) are produced by blood vessel endothelial cells in response to injury. Bleil et al. examined the sera of 61 patients with various types of systemic vasculitis, the sera of 13 patients with retinal vasculitis, and the sera of 199 patients with rheumatic diseases (Bleil et al. 1991) and found significantly elevated levels of FN and vWfAg in almost all patients with vasculitis syndromes. Therefore, we consider C-ANCA a marker specific for the diagnosis of WG or polyarteritis nodosa, whereas FN and vWfAg are nonspecific but sensitive markers of vascular damage.

Interestingly, FN may be indicative of vascular injury and/or inflammation in RV (Voskuyl et al. 1998). RA patients with RV and RA patients with EAMs have a five-fold and two-fold increase in the serum levels of FN, respectively, compared with patients with uncomplicated RA. These findings suggest that increased levels of FN are more frequently observed in RA patients with EAMs and, in particular, in patients with RV. The mechanisms by which FN is increased in RV patients remain to be defined. The release of FN into the circulatory systems has been observed after experimental pulmonary injury, and inflammation is considered the result of local blood vessel injury. The high FN levels in RV patients compared with RA patients might be an indicator of undiagnosed vasculitis in RA patients or may support the hypothesis that vasculopathy underlies EAMs in RA. These studies reflect the various levels of tissue inflammation and stimulation of vascular ECs that could ultimately lead to an enhanced release of FN into circulation. Serum FN, in combination with other molecules, such as adhesion molecules and cytokines, may be of significant clinical value as serological markers for vasculitis, including RV.

5. Conclusions

Despite outstanding progress made in recent years, the pathophysiology of systemic vasculitis and vasculitic complications has not yet been fully elucidated. The orchestration of the cytokine network and cell-cell interactions may be critical for the development of vascular inflammation. Because subclinical EC damage and vasculitis are occasionally seen in inflammatory rheumatic diseases, it will be important to clinically evaluate and diagnose the complications of systemic and localized vasculitis. Table 1 summarizes the cytokines and inflammatory molecules based on systemic vasculitic diseases.

Diseases	Cytokines	Chemokines	Adhesion molecules
ANCA-associated vasculitis and/or Microscopic polyangiitis	IL-17, IL-23 MIF, IL-18	CX3CL1	ICAM-1, VCAM-1 ELAM-1
Wegener's granulomatosis	TNF, IL-12, IL-17	CCL2, CCL3 CCL4, CCL5 XCL1, CX3CL1	ICAM-1
Churg-Strauss syndrome	IL-4, IL-13, IL-5 IL-2, IFN-α IL-25	CCL26, CCL17	
Kawasaki disease	IL-6, IL-17, IL-23	CCL2, CXCL8 CXCL10	CD40L
Takayasu arteritis	IL-6, IL-18	CCL2, CCL5 CXCL8	E-selectin
Giant cell arteritis	IL-6, IL-18	CCL5	
Rheumatoid vasculitis	TNF, IL-6, sIL-6R	CX3CL1	ICAM-1, ICAM-3 VCAM-1, E-selectin CD40L, CD44, FN
Cryoglobulinemic vasculitis		CCL2, CXCL10 CXCL13	

Table 1. Detectable cytokines, chemokines and adhesion molecules involved in several vasculitis diseases

Taken together, the results of multiple studies indicate that the assessment of serum concentrations of cytokines and inflammatory molecules will provide useful clinical information and a method to monitor therapeutic interventions. Further elucidation of the complex molecular networks will be helpful in understanding the immunopathology of systemic vasculitis and related conditions.

6. Acknowledgement

We thank Mrs. Hiroko T. Takeuchi and Kyoko Nohtomi for their excellent helps with the experiments. This study was supported, in part, by grant from the Ministry of Health, Labour and Welfare of Japan.

7. References

Abdulahad, W. H., Stegeman, C. A., Limburg, P. C. & Kallenberg, C. G. (2008). Skewed distribution of Th17 lymphocytes in patients with Wegener's granulomatosis in remission. *Arthritis and Rheumatism*, 58(7): pp. 2196-2205.

Ahn, S. Y., Cho, C. H., Park, K. G., Lee, H. J., Lee, S., Park, S. K., Lee, I. K. & Koh, G. Y. (2004). Tumor necrosis factor-alpha induces fractalkine expression preferentially in arterial endothelial cells and mithramycin A suppresses TNF-alpha-induced fractalkine expression. *American Journal of Pathology*, 164(5): pp. 1663-1672.

Akira, S., Taga, T. & Kishimoto, T. (1993). Interleukin-6 in biology and medicine. *Advances in Immunology*, 54: pp. 1-78.

Angiolillo, A. L., Sgadari, C., Taub, D. D., Liao, F., Farber, J. M., Maheshwari, S., Kleinman, H. K., Reaman, G. H. & Tosato, G. (1995). Human interferon-inducible protein 10 is a potent inhibitor of angiogenesis in vivo. *Journal of Experimental Medicine*, 182(1): pp. 155-162.

Angkasekwinai, P., Park, H., Wang, Y. H., Chang, S. H., Corry, D. B., Liu, Y. J., Zhu, Z. & Dong, C. (2007). Interleukin 25 promotes the initiation of proallergic type 2 responses. *Journal of Experimental Medicine*, 204(7): pp. 1509-1517.

Antonelli, A., Ferri, C., Fallahi, P., Ferrari, S. M., Sebastiani, M., Ferrari, D., Giunti, M., Frascerra, S., Tolari, S., Franzoni, F., Galetta, F., Marchi, S. & Ferrannini, E. (2008). High values of CXCL10 serum levels in mixed cryoglobulinemia associated with hepatitis C infection. *American Journal of Gastroenterology*, 103(10): pp. 2488-2494.

Aoki, S., Imai, K. & Yachi, A. (1993). Soluble intercellular adhesion molecule-1 (ICAM-1) antigen in patients with rheumatoid arthritis. *Scandinavian Journal of Immunology*, 38(5): pp. 485-490.

Ara, J., Mirapeix, E., Arrizabalaga, P., Rodriguez, R., Ascaso, C., Abellana, R., Font, J. & Darnell, A. (2001). Circulating soluble adhesion molecules in ANCA-associated vasculitis. *Nephrology, Dialysis, Transplantation*, 16(2): pp. 276-285.

Arimilli, S., Ferlin, W., Solvason, N., Deshpande, S., Howard, M. & Mocci, S. (2000). Chemokines in autoimmune diseases. *Immunological Review*, 177: pp. 43-51.

Asano, T. & Ogawa, S. (2000). Expression of IL-8 in Kawasaki disease. *Clinical and Experimental Immunology*, 122(3): pp. 514-519.

Autieri, M. V., Carbone, C. & Mu, A. (2000). Expression of allograft inflammatory factor-1 is a marker of activated human vascular smooth muscle cells and arterial injury. *Arteriosclerosis, Thrombosis, and Vascular Biology*, 20(7): pp. 1737-1744.

Ayoub, S., Hickey, M. J. & Morand, E. F. (2008). Mechanisms of disease: macrophage migration inhibitory factor in SLE, RA and atherosclerosis. *Nature Clinical Practice. Rheumatology*, 4(2): pp. 98-105.

Bacher, M., Metz, C. N., Calandra, T., Mayer, K., Chesney, J., Lohoff, M., Gemsa, D., Donnelly, T. & Bucala, R. (1996). An essential regulatory role for macrophage migration inhibitory factor in T-cell activation. *Proceedings of the National Academy of Sciences of the United States of America*, 93(15): pp. 7849-7854.

Bacon, P. A. (2005). Endothelial cell dysfunction in systemic vasculitis: new developments and therapeutic prospects. *Current Opinion in Rheumatology*, 17(1): pp. 49-55.

Baggiolini, M. (1998). Chemokines and leukocyte traffic. *Nature*, 392(6676): pp. 565-568.

Bazan, J. F., Bacon, K. B., Hardiman, G., Wang, W., Soo, K., Rossi, D., Greaves, D. R., Zlotnik, A. & Schall, T. J. (1997). A new class of membrane-bound chemokine with a CX3C motif. *Nature*, 385: pp. 640-644.

Becker, H., Maaser, C., Mickholz, E., Dyong, A., Domschke, W. & Gaubitz, M. (2006). Relationship between serum levels of macrophage migration inhibitory factor and the activity of antineutrophil cytoplasmic antibody-associated vasculitides. *Clinical Rheumatology*, 25(3): pp. 368-372.

Bisset, L. R. & Schmid-Grendelmeier, P. (2005). Chemokines and their receptors in the pathogenesis of allergic asthma: progress and perspective. *Current Opinion in Pulmonary Medicine*, 11(1): pp. 35-42.

Bjerkeli, V., Damas, J. K., Fevang, B., Holter, J. C., Aukrust, P. & Froland, S. S. (2007). Increased expression of fractalkine (CX3CL1) and its receptor, CX3CR1, in Wegener's granulomatosis possible role in vascular inflammation. *Rheumatology*, 46(9): pp. 1422-1427.

Blanchard, C., Wang, N., Stringer, K. F., Mishra, A., Fulkerson, P. C., Abonia, J. P., Jameson, S. C., Kirby, C., Konikoff, M. R., Collins, M. H., Cohen, M. B., Akers, R., Hogan, S. P., Assa'ad, A. H., Putnam, P. E., Aronow, B. J. & Rothenberg, M. E. (2006). Eotaxin-3 and a uniquely conserved gene-expression profile in eosinophilic esophagitis. *Journal of Clinical Investigation*, 116(2): pp. 536-547.

Blann, A. D., Herrick, A. & Jayson, M. I. (1995). Altered levels of soluble adhesion molecules in rheumatoid arthritis, vasculitis and systemic sclerosis. *British Journal of Rheumatology*, 34(9): pp. 814-819.

Blaschke, S., Brandt, P., Wessels, J. T. & Muller, G. A. (2009). Expression and function of the C-class chemokine lymphotactin (XCL1) in Wegener's granulomatosis. *Journal of Rheumatology*, 36(11): pp. 2491-2500.

Blaschke, S., Koziolek, M., Schwarz, A., Benohr, P., Middel, P., Schwarz, G., Hummel, K. M. & Muller, G. A. (2003). Proinflammatory role of fractalkine (CX3CL1) in rheumatoid arthritis. *Journal of Rheumatology*, 30(9): pp. 1918-1927.

Bleil, L., Manger, B., Winkler, T. H., Herrman, M., Burmester, G. R., Krapf, F. E. & Kalden, J. R. (1991). The role of antineutrophil cytoplasm antibodies, anticardiolipin antibodies, von Willebrand factor antigen, and fibronectin for the diagnosis of systemic vasculitis. *Journal of Rheumatology*, 18(8): pp. 1199-1206.

Bloom, B. R. & Bennett, B. (1966). Mechanism of a reaction in vitro associated with delayed-type hypersensitivity. *Science*, 153(731): pp. 80-82.

Bloom, B. R. & Shevach, E. (1975). Requirement for T cells in the production of migration inhibitory factor. *Journal of Experimental Medicine*, 142(5): pp. 1306-1311.

Bodolay, E., Koch, A. E., Kim, J., Szegedi, G. & Szekanecz, Z. (2002). Angiogenesis and chemokines in rheumatoid arthritis and other systemic inflammatory rheumatic diseases. *Journal of Cellular and Molecular Medicine*, 6(3): pp. 357-376.

Boehme, M. W., Schmitt, W. H., Youinou, P., Stremmel, W. R. & Gross, W. L. (1996). Clinical relevance of elevated serum thrombomodulin and soluble E-selectin in patients with Wegener's granulomatosis and other systemic vasculitides. *American Journal of Medicine*, 101(4): pp. 387-394.

Booth, A., Harper, L., Hammad, T., Bacon, P., Griffith, M., Levy, J., Savage, C., Pusey, C. & Jayne, D. (2004). Prospective study of TNFalpha blockade with infliximab in anti-neutrophil cytoplasmic antibody-associated systemic vasculitis. *Journal of the American Society of Nephrology*, 15(3): pp. 717-721.

Boyle, D. L., Shi, Y., Gay, S. & Firestein, G. S. (2000). Regulation of CS1 fibronectin expression and function by IL-1 in endothelial cells. *Cellular Immunology*, 200(1): pp. 1-7.

Bradley, J. R., Lockwood, C. M. & Thiru, S. (1994). Endothelial cell activation in patients with systemic vasculitis. *QJM*, 87(12): pp. 741-745.

Broglio, L., Erne, B., Tolnay, M., Schaeren-Wiemers, N., Fuhr, P., Steck, A. J. & Renaud, S. (2008). Allograft inflammatory factor-1: a pathogenetic factor for vasculitic neuropathy. *Muscle and Nerve*, 38(4): pp. 1272-1279.

Brown, K. L., Maiti, A. & Johnson, P. (2001). Role of sulfation in CD44-mediated hyaluronan binding induced by inflammatory mediators in human CD14(+) peripheral blood monocytes. *Journal of Immunology*, 167(9): pp. 5367-5374.

Bruhl, H., Vielhauer, V., Weiss, M., Mack, M., Schlondorff, D. & Segerer, S. (2005). Expression of DARC, CXCR3 and CCR5 in giant cell arteritis. *Rheumatology*, 44(3): pp. 309-313.

Buckley, C. D., Rainger, G. E., Nash, G. B. & Raza, K. (2005). Endothelial cells, fibroblasts and vasculitis. *Rheumatology*, 44: pp. 860-863.

Calandra, T., Bernhagen, J., Mitchell, R. A. & Bucala, R. (1994). The macrophage is an important and previously unrecognized source of macrophage migration inhibitory factor. *Journal of Experimental Medicine*, 179(6): pp. 1895-1902.

Calandra, T. & Roger, T. (2003). Macrophage migration inhibitory factor: a regulator of innate immunity. *Nature Reviews. Immunology*, 3(10): pp. 791-800.

Charo, I. F. & Taubman, M. B. (2004). Chemokines in the pathogenesis of vascular disease. *Circulation Research*, 95(9): pp. 858-866.

Chen, S., Bacon, K. B., Li, L., Garcia, G. E., Xia, Y., Lo, D., Thompson, D. A., Siani, M. A., Yamamoto, T., Harrison, J. K. & Feng, L. (1998). In vivo inhibition of CC and CX3C chemokine-induced leukocyte infiltration and attenuation of glomerulonephritis in Wistar-Kyoto (WKY) rats by vMIP-II. *Journal of Experimental Medicine*, 188(1): pp. 193-198.

Cichy, J. & Pure, E. (2000). Oncostatin M and transforming growth factor-beta 1 induce post-translational modification and hyaluronan binding to CD44 in lung-derived epithelial tumor cells. *Journal of Biological Chemistry*, 275(24): pp. 18061-18069.

Cid, M. C., Segarra, M., Garcia-Martinez, A. & Hernandez-Rodriguez, J. (2004). Endothelial cells, antineutrophil cytoplasmic antibodies, and cytokines in the pathogenesis of systemic vasculitis. *Current Rheumatology Reports*, 6(3): pp. 184-194.

Cid, M. C. & Vilardell, C. (2001). Tissue targeting and disease patterns in systemic vasculitis. *Best practice & research. Clinical Rheumatology*, 15(2): pp. 259-279.

Cross, J. T. & Benton, H. P. (1999). The roles of interleukin-6 and interleukin-10 in B cell hyperactivity in systemic lupus erythematosus. *Inflammation Research*, 48(5): pp. 255-261.

Dallos, T., Heiland, G. R., Strehl, J., Karonitsch, T., Gross, W. L., Moosig, F., Holl-Ulrich, C., Distler, J. H., Manger, B., Schett, G. & Zwerina, J. (2010). CCL17/thymus and activation-related chemokine in Churg-Strauss syndrome. *Arthritis and Rheumatism*, 62(11): pp. 3496-3503.

Daly, C. & Rollins, B. J. (2003). Monocyte chemoattractant protein-1 (CCL2) in inflammatory disease and adaptive immunity: therapeutic opportunities and controversies. *Microcirculation*, 10(3-4): pp. 247-257.

de Jong, Y. P., Abadia-Molina, A. C., Satoskar, A. R., Clarke, K., Rietdijk, S. T., Faubion, W. A., Mizoguchi, E., Metz, C. N., Alsahli, M., ten Hove, T., Keates, A. C., Lubetsky, J. B., Farrell, R. J., Michetti, P., van Deventer, S. J., Lolis, E., David, J. R., Bhan, A. K. & Terhorst, C. (2001). Development of chronic colitis is dependent on the cytokine MIF. *Nature Immunology*, 2(11): pp. 1061-1066.

Dean, D. C., Iademarco, M. F., Rosen, G. D. & Sheppard, A. M. (1993). The integrin alpha 4 beta 1 and its counter receptor VCAM-1 in development and immune function. *American Review of Respiratory Disease*, 148(6 Pt 2): pp. S43-46.

Dhawan, V., Mahajan, N. & Jain, S. (2006). Role of C-C chemokines in Takayasu's arteritis disease. *International Journal of Cardiology*, 112(1): pp. 105-111.

Di Lorenzo, G., Pacor, M. L., Mansueto, P., Lo Bianco, C., Di Natale, E., Rapisarda, F., Pellitteri, M. E., Ditta, V., Gioe, A., Giammarresi, G., Rini, G. B. & Li Vecchi, M. (2004). Circulating levels of soluble adhesion molecules in patients with ANCA-associated vasculitis. *Journal of Nephrology*, 17(6): pp. 800-807.

Eardley, K. S., Smith, S. W. & Cockwell, P. (2009). Chemokines in vasculitis. *Frontiers in Bioscience (Elite Ed)*, 1: pp. 26-35.

Emilie, D., Liozon, E., Crevon, M. C., Lavignac, C., Portier, A., Liozon, F. & Galanaud, P. (1994). Production of interleukin 6 by granulomas of giant cell arteritis. *Human Immunology*, 39(1): pp. 17-24.

Feldmann, M. & Pusey, C. D. (2006). Is there a role for TNF-alpha in anti-neutrophil cytoplasmic antibody-associated vasculitis? Lessons from other chronic inflammatory diseases. *Journal of the American Society of Nephrology*, 17(5): pp. 1243-1252.

Filer, A. D., Gardner-Medwin, J. M., Thambyrajah, J., Raza, K., Carruthers, D. M., Stevens, R. J., Liu, L., Lowe, S. E., Townend, J. N. & Bacon, P. A. (2003). Diffuse endothelial dysfunction is common to ANCA associated systemic vasculitis and polyarteritis nodosa. *Annals of the Rheumatic Diseases*, 62(2): pp. 162-167.

Firestein, G. S. (2003). Evolving concepts of rheumatoid arthritis. *Nature*, 423(6937): pp. 356-361.

Flipo, R. M., Cardon, T., Copin, M. C., Vandecandelaere, M., Duquesnoy, B. & Janin, A. (1997). ICAM-1, E-selectin, and TNF alpha expression in labial salivary glands of patients with rheumatoid vasculitis. *Annals of the Rheumatic Diseases*, 56(1): pp. 41-44.

Fong, A. M., Robinson, L. A., Steeber, D. A., Tedder, T. F., Yoshie, O., Imai, T. & Patel, D. D. (1998). Fractalkine and CX3CR1 mediate a novel mechanism of leukocyte capture, firm adhesion, and activation under physiologic flow. *Journal of Experimental Medicine*, 188(8): pp. 1413-1419.

Foote, A., Briganti, E. M., Kipen, Y., Santos, L., Leech, M. & Morand, E. F. (2004). Macrophage migration inhibitory factor in systemic lupus erythematosus. *Journal of Rheumatology*, 31(2): pp. 268-273.

Foster, C. A. (1996). VCAM-1/alpha 4-integrin adhesion pathway: therapeutic target for allergic inflammatory disorders. *Journal of Allergy and Clinical Immunology*, 98(6 Pt 2): pp. S270-277.

Gearing, A. J., Hemingway, I., Pigott, R., Hughes, J., Rees, A. J. & Cashman, S. J. (1992). Soluble forms of vascular adhesion molecules, E-selectin, ICAM-1, and VCAM-1: pathological significance. *Annals of the New York Academy of Sciences*, 667: pp. 324-331.

Gerard, C. & Rollins, B. J. (2001). Chemokines and disease. *Nature Immunology*, 2: pp. 108-115.

Gesualdo, L., Grandaliano, G., Ranieri, E., Monno, R., Montinaro, V., Manno, C. & Schena, F. P. (1997). Monocyte recruitment in cryoglobulinemic membranoproliferative glomerulonephritis: a pathogenetic role for monocyte chemotactic peptide-1. *Kidney International*, 51(1): pp. 155-163.

Grau, G. E., Roux-Lombard, P., Gysler, C., Lambert, C., Lambert, P. H., Dayer, J. M. & Guillevin, L. (1989). Serum cytokine changes in systemic vasculitis. *Immunology*, 68(2): pp. 196-198.

Grewal, I. S. & Flavell, R. A. (1998). CD40 and CD154 in cell-mediated immunity. *Annual Review of Immunology*, 16: pp. 111-135.

Hanaoka, R., Kasama, T., Muramatsu, M., Yajima, N., Shiozawa, F., Miwa, Y., Negishi, M., Ide, H., Miyaoka, H., Uchida, H. & Adachi, M. (2003). A novel mechanism for the regulation of IFN-gamma inducible protein-10 expression in rheumatoid arthritis. *Arthritis Research & Therapy*, 5(2): pp. R74-81.

Haringman, J. J., Ludikhuize, J. & Tak, P. P. (2004). Chemokines in joint disease: the key to inflammation? *Annals of the Rheumatic Diseases*, 63(10): pp. 1186-1194.

Hasegawa, M., Sato, S., Echigo, T., Hamaguchi, Y., Yasui, M. & Takehara, K. (2005). Up regulated expression of fractalkine/CX3CL1 and CX3CR1 in patients with systemic sclerosis. *Annals of the Rheumatic Diseases*, 64(1): pp. 21-28.

Haynes, B. F., Hale, L. P., Patton, K. L., Martin, M. E. & McCallum, R. M. (1991). Measurement of an adhesion molecule as an indicator of inflammatory disease activity. Up-regulation of the receptor for hyaluronate (CD44) in rheumatoid arthritis. *Arthritis and Rheumatism*, 34(11): pp. 1434-1443.

Hellmich, B., Csernok, E. & Gross, W. L. (2005). Proinflammatory cytokines and autoimmunity in Churg-Strauss syndrome. *Annals of the New York Academy of Sciences*, 1051: pp. 121-131.

Hergesell, O., Andrassy, K. & Nawroth, P. (1996). Elevated levels of markers of endothelial cell damage and markers of activated coagulation in patients with systemic necrotizing vasculitis. *Thrombosis and Haemostasis*, 75(6): pp. 892-898.

Hewins, P., Morgan, M. D., Holden, N., Neil, D., Williams, J. M., Savage, C. O. & Harper, L. (2006). IL-18 is upregulated in the kidney and primes neutrophil responsiveness in ANCA-associated vasculitis. *Kidney International*, 69(3): pp. 605-615.

Hoi, A. Y., Morand, E. F. & Leech, M. (2003). Is macrophage migration inhibitory factor a therapeutic target in systemic lupus erythematosus? *Immunology and Cell Biology*, 81(5): pp. 367-373.

Holcombe, R. F., Baethge, B. A., Wolf, R. E., Betzing, K. W., Stewart, R. M., Hall, V. C. & Fukuda, M. (1994). Correlation of serum interleukin-8 and cell surface lysosome-associated membrane protein expression with clinical disease activity in systemic lupus erythematosus. *Lupus*, 3(2): pp. 97-102.

Hruskova, Z., Mareckova, H., Rihova, Z., Rysava, R., Jancova, E., Merta, M. & Tesar, V. (2008). T cells in the pathogenesis of ANCA-associated vasculitis: current knowledge. *Folia Biologica*, 54(3): pp. 81-87.

Huugen, D., Tervaert, J. W. & Heeringa, P. (2006). TNF-alpha bioactivity-inhibiting therapy in ANCA-associated vasculitis: clinical and experimental considerations. *Clinical Journal of the American Society of Nephrology*, 1(5): pp. 1100-1107.

Imai, T., Hieshima, K., Haskell, C., Baba, M., Nagira, M., Nishimura, M., Kakizaki, M., Takagi, S., Nomiyama, H., Schall, T. J. & Yoshie, O. (1997). Identification and molecular characterization of fractalkine receptor CX3CR1, which mediates both leukocyte migration and adhesion. *Cell*, 91: pp. 521-530.

Jennette, J. C., Wieslander, J., Tuttle, R. & Falk, R. J. (1991). Serum IgA-fibronectin aggregates in patients with IgA nephropathy and Henoch-Schonlein purpura: diagnostic value and pathogenic implications. The Glomerular Disease Collaborative Network. *American Journal of Kidney Diseases*, 18(4): pp. 466-471.

Jia, S., Li, C., Wang, G., Yang, J. & Zu, Y. (2010). The T helper type 17/regulatory T cell imbalance in patients with acute Kawasaki disease. *Clinical and Experimental Immunology*, 162(1): pp. 131-137.

Johnson, B. A., Haines, G. K., Harlow, L. A. & Koch, A. E. (1993). Adhesion molecule expression in human synovial tissue. *Arthritis and Rheumatism*, 36: pp. 137-146.

Johnson, P. A., Alexander, H. D., McMillan, S. A. & Maxwell, A. P. (1997). Up-regulation of the endothelial cell adhesion molecule intercellular adhesion molecule-1 (ICAM-1) by autoantibodies in autoimmune vasculitis. *Clinical and Experimental Immunology*, 108(2): pp. 234-242.

Kaneider, N. C., Leger, A. J. & Kuliopulos, A. (2006). Therapeutic targeting of molecules involved in leukocyte-endothelial cell interactions. *FEBS Journal*, 273: pp. 4416-4424.

Kasama, T., Miwa, Y., Isozaki, T., Odai, T., Adachi, M. & Kunkel, S. L. (2005). Neutrophil-derived cytokines: potential therapeutic targets in inflammation. *Curr Drug Targets. Inflamm Allergy*, 4(3): pp. 273-279.

Kasama, T., Muramatsu, M., Kobayashi, K., Yajima, N., Shiozawa, F., Hanaoka, R., Miwa, Y., Negishi, M., Ide, H. & Adachi, M. (2002). Interaction of monocytes with vascular endothelial cells synergistically induces interferon gamma-inducible protein 10 expression through activation of specific cell surface molecules and cytokines. *Cellular Immunology*, 219(2): pp. 131-139.

Kasama, T., Wakabayashi, K., Sato, M., Takahashi, R. & Isozaki, T. (2010). Relevance of the CX3CL1/fractalkine-CX3CR1 pathway in vasculitis and vasculopathy. *Translational Research*, 155(1): pp. 20-26.

Katoh, S., McCarthy, J. B. & Kincade, P. W. (1994). Characterization of soluble CD44 in the circulation of mice. Levels are affected by immune activity and tumor growth. *Journal of Immunology*, 153(8): pp. 3440-3449.

Kim, S. H., Kim, T. B., Yun, Y. S., Shin, J. I., Oh, I. Y., Sir, J. J., Kim, K. M., Park, H. K., Kang, H. R., Chang, Y. S., Kim, Y. K., Cho, S. H., Song, Y. W., Choi, D. C., Min, K. U. & Kim, Y. Y. (2005). Hypereosinophilia presenting as eosinophilic vasculitis and multiple peripheral artery occlusions without organ involvement. *Journal of Korean Medical Science*, 20(4): pp. 677-679.

Kunkel, S. L., Lukacs, N., Kasama, T. & Strieter, R. M. (1996). The role of chemokines in inflammatory joint disease. *Journal of Leukocyte Biology*, 59(1): pp. 6-12.

Kuryliszyn-Moskal, A. (1998). Cytokines and soluble CD4 and CD8 molecules in rheumatoid arthritis: relationship to systematic vasculitis and microvascular capillaroscopic abnormalities. *Clinical Rheumatology*, 17(6): pp. 489-495.

Kuryliszyn-Moskal, A., Bernacka, K. & Klimiuk, P. A. (1996). Circulating intercellular adhesion molecule 1 in rheumatoid arthritis--relationship to systemic vasculitis and microvascular injury in nailfold capillary microscopy. *Clinical Rheumatology*, 15(4): pp. 367-373.

Lamprecht, P., Bruhl, H., Erdmann, A., Holl-Ulrich, K., Csernok, E., Seitzer, U., Mack, M., Feller, A. C., Reinhold-Keller, E., Gross, W. L. & Muller, A. (2003). Differences in CCR5 expression on peripheral blood CD4+CD28- T-cells and in granulomatous lesions between localized and generalized Wegener's granulomatosis. *Clinical Immunology*, 108(1): pp. 1-7.

Lamprecht, P., Kumanovics, G., Mueller, A., Csernok, E., Komocsi, A., Trabandt, A., Gross, W. L. & Schnabel, A. (2002). Elevated monocytic IL-12 and TNF-alpha production in Wegener's granulomatosis is normalized by cyclophosphamide and corticosteroid therapy. *Clinical and Experimental Immunology*, 128(1): pp. 181-186.

Leech, M., Metz, C., Hall, P., Hutchinson, P., Gianis, K., Smith, M., Weedon, H., Holdsworth, S. R., Bucala, R. & Morand, E. F. (1999). Macrophage migration inhibitory factor in rheumatoid arthritis: evidence of proinflammatory function and regulation by glucocorticoids. *Arthritis and Rheumatism*, 42(8): pp. 1601-1608.

Lesley, J., Hyman, R. & Kincade, P. W. (1993). CD44 and its interaction with extracellular matrix. *Advances in Immunology*, 54: pp. 271-335.

Levesque, M. C. & Haynes, B. F. (1997). Cytokine induction of the ability of human monocyte CD44 to bind hyaluronan is mediated primarily by TNF-alpha and is inhibited by IL-4 and IL-13. *Journal of Immunology*, 159(12): pp. 6184-6194.

Libby, P. (2002). Inflammation in atherosclerosis. *Nature*, 420(6917): pp. 868-874.

Lin, S. G., Yu, X. Y., Chen, Y. X., Huang, X. R., Metz, C., Bucala, R., Lau, C. P. & Lan, H. Y. (2000). De novo expression of macrophage migration inhibitory factor in atherogenesis in rabbits. *Circulation Research*, 87(12): pp. 1202-1208.

Luster, A. D. (1998). Chemokines--chemotactic cytokines that mediate inflammation. *New England Journal of Medicine*, 338: pp. 436-445.

Lyakh, L., Trinchieri, G., Provezza, L., Carra, G. & Gerosa, F. (2008). Regulation of interleukin-12/interleukin-23 production and the T-helper 17 response in humans. *Immunological Reviews*, 226: pp. 112-131.

Mackay, C. R. & Imhof, B. A. (1993). Cell adhesion in the immune system. *Immunology Today*, 14: pp. 99-102.

Mantovani, A. & Dejana, E. (1989). Cytokines as communication signals between leukocytes and endothelial cells. *Immunology Today*, 10: pp. 370-375.

Matsunawa, M., Isozaki, T., Odai, T., Yajima, N., Takeuchi, H. T., Negishi, M., Ide, H., Adachi, M. & Kasama, T. (2006). Increased serum levels of soluble fractalkine (CX3CL1) correlate with disease activity in rheumatoid vasculitis. *Arthritis and Rheumatism*, 54(11): pp. 3408-3416.

Matsunawa, M., Odai, T., Wakabayashi, K., Isozaki, T., Yajima, N., Miwa, Y., Nohtomi, K., Takeuchi, H. & Kasama, T. (2009). Elevated serum levels of soluble CX3CL1 in patients with microscopic polyangiitis. *Clinical and Experimental Rheumatology*, 27(1): pp. 72-78.

Matsuyama, T. & Kitani, A. (1996). The role of VCAM-1 molecule in the pathogenesis of rheumatoid synovitis. *Human Cell*, 9(3): pp. 187-192.

McInnes, I. B. & Schett, G. (2007). Cytokines in the pathogenesis of rheumatoid arthritis. *Nature Reviews. Immunol*, 7(6): pp. 429-442.

Middleton, J., Americh, L., Gayon, R., Julien, D., Aguilar, L., Amalric, F. & Girard, J. P. (2004). Endothelial cell phenotypes in the rheumatoid synovium: activated, angiogenic, apoptotic and leaky. *Arthritis Research & Therapy*, 6(2): pp. 60-72.

Miller, D. L., Yaron, R. & Yellin, M. J. (1998). CD40L-CD40 interactions regulate endothelial cell surface tissue factor and thrombomodulin expression. *Journal of Leukocyte Biology*, 63: pp. 373-379.

Moser, B. & Loetscher, P. (2001). Lymphocyte traffic cotrol by chemokines. *Nature Immunology*, 2: pp. 123-128.

Moser, B., Wolf, M., Walz, A. & Loetscher, P. (2004). Chemokines: multiple levels of leukocyte migration control. *Trends in immunology*, 25(2): pp. 75-84.

Muller-Ladner, U., Pap, T., Gay, R. E., Neidhart, M. & Gay, S. (2005). Mechanisms of disease: the molecular and cellular basis of joint destruction in rheumatoid arthritis. *Nature Clinical Practice. Rheumatology*, 1(2): pp. 102-110.

Muller Kobold, A. C., van Wijk, R. T., Franssen, C. F., Molema, G., Kallenberg, C. G. & Tervaert, J. W. (1999). In vitro up-regulation of E-selectin and induction of interleukin-6 in endothelial cells by autoantibodies in Wegener's granulomatosis and microscopic polyangiitis. *Clinical and Experimental Rheumatology*, 17(4): pp. 433-440.

Naka, T., Nishimoto, N. & Kishimoto, T. (2002). The paradigm of IL-6: from basic science to medicine. *Arthritis Research*, 4 Suppl 3: pp. S233-242.

Neville, L. F., Mathiak, G. & Bagasra, O. (1997). The immunobiology of interferon-gamma inducible protein 10 kD (IP-10): a novel, pleiotropic member of the C-X-C chemokine superfamily. *Cytokine and Growth Factor Reviews*, 8(3): pp. 207-219.

Nishihira, J., Koyama, Y. & Mizue, Y. (1998). Identification of macrophage migration inhibitory factor (MIF) in human vascular endothelial cells and its induction by lipopolysaccharide. *Cytokine*, 10(3): pp. 199-205.

Noguchi, S., Numano, F., Gravanis, M. B. & Wilcox, J. N. (1998). Increased levels of soluble forms of adhesion molecules in Takayasu arteritis. *International Journal of Cardiology*, 66 Suppl 1: pp. S23-33; discussion S35-26.

Nogueira, E., Hamour, S., Sawant, D., Henderson, S., Mansfield, N., Chavele, K. M., Pusey, C. D. & Salama, A. D. (2010). Serum IL-17 and IL-23 levels and autoantigen-specific Th17 cells are elevated in patients with ANCA-associated vasculitis. *Nephrology, Dialysis, Transplantation*, 25(7): pp. 2209-2217.

Nolan, S. L., Kalia, N., Nash, G. B., Kamel, D., Heeringa, P. & Savage, C. O. (2008). Mechanisms of ANCA-mediated leukocyte-endothelial cell interactions in vivo. *Journal of the American Society of Nephrology*, 19(5): pp. 973-984.

Noris, M., Daina, E., Gamba, S., Bonazzola, S. & Remuzzi, G. (1999). Interleukin-6 and RANTES in Takayasu arteritis: a guide for therapeutic decisions? *Circulation*, 100(1): pp. 55-60.

Ohlsson, S., Bakoush, O., Tencer, J., Torffvit, O. & Segelmark, M. (2009). Monocyte chemoattractant protein 1 is a prognostic marker in ANCA-associated small vessel vasculitis. *Mediators of Inflammation*, 2009: pp. 584916.

Ohta, N., Fukase, S. & Aoyagi, M. (2001). Serum levels of soluble adhesion molecules ICAM-1, VCAM-1 and E-selectin in patients with Wegener's granulomatosis. *Auris, Nasus, Larynx*, 28(4): pp. 311-314.

Ohwatari, R., Fukuda, S., Iwabuchi, K., Inuyama, Y., Onoe, K. & Nishihira, J. (2001). Serum level of macrophage migration inhibitory factor as a useful parameter of clinical course in patients with Wegener's granulomatosis and relapsing polychondritis. *Annals of Otology, Rhinology and Laryngology*, 110(11): pp. 1035-1040.

Okamura, H., Tsutsui, H., Kashiwamura, S., Yoshimoto, T. & Nakanishi, K. (1998). Interleukin-18: a novel cytokine that augments both innate and acquired immunity. *Advances in Immunology*, 70: pp. 281-312.

Onodera, S., Nishihira, J., Koyama, Y., Majima, T., Aoki, Y., Ichiyama, H., Ishibashi, T. & Minami, A. (2004). Macrophage migration inhibitory factor up-regulates the expression of interleukin-8 messenger RNA in synovial fibroblasts of rheumatoid arthritis patients: common transcriptional regulatory mechanism between interleukin-8 and interleukin-1beta. *Arthritis and Rheumatism*, 50(5): pp. 1437-1447.

Palomino-Morales, R. J., Vazquez-Rodriguez, T. R., Torres, O., Morado, I. C., Castaneda, S., Miranda-Filloy, J. A., Callejas-Rubio, J. L., Fernandez-Gutierrez, B., Gonzalez-Gay, M. A. & Martin, J. (2010). Association between IL-18 gene polymorphisms and biopsy-proven giant cell arteritis. *Arthritis Research & Therapy*, 12(2): pp. R51.

Pan, Y., Lloyd, C., Zhou, H., Dolich, S., Deeds, J., Gonzalo, J.-A., Vath, J., Gosselin, M., Ma, J., Dussault, B., Woolf, E., Alperin, G., Culpepper, J., Gutierrez-Ramos, J. C. & Gearing, D. (1997). Neurotactin, a membrane-anchored chemokine upregulated in brain inflammation. *Nature*, 387: pp. 611-617.

Panzer, U., Steinmetz, O. M., Reinking, R. R., Meyer, T. N., Fehr, S., Schneider, A., Zahner, G., Wolf, G., Helmchen, U., Schaerli, P., Stahl, R. A. & Thaiss, F. (2006). Compartment-specific expression and function of the chemokine IP-10/CXCL10 in a model of renal endothelial microvascular injury. *Journal of the American Society of Nephrology*, 17(2): pp. 454-464.

Park, M. C., Lee, S. W., Park, Y. B. & Lee, S. K. (2006). Serum cytokine profiles and their correlations with disease activity in Takayasu's arteritis. *Rheumatology*, 45(5): pp. 545-548.

Peters, J. H., Ginsberg, M. H., Bohl, B. P., Sklar, L. A. & Cochrane, C. G. (1986). Intravascular release of intact cellular fibronectin during oxidant-induced injury of the in vitro perfused rabbit lung. *Journal of Clinical Investigation*, 78(6): pp. 1596-1603.

Peters, J. H., Maunder, R. J., Woolf, A. D., Cochrane, C. G. & Ginsberg, M. H. (1989). Elevated plasma levels of ED1+ ("cellular") fibronectin in patients with vascular injury. *The Journal of Laboratory and Clinical Medicine*, 113(5): pp. 586-597.

Polzer, K., Karonitsch, T., Neumann, T., Eger, G., Haberler, C., Soleiman, A., Hellmich, B., Csernok, E., Distler, J., Manger, B., Redlich, K., Schett, G. & Zwerina, J. (2008). Eotaxin-3 is involved in Churg-Strauss syndrome--a serum marker closely correlating with disease activity. *Rheumatology*, 47(6): pp. 804-808.

Riedemann, N. C., Guo, R. F., Gao, H., Sun, L., Hoesel, M., Hollmann, T. J., Wetsel, R. A., Zetoune, F. S. & Ward, P. A. (2004). Regulatory role of C5a on macrophage migration inhibitory factor release from neutrophils. *Journal of Immunology*, 173(2): pp. 1355-1359.

Roche, N. E., Fulbright, J. W., Wagner, A. D., Hunder, G. G., Goronzy, J. J. & Weyand, C. M. (1993). Correlation of interleukin-6 production and disease activity in polymyalgia rheumatica and giant cell arteritis. *Arthritis and Rheumatism*, 36(9): pp. 1286-1294.

Rossi, D. & Zlotnik, A. (2000). The biology of chemokines and their receptors. *Annual Review of Immunology*, 18: pp. 217-242.

Rot, A. & von Andrian, U. H. (2004). Chemokines in innate and adaptive host defense: basic chemokinese grammar for immune cells. *Annual Review of Immunology*, 22: pp. 891-928.

Rovin, B. H., Lu, L. & Zhang, X. (2002). A novel interleukin-8 polymorphism is associated with severe systemic lupus erythematosus nephritis. *Kidney International*, 62(1): pp. 261-265.

Rovin, B. H., Rumancik, M., Tan, L. & Dickerson, J. (1994). Glomerular expression of monocyte chemoattractant protein-1 in experimental and human glomerulonephritis. *Laboratory Investigation*, 71(4): pp. 536-542.

Ruoslahti, E. (1988). Fibronectin and its receptors. *Annual Review of Biochemistry*, 57: pp. 375-413.

Ruth, J. H., Volin, M. V., Haines, G. K., 3rd, Woodruff, D. C., Katschke, K. J., Jr., Woods, J. M., Park, C. C., Morel, J. C. & Koch, A. E. (2001). Fractalkine, a novel chemokine in rheumatoid arthritis and in rat adjuvant-induced arthritis. *Arthritis and Rheumatism*, 44(7): pp. 1568-1581.

Salih, A. M., Nixon, N. B., Dawes, P. T. & Mattey, D. L. (1999). Soluble adhesion molecules and anti-endothelial cell antibodies in patients with rheumatoid arthritis complicated by peripheral neuropathy. *Journal of Rheumatology*, 26(3): pp. 551-555.

Sallusto, F., Lenig, D., Mackay, C. R. & Lanzavecchia, A. (1998). Flexible programs of chemokine receptor expression on human polarized T helper 1 and 2 lymphocytes. *Journal of Experimental Medicine*, 187: pp. 875-883.

Sansonno, D., Tucci, F. A., Troiani, L., Lauletta, G., Montrone, M., Conteduca, V., Sansonno, L. & Dammacco, F. (2008). Increased serum levels of the chemokine CXCL13 and up-regulation of its gene expression are distinctive features of HCV-related cryoglobulinemia and correlate with active cutaneous vasculitis. *Blood*, 112(5): pp. 1620-1627.

Schneeweis, C., Rafalowicz, M., Feist, E., Buttgereit, F., Rudolph, P. E., Burmester, G. R. & Egerer, K. (2010). Increased levels of BLyS and sVCAM-1 in anti-neutrophil cytoplasmatic antibody (ANCA)-associated vasculitides (AAV). *Clinical and Experimental Rheumatology*, 28(1 Suppl 57): pp. 62-66.

Schwarzbauer, J. E. (1991). Alternative splicing of fibronectin: three variants, three functions. *Bioessays.*, 13(10): pp. 527-533.

Seiter, S., Schadendorf, D., Tilgen, W. & Zoller, M. (1998). CD44 variant isoform expression in a variety of skin-associated autoimmune diseases. *Clinical Immunology and Immunopathology*, 89(1): pp. 79-93.

Selvi, E., Tripodi, S. A., Catenaccio, M., Lorenzini, S., Chindamo, D., Manganelli, S., Romagnoli, R., Ietta, F., Paulesu, L., Miracco, C., Cintorino, M. & Marcolongo, R. (2003). Expression of macrophage migration inhibitory factor in diffuse systemic sclerosis. *Annals of the Rheumatic Diseases*, 62(5): pp. 460-464.

Sfikakis, P. P. & Tsokos, G. C. (1997). Clinical use of the measurement of soluble cell adhesion molecules in patients with autoimmune rheumatic diseases. *Clinical and Diagnostic Laboratory Immunology*, 4(3): pp. 241-246.

Shikishima, Y., Saeki, T. & Matsuura, N. (2003). Chemokines in Kawasaki disease: measurement of CCL2, CCL22 and CXCL10. *Asian Pacific Journal of Allergy and Immunology*, 21(3): pp. 139-143.

Sinico, R. A., Radice, A., Corace, C., L, D. I. T. & Sabadini, E. (2005). Value of a new automated fluorescence immunoassay (EliA) for PR3 and MPO-ANCA in monitoring disease activity in ANCA-associated systemic vasculitis. *Annals of the New York Academy of Sciences*, 1050: pp. 185-192.

Sivalingam, S. P., Yoon, K. H., Koh, D. R. & Fong, K. Y. (2003). Single-nucleotide polymorphisms of the interleukin-18 gene promoter region in rheumatoid arthritis patients: protective effect of AA genotype. *Tissue Antigens*, 62(6): pp. 498-504.

Sneller, M. C. & Fauci, A. S. (1997). Pathogenesis of vasculitis syndromes. *Medical Clinics of North America*, 81(1): pp. 221-242.

Sohn, M. H., Noh, S. Y., Chang, W., Shin, K. M. & Kim, D. S. (2003). Circulating interleukin 17 is increased in the acute stage of Kawasaki disease. *Scandinavian Journal of Rheumatology*, 32(6): pp. 364-366.

Springer, T. A. (1990). Adhesion receptors of the immune system. *Nature*, 346: pp. 425-434.

Strieter, R. M., Polverini, P. J., Arenberg, D. A. & Kunkel, S. L. (1995). The role of CXC chemokines as regulators of angiogenesis. *Shock*, 4(3): pp. 155-160.

Sundy, J. S. & Haynes, B. F. (2000). Cytokines and adhesion molecules in the pathogenesis of vasculitis. *Current Rheumatology Reports*, 2(5): pp. 402-410.

Szekanecz, Z., Szucs, G., Szanto, S. & Koch, A. E. (2006). Chemokines in rheumatic diseases. *Current Drug Targets*, 7(1): pp. 91-102.

Takahashi, H., Soderstrom, K., Nilsson, E., Kiessling, R. & Patarroyo, M. (1992). Integrins and other adhesion molecules on lymphocytes from synovial fluid and peripheral blood of rheumatoid arthritis patients. *European Journal of Immunology*, 22(11): pp. 2879-2885.

Takatori, H., Kanno, Y., Chen, Z. & O'Shea, J. J. (2008). New complexities in helper T cell fate determination and the implications for autoimmune diseases. *Modern Rheumatology*, 18(6): pp. 533-541.

Terrier, B., Bieche, I., Maisonobe, T., Laurendeau, I., Rosenzwajg, M., Kahn, J. E., Diemert, M. C., Musset, L., Vidaud, M., Sene, D., Costedoat-Chalumeau, N., Le Thi-Huong, D., Amoura, Z., Klatzmann, D., Cacoub, P. & Saadoun, D. (2010). Interleukin-25: a cytokine linking eosinophils and adaptive immunity in Churg-Strauss syndrome. *Blood*, 116(22): pp. 4523-4531.

Thienel, U., Loike, J. & Yellin, M. J. (1999). CD154 (CD40L) induces human endothelial cell chemokine production and migration of leukocyte subsets. *Cellular Immunology*, 198: pp. 87-95.

Tripathy, N. K., Chandran, V., Garg, N. K., Sinha, N. & Nityanand, S. (2008). Soluble endothelial cell adhesion molecules and their relationship to disease activity in Takayasu's arteritis. *Journal of Rheumatology*, 35(9): pp. 1842-1845.

Tripathy, N. K., Sinha, N. & Nityanand, S. (2004). Interleukin-8 in Takayasu's arteritis: plasma levels and relationship with disease activity. *Clinical and Experimental Rheumatology*, 22(6 Suppl 36): pp. S27-30.

Turesson, C., Englund, P., Jacobsson, L. T., Sturfelt, G., Truedsson, L., Nennesmo, I. & Lundberg, I. E. (2001). Increased endothelial expression of HLA-DQ and interleukin 1alpha in extra-articular rheumatoid arthritis. Results from immunohistochemical studies of skeletal muscle. *Rheumatology*, 40(12): pp. 1346-1354.

Umehara, H., Bloom, E., Okazaki, T., Domae, N. & Imai, T. (2001). Fractalkine and vascular injury. *Trends in Immunology*, 22(11): pp. 602-607.

Utans, U., Arceci, R. J., Yamashita, Y. & Russell, M. E. (1995). Cloning and characterization of allograft inflammatory factor-1: a novel macrophage factor identified in rat cardiac allografts with chronic rejection. *Journal of Clinical Investigation*, 95(6): pp. 2954-2962.

van Dinther-Janssen, A. C., Horst, E., Koopman, G., Newmann, W., Scheper, R. J., Meijer, C. J. & Pals, S. T. (1991). The VLA-4/VCAM-1 pathway is involved in lymphocyte adhesion to endothelium in rheumatoid synovium. *Journal of Immunology*, 147(12): pp. 4207-4210.

Verschueren, P. C., Voskuyl, A. E., Smeets, T. J., Zwinderman, K. H., Breedveld, F. C. & Tak, P. P. (2000). Increased cellularity and expression of adhesion molecules in muscle biopsy specimens from patients with rheumatoid arthritis with clinical suspicion of vasculitis, but negative routine histology. *Annals of the Rheumatic Diseases*, 59(8): pp. 598-606.

Voskuyl, A. E., Emeis, J. J., Hazes, J. M. W., van Hogezand, R. A., Biemond, I. & Breedveld, F. C. (1998). Levels of circulating cellular fibronectin are increased in patients with rheumatoid vasculitis. *Clinical and Experimental Rheumatology*, 16: pp. 429-434.

Voskuyl, A. E., Martin, S., Melchers, L., Zwinderman, A. H., Weichselbraun, I. & Breedveld, F. C. (1995). Levels of circulating intercellular adhesion molecule-1 and -3 but not circulating endothelial leucocyte adhesion molecule are increased in patients with rheumatoid vasculitis. *British Journal of Rheumatology*, 34(4): pp. 311-315.

Wang, C. L., Wu, Y. T., Liu, C. A., Lin, M. W., Lee, C. J., Huang, L. T. & Yang, K. D. (2003). Expression of CD40 ligand on CD4+ T-cells and platelets correlated to the coronary artery lesion and disease progress in Kawasaki disease. *Pediatrics*, 111(2): pp. E140-147.

Weyand, C. M., Fulbright, J. W., Hunder, G. G., Evans, J. M. & Goronzy, J. J. (2000). Treatment of giant cell arteritis: interleukin-6 as a biologic marker of disease activity. *Arthritis and Rheumatism*, 43(5): pp. 1041-1048.

Weyand, C. M., Ma-Krupa, W., Pryshchep, O., Groschel, S., Bernardino, R. & Goronzy, J. J. (2005). Vascular dendritic cells in giant cell arteritis. *Annals of the New York Academy of Sciences*, 1062: pp. 195-208.

Witkowska, A. M., Kuryliszyn-Moskal, A., Borawska, M. H., Hukalowicz, K. & Markiewicz, R. (2003). A study on soluble intercellular adhesion molecule-1 and selenium in patients with rheumatoid arthritis complicated by vasculitis. *Clinical Rheumatology*, 22(6): pp. 414-419. Epub 2003 Nov 2011.

Yajima, N., Kasama, T., Isozaki, T., Odai, T., Matsunawa, M., Negishi, M., Ide, H., Kameoka, Y., Hirohata, S. & Adachi, M. (2005). Elevated levels of soluble fractalkine in active systemic lupus erythematosus: Potential involvement in neuropsychiatric manifestations. *Arthritis and Rheumatism*, 52: pp. 1670-1675.

Yang, Y., Degranpre, P., Kharfi, A. & Akoum, A. (2000). Identification of macrophage migration inhibitory factor as a potent endothelial cell growth-promoting agent released by ectopic human endometrial cells. *Journal of Clinical Endocrinology and Metabolism*, 85(12): pp. 4721-4727.

Yang, Z. F., Ho, D. W., Lau, C. K., Lam, C. T., Lum, C. T., Poon, R. T. & Fan, S. T. (2005). Allograft inflammatory factor-1 (AIF-1) is crucial for the survival and pro-inflammatory activity of macrophages. *International Immunology*, 17(11): pp. 1391-1397.

Zhou, Y., Huang, D., Farver, C. & Hoffman, G. S. (2003). Relative importance of CCR5 and antineutrophil cytoplasmic antibodies in patients with Wegener's granulomatosis. *Journal of Rheumatology*, 30(7): pp. 1541-1547.

Zimmerman, G. A., Mcintyre, T. M. & Prescott, S. M. (1996). Perspectives series: Cell adhesion in vascular biology. *Journal of Clinical Investigation*, 98: pp. 1699-1702.

Zwerina, J., Axmann, R., Jatzwauk, M., Sahinbegovic, E., Polzer, K. & Schett, G. (2009). Pathogenesis of Churg-Strauss syndrome: recent insights. *Autoimmunity*, 42(4): pp. 376-379.

Part 3

General Overviews in Vasculitis

11

Wegener's Granulomatosis

Lígia Peixoto, Patrício Aguiar, Filipe Veloso Gomes, João Espírito Santo, Nuno Marques, Ilídio Jesus and J. M. Braz Nogueira
Centro Hospital Lisboa Norte - Hospital de Santa Maria
Portugal

1. Introduction

Wegener's granulomatosis (WG) is a rare multisystemic autoimmune disease of unknown aetiology, characterized by necrotizing granulomatous inflammatory and pauci-immune vasculitis in small- and medium-sized blood vessels (capillaries, venules, arterioles and arteries) associated with antineutrophil cytoplasmic antibodies ($ANCA_S$) directed against proteinase 3 (PR3), a neutrophil serine protease, presented in primary azurophil granules of polymorphonuclear neutrophils (PMN) and lysosomes of monocytes. It typically produces granulomatous inflammation of the upper and lower respiratory tracts, and a segmental necrotizing glomerulonephritis (classic triad of disease), although any organ can be involved.

2. History and epidemiology

In 1897, Peter McBride described the first patient with this condition. Later, in 1931, Klinger [(1)] reported a case of this disease, a 70-year-old physician with constitutional symptoms, inflammation of the upper respiratory tract leading to saddle nose deformity, glomerulonephritis and pulmonary lesions. In 1936, the German pathologist, Friedrich Wegener [(2)] published three cases with similar clinical features. Goodman and Churg, in 1954, described a triad of pathological features of the disease: 1) systemic necrotizing angiitis, 2) necrotizing granulomatous inflammation of the respiratory tract, and 3) necrotizing glomerulonephritis.
WG is an uncommon disease with an estimated prevalence, in the United States, of 3 per 100,000 [(3)]. The incidence and prevalence of WG in the United Kingdom is estimated at 10,2 cases and 250 cases per million population, respectively. It is extremely rare in blacks compared with whites; the male-to-female ratio is 1:1 and, although the disease can be seen at any age, the mean age of diagnosis is 40 years [(3, 4)].

3. Pathology and pathogenesis

The histopathologic characteristics of WG are necrotizing vasculitis of small- and medium-sized blood vessels with granuloma formation, with an important triad of granulomatous inflammation, vasculitis and necrosis.
Lung biopsy shows the typical necrotizing granulomatous vasculitis, almost always with multiple and bilateral nodules (50% are cavitated) or diffuse infiltrates, composed of neutrophils, lymphocytes, plasma cells, histiocytes and eosinophils.

Upper respiratory tract tissue reveals acute and chronic inflammation, necrosis and granulomatous lesions, with or without vasculitis (4), being the triad of pathological features present in only about 15% of cases.
Renal involvement is manifested by segmental and focal necrotizing glomerulonephritis, often with crescents and mononuclear tubulointerstitial infiltrates, without evidence of immune complex deposition (pauci-immune on immunofluorescence or electron microscopy). However granulomas are infrequently found in renal biopsy specimens (5).
The immunopathogenesis of this disease is still unclear, although the knowledge has suffered substantial progress in recent years, with both cellular and humoral immunity thought to be involved. Also, genetic background and environmental factors may play an important role in WG.
Autoimmune responses to PR3 (Wegener autoantigen) plays a central role in disease development, according to in vitro and in vivo experimental data (6). Activated PMNs release PR3, which interacts with dendritic cells and induces their maturation into antigen-presenting cells, able to induce an unbalanced Th1 response, and leading to granuloma formation (7). Nowadays, the latter is accepted to be the place of ANCA production, essential to the onset of vasculitis, since PR3-ANCA activates PMNs and monocytes to develop a respiratory burst, adhere and migrate across the endothelium. The activated PMN and monocytes release pro-inflammatory mediators, such as TNF-α, IL-1, IL-8 (8). This process is reinforced by activation of the alternative complement pathway (6). The presence of ANCAs suggests the role of humoral autoimmunity (Figure 1).

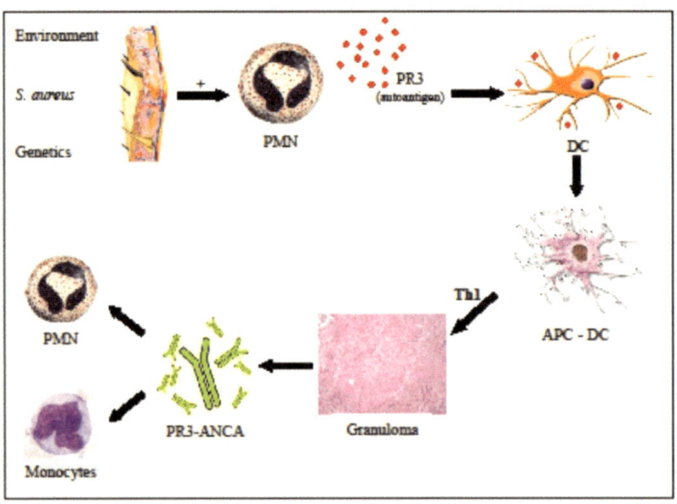

Fig. 1. Pathogenesis of WG. PMN: polymorphonuclear DC: Dentric cell; APC: Antigen-presenting cell

It is common to see WG progressing from a localized stage, restricted to the respiratory tract, to a systemic disease (generalized), and this transition may be influenced by a number of genetic risk factors. There is evidence that the human leukocyte antigen (HLA) system is involved both in WG development (9, 10), and other ANCA-positive vasculitides. Research is being carried out to confirm this association, for instance, to confirm the possible relation between WG and a region on chromosome 6p21.3 (11), although further investigation is needed. Indeed, this autoimmune disease is genetically associated with the class II region of the major histocompatibility complex (MHC), such as HLA-DPB1*0401 allele [12, 13]. Similarly to other autoimmune diseases, the functional polymorphism, 620W, in the intracellular tyrosine phosphatase gene PTPN 22, is a predisposing factor for WG in the presence of ANCA. This is due to loss of function of the PTPN 22 protein, which is important in T-cell receptor (TCR) signaling, via inhibition of key molecules in the receptor pathway, resulting in activation and proliferation of T cells and, subsequently, in humoral alterations [14]. Another genetic risk factor for WG is the CTLA-4 (cytotoxic T-lymphocyte antigen 4) polymorphism [15].

Environmental exposure to solvents or silica, farming and living in northern latitudes has been associated to the development of this autoimmune disease [16].

The relationship between WG and infectious diseases was first described by Friedrich Wegener in 1936 in its original descriptions, when he proposed that infectious agents are implicated in the disease pathogenesis [17]. Chronic nasal carriage of *Staphylococcus aureus* (the frequency in a healthy population varies from 20-35%) has been associated with a higher relapse rate of WG, suggesting a role of these bacteria in its pathophysiology [18]. Several toxins of this pathogen stimulate B-cell and probably T-cell activity. Also, direct stimulation of neutrophils in vitro has been documented [19], with *Staphylococcus aureus* producing proteinases with activity against human proteinase inhibitors, like α_1-antiprotease, which is the main inhibitor of proteinase-3, resulting in persistent inflammatory activity [20]. Additionally, several reports have noted that antibiotic therapy with sulfamethoxazole-trimethoprim has been beneficial in the treatment of refractory or limited WG localized to the respiratory tract [21].

4. Clinical manifestations

WG has a spectrum of clinical presentations. While the disease is active, most patients have nonspecific symptoms and signs such as malaise, weakness, migratory arthralgias, anorexia, weight loss, night sweats and fever. It is important to exclude secondary infection when fever is present. These constitutional symptoms may last for weeks to months without evidence of specific organ involvement.

Ear, nose and throat (ENT) manifestations are frequent in WG [22]. Involvement of the upper airways occurs in 95% of the patients, being chronic sinusitis the most common initial complaint (67%). Other frequent manifestations include saddle nose deformity by collapse of nasal support with bone and cartilage destruction, subglottic tracheal stenosis (16%) causing stridor, rhinitis, epistaxis, oral and/or nasal ulcers, serous otitis media, otorrhea and hearing loss (conductive and neurosensorial) [23].

Lung involvement is also common and may be manifested as asymptomatic diffuse pulmonary infiltrates (71%), nodules, atelectasis, consolidation and/or pleural effusion or may be clinically expressed as cough (34%), hemoptysis (18%) due to bronchiectasis, cavitated pulmonary parenchymal lesions or diffuse alveolar hemorrhage (DAH), dyspnoea (7%), pleuritic pain and chest discomfort (8%) [24]. The development of pulmonary fibrosis and pulmonary arterial hypertension may also occur. Chest radiography and computerized tomography (CT) scan are important investigations that must be included in the workup of these patients.

WG can also be recognized as tumor-like masses outside the lung, being the breast and kidney the most common extra-thoracic locations, although such cases are rare [25].

Another typical complication is **renal disease**, which is present in 17% at initial diagnosis and in 77% throughout the course of the disease, manifesting itself with acute renal failure, hematuria, red blood cell casts and proteinuria.

Eye involvement (52%) is manifested as conjunctivitis, dacryocystitis, keratitis, uveitis, scleritis, optic nerve vasculitis, retinal artery occlusion, diplopia and proptosis caused by retroorbital mass (26).

Cutaneous manifestations, present in 45% of patients, are nonspecific findings and usually affect the lower extremities. Palpable purpura, papules, subcutaneous nodules, ulcerations, livedo reticularis and urticaria are frequent, being leukocytoclastic angiitis (purpura, focal necrosis and ulceration) the most common skin lesion (27).

Musculoskeletal system is also often involved by the vasculitic process, with myalgias, polyarticular and symmetric arthralgias, and non-deforming arthritis of the large joints, being present in 32% of patients at initial diagnosis and in 67% throughout the course of the disease.

Cerebral manifestations (23%) include cranial nerve neuropathy, cerebral vasculitis, mononeuritis multiplex, pachymeningitis, central nervous system mass lesions, among other less frequent manifestations. Peripheral neuropathy is, however, more common than central nervous system involvement.

In patients with WG has been documented a high incidence of venous thrombotic events (VTEs). According to WeCLOT study (27) the incidence of VTEs was 7/100 person-years, but rotine anticoagulation for all patients is not recommended. Antiplasminogen antibodies were higher in PR3-ANCA patients than healthy control subjects (five in nine patients with VTE were positive for antiplasminogen antibodies) (28).

Less frequently, involvement of the heart (present in 6-44% of the patients with pericarditis, myocarditis, conduction system abnormalities and coronary vasculitis) (29); gastrointestinal tract (splanchnic vasculitis, abdominal pain); oral cavity ("strawberry gingival hyperplasia"); lower genitourinary tract (urethra, ureters, cervix, vagina, testicular and prostate), parotid glands, thyroid gland (hyperthyroidism), liver or breast is seen.

Organ involvement	Percent at initially of the disease	Percent during the course of disease
ENT	73	92
Lung	45	85
Kidney	18	77
Ocular	15	52
Skin lesions	13	46

Table 1. Percent of organ involvement in WG (22)

5. Laboratory findings

Characteristic laboratory findings are nonspecific and include elevated sedimentation rate and C-reactive protein, mild normocitic, normochromic anemia (50%), leukocytosis with neutrophil predominance, thrombocytosis (>400,000/microL) as an acute phase reactant, elevated blood urea nitrogen and creatinine levels, hypoalbuminemia, hypergammaglobulinemia (essentially of the IgA class), antinuclear antibody may be positive and slightly elevated rheumatoid factor levels. Patients should have a urinalysis, including microscopic analysis of urinary sediment, to determine the presence of hematuria and proteinuria.

Almost 90% of the patients with active WG have a positive anti-PR3 ANCA and only a small percentage of patients may have anti-myeloperoxidase (anti-MPO) ANCA.

ANCAs can be detected by two methods: immunofluorescence (IF) and enzyme-linked immunosorbent assay (ELISA). The former is a qualitative ANCA assay and there are three IF patterns recognized: cytoplasmic (C-ANCA), perinuclear (P-ANCA) and atypical. However, this technique has significant inter-reader variability unlike ELISA. The latter provides target antigen-specific characterization of ANCA. Only ANCA directed against PR3 or MPO have been associated with primary vasculitic syndromes. False positive ANCA titers appear in certain infectious and neoplastic diseases. Together, IF and ELISA confer 96% of sensitivity and 98,5% of specificity for the diagnosis of WG (30).

C-ANCA directed against PR3 is most specific for WG, especially if active glomerulonephritis is present. Rising C-ANCA titers may herald a relapse in some patients with WG, but this relationship is unreliable (31).

The measurement of PR3 membrane expression on neutrophils by flow cytometry (an increase is predictive of relapse) is a promissory marker for the activation of WG, but more research is needed (30).

6. Diagnosis

In a patient with the clinical features described above, the diagnosis of WG requires the demonstration of necrotizing granulomatous vasculitis on tissue biopsy, often from a site of active disease, being lung and kidney biopsies the most specific (lung biopsy is performed in the absence of renal involvement).

WG can be classified according to the nomenclature of the Chapel Hill Consensus (CHC) Conference for primary systemic vasculitis (table 2) (32) and according to the classification criteria defined by the American College of Rheumatology (ACR) (table 3) in 1990 (33).

- Granulomatous inflammation involving the respiratory tract and
- Necrotizing vasculitis affecting small- to medium-sized vessels (capillaries, venules, arterioles and arteries)
- Necrotizing glomerulonephritis is common
- Cytoplasmic pattern ANCAs (C-ANCA) with antigen specificity for proteinase 3 (PR3) are a very sensitive marker for WG

Table 2. Definition of WG according to the Chapel Hill Consensus Conference

1. Nasal or oral inflammation: oral ulcers or purulent or bloody nasal discharge
2. Abnormal chest radiograph: nodules, fixed infiltrates or cavities
3. Nephritic urinary sediment: microhematuria or red blood cells casts
4. Granulomatous inflammation on biopsy
5. For the diagnosis of WG the patient must have, at least, 2 or more of these 4 criteria (sensitivity of 88,2% and specificity of 92%)

Table 3. American College of Rheumatology Classification Criteria

The European Vasculitis Study Group (EUVAS) has developed a definition of the disease stage including localized disease (table 4) (34). WG can also be divided in limited (absence of disease features that pose immediate threats to either a critical individual organ or to the patient's life) or severe disease.

Disease Stages	Organ involvement	Detection of ANCA
Localized	Upper and lower airways	- / +
Early systemic	Any, but no imminent organ failure, creatinine < 150μmol/L	+
Generalized	Any, creatinine < 500μmol/L	+
Rapid progressive GN	Creatinine > 500μmol/L	+
Refractory	Progress in spite of therapy	+

Table 4. Disease stages according to the European Vasculitis Study Group (EUVAS)

7. Differential diagnosis

The differential diagnosis includes pathologies with related clinical features, mainly lung - kidney syndrome, or with similar laboratory findings (ANCA positive). The following table lists the most relevant disorders (table 5).

Churg - Strauss Syndrome	NK nasal type lymphoma
Microscopic polyangiitis	Cocain induced
Goodpasture's syndrome	Lymphomatoid granulomatosis (EBV)
Relapsing polycondhritis	Hemolytic- Uraemic syndrome
Upper airways or lung tumors	Infective endocarditis
Glomerulonephritis	Polyarteritis nodosa
Histoplasmosis	Sarcoidosis
Rhinoscleroma	Systemic Lupus Erythematosus

Table 5. WG´s differential diagnosis

8. Treatment

Therapy is adapted according to disease stage and activity [35] and requires remission induction with initial immunosuppressive therapy, followed by maintenance immunosuppressive therapy to prevent relapse and control the disease.

8.1 Remission induction

Patients with **limited disease** (localized/early systemic) should be treated with oral steroids 1mg/Kg/day in combination with oral or subcutaneous methotrexate (20-25mg/week), according to the NORAM study [36]. Daily folic acid 1mg/day is recommended. In these cases cyclophosphamide should be avoided due to associated toxicity. Methotrexate is equal to cyclophosphamide in inducing remisson [36], although the former was associated with more relapses at 18 months, compared to cyclophosphamide, 69,5% vs 46,5% , respectively.

Patients with **generalized disease or severe disease** (threatened vital organ function) should be treated with cyclophosphamide in combination with steroids (FAUCI scheme, introduced in 1970s).

Cyclophosphamide can be given orally (2mg/Kg/day and the maximum dosage is 200mg/day) or intravenously (15mg/Kg every 2 weeks for the first 3 pulses, then every 3 weeks for the next 3-6 pulses, being the maximum dose 1500mg) and must be adjusted to renal function and age (table 6). The total duration of treatment should not exceed 6 months

[37]. Pulsed cyclophosphamide has fewer side effects (lower rate of leucopenia) than oral doses, with equal efficacy [38] for remission induction. However, higher relapse rates in the maintenance phase, following the pulsed scheme, have been reported, and more studies are needed to assess this [35].

Age (years)	Creatinine 150-300µmol/l	Creatinine 300-500µmol/l
< 60	15mg/Kg/pulse	12,5mg/Kg/pulse
> 60 and <70	12,5mg/Kg/pulse	10mg/Kg/pulse
>70	10mg/Kg/pulse	7.5mg/Kg/pulse

Table 6. Pulsed cyclophosphamide reductions for renal function and age

Steroids were always considered the cornerstone of therapy. Although their use has not been evaluated in randomized controlled trials, every clinical trial has used this therapy in combination with another immunosuppressant. The ideal dose and duration of steroid therapy is unknown and further studies are needed. They are usually given orally (1mg/Kg/day of prednisolone during 1 month and then tapering slowly), but in the set of rapidly progressive glomerulonephritis and/or alveolar hemorrhage intravenous pulse methylprednisolone (0,5-1g/day for 3 consecutive days) can be used. In these two settings, plasma exchange can also be considered as adjuvant, although it has not been shown to improve overall survival.

Patients treated with cyclophosphamide and corticosteroids should receive prophylaxis against *Pneumocystis jiroveci* pneumonia with trimethoprim/sulfamethoxazole 960mg 3 times per week or, in cases with allergy to this antibiotic, dapsone 100mg daily.

8.2 Remission maintenance

In order to minimize exposure to the side effects of treatment with cyclophosphamide, alternative therapies have been proposed in recent years.

In the remission maintenance three agents can be used: azathioprine (2mg/Kg/day), methotrexate (20-25mg/week) and leflunomide. According to the CYCAZAREM trial [40], the former is safer than and as effective as cyclophosphamide. In a trial published in New England Journal of Medicine in December 2008, methotrexate has been shown to be similar to azathioprine in security and efficacy in maintaining remission [41]. Leflunomide was compared with methotrexate in a small trial and the results showed a trend to lower relapse rates with the first agent, but with more adverse effects [42]. In this study the dose of leflunomide was 30mg/day.

Mycophenolate mofetil (2g/day) can also be considered for maintenance therapy when there is intolerance or lack of efficacy with azathioprine or methotrexate, although more studies are needed.

8.3 Alternative therapies

Alternative therapies have increasingly been investigated, some of them with promise results.

Several studies showed clinical improvement or remission with **rituximab** (375mg/m^2 per week for four weeks). This data was confirmed by two recent trials, RAVE [43] and RITUXVAS [44], which showed non inferiority of rituximab compared with cyclophosphamide for induction of remission for the first study and remission of severe disease (renal involvement) for the second trial, with the former study reporting a possible superiority of rituximab in relapsing disease and in the RITUXVAS trial the rituximab group was associated with high rate of severe adverse events.

Etanercept studies, namely the Wegener´s granulomatosis etanercept (WGET) trial (45) didn´t find improvement in the maintenance of remission, with either severe or nonlifethreatening disease activity, when added to standard therapy, with a possible risk to increase infections and malignancies. This study didn´t evaluated this drug per se.
Infliximab, antithymocyte globulins and alentuzumab (CAMPATH-1H study) (46) are under investigation and further studies are needed to define their role in therapy.
Some studies suggest the use of intravenous immunoglobulin for refractory vasculitis, when conventional therapy is contra-indicated or for relapsed disease. However more studies are needed.

9. Prognosis

Patients with WG should have a closely follow-up, with regularly visits to her/his physician, involving multidisciplinary approach, and frequents exams to monitored the disease.
Relapse is common (50% within 5 years), being ANCA status at diagnosis, target organ involvement (lung, renal, heart and chronic nasal carriage of *Staphylococcus aureus*) and treatment with <10g of cyclophosphamide in the first 6 months, maintaining prednisone >20mg/day for <2, 75 months and/or goal of zero dose of glucocorticoids factors associated to high risk of relapse (47).
Untreated generalized or severe disease has a poorer prognosis, with a mortality rate up to 90% within 2 years, but the introduction of immunosuppressive therapy increases the lifelong of these patients, being the overall 10-year survival rate 75-88% (48). Renal involvement is associated with a bad prognosis.
The leading causes of death are infection, respiratory and renal failure, malignancy and cardiovascular disease, being the first one the major responsible for the mortality and morbidity in WG.

10. References

[1] Klinger H. Grenzformen der Pericarditis nodosa. Frankfurt Zeitschr Pathol 1931; 42: 455-480.
[2] Fauci AS, Wolff SM. Wegener´s granulomatosis: studies in eighteen patients and a review of the literature. Medicine (Baltimore) 1973; 52: 535-561.
[3] Duna GF, Galperin C, Hoffman GS: Wegener´s granulomatosis. *Rheum Dis Clin* North Am 1995; 21: 949-986.
[4] Carol A. Langford, Anthony S. Fauci. The vasculitis syndromes. In: Fauci A. et all. *Harrison´s – Principles of Internal Medicine*; 17th edition; Mc Graw Hill, 2008; 2119-2124.
[5] Haas, M, Eustace, JA. Immune complex deposits in ANCA-associated crescentic glomerulonephritis: a study of 126 cases. *Kidney Int* 2004; 65: 2145.
[6] Kallenberg CG. Pathogenesis of ANCA-associated vasculitides. Ann Rheum Dis 2011; 70 (suppl 1): 59-63
[7] Csernok E, Ai M, Gross WL, Wicklein D, et al. Wegener´s autoantigen induces maturation of dendritic cells and licenses them for Th1 priming via the protease-activated receptor-2 pathway. *Blood* 2006; 107 (11): 4440-8.
[8] Moosig F, Csernok E, Kumanovics G, Gross WL (2000) Clin Exp Immunol 122:499-503.
[9] Spence SJ, Burns A, Gaskin G, et al: HLA class II specificities in vasculitis with antibodies to neutrophil cytoplasmic antigens. *Kidney Int* 1992, 41 (4): 1059-1063.

[10] Cotch MF, Fauci AS, Hoffman GS: HLA typing in patients with Wegener granulomatosis. *Ann Intern Med* 1995, 122 (8): 635.
[11] Szyld P, Jagiello P, Csernok E, et al. On the Wegener granulomatosis associated region on chromosome 6p21.3. BMC *Med Genet* 2006; 7: 21.
[12] Jagiello P, Gencik M, Arning L, et al. New genomic region for Wegener´s granulomatosis as revealed by an extended association screen with 202 apoptosis related genes. *Hum Genet* 2004; 114: 468-77.
[13] Heckmann M, Holle JU, Arning L, et al (2007) *Ann Rheum Dis* (in press).
[14] Jagiello P, Aries P, Arning L, et al. The PTPN22 620 W allele is a risk factor for Wegener´s granulomatosis. *Arthritis Rheum* 2005; 52 (12): 4039-43.
[15] Zhou Y, Huang D, Paris PL, Sauter CS, Prock KA, Hoffman GS (2004) Arthritis Rheum 50:2645-2650.
[16] Spagnolo P, Richeldi L, DuBois RM. Environmental triggers and susceptibility factors in idiopathic granulomatous diseases. *Semin Respir Crit Care Med.* December 2008; 29:610-619.
[17] Wegener F. Über generalisierte, septische GefäBerkrankungen [Regarding generalized, septic vascular diseases]. Verh Dtsch Pathol Gesellsch. 1936; 26:202-10.
[18] Stegemann CA, Tervaert JW, Sluiter WJ, et al. Association of nasal carriage of *S. aureus* and higher relapse rates in Wegener´s Granulomatosis. *Ann Intern Med* 1994; 120: 12-17.
[19] Bates EJ, Ferrante A, Beard LJ. Characterization of the major neutrophil stimulating activity present in culture medium conditioned by *Staphylococcus aureus*-stimulated mononuclear leucocytes. Immunology 1991; 72:448-50.
[20] Potempa J, Watorek W, Travis J. The inactivation of human plasma a1-proteinase inhibitor by proteinases from Staphylococcus aureus. J Biol Chem. 1986; 261:14330-4.
[21] Valeriano- Marcet J, Spiera H. Treatment of Wegener´s granulomatosis with sulfamethoxazole-trimethoprim. Arch Intern Med. 1991; 151:1649-52.
[22] Hoffman, GS, Kerr, GS, Leavitt, RY, et al. Wegener granulomatosis: an analysis of 158 patients. *Ann Intern Med* 1992; 116:488.
[23] Jayne D. The diagnosis of vasculitis. Best Practice & Research Clinical Immnunology 2009; 23:445.
[24] Manganelli P, Fietta P, Carotti M, et al. Respiratory system involvement in systemic vasculitis. Clin Exp Rheumatol. March-April 2006; 24:S48-S59.
[25] Kariv, R, Sidi, Y, Gur, H. Systemic vasculitis presenting as a tumorlike lesion. Four case reports and an analysis of 79 reported cases. Medicine (Baltimore) 2000; 79:349.
[26] Harper, SL, Letko, E, Samson, CM, et al. Wegener´s granulomatosis: the relationship between ocular and systemic disease. J Rheumatol 2001; 28:1025.
[27] Merkel PA, Lo GH, Holbrook JT, et al. Brief communication: high incidence of venous thrombotic events among patients with Wegener granulomatosis: the Wegener´s Clinical Occurrence of Thrombosis (WeCLOT) Study. Ann Intern Med 2005; 142:620.
[28] David J. Bautz, Gloria A. Preston, Sofia Lionaki, et al. Antibodies with Dual Reactivity to Plamonogen and Complementary PR3 in PR3-ANCA Vasculitis. *J Am Soc Nephrol* 2008; 19:2421-2429.
[29] Marques N, Mimoso J, et al. Unstable angina as initial manifestation of Wegener granulomatosis: case report. Rev Port Cardiol 2008, 27: 1469-77.
[30] Moosig F, Lamprecht P, Gross WL. Wegener´s Granulomatosis: the current view. Clin Rev Allergy Immunol. October 2008; 35(1-2):19-21.

[31] Sanders JS, Huitma MG, Kallenberg CG, Stegeman CA. Prediction of relapses in PR3-ANCA-associated vasculitis by assessing responses of ANCA titers to treatment. *Rheumatology* (2006); 45(6):724-9.

[32] Jennette JC, Falk RJ, Andrassy K, Bacon PA, Churg J, Gross WL, Hagen EC, Hoffman GS, Hunder GG, Kallemberg CG. Nomenclature of systemic vasculitides. Proposal of an internacional consensus conference. Arthritis Rheum 1994; 37:187-92.

[33] Leavitt, RY, Fauci, AS, Bloch, DA, et al. The American College of Rheumatology 1990 criteria for the classification of Wegener´s granulomatosis. *Arthritis Rheum* 1990; 33:1101-7.

[34] Jayne D for the European Vasculitis Study Group (EUVAS). Update on the European Vasculitidis Study Group trials. Curr Opin Rheumatol 2001; 13:541-9.

[35] Mukhtyar C, Guillevin L, Cid MC, et al. EULAR recommendations for the management of primary small and medium vessel vasculitis. *Ann Rheum Dis.* March 2009; 68:310-317.

[36] Stone J, Hoffman G, Merkel P, et al. A disease-specific activity index for Wegener´s Granulomatosis: modification of the BVAS. Arthritis & Rheumatism 2001; 44:912-920.

[37] De Groot K, Rasmussen N, Bacon P, et al. Randomised trial of cyclophosphamide versus methotrexate for induction of remission in early systemic antineutrophil cytoplasmic antibody associated vasculitis. Arthritis Rheum 2005; 52:2462-8.

[38] C. Lapraik, R. Watts, P. Bacon, et al. BSR and BHPR guidelines for the management of adults with ANCA associated vasculitis. Rheumatology 2007; 46:1-11.

[39] DeGroot K, Harper L, Jayne DRW, et al. Pulse versus daily oral cyclophosphamide for induction of remission in antineutrophil cytoplasmic antibody-associated vasculitis: a randomized trial. Ann Intern Med. May 2009; 150:670-680.

[40] Jayne D, Rasmussen N, Andrassy K, Bacon P, et al. A randomized trial of maintenance therapy for vasculitis associated with antineutrophil cytoplasmic antibodies. *NEJM* July 2003; 349:36-44.

[41] Pagnoux C, Mahr A, Hamidou MA, et al. Azathioprine or methotrexate maintenance for ANCA-associated vasculitis. N Engl J Med. December 2008; 359:2790-2803.

[42] Metzler C, Miehle N, Manger K, et al. Elevated relapse rate under oral methotrexate versus leflunomide for maintenance of remissionin Wegener´s granulomatosis. Rheumatology (Oxford). July 2007; 46 (7):1087-1091.

[43] Stone JH, Merkel PA, Spiera R, et al. Rituximab versus cyclophosphamide for ANCA-associated vasculitis. N Engl J Med. Jul 15 2010; 363 (3):221-32.

[44] Jones, RB, Tervaert, JW, Hauser, T, et al. Rituximab versus cyclophosphamide in ANCA-associated renal vasculitis. N Engl J Med 2010; 363:211.

[45] Wegener´s Granulomatosis Etanercept Trial (WGET) Research Group (2005) *N Engl J Med* 352:351-361.

[46] Walsh M, Chaudhry A, Jayne D. Long-term-follow-up of relapsing/refractory anti-neutrophil cytoplasm antibody associated vasculitis treated with the lymphocyte depleting antibody alemtuzumab (CAMPATH-1H). *Ann Rheum Dis.* September 2008; 67 (9):1322-1327.

[47] Walsh M, Merkel PA, Mahr A, et al. Effects of duration of glucocorticoid therapy on relapse rate in antineutrophil cytoplasmic antibody-associated vasculitis: A meta-analyses. Arthritis Care Res (Hoboken). Aug 2010; 62 (8):1166-73.

[48] Phillip R, Lugman R. Mortality in systemic vasculitis: a systematic review. *Clin Exp Rheumatol*. September-October 2008; 26:S94-S104.

12

The Etiology, Mechanisms, and Treatment of Churg-Strauss Syndrome

Tsurikisawa N., Saito H., Oshikata C., Tsuburai T. and Akiyama K.
Clinical Research Center for Allergy and Rheumatology, National Hospital Organization Sagamihara National Hospital, Japan

1. Introduction

Churg–Strauss syndrome (CSS) is a rare disease characterized by allergic granulomatosis and necrotizing vasculitis following peripheral blood eosinophilia and eosinophilic tissue infiltration (Churg & Strauss, 1951). CSS is classified as a vasculitis of small and medium-sized arteries (Jennette & Falk, 1995), although the vasculitis is not often apparent in the initial phases of the disease. It occurs mainly in adults, almost always in patients with a history of bronchial asthma, and is associated with chronic rhinosinusitis. The most frequently affected organs are the lungs and the ear, nose, and throat (ENT) system, followed by the skin. Involvement of the cardiac and gastrointestinal tract systems determines the prognosis. Nonspecific immunosuppressive therapy with corticosteroids (CSs), cyclophosphamide (CYC) and other drugs produces good responses initially in most patients, but relapses are frequent, especially in the early disease phase, and morbidity and mortality remain important problems. Our research has explored the etiology of CSS by use of HLA analysis and has shown that the clinical and immunological manifestations of asthma occur in the pre-vasculitic phase of the disease. Our work further indicates that treatment, especially in the form of intravenous immunoglobulin (IVIG), is beneficial.

2. Clinical manifestations, mechanisms, and treatment

2.1 Etiology and genetic factors

The precise etiologies of CSS and the role played by genetic factors remain unknown. In some CSS patients, vasculitis is apparent within a few weeks or months of exposure to putative triggers, such as rapid discontinuation of oral corticosteroids, vaccination, desensitization, viral infection, or medication with leukotriene receptor antagonists. Although there are some reports of genetic factors, such as the IL10.2 haplotype (Vaglio et al., 2007) and HLA (human leukocyte antigen)-DPB1 (Wieczorek et al., 2008), influencing susceptibility to CSS, to date there is no compelling evidence supporting the involvement of such factors. Familial cases of systemic vasculitis associated with p-ANCA (p-antineutrophil cytoplasmic antibody)-positive vasculitis or Wegener's granulomatosis (WG) have been reported, but there have been no reports of familial CSS, excluding cases of familial vasculitis with CSS and WG in two first-degree relatives. We presented the first case of familial CSS in two sisters with atopic-type bronchial asthma and negativity for p-ANCA

(Tsurikisawa et al., 2007). The two sisters had seven siblings, for a total of four females and five males. Eight were still alive, but both parents were dead. The parents had no known history of atopy, and of the siblings only another sister, the oldest, also had bronchial asthma and atopy. We analyzed human leukocyte antigen (HLA)-A, HLA-B, HLA-DRB1, HLA-DQA1, HLA-DQB1, and HLA-DPB1 in the two CSS sisters and their six living siblings (Table 1). All four sisters, including the two CSS sisters, had HLA-A02, HLA-B48, DRB1-15, DQA1-01, DQB1-06, and DPB1-20; all four brothers had HLA-A20, HLA-B39, DRB1-04, DQA1-03, DQB1-03, and DPB1-04. Testing revealed no significant differences in the frequencies of any of the HLAs (P = 0.102–0.67). Our results and accumulated clinical evidence indicate that CSS is not a heritable disease.

	HLA-A		HLA-B		DRB1		DQA1		DQB1		DPB1	
Patient 1	02	24	48	52	15	15	01	01	06	06	20	09
Patient 2	02	02	48	40	15	09	01	03	06	03	20	05
Sister 1	02	24	48	52	15	15	01	01	06	06	20	09
Sister 2	02	02	48	40	15	90	01	03	06	30	20	05
Brother 1	20	24	39	52	15	04	01	03	06	03	05	09
Brother 2	20	24	39	52	15	04	01	03	06	03	05	09
Brother 3	20	02	39	40	90	04	03	03	30	03	05	05
Brother 4	20	24	39	52	15	04	01	03	06	03	05	09

Table 1. HLA typing of two CSS patients and their siblings.

2.2 Clinical manifestation of vasculitis

CSS is a rare disorder characterized by an incidence of 0.11 to 2.66 new cases per million population per year and an overall prevalence of 10.7 to 14 per 1,000,000 adults (Gatenby, 2009; Mahr, 2004; Mohammad 2007). The male-to-female ratio ranges from 0.3 to 2.3 and the mean age at onset reported in the literature varies from 38 to 52 years (range 7–74 years) (Kahn 2008; Sinico & Bottero, 2009). Nonetheless, there is a generally agreed-upon clinical description of the disease. The frequencies of organ involvement and other clinical features of CSS previously reported by others and observed at our hospital are summarized in Table 2. CSS has been traditionally induced in ANCA-associated vasculitis, WG, and microscopic polyangiitis (MPA). The prevalence of ANCAs in CSS is less consistent than in WG or MPA, being reported in approximately 40% of cases (Guillevin et al., 1999; Kahn et al., 2008; Pagnoux & Guillevin, 2010; Sinico & Bottero, 2009). Recently, it was shown that different clinical phenotypes could be observed according to the presence or absence of ANCA, thereby suggesting that there are varying disease mechanisms in the pathogenesis of CSS. Increased prevalence of central nervous system involvement (Keogh & Speck, 2003), renal involvement, peripheral neuropathy, and pulmonary hemorrhage (Sinco et al., 2005) has been reported among ANCA-positive patients. Negative ANCA status is associated with heart disease and lung involvement (Sinco et al., 2005). From these findings, it has been hypothesized that, as in WG and MPA, ANCAs may contribute directly to the endothelial vasculitic damage seen in ANCA-positive patients, whereas in ANCA-negative patients eosinophils may be directly responsible for the release of cationic proteins and eosinophil-derived neurotoxin (Kallenberg, 2005). These data suggest that CSS, when presenting as a form of necrotizing small-vessel vasculitis, is a true ANCA-associated disease, characterized by positivity for myeloperoxidase (MPO)-ANCAs. Alternatively, ANCA-negative patients may be clinically characterized by tissue infiltration by eosinophils that results in fibrotic organ damage; their disease may belong more to the spectrum of hypereosinophilic syndromes rather than to the spectrum of ANCA vasculitis. The existence of two clinical phenotypes may reveal different pathways of pathogenicity in CSS.

	Churg	Chumbley	Lanham	Hashimoto	Guillevin	Our cases
	USA	USA	UK	Japan	France	Japan
	1951	1977	1984	1994	1999	2011
Cases	13	30	138	87	96	86
M/F	4/9	21/9	72/66	41/46	45/51	27/59
Age mean	33	47	38	47	48	53.4
Age range	(7-62)	(15-69)		(17-79)	(17-74)	(19-83)
Clinical manifestations(%)						
Asthma	100	100	100	93	100	100
Pulmonary infiltrates	39	27	74	33	38	80
Nose, ear, throat	77	70	69		48	91
Multiplex mononeuritis	69	63	64	65	78	99
Gastrointestinal	92	17	62	19	33	85
Heart	54	16	52	33	30	74
Arthritis	31	20	46	52	41	42
Myalgias			33	51	54	25
Skin		66	51			
Purpura	62		46	44	31	67
Nodules	54	27	33	27	19	6
Renal	31	20	46	46	16	58
Central nervous system	61		27		8	18

Table 2. Clinical manifestation of vasculitis

2.3 Mechanisms and clinical manifestations of the pre-vasculitic phase of CSS as an asthmatic phase

Asthma is present in 96% to 100% of CSS patients and is the cardinal feature of CSS. Asthma may precede systemic vasculitis by approximately 8 years and, in some cases, by more than 30 years (Chumbley et al., 1977; Churg & Strauss, 1951; Guillevin et al., 1999; Lhote & Guillevin, 1995). The precise etiology of CSS and the asthmatic phase that precedes it, as well as the role of genetic factors, remains unknown. We demonstrated in a retrospective cohort study that the clinical manifestations of asthma occur in the pre-vasculitic phase of the disease (Tsurikisawa et al., 2007). The asthma of 87.5% of 24 patients in the pre-vasculitic phase of CSS at their first hospital visit was severe. It was characterized in 42.9% of these patients by a need for treatment with systemic steroids and mechanical ventilation and by the presence of sinusitis in 57.1% during the period from the first hospital visit to the onset of CSS (*P* < 0.0001) (Table 3).

Characteristic	Non-CSS severe asthma N = 130 (44.2%)	Severe asthma pre-CSS N = 21 (87.5%)	*P*-value
Systemic corticosteroid treatment	N = 9 (6.9%)	N = 9 (42.9%)	<0.0001
Corticosteroid dose (in mg, converted to the prednisolone equivalent)	5.3±2.0	7.2±3.6	N.S
Inhaled corticosteroid dose (in µg, converted to the beclomethasone equivalent)	1194.7±575.1	1371.4±721.9	N.S
Intubation	N = 2 (1.5%)	N = 3 (14.3%)	0.0018
Sinusitis	N = 40 (30.8%)	N = 12 (57.1%)	<0.0001

Table 3. Differences between non-CSS (Churg-Strauss syndrome) severe asthma and severe asthma in the pre-vasculitic phase of CSS.

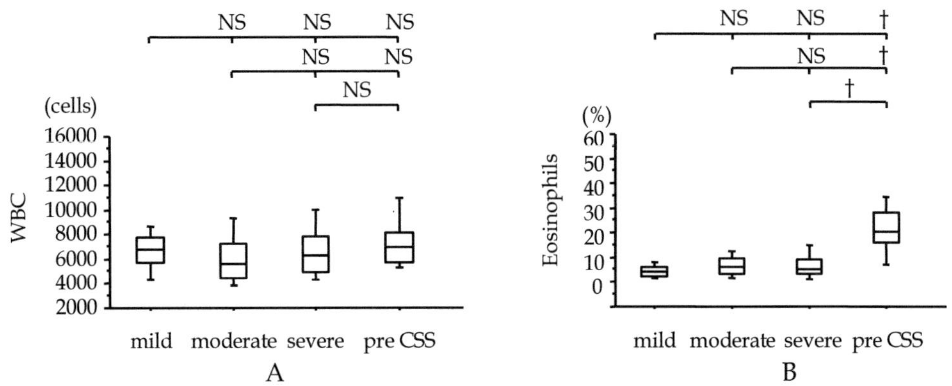

Fig. 1. Total numbers of white blood cells (WBC) (A)s and percentages of eosinophils (B) in the peripheral blood of all patients at the first hospital visit. The percentage of eosinophils in the peripheral blood of pre-CSS asthma patients was significantly higher than that in other asthma patients. † $P < 0.01$. NS: not significant.

The percentage of eosinophils in the peripheral blood of pre-CSS asthmatics at the first hospital visit was also significantly higher than that in non-CSS asthmatics (P < 0.01) (Fig. 1).Receiver operating characteristic (ROC) analysis was used to evaluate the diagnostic value of the percentage of eosinophils in the peripheral blood for predicting future onset of CSS. The area under the curve was 0.8992 (95% CI = 0.825–0.973). A reasonably high specificity (99.4%) and a high sensitivity (66.7%), with a cut-off point of 20%, were obtained (Fig. 2).

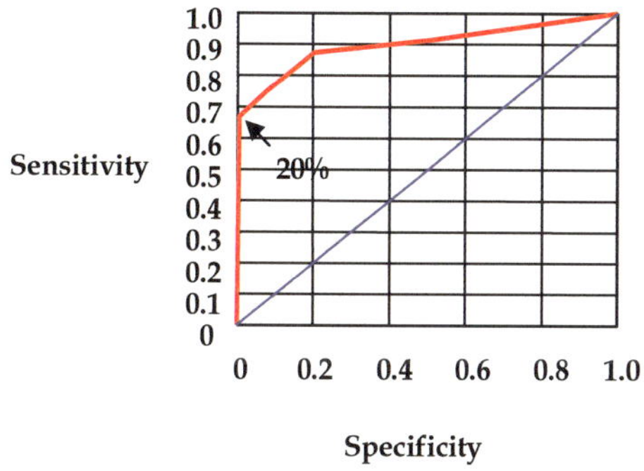

Fig. 2. ROC curve for evaluating the value of the percentage of eosinophils in the peripheral blood as a predictor of future onset of CSS

The percentage forced expiratory volume (%FEV1) in the severe asthmatics and the asthmatic patients who later developed CSS was lower than that in patients with mild or moderate asthma (p < 0.01). The %FEV1 in the asthmatic patients who later developed CSS was the same as that in patients with severe asthma (Fig. 3). However, bronchial hyperresponsiveness (BHR) to acetylcholine (ACh) in the pre-vasculitic patients was significantly less severe than that in the non-CSS patients with severe asthma (P < 0.01) and was as mild as that in patients with mild asthma (Fig. 4). Thus, asthma severity in the pre-vasculitic phase of CSS is related to airflow limitation and to eosinophilic inflammation in the peripheral blood, but not to BHR, which may occur as a result of airway vasculitis. We propose that asthma patients who develop CSS differ from other asthma patients, from whom they can be differentiated at the first hospital visit by evaluating these factors.

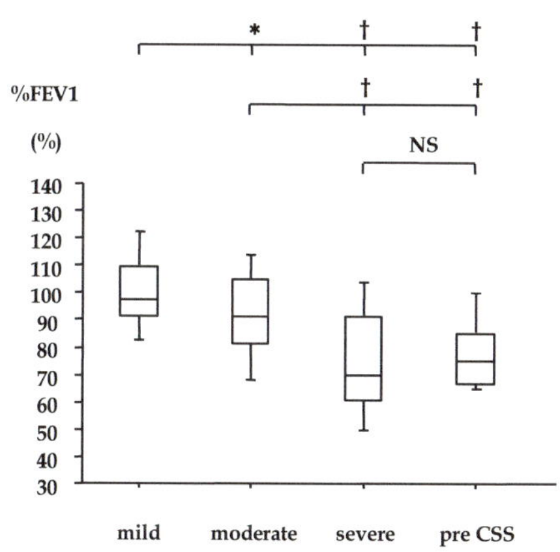

Fig. 3. FEV1 (% predicted) at the first hospital visit in all patients.

The %FEV1 was measured at the first hospital visit in asthmatic patients (mild, moderate, severe) and in those who later developed CSS. The %FEV1 in the severe asthmatics and the asthmatic patients who later developed CSS was lower than in patients with mild asthma ($P < 0.01$). However, the %FEV1 in the asthmatic patients who later developed CSS was the same as that in patients with severe asthma.† $P < 0.01$. * $P < 0.05$. NS: not significant.

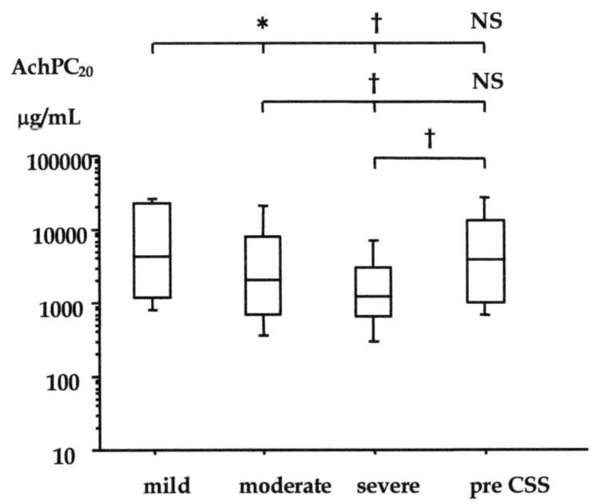

Fig. 4. Bronchial hyperresponsiveness (BHR) to inhaled Ach in all patients within 1 month of the first hospital visit.

Modified box plots represent the distribution of BHR to inhaled Ach in asthmatic patients (mild, moderate, severe) and pre-CSS asthma patients within 1 month of the first hospital visit. † Mann-Whitney Test, $P < 0.01$. NS: not significant.

Eosinophilic infiltrations, such as those found in chronic eosinophilic pneumonia (CEP) and eosinophilic gastroenteritis, precede systemic vasculitis in half of all patients with CSS (Lhote & Guillevin, 1995; Steinfeld et al., 1994). Some clinicians suggest that patients with CEP following asthma are more likely to develop CSS if the CEP is left untreated (Churg, 2001). However, some patients in whom asthma is complicated by CEP do not develop CSS. There is no clear mechanism that explains why some CEP patients with asthma develop CSS, whereas others do not. The etiology of idiopathic CEP is not understood, although in some cases CEP is caused by infection with a parasite, virus, or fungus or by drugs, toxic agents, or radiation therapy (Cottin & Cordier, 2005; Marchand & Cordier, 2006). Asthma occurs before CEP in about half to two-thirds of CEP patients (Cottin & Cordier, 2005; Marchand & Cordier 2006). Increasing numbers of eosinophils and lymphocytes in the peripheral blood and bronchoalveolar lavage fluid (BALF) contribute to the development of CEP. There are many mediators of eosinophilia in CEP, including regulated upon activation normal T-cell-expressed and -secreted (RANTES), eotaxin, thymus- and activation-regulated chemokine (TARC/CCL17), and cytokines, including IL-2, IL-3, IL-5, IL-10, IL-13, and IL-18. The number of $CD4^+CD25^+$ T cells in the BALF and peripheral blood is increased in patients with CEP (Albera, 1995). By contrast, peripheral blood mononuclear cells in patients with CSS secrete not only the type 1 cytokine IFN-γ, but also type 2 cytokines, such as IL-4, IL-13, and, in particular, IL-5.

T-regulatory (T_{reg}) cells play essential roles in maintaining immunologic homeostasis, preventing autoimmunity, and providing peripheral tolerance to antigens, including autoantigens and allergens. T_{reg} cells, including Tr1 (T-regulatory cells type 1), $CD4^+CD25^+$, Th3, and natural killer (NK) T cells, all suppress effector T cells of either the Th1 or Th2 phenotype, which are involved in mediating inflammation (Jonuleit et al., 2002; Sakaguchi, 2000; Weiner, 2001). $CD4^+CD25^+$ cells are naturally occurring T-regulatory (nT_{reg}) cells that are defined as $CD25^{hi}$ $CD127^{low}$ $FOXP3^+$ (Roncarolo & Battaglia, 2007). nT_{reg} cells mediate their suppressive effects through cell contact. Tr1 cells are antigen-specific populations derived from conventional $CD4^+CD25^-$ naïve precursors following exposure to antigen under conditions of limiting costimulation, such as with IL-10, immature dendritic cells, or dexamethasone. The mechanism by which Tr1 cells exert suppression appears to be mediated by secretion of suppressor cytokines, such as IL-10 and TGF-β. Recent studies have focused on the role of T_{reg} cells in human diseases such as systemic lupus erythematosus, rheumatoid arthritis, cancer, Guillain–Barré syndrome, multiple sclerosis, infection, and asthma. However, whether T_{reg} cell activity is involved in the mechanism and etiology of CSS is not known. We examined the phenotypes and functions of $CD4^+CD25^+$ T cells from asthma patients with CEP and from CSS patients at disease onset and after therapy, and we compared our findings with those in patients with general asthma. We found that, at disease onset, CSS patients, unlike CEP patients, had significantly fewer $CD4^+CD25^+$ T cells than patients with any type of asthma (steps 1–4) (Saito et al., 2008;

	Normal controls (n = 9)	Bronchial asthma				CSS at onset	CEP at onset
		Step 1	Step 2	Step 3	Step 4		
Blood eosinophils (no. of cells)	161.9± 65.0	209.4± 168.3	290.6± 209.8	357.3± 215.5	380.0± 517.0	8042.6± 6559.3†&††	3762.6± 2310.3†
$CD4^+CD25^+$ (%)	31.4± 8.2‡	52.2± 12.2	52.6± 11.8	46.2± 6.6	42.7± 10.3*	34.9± 15.6†&††	48.1± 11.6
IL-5 in $CD4^+CD25^+$ (%)	0.0± 0.0	4.4± 6.6	5.2± 10.1	6.2± 10.8	4.1± 7.4	14.6± 11.9†††	11.2± 12.5††††
IL-10 in $CD4^+CD25^+$ (%)	0.0± 0.0	4.7± 7.5	4.9± 6.3	1.1± 2.2	2.7± 4.4	0.3± 1.0**	20.9± 17.0†&††
IL-10 in $CD4^+CD25^-$ (%)	0.5± 1.2	0.5± 1.5	0.4± 0.6	0.2± 0.5	0.3± 0.5	0.1± 0.1	6.6± 11.4†&††
TGF-β in $CD4^+CD25^+$ (%)	0.0± 0.0‡‡	6.7± 10.0	4.4± 6.9	2.8± 5.0	2.6± 5.9	1.0± 0.9‡‡‡	6.7± 10.5††
IL-2 in $CD4^+CD25^-$ (%)	26.3± 25.8	35.1± 17.9	32.4± 22.3	23.1± 21.2	17.0± 16.5***	7.6± 7.2‡‡‡	22.0± 17.0††

Table 4. Eosinophil counts and cytokines in $CD25^+$ or $CD25^-$ $CD4^+$ T cells in normal controls, patients with asthma (as classified by the US National Institutes of Health and National Asthma Education and Prevention Program), patients with chronic eosinophilic pneumonia (CEP), and patients with Churg-Strauss syndrome (CSS)

† CSS or CEP vs. control and Step 1 and Step 2 and Step 3 and Step 4: $P < 0.01$; †† CSS vs. CEP: $P < 0.01$; ††† CSS vs. control and Step 1 and Step 2 and Step 4: $P < 0.01$, vs. Step 3: $P < 0.05$; †††† CEP vs. control: $P < 0.01$, vs. Step 1 and Step 2 and Step 4: $P < 0.05$; * Step 4 vs. Step 1 and Step 2: $P < 0.01$; **: CSS vs. Step 1 and Step 2: $P < 0.05$;

*** Step 4 vs. Step 1: $P < 0.01$, vs. Step 2: $P < 0.05$; ‡ control vs. Step 1 and Step 2 and Step 3 and CEP: $P < 0.01$, vs. Step 4: $P < 0.05$; ‡‡ control vs. Step 1 and Step 2 and Step 3 and Step 4 and CEP: $P < 0.01$; ‡‡‡ CSS vs. Step 1 and Step 2: $P < 0.01$

Tsurikisawa et al., 2008)(Table 4). $CD4^+CD25^+$ T cells producing IL-10 were rarely detected in CSS patients at disease onset or relapse, whereas the numbers of IL-10–producing T cells in CEP patients were high at disease onset. Fewer $CD4^+CD25^-$ T cells producing IL-2 were found in CSS patients before treatment than were found in CEP patients at disease onset ($P < 0.01$) (Table 4). The proportions of $CD4^+CD25^+$ T cells producing IL-10 and of $CD4^+CD25^-$ T cells producing IL-2 in CSS patients significantly increased at remission after treatment ($P < 0.01$) (Fig 5). We confirmed that maintenance of the numbers of T_{reg} cells in asthma patients with CEP may inhibit CSS development via the action of cytokines, such as IL-10 and IL-2, produced by $CD4^+CD25^+$ and $CD4^+CD25^-$ T cells, respectively.
In contrast, the $CD4^+CD25^+$ T cell count in patients with CEP at onset was the same as that in asthmatics at every step of asthma (Table 4) and did not change even with improvement of the disease (Fig. 5). The $CD4^+CD25^+$ T cell count in patients with CSS significantly increased with either relapse or remission after treatment, and this increase was significantly greater in patients in remission than in those who relapsed ($P < 0.01$) (Fig. 5). Moreover, when we compared the intracellular cytokine levels of IL-10 and TGF-β with the serum levels of IL-10 (all patients assayed: <2.0 pg/mL) and TGF-β (all patients assayed: <8.0 pg/mL) , we found that the serum IL-10 levels were extremely low in all patients with asthma, CSS, and CEP. There was not significant the serum IL-10 level among three groups. It is not clear why there were no significant differences among the serum levels of these cytokines yet there were significant differences among the intracellular levels.

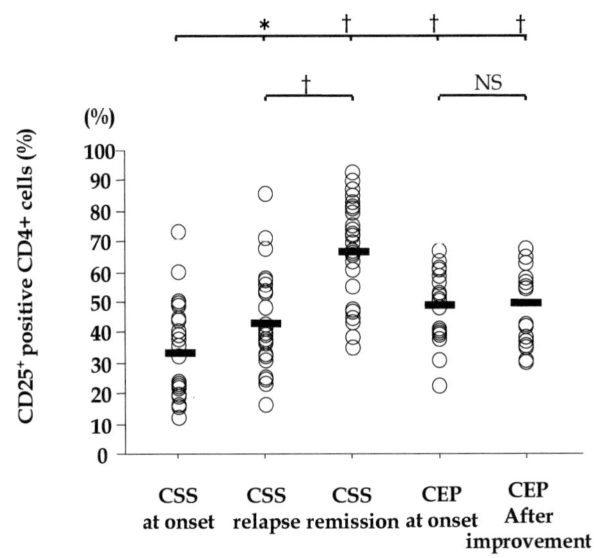

Fig. 5. Percentages of $CD4^+$ among $CD25^+$ T cells in patients with CSS and CEP at disease onset and after treatment. Median values are shown by horizontal bars. Differences between patient groups were evaluated by using the Mann–Whitney U test. † $P < 0.01$. * $P < 0.05$. NS: not significant.

The number of $CD4^+CD25^+$ T cells producing IL-5, which causes eosinophilia in peripheral blood cells and lung tissue, was high in CSS and CEP patients at disease onset and decreased significantly after treatment of CSS and improvement of CEP (Fig. 6a).

$CD4^+CD25^+$ T cells producing IL-10 were rarely detected in patients with CSS at onset or in those who relapsed. However, when patients with CSS achieved clinical remission after treatment, the number of $CD4^+CD25^+$ T cells producing IL-10 significantly increased compared with the number at onset. The number of $CD4^+CD25^+$ T cells producing IL-10 in patients with CEP was high at disease onset and decreased significantly after improvement of eosinophilic pneumonia (Fig. 6(b)). The number of $CD4^+CD25^-$ T cells producing IL-2 in patients with CSS at onset was significantly less than that in patients with CEP at onset.

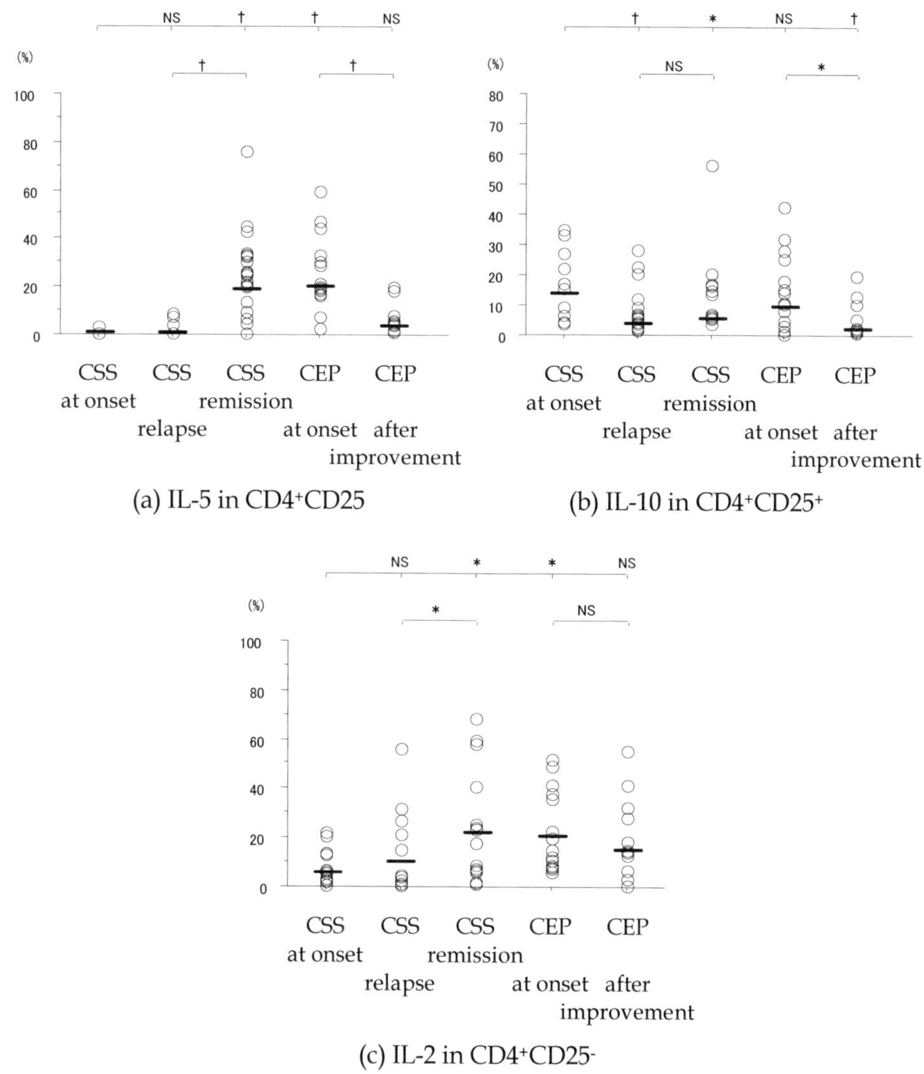

Fig. 6. (a) Percentages of $CD4^+CD25^+$ T cells producing IL-5; (b) $CD4^+CD25^+$ T cells producing IL-10; and (c) $CD4^+CD25^-$ T cells producing IL-2 in patients with CSS or CEP at disease onset and after treatment. Median values are shown by horizontal bars. Differences between patient groups were evaluated by using the Mann–Whitney U test. † $P < 0.01$. * $P < 0.05$. NS: not significant.

After treatment, CSS patients who achieved remission showed a significant increase in the number of $CD4^{+}CD25^{-}$ T cells producing IL-2, to the level seen in CEP patients at disease onset, but there was no change in the count of $CD4^{+}CD25^{-}$ T cells producing IL-2 in patients with CEP between disease onset and improvement (Fig. 6c). The number of organs involved was significantly negatively correlated with the percentage of $CD4^{+}CD25^{+}$ T cells at onset, remission, and relapse in CSS patients ($r = -0.51$, $P < 0.01$, Fig. 7). The percentage of $CD25^{+}$ $CD4^{+}$ T cells was correlated with IL-10 production in all patients with stable asthma and in those with CSS or CEP at onset ($R = 0.42$, $P < 0.01$; data not shown). These results show that the $CD4^{+}CD25^{+}$ T cells producing IL-10 were Tr1 cells.

Dysregulated production of IL-17 is associated with human autoimmune diseases, including multiple sclerosis, inflammatory bowel disease, and psoriasis. $CD4^{+}$ T cells that produce IL-17 represent a distinct lineage (Th17) that produces neither IL-4 nor IFN-γ. Recently, a relationship between T_{reg} cells and Th17 in the pathogenesis of some human autoimmune diseases was reported (Lock C et al 2002, Fujino et al 2003, Vaknin-Dembinsky A et al 2006, Zheng et al 2007).

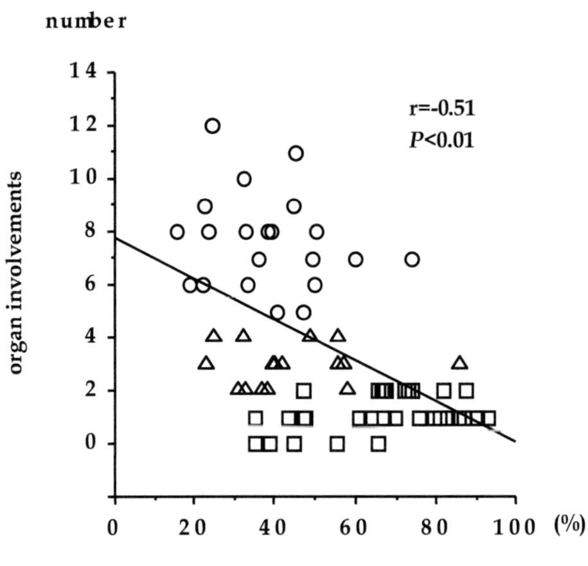

Fig. 7. Correlation between percentage of $CD25^{+}$ $CD4^{+}$ T cells and the degree of organ involvement. "Organ involvement" included asthma, sinusitis, pulmonary infiltration, mononeuritis multiplex or polyneuropathy, arthritis, tympanitis, lymphadenitis, mastitis, or involvement of the myocardium, gastrointestinal tract, kidney, skin, central nervous system, eye, gallbladder, or liver. Open circles represent patients with CSS at onset, open triangles represent patients with CSS who relapsed after an initial remission, and open squares represent patients with CSS in remission after treatment. A significant linear relationship is evident ($r = -0.51$, $P < 0.01$) for all patient groups.

We confirmed that the percentage of CD4+ T cells producing IL-17 was significantly greater in patients with active CSS than in healthy control patients or in patients with asthma, BA + CEP, or inactive CSS (Fig. 8) (Saito et al., 2009). Moreover, the percentage of CD4+ T cells

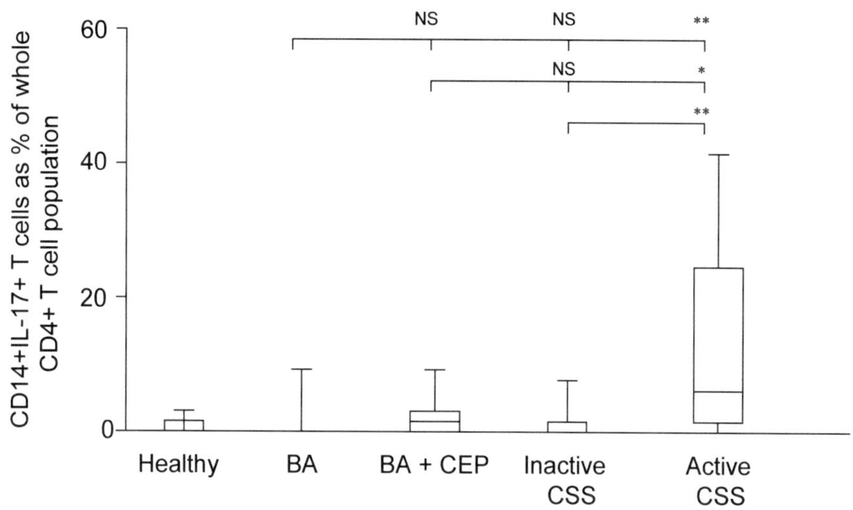

Fig. 8. Increased ability of $CD4^+$ T cells from active CSS patients to produce IL-17.

producing IL-17 in active CSS who were at onset or at relapse was significantly greater than those in inactive CSS and the percentage of CD4+CD25+ T cells producing IL-10 (Tr1 cells) in active CSS significantly decreased than those in inactive CSS who achieved remission after treatment (Tr 1) (Fig. 9) (Saito et al., 2009). Th17 cells were identified as CD4+ T cells that produced mainly IL-17 and IL-22. Eosinophilia is a characteristic of CSS, and some reports suggest that the IL-25 produced by eosinophils promotes innate adaptive immunity by enhancing Th2 cytokine production (Terrier et al., 2010). We showed that the number of CD4+ T cells producing IL-17 or IL-22 in the peripheral blood of CSS patients increased at

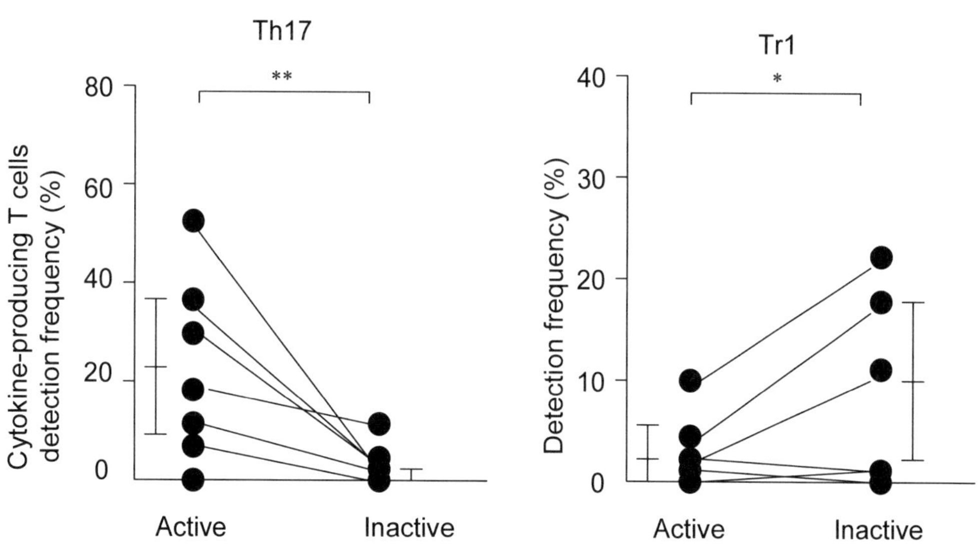

Fig. 9. Th17 or Tr1 cells representing $CD4^+CD25^+$ T cells that produce IL-17 or IL-10 in relation to disease activity in CSS patients. ** $P < 0.01$, * $P < 0.05$.

relapse and that the numbers of these CD4+ T cells were correlated with the number of CD4+ T cells producing IL-25 (Fig.10) (Saito et al., 2011). Indoleamine 2, 3-dioxygenase (IDO) expression in monocytes from all CSS patients was positively correlated with the percentage of CD4+CD25+ Treg cells producing IL-10 and inversely correlated with the percentage of Th17 cells (Fig. 11) (Saito et al., 2011). Thus CSS relapse may be linked to elevated levels of CD4+ T cells producing IL-25, which promote Th2 inflammation and reduce Tr1 cell subpopulations, which also result from lower IDO expression in monocytes. Thus, the percentages of CD4+CD25+ Treg cells producing IL-10 and of Th17 cells reflect the disease activity of CSS (Fig. 11).

Mononuclear leukocytes derived from patients from each group were stimulated with PMA and ionomycin in the presence of 10 μg/mL of brefeldin A to generate and accumulate IL-17. Statistical significance was tested using the Mann-Whitney U test. * * P < 0.01, * P < 0.05, NS: not significant.

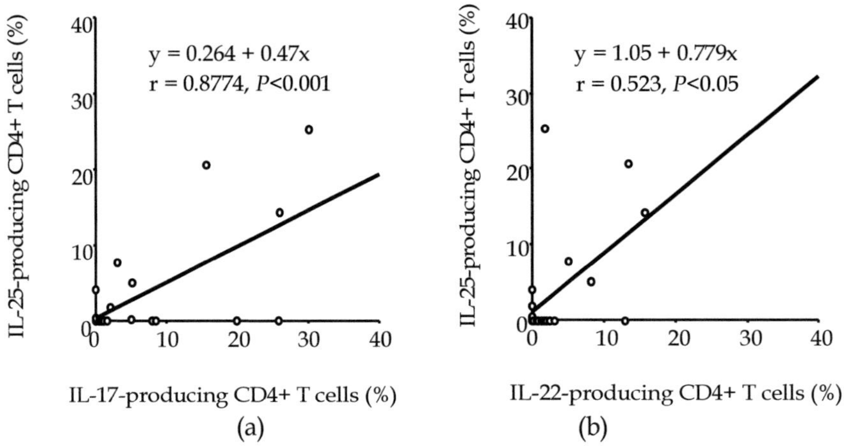

Fig. 10. Correlation between IL-25 and Th17 cell generation.

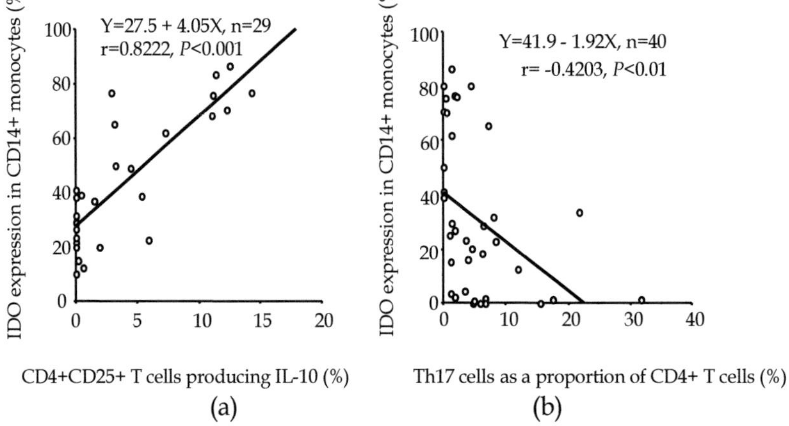

Fig. 11. Monocyte IDO expression and CD4+CD25+ T cells that producing IL-10 and Th17 cell detection.

We found a positive correlation between the percentage of $CD4^+$ T cells producing IL-25 and the percentage of $CD4^+$ T cells producing IL-17 (a) or IL-22 (Fig. 9b) in relapsed CSS patients. The increase in IL-25 may be linked to increased Th17 cell generation.
IDO expression in monocytes from all CSS patients was positively correlated with the detection frequency of $CD4^+CD25^+$ T cells that producing IL-10and inversely correlated with the detection frequency of Th17 cells.

2.4 Treatment

The mainstay of treatment for CSS is systemic CS therapy. Additional treatments with immunosuppressive agents, such as CYC or azathioprine, may be used in some patients. Other treatment options include methotrexate, mycophenolate mofetil, rituximab, interferon-alpha, anti-IgE therapy, anti-IL-5 antibodies, anti-TNF-alpha (infliximab, etanercept, adalimumab), plasma exchange, and intravenous immunoglobulin (IVIG). Corticosteroids and immunosuppressants, especially CYC, have improved considerably most symptoms of vasculitis, particularly those involving the gastrointestinal system, skin, and lungs, as well as constitutional symptoms. However mononeuritis multiplex and heart failure in patients with CSS or ANCA-associated systemic vasculitis do not respond to combination therapy with CS and CYC (Abril et al., 2003; Hattori et al., 1999; Renaldini et al., 1993; Sehgal et al., 1995). IVIG therapy has been used to treat various diseases, including MPA, WG, and ANCA-associated systemic vasculitis (Jayne et al., 1991; Lockwood, 1996; Richter et al., 1995). Hamilos and Christensen were the first to report that eosinophilia in CSS is improved by treatment with IVIG (Hamilos & Christensen, 1991), and other investigators have since described successful treatment with IVIG of CSS itself (Armentia et al., 1993; Levy et al., 1999). We previously reported (Tsurikisawa et al., 2004) that IVIG therapy improved mononeuritis multiplex or heart failure in 14 of 15 patients with CSS who did not respond to combination therapy with CS and CYC. IVIG (400 mg) was given daily for 5 days. Neuropathy was evaluated by assessing manual muscle strength and skin temperature at affected sites. Cardiac function was evaluated by using ejection fraction assessment with echocardiography and two imaging tests of the myocardium (^{123}I-meta-iodobenzylguanidine (MIBG) and ^{201}Tl). Peripheral eosinophil counts and CD69 expression on the surfaces of eosinophils were also examined. We found that manual muscle strength improved and the skin temperature of both hands and legs significantly increased on IVIG therapy (Fig. 12). In the five patients with heart failure, the ejection fraction of the left ventricle significantly increased from 35.2% to 61.0% (Fig. 13). Myocardial uptake of ^{123}MIBG significantly increased, indicating improved myocardial viability (Fig. 14). ^{201}Tl images showed a perfusion defect and, following IVIG therapy, improved blood perfusion. IVIG therapy did not, however, affect the peripheral blood eosinophil count, but it did downregulate the expression of CD69 (Fig. 15). This finding suggests that, in CSS, activated eosinophils survive even after CS or CYC treatment, and that IVIG therapy decreases the number of activated eosinophils that express early activation markers such as CD69. The progression of CSS may, therefore, be related more to the abundance of CD69-expressing eosinophils than to the total number of eosinophils. Thus, one mechanism by which IVIG therapy acts on CSS may be the inactivation of eosinophils. IVIG therapy may induce remission by ameliorating neuropathy and heart failure in those patients who are unresponsive to treatment with CSs or CYC.

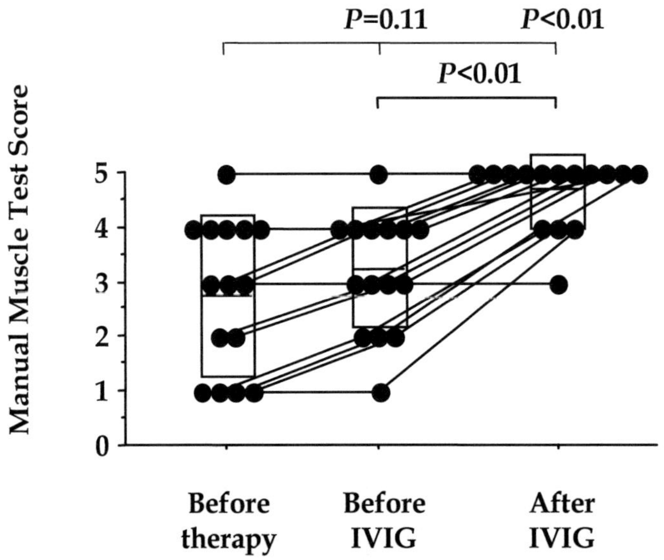

Fig. 12. Manual muscle test. "Before therapy" indicates before treatment with corticosteroid or cyclophosphamide or both; before IVIG and after IVIG indicate before and after high-dose intravenous immunoglobulin therapy, respectively.

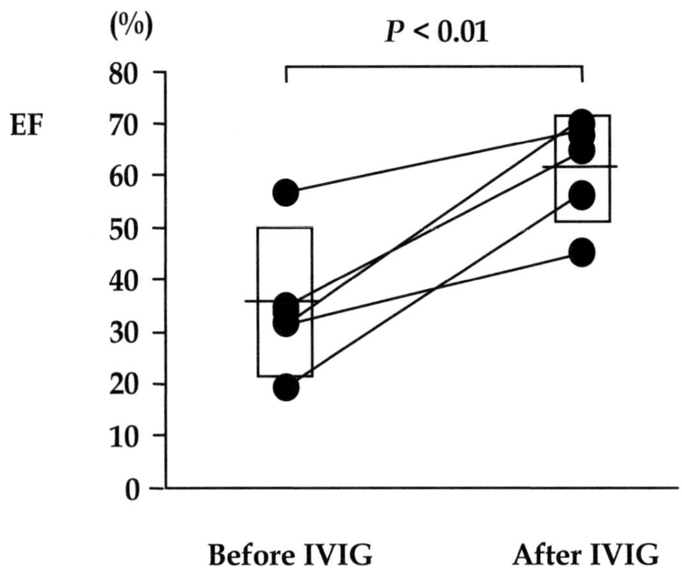

Fig. 13. Ejection fraction as measured by using echocardiography. EF, ejection fraction

Image analysis of MIBG was performed on the regions over the whole left ventricular myocardium and the upper mediastinal area. The heart to mediastinum (H/M) ratio was then determined from the cardiac ^{123}I-MIBG images. The washout rate of MIBG within the myocardium was measured as a percent change in the left ventricular activity from early to delayed images within the left ventricular regions.

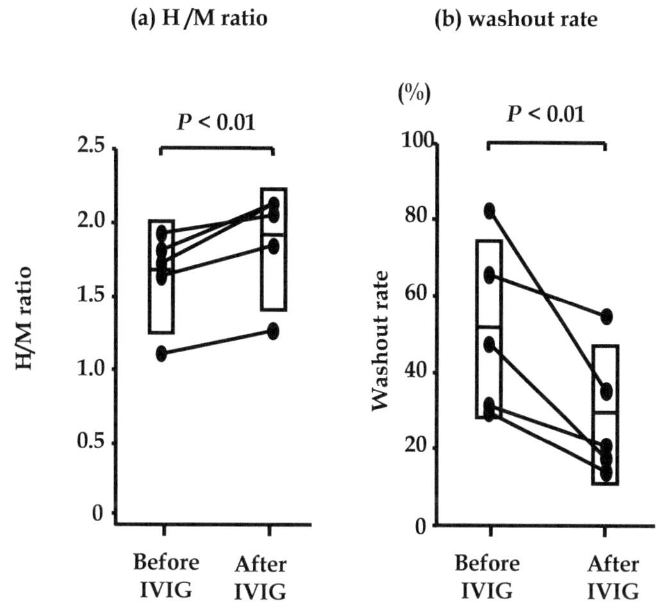

Fig. 14. The heart to mediastinum (H/M) ratio (A) and washout rate (B) of ^{123}I-MIBG in patients with heart failure.

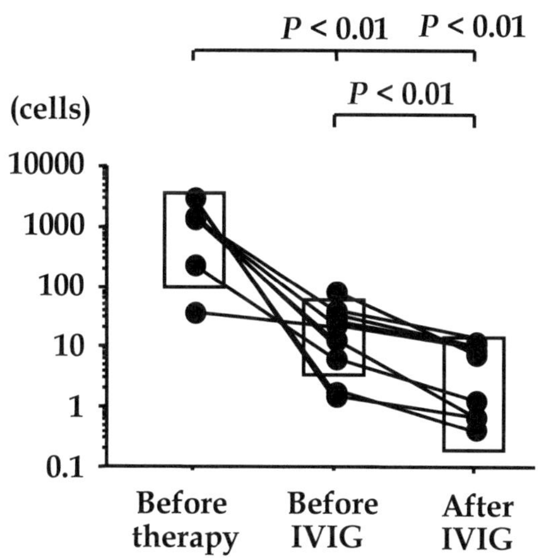

Fig. 15. Effect of intravenous immunoglobulin (IVIG) on CD69$^+$ eosinophil production.

However, administration of IVIG alone, without concomitant treatment with CSs and CYC as an initial treatment approach for CSS, did not improve vasculitic symptoms in various organs, including the digestive tract, skin and pulmonary infiltration. Furthermore, it had no effect on peripheral nerve damage, cardiac dysfunction, the number of eosinophils (including CD69$^+$CCR3$^+$-activated eosinophils), or the proportion of eosinophils with vacuole formation in white blood cells. This suggests that CS administration reduces eosinophil counts but does not reduce the percentage of activated eosinophils, and that IVIG administered with CSs may exhibit an adjuvant effect. IVIG should, therefore, not be used in place of conventional therapy with CSs or immunosuppressants such as CYC, except when patients are resistant to CS and CYC therapy (Guillevin & Pagnoux, 2003).

After treatment with CSs, immunosuppressants, or IVIG therapy, paralysis—presenting as multiple mononeuropathy—often remains. We consider rehabilitation for multiple mononeuropathy just as important as the therapeutic management of these patients. We found that application of transdermal isosorbide dinitrate (ISDN) patches to the toes of the affected leg or hand produced warming and improved numbness (Fig. 16) (Tsurikisawa et al., 2003). Application of ISDN patches to the affected leg or hand also increased the skin temperature, not only on the affected side but also on the contralateral site. The mechanism involves an increase in blood flow, via local and systemic vasodilating effects, in the region where the ISDN patches are applied; this reduces hyperalgesia and blocks neurogenic inflammation, leading to improved nerve conduction by increasing neuronal postsynaptic cyclic GNP levels.

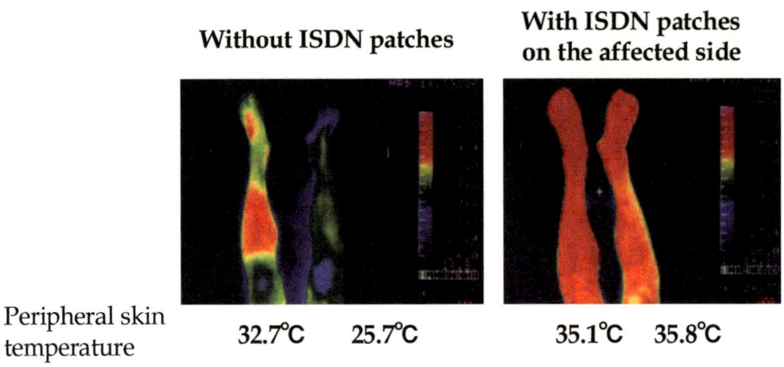

Fig. 16. Skin temperature after application of ISDN patches to an affected leg. The skin temperature increased not only in the affected leg, but also on the contralateral side.

2.5 Prognosis

Before the use of CSs, the mortality rate of CSS was approximately 50% within 3 months of diagnosis (Gayraud et al., 2001; Guillevin et al., 1999). Other reports suggest a 5-year survival rate for CSS of 62% to 80% (Chumbley et al., 1977; Gayraud et al., 2001; Guillevin et al., 1996; Lane et al., 2005). Most deaths result from complications of the vasculitic phase of the disease and are due to cardiac failure or myocardial infarction, cerebral hemorrhage, renal failure, gastrointestinal bleeding, or status asthmaticus. The presence or absence of the features that make up the five-factor score (FFS) [cardiac involvement, gastrointestinal disease (bleeding, perforation, infarction or pancreatitis), renal insufficiency (creatinine concentration >1.6 mg/dl; proteinuria >1 g/day), and central nervous system involvement] has been used to predict survival in CSS (Gayraud et al., 2001; Guillevin et al., 1996). Of the five elements of the FFS, cardiac involvement and gastrointestinal disease appear to be the strongest indicators of poor prognosis (Guillevin et al., 1999). According to published reports, the remission rate in CSS ranges from 81% to 91% and the relapse rate ranges from 20% to 60% (Mukhtyar et al., 2008; Pavone et al., 2006. Gastrointestinal involvement, ANCA persistent positivity, and a rise in ANCA titer are also risk factors for relapse. We reported that cardiac sympathetic nerve function was damaged in CSS patients with cardiac involvement and that ^{123}I-MIBG scintigraphy was useful for detecting cardiac involvement and predicting cardiac events (Horiguchi et al., 2011). ^{123}I-MIBG scintigraphy was performed in 28 patients with CSS, 12 of whom had cardiac involvement, and the early and delayed heart to mediastinum ratio (early H/M and delayed H/M) and washout rate were calculated. We found that early H/M and delayed H/M were significantly lower, and the washout rate was significantly higher, in patients with cardiac involvement than in control patients and those without cardiac involvement (early H/M, $P = 0.0024$, $P = 0.0001$; delayed H/M, $P = 0.0002$, $P = 0.0001$; washout rate, $P = 0.0012$, $P = 0.0052$; vs. those without cardiac involvement and vs. control patients, respectively). Accuracy in detecting cardiac involvement was 86% for delayed H/M and the washout rate and 79% for early H/M and B-type natriuretic peptide (BNP). Kaplan-Meier analysis showed significantly lower cardiac-event-free rates in patients with early H/M ≤2.18 and BNP >21.8 pg/mL than in patients with early H/M >2.18 and BNP ≤21.8 pg/mL (log rank test $P = 0.006$).

3. Conclusion

A prognosis of CSS suggests a 5-year survival rate in the range of 62% to 80%, which is far from ideal. CSS involves multilateral systemic vasculitis that shares many clinical characteristics with other ANCA-associated vasculitides, potentially causing a necrotizing process that can involve any organ or system. The clinical features of CSS reflect the pathogenic role of peripheral blood and tissue hypereosinophilia, which can directly contribute to damage of primary organs. These two aspects of the disease complicate diagnosis and the initiation of pharmacologic treatment. The mainstay of treatment for CSS is CSs or CYC or both; however, patients with CSS who experience mononeuritis multiplex or heart failure do not respond to combination therapy with CSs and CYC. We recommended IVIG therapy, in addition to conventional therapy, for CSS patients with severe neuropathy or heart failure who fail to respond to combination therapy with CSs and CYC. IVIG treatment not only decreases the number of activated eosinophils expressing $CD69^{+}CCR3^{+}$ but also could reduce the amount of CS needed for maintenance of remission in CSS (Danieli et al. 2004). Increased availability of novel therapies for CSS, together with a better understanding of the pathogenesis of the disease, should improve the long-term management of this condition.

4. Acknowledgment

We thank Drs. Hiroyuki Mitomi, Miyako Ishiyama, Ayako Horita, and Ikuo Saito for their suggestions in the discussion of the pathology of CSS; Drs. Yoriko Horiguchi, Akihiko Ishibashi, Yukiko Morita, and Hideo Himeno for their suggestions in the discussion of cardiac involvement; Dr. Shunsuke Suzuki for his suggestions in the discussion of clinical manifestation; and Dr. Akemi Saito for performing the assays on the serum samples.

5. References

Churg, J. & Strauss, L. (1951). Allergic granulomatosis, allergic angiitis, and periarteritis nodosa. *American Journal of Pathology*, vol. 27, 277-301

Jennette, J.C. & Falk R.J. (1995) Clinical and pathological classification of ANCA associated vasculitis: what are the controversies? *Clinical Experimental Immunology*, vol. 101: 18–22

Vaglio, A., Martorana D., Maggiore, U., Grasselli, C., Zanetti, A., Pesci, A., Garini, G., Manganelli, P., Bottero, P., Tumiati, B., Sinco, R.A., Savi, M., Buzio, C., & Neri, T.M. (2007) HLA-DRB4 as a genetic risk factor for Churg-Strauss Syndrome. *Arthritis & Rheumatism* vol. 56, 3159–66

Wieczorek S, Hellmich B, Arning L, Moosig F, Lamprecht P, Gross WL & Epplen JT. (2008) Functionally relevant variations of the interleukin-10 gene associated with antineutrophil cytoplasmic antibody-negative Churg-Strauss Syndrome, but not with Wegener's granulomatosis. Arthritis Rheum 58: 1839-48

Tsurikisawa N, Morita S, Tsuburai T, Oshikata C, Ono E, Saito H, Yanagihara Y & Akiyama K. (2007) Familial Churg-Strauss Syndrome in Two Sisters.Chest 131:592-4

Gatenby PA, Lucas RM, Engelsen O, Ponsonby AL & Clements M. (2009) Antineutrophil cytoplasmic antibody-associated vasculitis: could geographic pattern be explained by ambient ultraviolet radiation? Arthritis Rheum 61: 1417-24

Mohammad AJ, Jacobsson LT, Mahr AD Sturfelt G & Segelmark M. (2007) Prevalence of Wegener's granulomatosis, microscopic polyangiitis, polyarteritis nodosa and Churg-Strauss Syndrome within a defined population in southern Sweden. Rheumatology (Oxford) 46: 1329-37

Mahr A, Guillevin L, Poissonnet M & Ayme S. (2004) Prevalence of polyarteritis nodosa, microscopic polyangiitis, Wegener's granulomatosis, and Churg-Strauss Syndrome in a French urban multiethnic population in 2000: a capture-recapture estimate. Arthritis Rheum 51: 92-9

Sinico RA & Bottero P. (2009) Churg-Strauss angiitis. Best Pract Res Clin Rheumatol 23: 355-66

Kahn JE, Bletry O & Guillevin L. (2008) Hypereosinophilic syndromes. Best Pract Res Clin Rheumatol 22: 863-82

Lanham J, Elkon K, Pusey C, Hughes G. (1984) Systemic vasculitis with asthma and eosinophilia: A clinical approach to the Churg-Strauss syndrome. Medicine 63: 65-81

Mukhtyar C, Flossmann O, Hellmich B, Bacon P, Cid M, Cohen-Tervaert JW, Gross WL, Guillevin L, Jayne D, Mahr A, Merkel PA, Raspe H, Scott D, Witter J, Yazici H & Luqmani RA. (2008) European Vasculitis Study Group (EUVAS). Outcomes from studies of antineutrophil cytoplasm antibody associated vasculitis: a systemic review by the European League Against Rheumatism systemic vasculitis task force. Ann Rheum Dis 67: 1004-10

Guillevin L & Pagnoux C. (2003) When should immunosuppressants be prescribed to treat systemic vasculitides? Internal Med 42: 313–317

Pagnoux C & Guillevin L. (2010) Churg-Strauss Syndrome: evidence for disease subtypes? Curr Opin Rheumatol 22:429-43

Keogh KA & Specks U. (2003) Churg-Strauss Syndrome: clinical presentation, antineutrophil cytoplasmic antibodies, and leukotriene receptor antagonists. Am J Med 115: 632-8

Kallenberg CG. (2005) Churg-Strauss Syndrome: just one disease entity? Arthritis Rheum 52: 2589-93

Guillevin L, Cohen P, Gayraud M, Lhote F, Jarrousse B & Casassus P. (1999) Churg-Strauss syndrome. Clinical study and long-term follow-up of 96 patients. Medicine. 78: 26-37

Chumbley LC, Harrison EG & DeRemee RA. (1977) Allergic granulomatosis and angiitis (Churg-Strauss syndrome). Mayo Clin Proc 52: 477-84

Tsurikisawa N, Tsuburai T, Saito H, Morita S, Horiguchi Y, Mitomi H & Akiyama K. (2007) A retrospective study of bronchial hyperresponsiveness in asthmatic patients prior to the onset of Churg-Strauss Syndrome. Allergy Asthma Proc 28:336-43

Steinfeld S, Golstein M & De Vuyst P. (1994) Chronic eosinophilic pneumonia (CEP) as a presenting feature of Churg-Strauss syndrome (CSS). Eur Respir J 7: 2098

Lhote F & Guillevin L. (1995) Polyarteritis nodosa, microscopic polyangiitis, and Churg-Strauss syndrome. Clinical aspects and treatment. Rheum Dis Clin North Am 21:911-47

Marchand E & Cordier JF. (2006) Idiopathic chronic eosinophilic pneumonia. Semin Respir Crit Care Med 27:134–41.

Cottin V & Cordier JF. (2005) Eosinophilic pneumonias. Allergy 60:841–57

Albera C, Ghio P, Solidoro P, Mabritto I, Marchetti L & Pozzi E. (1995) Activated and memory alveolar T-lymphocytes in idiopathic eosinophilic pneumonia. Eur Respir J 8:1281–5

Sakaguchi S. (2000) Regulatory T cells: key controllers of immunologic self-tolerance. Cell 101:455–8.

Jonuleit H, Schmitt E, Kakirman H, Stassen M, Knop J & Enk AH. (2002) Infectious tolerance: human CD25(+) regulatory T cells convey suppressor activity to conventional CD4(+) T helper cells. J Exp Med 196:255–60.

Weiner HL. (2001) Induction and mechanism of action of transforming growth factor-beta-secreting Th3 regulatory cells. Immunol Rev 182:207–14.

Roncarolo MG & Battaglia M. (2007) Regulatory T-cell immunotherapy for tolerance to self antigens and alloantigens in humans. Nat Rev Immunol 7:585–98.

Tsurikisawa N, Saito H, Tsuburai T, Oshikata C, Ono E, Mitomi H & Akiyama K. (2008) Differences in regulatory T cells between Churg-Strauss syndrome and chronic eosinophilic pneumonia with asthma. J Allergy Clin Immunol 122:610-6

Saito H, Tsurikisawa N, Tsuburai T & Akiyama K. (2008) Involvement of regulatory T cells in the pathogenesis of Churg-Strauss syndrome. Int Arch Allergy Immunol 146: 73-6

Lock C, Hermans G, Pedotti R, Brendolan A, Schadt E, Garren H, Langer-Gould A, Strober S, Cannella B, Allard J, Klonowski P, Austin A, Lad N, Kaminski N, Galli SJ, Oksenberg JR, Raine CS, Heller R, Steinman L. (2002) Gene-microarray analysis of multiple sclerosis lesions yields new targets validated in autoimmune encephalomyelitis. Nat Med 8: 500-508

Fujino S, Andoh A, Bamba S, Ogawa A, Hata K, Araki Y, Bamba T, Fujiyama Y. (2003) Increased expression of interleukin 17 in inflammatory bowel disease. Gut Jan;52(1):65-70.

Vaknin-Dembinsky A, Balashov K, Weiner HL. (2006) IL-23 is increased in dendritic cells in multiple sclerosis and down-regulation of IL-23 by antisense oligos increases dendritic cell IL-10 production. J Immunol Jun 15;176(12):7768-74.

Zheng Y, Valdez PA, Danilenko DM, Hu Y, Sa SM, Gong Q, Abbas AR, Modrusan Z, Ghilardi N, de Sauvage FJ, Ouyang W. (2008) Interleukin-22 mediates early host defense against attaching and effacing bacterial pathogens.Nat Med. Mar;14(3):282-9.

Saito H, Tsurikisawa N, Tsuburai T, Oshikata C & Akiyama K. (2009) Cytokine production profile of CD4+ T cells from patients with active Churg-Strauss syndrome tends toward Th17. Int Arch Allergy Immunol. 149 Suppl 1:61-5.

Terrier B, Bièche I, Maisonobe T, Laurendeau I, Rosenzwajg M, Kahn JE, Diemert MC, Musset L, Vidaud M, Sène D, Costedoat-Chalumeau N, Le Thi-Huong D, Amoura Z, Klatzmann D, Cacoub P, Saadoun D. (2010) Interleukin-25: a cytokine linking eosinophils and adaptive immunity in Churg-Strauss syndrome. Blood. Nov 25;116(22):4523-31.

Saito H, Tsurikisawa N, Tsuburai T, Oshikata C & Akiyama K. (2011) The proportion of regulatory T cells in the peripheral blood reflects the relapse or remission status of patients with Churg-Strauss syndrome. Int Arch Allergy Immunol 155 Suppl; 46-52

Abril A, Calamia KT & Cohen MD. (2003) The Churg Strauss syndrome (allergic granulomatous angiitis): review and update. Semin Arthritis Rheum 33: 106-14

Hattori N, Ichimura M, Nagamatsu M, Li M, Yamamoto K, Kumazawa K, Mitsuma T & Sobue G. (1999) Clinicopathological features of Churg-Strauss syndrome-associated neuropathy. Brain 122, 427-39

Sehgal M, Swanson JW, DeRemee RA & Colby TV. (1995) Neurological manifestations of Churg-Strauss syndrome. Mayo Clin Proc. 70: 337-341

Renaldini E, Spandrio S, Cerudelli A, Affatato A & Balestrieri GP. (1993) Cardiac involvement in Churg-Strauss syndrome: a follow-up of three cases. Eur Heart J. 14: 1712-1716

Hamilos D.L & Christensen J. (1991) Treatment of Churg-Strauss syndrome with high-dose intravenous immunoglobulin. J. Allergy Clin Immunol. 88: 823-4

Tsurikisawa N, Taniguchi M, Saito H, Himeno H, Ishibashi A, Suzuki S & Akiyama K. (2004) Treatment of Churg-Strauss syndrome with high-dose intravenous immunoglobulin. Annals Allergy Asthma Immunol, 92: 80-7

Tsurikisawa N, Taniguchi M, Suzuki S & Akiyama K. (2003) Effects of a nitro compound patch on neuropathy in Churg-Strauss syndrome. Allergy 58:686-7

Gayraud M, Guillevin L, Toumelin P, Cohen P, Lhote F, Casassus P & Jarrousse B. (2001) Long-term followup of polyarteritis nodosa, microscopic polyangiitis, and Churg-Strauss syndrome. Arthritis Rheumatism. 44: 666-75

Guillevin L, Lhote F, Gayraud M, Cohen P, Jarrousse B, Lortholary O, Thibult N & Casassus P. (1996) Prognostic factors in polyarteritis nodosa and Churg-Strauss syndrome: a prospective study in 342 patients. Medicine (Baltimore) 75: 17-28

Lane SE, Watts RA, Shepstone L & Scott DGI. (2005) Primary systemic vasculitis: clinical features and mortality. Q J Med 98:97-111

Pavone L, Grasselli C, Chierici E, Maggiore U, Garini G, Ronda N, Manganelli P, Pesci A, Rioda WT, Tumiati B, Pavesi G, Vaglio A & Buzio C. (2006) Outcome and prognostic factors during the course of primary small-vessel vasculitides. J. Rheumatology 33: 1299-306

Horiguchi Y, Morita Y, Tsurikisawa N & Akiyama K. (2011) 123I-MIBG imaging detects cardiac involvement and predicts cardiac events in Churg-Strauss syndrome. Eur J Nucl Med Mol Imaging 38: 221-9

Sinco RA, Di Toma L, Maggiore U, Bottero P, Radice A, Tosoni C, Gregorini G, Monti S, Frassi M, Vecchio F, Corace C, Venegoni E & Buzio C. (2005) Prevalence and clinical significance of antineutrophil cytoplasmic antibodies in Churg-Strauss syndrome. Arthritis Rheum 52: 2926-35

Danieli MG, Cappelli M, Malcangi G, Logullo F, Salvi A, Danieli G. (2004) Long term effectiveness of intravenous immunoglobulin in Churg-Strauss syndrome. *Ann Rheum Dis* 63: 1649-54

13

Churg-Strauss Syndrome: Clinical and Immunological Features

Khrystyna Lishchuk-Yakymovych, Valentyna Chopyak and Roman Pukalyak
Danylo Halytskyy Lviv National Medical University
Ukraine

1. Introduction

The vasculitides include a broad spectrum of disorders that span a clinical spectrum from benign, self-limited disease to fulminant conditions that are fatal in the absence of therapy. Whereas the large-vessel vasculitides consist of 2 principal disorders, giant cell arteritis and Takayasu arteritis, the medium- and small-vessel vasculitides are much more diverse, including multiple diseases that can affect nearly every organ system (Seo & Stone, 2007). This article is the second of a 2-part series that focuses on the challenges faced by clinicians who care for patients with vasculitis. The first article in this series discussed the large-vessel vasculitides. The problem of systemic autoimmune diseases such as systemic vasculitis with vascular lesions of medium and small vessels, including: Wegener granulomatosis, Churg-Strauss syndrome, microscopic poliangiitis, nodose poliarteriitis, attracts every year more attention of doctors, due to the worldwide relentless increase of patients with these diseases (Lhote & Guillevin, 2009; Tsukadaira, 2009). Recently, several reports have suggested that vasculitis is becoming more common.

Systemic vasculitis is a group of heterogeneous diseases (syndromes), characterized by inflammation and damage to blood vessels and which compromises or destroys the vessel wall leading to haemorrhagic and / or ischaemic events, giving impetus to the development of a wide spectrum of symptoms and signs. The forms of vasculitis may be varied: primary [idiopathic, e.g. cutaneous leukocytoclastic angiitis, Wegener's granulomatosis, Churg–Strauss syndrome and microscopic polyangiitis] and secondary [a manifestation of connective tissue disease, infection, adverse drug eruption, or a paraneoplastic phenomenon], local and generalized, transient, recurrent and chronic; included group of diseases in which vasculitis is a primary characteristic. They are general in nature, though sometimes a local clinic can manifest symptoms. General damage of blood vessels may occasionally appear and disappear, but in most cases there are long-term. Each new escalation leads to the increase of clinical symptoms. Clinical implications of SV course depend on a number of factors, including etiology, location, size and number of blood vessels, the extent and severity of disease, its activity and nature of treatment.

Systemic vasculitis as the existing disease was first described by A. Cussmaul and I. Maier, when they reported a case of necrotizing arteritis and called it nodose periarteriitis. There are over twenty different forms of Systemic vasculitis. One of the first classification was their classification by P. Zeek's, which included five categories of Systemic vasculitis: nodose periarteriitis, hypersensitivity angiitis, allergic granulomatous angiitis, rheumatic angiitis, temporal arteritis. It was based on pathological data and damage and on their sizes. On the basis of etiologic and pathogenetic, clinical and pathomorphological criteria has been done many classifications of SV. But they are all flawed, because there are several factors that may affect the objectivity of classification opinions. They include: location and technology collection of fabrics, including various vascular pools, the possibility of angiography, variability in cellular composition depending on the morphogram stage, previous treatment options etc.

Primary systemic vasculitis has an incidence of more than 100 new cases per million. Currently, the most widely adopted vasculitis classification system is that of Chapel Hill Consensus Conference (CHCC), which is based on pathological criteria. The other widely used system is that of the American College of Rheumatology (ACR), which is based predominately on clinical findings.

The etiology of the systemic vasculitis is largely unknown, although they are widely believed to be autoimmune in origin, triggered by different environmental events. Epidemiologic studies have indicated factors, including silica exposure, infection, seasonal variation in occurrence, drugs, ultraviolet radiation and vitamin D, latitudinal gradient and etc.

Pathogenic mechanisms remain uncertain. In the modern literature widely discusses the pathogenic role in the development of systemic vasculitis of neutrophils, eosinophils, antineutrophil cytoplasmic antibodies, circulating immune complexes, lymphocytes, cytokines, total IgE and etc.

In general, systemic symptoms accompany all cutaneous vasculitic syndromes, and these symptoms include fever, malaise, weight loss, arthritis and/or arthralgias. In the majority of patients, vasculitic lesions will affect the lower extremities, mostly at dependent sites or underlying tight-fitting clothes. Upper extremity, trunk and head and neck involvement are infrequent and often signal the presence of more severe disease or coexisting systemic vasculitis. The subtlety and diversity of symptoms in the initial phase of vasculitis can be a real diagnostic problem, and thus early recognition of a vasculitic condition relies on the experience of a team of dedicated professionals from several different subspecialties, including laboratory medicine. The initial assessment will be to make a diagnosis, categorize disease severity and formulate a management plan. A structured approach, based on careful disease staging and evaluation, is the cornerstone of good disease management. Initial evaluation includes a comprehensive clinical assessment, serological tests, radiology and histology. The first step in the patients management is clinical history and examination, the second one of the initial investigations include full blood count, inflammatory markers [C-reactive protein (CRP) and erythrocyte sedimentation rate (ESR)], renal function such as epidermal growth factor receptor (eGFR) and serology to include antiglomerular basement membrane antibodies. Inflammatory markers provide a non-specific tool for assessing inflammatory activity and monitoring treatment. Urinalysis detects proteinuria and haematuria.

Specific diadnostic is based on detection of specific markers: characteristic autoantibodies are formed towards enzymes and bactericidal proteins within the cytoplasmic granules of neutrophils and monocytes in a substantial proportion of patients with systemic vasculitis manifesting as Wegener's granulomatosis, microscopic polyangiitis and Churg-Strauss syndrome, as well as in patients with limited forms of these conditions. Histological examination of biopsy material is useful in confirming a diagnosis in the context of clinical findings and laboratory data. Also, skin biopsy is the gold standard for the diagnosis of vasculitis type. For subsequent evaluations, it is effective and practical to measure clinical disease status for most patients with small and medium vessel vasculitis. Therapy is based on the pattern of vasculitis and on careful evaluation of the extent and activity of disease. The treatment of vasculitis comprises induction of remission followed by maintenance. Remission should be induced rapidly, balancing potential target organ damage against drug toxicity. Maintenance with immunosuppression should limit the amount of corticosteroid use and prevent relapse. Concomitant medication is used to treat or prevent adverse events from immunosuppressive treatment.

2. Connection between systemic vasculitis, bronchial asthma, eosinophilic syndrome and churg-strauss syndrome

The unreleased question of eiosinophilic background in patients with systemic vasculitis and its influence on the disease activity, is very actual today. The most important eosinophilic-associated systemic vasculitis between all vascular processes is Churg-Strauss syndrome, that occur with eosinophilia asdiagnostic criterion due to ACR,1990. Since its first description as allergic granulomatous angiitis in 1951 (Churg and Strauss, 1951), and subsequently its affiliation with the small-sized vessel systemic necrotizing vasculitides and, more specifically, the so-called subgroup of antineutrophil cytoplasmic antibody (ANCA)-associated vasculitides in the early 1990s, knowledge about the pathophysiological mechanisms of Churg-Strauss syndrome has greatly improved. Its natural clinical history and progression are better understood, but the syndrome's potential subsets are not yet totally elucidated. Major advances have also been made in the therapeutic management of affected patients, but much remains to be done because sustained off-treatment remissions are quite rare and patients often require a long-term low-dose corticosteroid therapy (Cohen et al., 2007; Ribi et al., 2008). International studies and workshops on vasculitis classification, immunology, genetics, and treatments are ongoing or planned. Here, we review the current known aspects of Churg-Strauss syndrome (Pagnoux, 2010). Churg-Strauss syndrome is a rare disease, with an annual incidence ranging between 0.5 and 6.8 per million inhabitants and a prevalence of 10.7-14 per million inhabitants (Pagnoux et al., 2007; Watts et al., 2005), with a mean age at onset around 50 years and no sex preponderance. No strong evidence of a differential geographical distribution pattern has been reported so far, nor a blatant change in its frequency over the past decades. However, some studies reported a slightly higher prevalence in northern, as opposed to southern, Europe, and in urban, as compared to rural, regions.

Several exogenous triggering factors for disease onset or flares have been identified or, more cautiously, suspected in some European or North American studies. They include vaccinations, desensitizations, and drugs, such as macrolides, carbamazepine, quinine, and also anti-asthma agents, like leukotriene-receptor antagonists and, more recently, omalizumab, a recombinant monoclonal anti-immunoglobulin E (IgE) antibody (Bibby et al., 2010; Pagnoux et al., 2007). These latter two often provide the opportunity for substantial tapering or withdrawal of corticosteroids in asthmatic patients, thereby unmasking an underlying 'forme fruste' of Churg-Strauss syndrome, which had so far been controlled by corticosteroids, but a direct triggering role of these agents cannot be excluded (Bibby et al., 2010). Whether or not "common" asthma represents a risk factor for Churg-Strauss syndrome *per se* has not been clearly determined, because both conditions share some underlying mechanisms. The earliest studies reported a higher annual incidence of Churg-

Strauss syndrome in asthmatic patients treated with non-leukotriene-modifying asthma drugs (64.4 per million asthmatics) or a leukotriene-receptor antagonist (about 60 per million asthmatics). A more recent study reported a somewhat lower Churg-Strauss syndrome incidence of 34.6 per million asthmatics per year (Harrold et al., 2005), which remains higher than in the general population; but other reported incidences varied from 0 to 67 according to disease definition. Whereas asthma often clusters in families, familial cases of Churg-Strauss syndrome are exceptional, diminishing the gene and environmental factor impact on the latter. However, results of several genetic studies suggested some predisposing hereditary factors, like the HLA-DRB1*04 and HLA-DRB1*07 alleles and the HLA-DRB4 gene, which are more frequent in Churg-Strauss syndrome patients than healthy controls, the interleukin IL10.2 haplotype, which is associated with enhanced IL-10 expression, and possibly the CD226 Gly307Ser polymorphism (Wieczorek et al., 2010).

Its most typical presentation consists of the appearance, in a patient with late-onset asthma, of vasculitic manifestations, like fever, cutaneous purpura and mononeuritis multiplex. In such a setting, the combination of blood eosinophilia and inflammatory syndrome is highly suggestive of the diagnosis, which can be further supported by the detection of antineutrophil cytoplasmic antibodies (ANCA), especially P-ANCA (perinuclear-ANCA) with anti-myeloperoxidase specificity and the presence of eosinophilic granulomas and/or necrotizing vasculitis in an affected-tissue biopsy. Asthma is the most common sign of Churg-Strauss syndrome, but Churg-Strauss syndrome can cause a variety of problems, ranging from hay fever, rash and gastrointestinal bleeding, to severe pain and numbness in your hands and feet. The wide range of symptoms — and their similarity to symptoms of other disorders — make Churg-Strauss syndrome challenging to diagnose. Biological phenotypes of interest for assessing severity of Churg-Strauss syndrome may be IgE level, ANCA, cytokines (IL-2, 4, 5, 10) and eosinophilia. Phenotypes other than usual Churg-Strauss syndrome need to be considered. Phenotypic heterogeneity may help to disentangle etiologic heterogeneity. Churg-Strauss syndrome, its verification and activity could be mediated by different pathogenetic mechanisms and realized mediators, such as ANCA, eosinophils, cytokines, total IgE etc. Severity of eosinophilia in patients with Churg-Strauss syndrome represents a clinical subphenotype of interest, and studying severe eosinophilia (extreme phenotype) may increase the power to detect linkage. It would be useful to define Churg-Strauss syndrome phenotypes unencumbered by the activity of disease, which may depend heavily on nongenetic factors, and free of gene-trigger interactions. Besides the activity, environmental factors and inadequate treatment can modify the severity of the Churg-Strauss syndrome phenotype. Consideration of treatment as a marker of severity implies that the relevant phenotype for etiological research is masked by the treatment.

Intermediate Phenotypes

Intermediate phenotypes are important with respect to pleiotropy and etiological heterogeneity. Bronchial hyperresponsiveness, total IgE, eosinophilia, ANCA-presence and vacular involvement are usually considered intermediate phenotypes for Churg-Strauss syndrome.

Refinement of Phenotypes

Considering environmental factors and potential interactions with genetic factors may increase our ability to detect genetic factors in multifactorial diseases such as Churg-Strauss syndrome.

There is increasing evidence that the associations of ANCAs, total IgE, and eosinophilia with environmental and clinical factors are different in patients with Churg-Strauss syndrome and different eosinophilia severity.

The most typical clinical presentation of Churg-Strauss syndrome is the appearance of vasculitic manifestations in a patient with known allergic rhinitis, nasal and sinus polyposis, and late-onset asthma (almost constant, and usually preexisting for 5-10 years). General symptoms (i.e., fever or weight loss), mononeuritis multiplex, and/or necrotic cutaneous purpura are the most frequent manifestations at disease onset, in combination with elevated blood eosinophilia and inflammatory syndrome. The detection of ANCA, especially P-ANCA (with perinuclear labeling pattern in indirect immunofluorescence) with anti-myeloperoxidase (antiMPO) specificity (in enzyme-linked immunosorbent assay), strongly supports the diagnosis, but they are present in only 35-40% of the patients (Sablé-Fourtassou et al., 2005; Sinico &Bottero, 2009). While Lanham et al. (1984) commendably described in the 1980s that Churg-Strauss disease most typically emerges through 3 successive phases (prodromic phase, with asthma and allergic manifestations; then, eosinophil infiltration into tissues, especially lung and/or myocardium; and eventually, systemic and vasculitic phase), not all patients experience this clear-cut stepwise progression and many have overlapping manifestations from these different phases.

In addition to almost constant asthma and airflow obstruction, lung manifestations include patchy and transient alveolar (eosinophilic) infiltrates and/or pleurisy, and, rarely, lung non-excavated nodules or alveolar hemorrhage. Allergic rhinitis, sinusitis, and/or nasal polyposis can be observed in 60-80% of the patients. Notably, Churg-Strauss syndrome patients must be evaluated for heart involvement, because it carries a poor prognosis, has therapeutic implications, and can be paucisymptomatic. In the earliest studies, heart involvement was reportedly occurring in up to 50-60% of the patients (Pagnoux, 2010) and represented the major cause of mortality, accounting for 48% of patient deaths (Pagnoux, 2010). In more recent reports, outcomes were better. For instance, Neumann et al. (2009) reported that there were "only" two deaths from severe endomyocarditis among the 22 patients with cardiac involvement, with recovery of nearly normal cardiac function in almost all of the survivors.

However, the reported cardiac manifestations and their frequencies are strongly dependent on which cardiac investigations were done. Cardiac magnetic resonance imaging might reveal clinically silent and echographically undisclosed myocardial involvement, whose clinical significance is uncertain today (Bhagirath et al., 2009; Neumann et al., 2009). Cardiac screening with magnetic resonance imaging can better delineate inflammatory pericardial involvement and reveal microvasculitis of the epi- and myocardial vessels, endo- and/or myocardial inflammation, and/or less reversible fibrosis. These are supposedly attributable to eosinophil infiltration and/or ischemic lesions due to coronary artery vasculitis, which, nonetheless, is rare in Churg-Strauss syndrome (Bhagirath et al., 2009). Intraventricular thrombi are other, but rare, possible cardiovascular abnormalities, usually also visible on echocardiography. Positron-emission tomography has also been used to evaluate cardiac involvement, with some interesting results.

The aim of this study was to analyze clinical, morphological and immunological features in patients with Churg-Strauss syndrome in comparison to the patients with bronchial asthma and systemic vasculitis with eosinophilia and to study eosinophils influence on vasculitis, especially Churg-Strauss, progression and complication.

The recognition of eosinophils as complex immunomodulatory cells has been increasing in recent years. Eosinophils are derived from hematopoietic stem cells that are committed initially to the myeloid and subsequently to the basophil-eosinophil granulocyte lineage (Tefferi, 2005). The material in these granules includes cationic proteins major basic protein, eosinophilic cationic protein, eosinophil-derived neurotoxin, eosinophil peroxidase), cytokines (interleukins [ILs], tumor necrosis factor), and lipid mediators (leukotriene C4) (Rothenberg, 1998). Interleukin 5 is considered the major eosinophil growth and survival factor, whereas chemokines (eotaxin, platelet-activating factor, RANTES [regulated on activation, normal T expressed and secreted]) and endothelial adhesion molecules (integrins, vascular cell adhesion molecules) contribute to eosinophil trafficking (Elsner & Kapp, 2001; Tefferi, 2005). Major basic protein, eosinophil cationic protein, and eosinophil-derived neurotoxin are the primary mediators of eosinophil-associated toxicity to microbes (parasites, protozoa, bacteria, viruses) and human tissue (myocarditis, pneumonitis, dermatitis, neuropathy, vasculitis) (Gleich, 2009). The lung and gastrointestinal systems constitute the main residence for eosinophils. Blood eosinophilia (absolute eosinophil count [AEC] ≥600 cells/µL) is the usual initial clue for the presence of an eosinophilic disorder. The degree of blood eosinophilia, in the absence of active treatment, can be categorized into mild (AEC 600-1500 cells/µL), moderate (AEC 1500-5000 cells/µL), or severe (AEC >5000 cells/µL) (Brito-Babapulle, 2003; Tefferi, 2005). Target organ damage is unusual with mild eosinophilia, but its occurrence in association with moderate to severe eosinophilia does not appear to depend on the specific cause of eosinophilia. The eosinophil has been perceived as a terminal effector cell in allergic airway diseases. However, recent work has shown that this multifunctional cell could be more involved in the initial stages of allergic disease development than was previously thought, particularly with regard to the ability of the eosinophil to modulate T-cell responses. In this review, we discuss recent advances that suggest that eosinophils can present antigen to naïve as well as to antigen experienced T cells, induce T helper 2 cell development, cytokine production or both, and affect T-cell migration to sites of inflammation. These findings are changing the way that eosinophil function in disease is perceived, and represent a shift in the dogma of allergic disease development (Walsh & August, 2010).

The pathogenesis of eosinophilia and tissue damage in Churg-Strauss syndrome is yet unclear, but an unknown allergen or environmental trigger is thought to provoke fatal consequences in pre-sensitized asthma patients. On a cellular level, a strong shift towards a Th2-like response with massive T-cell activation is evident (Walsh & August, 2010). *In vitro*, T-cell lines from Churg-Strauss syndrome patients produce significant amounts of IL-4 and -13 (Rothenberg, 1998). This is underlined by the fact that active CSS patients have usually high serum levels of IgE and IgE-containing immune complexes (Gleich, 2009). In tissue biopsies, granulomatous vasculitic lesions filled with eosinophils, macrophages and lymphocytes are observed (Elsner & Kapp, 2001). Local activation with degranulation of eosinophils and subsequent release of granule proteins such as eosinophil-derived neurotoxin (EDN) and major basic protein (MBP) is thought to contribute to vasculitic damage.

However, the molecules specifically contributing to eosinophilia and subsequent degranulation in Churg-Strauss syndrome are enigmatic. Recently, animal and human studies have revealed the role of a chemokine family ('eotaxins') involved in tissue eosinophilia and eosinophil maturation in allergic asthma and eosinophilic oesophagitis (EO) (Gleich, 2009). To date, three members of the eotaxin family have been described: eotaxin-1 (CCL11), eotaxin-2 (CCL24) and eotaxin-3 (CCL26). All eotaxins bind to and activate chemokine receptor 3 (CCR3) but have little homology and seem to possess different physiological properties. We hypothesized that these eotaxins might play a role in eosinophilia in Churg-Strauss syndrome and thus compared serum levels of eotaxin-1, -2 and -3 in active and inactive Churg-Strauss syndrome patients with healthy controls (HC). Furthermore, we determined local expression of eotaxin-3 at sites of active disease in Churg-Strauss syndrome.

Skin biopsy is the gold standard for the diagnosis of cutaneous vasculitis, whose manifestations include urticaria, infiltrative erythema, petechiae, purpura, purpuric papules, haemorrhagic vesicles and bullae, nodules, livedo racemosa, deep (punched out) ulcers and digital gangrene. Skin biopsy, extending to subcutis and taken from the earliest, most symptomatic, reddish or purpuric lesion is crucial for obtaining a high-yielding diagnostic sample. Based on histology, vasculitis can be classified on the size of vessels affected and the dominant immune cell mediating the inflammation (e.g. neutrophilic granulomatous, lymphocytic, or eosinophilic).

Disruption of small vessels by inflammatory cells, deposition of fibrin within the lumen and / or vessel wall coupled with nuclear debris allows for the confident recognition of small vessel, mostly neutrophilic vasculitis (also known as leukocytoclastic vasculitis).

The main histopathological features in the cutaneous lesions of Churg-Strauss syndrome are dermal leukocytoclastic vasculitis with a variable eosinophilic infiltrate and non-vasculitic tissue eosinophilia with granuloma formation. This wide histopathological spectrum may account for the various skin manifestations of Churg-Strauss syndrome. However, the unique histopathological combination of dermal eosinophilic vasculitis and subcutaneous granulomatous phlebitis accompanied by bulla formation has not been previously described. We report an unusual Churg-Strauss syndrome case showing dermal necrotizing eosinophilic vasculitis and granulomatous phlebitis in purpuric lesions coupled with subepidermal blistering. The blisters showed dermal granulomatous dermatitis and eosinophilia without evidence of vasculitis. Dermal necrotizing eosinophilic vasculitis was characterized by fibrinoid alteration of the vessel wall, a prominent perivascular eosinophilic infiltrate, a few infiltrating histiocytes along the affected vessel wall, and the absence of neutrophilic infiltration. The underlying subcutaneous granulomatous phlebitis was characterized by an angiocentric histiocytic infiltrate surrounded by marked eosinophilic infiltrate. Deposition of cytotoxic proteins and radicals derived from eosinophils in the vessel walls and papillary dermis followed by a secondary granulomatous response may account for the unique clinical and histopathological features in this case (Gleich, 2009; Pagnoux, 2010).

3. Results of the research

We identified 30 unselected consecutive patients in whom Churg-Strauss syndrome (14 men and 16 women) aged from 19 to 78 years (40,35 ± 2,99 years) was diagnosed clinically at internal medicine departments (nephrology, clinical immunology and rheumatology, pulmonology, neurology, and others) in Lviv oblast clinical hospital and immunologicaly – at the department of clinical immunology and allegrology of Lviv national medical university and at West-Ukrainian medical center of clinical immunology and allergology in Ukraine between 2000 and 2010. There were observed 30 patients with bronchial asthma (15 men and 15 women) aged from 18 to 70 years (31,9 ± 4,4 years) and 19 patients with systemic vasculitis with eosinophilia (8 men and 11 women) aged from 19 to 78 years (37,6 ± 3,8 years) and consulted at the department of clinical immunology and allegrology of Lviv national medical university and at West-Ukrainian medical center of clinical immunology and allergology in Ukraine between 2000 and 2010. We examined the medical records of all these patients. Churg-Strauss syndrome was defined according to the Chapel Hill Consensus Conference nomenclature (Rothenberg, 1998). The classification criteria for

Churg-Strauss syndrome of the American College of Rheumatology (ACR) (Masi, 1990) as well as Lanham's (Hammersmith) criteria (Gleich, 2009) were retrospectively applied to the study population. All patients had direct (histologic) or indirect (using surrogate markers) evidence of vasculitis (Keogh, 2003). Systemic vasculitis with eosinophilia, bronchial asthma (according to Global Initiative for Asthma [GINA] guidelines) and eosinophilic syndrome (ES) were diagnosed according to approved medical diagnostic protocols too.

Sign	Patients with BA and eosinophilia (n = 30)		Patients with SV and eosinophilia (n = 19)		Patients with CSS (n = 30)		P_{1-2}	P_{1-3}	P_{2-3}
	1		2		3				
	Abs.	%	Abs.	%	Abs.	%			
1	**2**	**3**	**4**	**5**	**6**	**7**	**8**	**9**	**10**
Disease duration	9,6±2,9		8,3±2,1		7,0±2,3		NS	NS	NS
Complicated genetic (family) allergic anamnesis	19	63,3	10	52,6	23	76,7	NS	0,05	NS
Complicated ontogenetic allergic anamnesis	30	100	10	52,6	21	70	0,001	0,01	0,01
Polinosis	11	36,7	-	-	14	46,7	-	NS	-
Food allergy	4	13,3	-	-	6	20	-	NS	-
Insect allergy	14	46,7	-	-	2	6,7	-	0,001	-
Drug allergy	-	-	10	52,6	2	6,7	-	-	0,001
Allergic rhinitis	4	13,3		-	11	36,7	-	0,01	-
Allergic rhinitis and nasal poliposis	4	13,3		-	10	33,3	-	0,01	-
Bronchial asthma	30	100	-	-	26	86,7	0,001	NS	0,001
Bronchial asthma and nasal poliposis	-	-	-	-	7	23,3	-	0,001	0,001
Complicated genetic (family) autoimmune anamnesis	-	-	5	16,7	7	23,3	-	-	NS
Often pulmonary infection diseases: pharyngitis, laryngitis, bronchitis, pneumonia over the time of year	18	60,0	14	46,7	17	56,7	NS	NS	NS

Table 1. Main anamnesis features in patients with bronchial asthma with eosinophilia, systemic vasculitis with eosinophilia and with Churg-Strauss syndrome (M±m)

Clinical manifestations were usually confirmed by instrumental examinations as appropriate and/or tissue biopsy. One or more biopsy specimens from affected tissues were obtained when considered necessary by the clinicians. A biopsy specimen was considered consistent with a diagnosis of Churg-Strauss syndrome when eosinophilic tissue infiltration and/or vasculitis were found. Routine laboratory tests were performed in all cases at the time of diagnosis and at followup. The presence of ANCAs, IgE, CIC was determined in all patients at the time of diagnosis due to the necessity, using approved methods for each detection.

Statistical analysis. All analyses were performed using Stata statistical software, release 8.2 (Stata Corporation, College Station, TX). The differences between patients with Churg-Strauss syndrome and different eosinophilia severity in continuous variables were tested by the Mann-Whitney U test and in categorical variables by Fisher's exact test. All reported *P* values are 2-sided. *P* values less than 0.05 were considered significant.

In the result of this research it was observed some clinical features in patients with Churg-Strauss syndrome in the comparison with patients with bronchial asthma and systemic vasculitis with eosinophilia.

In patients with bronchial asthma and systemic vasculitis with eosinophilic syndrome, as well as Churg-Strauss syndrome have had a variety of anamnesis data(presented in the Table 1), severity of clinical symptoms (presented in the Table 2) and features of the course, activity and severity (presented in the Table 3).

The analysis of anamnesis data in the comparable groups of patients has showed in Table 1, which includes the following features as duration of the disease - we examined 30 patients with Churg-Strauss syndrome and it was fixed an average of 7,0 ± 2,3 years, and in 30 patients with bronchial asthma with eosinophilia - 9,6 ± 2,9 years and in 19 patients with systemic vasculitis with eosinophilia - 8,3±2,1 years.

NS- not significant

Ontogenetic history of allergy was loaded in 21 (70%) patients with Churg-Strauss syndrome, in 47,4% patients with SV with eosinophilia (p<0,01) and in 30% patients with bronchial asthma with eosinophilia (p<0,05). Pollen allergy, which manifested with pollinosis was found in 14 (46.7%) patients with Churg-Strauss syndrome, as compared with one (36,7%) patient with bronchial and eosinophilia (p< 0,05). Complicated genetic autoimmune anamnesis was found in 7 (23,3%) patients with Churg-Strauss syndrome and in 5 (16,7%) patients with systemic vasculitis with eosinohilia (P<0,05) and was not impeded in patients with bronchial asthma and eosinophilia.

Complicated immunodeficiency anamnesis (six or more respiratory diseases during the year) was established in 17 (56,7%) patients with Churg-Strauss syndrome, in 18 (60%) patients with bronchial asthma and eosinophilia and in 14 (73.6%) patients with systemic vasculitis with eosinophilia.

NS- not significant

In the Table 2, low level of productivity cough was recorded in 17 (56,7%) patients with Churg-Strauss syndrome and in 16 (53,3%) patients with bronchial asthma with eosinophilia (p<0,05). Complicated nasal breathing was found in 21 (70%) patients with Churg-Strauss syndrome and in 19 (63,3%) patients with bronchial asthma and eosinophilia (p<0,05). Typical night asthma attacks were noted in 5 (16,7%) patients with bronchial asthma with eosinophilia, in 14 (46,7%) patients with Churg-Strauss syndrome (p<0,01). Skin itching were found in 17 (56,7%) patients with Churg-Strauss syndrome and in 8 (26,7%) patients with bronchial asthma with eosinophilia ($p<0,05$) and in patients with systemic vasculitis with eosinophilia ($p<0,05$). Erythematous rash noted in 7 (23,3%) patients with Churg-Strauss syndrome, in 4 (21%) patients with systemic vasculitis with eosinophilia ($p<0,05$); multiform erythema - in 6 (20%) patients with Churg-Strauss syndrome and in 5 (26,3%) patients with systemic vasculitis with eosinophilia ($p<0,05$). These skin manifestations was not typical for patients with bronchial asthma.

Sign	Patients with BA and eosinophilia (n = 30)		Patients with SV and eosinophilia (n = 19)		Patients with CSS (n = 30)		P_{1-2}	P_{1-3}	P_{2-3}
	1		2		3				
	Abs.	%	Abs.	%	Abs.	%			
1	2	3	4	5	6	7	8	9	10
Complaints and clinical signs									
Underproductive cough	16	53,3	-	-	17	56,7	-	NS	-
Complicated nasal breathing	19	63,3	-	_	21	70	-	NS	-
Night attack of coughing	5	16,7	-	-	14	46,7	-	NS	-
Skin itching	8	26,6	11	31,6	17	56,7	NS	0,05	0,05
Erythematous rash	-	-	4	21,1	7	23,3	-	-	NS
Erythema multiforme	-	-	5	26,2	6	20	NS	NS	0,001
Non-palpable spot haemorrhagic rush		-	-	-	6	20,0	-	-	-
Palpable spot haemorrhagic rush	-	-	2	10,5	14	46,7	-	-	0,01
Haemorrhagic rash with confluence ability	-	-	1	5,3	18	60,0	-	-	0,001
Papular rash	3	10,0	4	21,1	14	46,7	NS	0,01	NS
Vesicular rash	-	-	6	31,6	19	63,3	NS	NS	0,01
Hyperpyrexia	-	-	8	42,1	17	56,7	-	-	0,05
Arthralgia	-	-	11	57,9	20	66,7	-	-	0,05
Arthritis	-	-	4	21,1	17	56,7	-	-	0,01
Myalgia	22	73,3	18	94,7	23	76,7	NS	NS	NS
Lymphadenopathy		-	-	-	8	26,7	-	-	-
Diarrhea	-	-	-	-	4	13,3	-	-	-
Polyneuropathy	-	-	-	-	14	46,7	-	-	-
Weakness	16	53,3	17	89,5	21	70,0	NS	NS	NS

Table 2. Main anamnesis features in patients with bronchial asthma with eosinophilia, systemic vasculitis witheosinophilia and with Churg-Strauss syndrome (M±m)

Sign		Patients with BA and eosinophilia (n = 30)		Patients with SV and eosinophilia (n = 19)		Patients with CSS (n = 30)		P 1-2	P 1-3	P 2-3
		1		2		3				
		Abs.	%	Abs.	%	Abs.	%			
1		2	3	4	5	6	7	1	2	3
Course character	exacerbation	-	-	5	26,3	10	33,3	-	-	0,05
	subacute	-	-	3	15,8	8	26,7	-	-	NS
	chronical	22	73,4	11	57,9	12	40	0,05	0,01	0,05
Disease activity	I degree	-	-	4	21,1	9	30	-	-	NS
	II degree	-	-	13	68,4	14	46,7	-	-	NS
	III degree	-	-	2	10,5	7	23,3	-	-	0,05
Severity stage	mild	8	26,7	4	21,1	3	10	0,05	0,05	NS
	intermittent / moderate	14	46,7	11	57,9	21	70	NS	0,05	0,05
	severe	8	26,7	4	21,1	6	20	0,05	NS	NS

Table 3. Trends of course, activity and severity of disease in patients with bronchial asthma with eosinophilia,, systemic vasculitis with eosinophilia and with Churg-Strauss syndrome (M±m)

In the same time, not-palpable hemorrhagic rash, was detected only in 6 (20%) patients with Churg-Strauss syndrome (p<0,001); palpating hemorrhagic spot rash - in 14 (46,7%) patients with Churg-Strauss syndrome, in 2 (10,5%) patients with systemic vasculitis with eosinophilia (p<0,01); hemorrhagic rash with a penchant of mergers - in 18 (60%) patients with Churg-Strauss syndrome, and only in one (5.3%) patient with systemic vasculitis with eosinophilia (p<0,001). Hemorrhagic eruption of different nature in patients with bronchial asthma and eosinophilia were not detected. Papular and vesicular rash were typical for patients with Churg-Strauss syndrome too. The common symptoms in examinated patients were distributed as follows: hyperthermia was found in 17 (56,7%) patients with Churg-Strauss syndrome and in 8 (42,1%) patients with systemic vasculitis and eosinophilia (p<0,05), arthralgic syndrome - in 20 (66,7%) patients with Churg-Strauss syndrome and in 11 (57,9%) patients with systemic vasculitis and eosinophoilia (p<0,05), arthritic syndrome - in 17 (56,7%) patients with Churg-Strauss syndrome and in four (21,1%) patients with systemic vasculitis and eosnophilia (p<0,01), mialgia - in 23 (76.7%) patients with Churg-Strauss syndrome, in 18 (94,7%) patients with systemic vasculitis (p<0,05) and in 22 (73,3%) patients with bronchial asthma and eosinophilia (p<0,05). Importantly, the lymphadenopathy was referred only in 8 (26,7%) patients with Churg-Strauss syndrome (p<0,001), diarrhea - in four (13.3%) patients with Churg-Strauss syndrome (p<0,001), polyneuropathy - in 14 (46 7%) patients with Churg-Strauss syndrome (p<0,001). These clinical signs were not identified in other groups of examined patients.

Weakness was recorded in 21 (70%) patients with Churg-Strauss syndrome and in 17 (89,7%) patients with systemic vasculitis with easinophilia (p<0,05) and in 16 (53,3%) patients with bronchial asthma and eosinophilia (p<0,05).

The most severe and active course of disease is more typical for patients with Churg-Strauss syndrome (p<0,05), that is presented in the Table 3.

Sign	Patients with CSS and mild eosinophilia (AEC 600-1500 cells/µL) (n=12)		Patients with CSS and moderate eosinophilia (AEC 1500-5000 cells/µL) (n = 13)		Patients with CSS and severe eosinophilia (AEC >5000 cells/µL) (n = 5)	
	1		2		3	
	Abs.	%	Abs.	%	Abs.	%
1	2	3	4	5	6	7
Polinosis	4	33,3	7	53,8	3	60,0
Allergic rhinitis	5	41,7	12	92,3	4	80,0
Allergic rhinitis and nasal poliposis	2	16,7	6	46,2	3	60,0
Bronchial asthma	9	75,0	12	92,3	5	100
Nasal poliposis						
Bronchial asthma and nasal poliposis	2	16,7	3	23,1	2	40,0
Underproductive cough	2	16,7	10	76,9	5	100
Complicated nasal breathing	4	33,3	12	92,3	5	100
Bronchial hyperreactivity	3	25,0	11	84,6	3	60,0
Skin itching	3	25	12	92,3	4	80,0
Erythematous rash	-	-	4	30,8	3	60,0
Erythema multiforme	-	-	3	23,1	3	60,0
Non-palpable spot haemorrhagic rush	4	33,3	2	15,4	-	-
Palpable spot haemorrhagic rush	6	50,0	4	30,8	4	80,0
haemorrhagic rash with confluence ability	2	16,7	11	84,6	5	100,0
Papular rash	8	66,7	5	38,5	1	20,0
Vesicular rash	3	25	12	92,3	4	80,0
Hyperpyrexia	6	50,0	7	53,8	4	80,0
Arthralgia	6	50,0	11	84,6	3	60,0
Arthritis	4	33,3	8	61,5	5	100,0
Myalgia	6	50,0	12	92,3	5	100,0
Lymphadenopathy	1	8,3	4	30,8	3	60,0
Diarrhea	1	8,3	1	8,3	2	40,0
Polyneuropathy	5	41,7	5	38,5	4	80,0
Weakness	4	33,3	13	92,3	4	80,0

Table 4. Main clinical signs in patients with Churg-Strauss syndrome depending of eosinophilia severity (M±m)

NS- not significant

There were found some clinical features, which were more typical for patients with Churg-Strauss syndrome and were more expressed in patients with Churg-Strauss syndrome: chronical disease course, III activity degree and moderate stage of severity are more typical for patients with Churg-Strauss syndrome compared with patients with bronchial asthma and systemic vasculitis with eosinophilia.
There were found some clinical signs in patients with Churg-Strausss syndrome depending of eosinophilia severity too, that is presented in the Table 4.

NS- not significant

For patients with Churg-Strauss syndrome and severe eosinophilia are more typical in anamnesis such signs as polinosis, allergic rhinitis, allergic rhinitis with nasal poliposis, bronchial asthma with nasal poliposis. Between clinical signs more typical for patients with severe eosinophilia are underproductive, complicated nasal breathing cough, erythematous rash, erythema multiforme, palpable spot haemorrhagic rush and haemorrhagic rash with confluence ability, hyperpyrexia, arthritis, lymphadenopathy, diarrhea and polyneuropathy.
There are many immunological peculiarities that play very important role in the opportunity of examined diseases development, activity, severity and complication. Some of such immunological peculiarities are presented in the Table 5.

Indexes		Patients with BA and eosinophilia (n = 30)	Patients with SV and eosinophilia (n = 19)	Patients with CSS (n = 30)	P_{1-2}	P_{1-3}	P_{2-3}
		1	2	3			
Lymphocytes	cells/µL)	1,70±0,23	1,86±0,19	1,89±0,12	NS	NS	NS
$CD3^+$	%	63,7±3,18	50,8±2,55	50,8±2,89	0,05	0,05	NS
	cells/µL)	1,08±0,12	1,11±0,27	0,96±0,13	NS	NS	NS
$CD4^+$	%	40,9±1,60	29,8±1,75	42,6±2,60	0,05	NS	0,05
	cells/µL)	0,43±0,04	0,31±0,03	0,41±0,10	0,05	NS	0,05
$CD8^+$	%	23,3±1,72	21,0±1,67	18,3±1,49	NS	NS	NS
	cells/µL)	0,24±0,03	0,24±0,09	0,18±0,04	NS	NS	NS
$CD16^+/56^+$	%	14,1±1,26	16,00±2,59	16,01±1,30	NS	NS	NS
	cells/µL)	0,25±0,05	0,30±0,07	0,30±0,05	NS	NS	NS
$CD19^+$	%	16,9±1,94	20,8±3,60	22,40±2,24	NS	0,05	NS
	cells/µL)	0,31±0,03	0,38±0,05	0,44±0,07	NS	0,05	NS
$CD25^+$	%	17,9±1,12	21,3±1,62	29,4±1,19	NS	0,01	0,05
	cells/µL)	0,34±0,02	0,40±0,05	0,56±0,05	NS	0,001	0,01
HLA DR^+	%	27,3±1,22	30,0±1,48	26,30±1,83	NS	NS	NS
	cells/µL)	0,48±0,02	0,53±0,02	0,50±0,07	NS	NS	NS
$CD95^+$	%	17,3±0,88	18,6±2,66	24,7±1,37	NS	0,05	0,05
	cells/µL)	0,29±0,05	0,35±0,03	0,47±0,05	NS	0,01	0,05

Table 5. Trends of lymphograme indexes and lymphocytes activity markers in patients with bronchial asthma, systemic vasculitis with eosinophilia and with Churg-Strauss syndrome (M±m)

NS- not significant

There were found some peculiarities of immunological parameters in patients with Churg-Strauss syndrome, such as significantly lower proportional level of CD3 +lymphocytes ($p<0,05$), higher proportional and absolute level of CD19 +-lymphocytes ($p<0,05$), intensively expressed proportional ($p<0,01$) and absolute ($p<0,001$) early count of lymphocyte activation marker (CD25 +) and significantly intensively proportional ($p<0,05$) and absolute ($p<0,01$) expression of CD95+ in patients with Churg-Struss syndrome compared with patients with bronchial asthma and eosinophilia. Compared with patients with systemic vasculitis with eosinophilia, patients with Churg-Strauss syndrome had a significantly higher proportional ($p<0,05$) and absolute ($p<0,05$) mean of CD4 +lymphocytes, intensively expressed proportional ($p<0,05$) and absolute ($p<0,01$) count of early lymphocyte activation marker (CD25 +) and significantly intensively proportional and absolute expression of CD95+ ($p<0,05$).
There were found some immunological signs in patients with Churg-Strausss syndrome depending of eosinophilia severity too, that is presented in the Table 6.

Indexes		Patients with CSS and mild eosinophilia (AEC 600-1500 cells/μL) (n=12)	Patients with CSS and moderate eosinophilia (AEC 1500-5000 cells/μL) (n = 13)	Patients with CSS and severe eosinophilia (AEC >5000 cells/μL) (n = 5)	P_{1-2}	P_{1-3}	P_{2-3}
		1	2	3			
1	2	3	4	5	6	7	8
Eosinophils	cells/μL)	0,59±0,05	3,58±0,82	5,81±0,92	0,001	0,001	0,05
Lymphocytes	cells/μL)	1,61±0,15	2,24±0,47	3,01±0,15	NS	0,05	NS
CD3+	%	56,7±1,66	48,53±2,26	46,50±1,18	0,05	0,05	NS
	cells/μL)	0,91±0,09	1,08±0,05	1,39±0,06	NS	0,05	NS
CD4+	%	36,5±2,16	41,20±3,97	50,30±4,21	NS	0,05	0,05
	cells/μL)	0,33±0,06	0,44±0,08	0,70±0,09	NS	0,01	0,01
CD8+	%	19,65±1,72	18,50±2,68	16,67±2,33	NS	NS	NS
	cells/μL)	0,18±0,03	0,20±0,07	0,23±0,07	NS	NS	NS
CD16+/56+	%	14,91±2,07	14,80±1,52	18,3±1,76	NS	NS	NS
	cells/μL)	0,24±0,03	0,33±0,05	0,55±0,08	NS	NS	NS
CD19+	%	20,05±1,86	22,03±2,61	25,0±2,12	NS	0,05	NS
	cells/μL)	0,32±0,05	0,49±0,03	0,75±0,09	NS	0,05	0,001
CD25+	%	28,33±2,73	29,82±1,89	30,4±1,58	NS	NS	NS
	cells/μL)	0,46±0,07	0,66±0,09	0,92±0,12	NS	0,01	0,05
HLA DR+	%	20,05±1,68	26,50±1,46	31,9±2,48	NS	0,05	NS
	cells/μL)	0,32±0,05	0,59±0,06	0,96±0,11	NS	0,001	0,05
CD95+	%	20,73±1,27	23,50±2,67	29,9±7,06	NS	NS	NS
	cells/μL)	0,33±0,03	0,52±0,05	0,89±0,1	NS	0,001	0,05

Table 6. Trends of lymphograme indexes and lymphocytes activity markers in patients with Churg-Strauss syndrome depending of eosinophilia severity (M±m).

NS- not significant

There were found some peculiarities of immunological markers in patients with Churg-Strauss syndrome and different eosinophilia severity, such as the highest eosinophils level in patients with Churg-Strauss syndrome and severe eosinophilia in comparison to the patients with mild eosinophilia ($p<0,001$) and moderate eosinophila ($p<0,05$), significantly lower absolute level of lymphocytes in patients with Churg-Strauss and severe eosinophilia $p<0,05$) in comparison to patients with mild eosinophilia; significantly lower proportional and absolute level of CD3 +lymphocytes ($p<0,05$), CD4 +lymphocytes ($p<0,05$), CD19 +lymphocytes ($p<0,05$), significantly intensively expressed early lymphocyte activation markers such as (CD25 +) ($p<0,01$), late lymphocyte activation markers such as (HLA DR +) ($p<0,001$) and significantly intensively expression of CD95+ ($p<0,001$) in patients with Churg-Struss syndrome and severe eosinophilia compared with patients with Churg-Strauss syndrome and mild eosinophilia. There were found some significantly lower proportional and absolute level of CD4 +lymphocytes ($p<0,05$), absolute level of CD19 +lymphocytes ($p<0,001$), significantly intensively expressed early lymphocyte activation markers such as (CD25 +) ($p<0,05$), late lymphocyte activation markers such as (HLA DR +) ($p<0,05$) and significantly intensively expression of CD95+ ($p<0,05$) in patients with Churg-Struss syndrome and severe eosinophilia compared with patients with Churg-Strauss syndrome and moderate eosinophilia.

No significant peculiarities were found in patients with Churg-Strauss syndrome and mild or moderate eosinophilia.

We have also analyzed the features of serum interleukins (IL-2, IL-4, IL-5, IL-10) in patients with Churg-Strauss syndrome and other examined groups, that is showed in the Table 7.

Interleukins		Patients with BA and eosinophilia (n = 30)	Patients with SV and eosinophilia (n = 19)	Patients with CSS (n = 30)	P_{1-2}	P_{1-3}	P_{2-3}
		1	2	3			
IL-2	pg/ml	3,79±0,98	6,31±0,75	8,78±0,26	0,05	0,05	0,01
IL-4	pg/ml	8,17±0,17	5,38±0,55	6,64±0,16	0,01	0,05	NS
IL-5	pg/ml	6,60±1,26	12,4±2,28	97,9±17,5	0,001	0,001	0,001
IL-10	pg/ml	2,88±0,19	3,27±0,29	2,12±0,14	NS	0,05	0,05

Table 7. Trends of pro-inflammatory (IL-2) and anti-inflammatory (IL-4, IL-5, IL-10) cytokines in patients with bronchial asthma, systemic vasculitis with eosinophilia and with Churg-Strauss syndrome (M±m)

NS- not significant

Comparing realizing possibility of pro- and anti-inflammatory mechanisms of cytokines such as IL-2, IL-4, IL-5 and IL-10 in patients with bronchial asthma with eosinophilia, systemic vasculitis with eosinophilia and Churg-Strauss syndrome it was found significant increase of IL-4 ($p<0,01$) and IL-5 ($p<0,001$) level in patients with bronchial asthma and eosinophilia, increase of IL-2 ($p<0,05$), IL-4 ($p<0,05$) and IL-5 ($p<0,05$) in patients with systemic vasculitis with eosinophilia, increase of IL-2 ($p<0,05$) and IL-5 ($p<0,001$) level and decrease of IL-10 ($p<0,05$) level in patients with Churg-Strauss syndrome.

There were found some cytokines production peculiarities in patients with Churg-Strausss syndrome depending of eosinophilia severity, that is presented in the Table 8.

Interleukins		Patients with CSS and mild eosinophilia (AEC 600-1500 cells/µL) (n=12)	Patients with CSS and moderate eosinophilia (AEC 1500-5000 cells/µL) (n = 13)	Patients with CSS and severe eosinophilia (AEC >5000 cells/µL) (n = 5)	P_{1-2}	P_{1-3}	P_{2-3}
		1	2	3			
IL-2	pg/ml	8,44±0,11	8,74±0,16	9,18±0,08	NS	0,05	NS
IL-4	pg/ml	5,7±0,13	6,8±0,11	7,42±0,09	NS	0,05	NS
IL-5	pg/ml	32,7±7,5	49,4±9,6	211,6±29,5	NS	0,001	0,001
IL-10	pg/ml	2,34±0,08	2,04±0,09	1,98±0,05	NS	0,05	NS

Table 8. Trends of pro-inflammatory (IL-2) and anti-inflammatory (IL-4, IL-5, IL-10) cytokines in patients with Churg-Strauss syndrome depending of eosinophilia severity (M±m)

NS- not significant

Analizing realizing possibility of pro- and anti-inflammatory cytokines such as IL-2, IL-4, IL-5 and IL-10 in patients with Churg-Strauss syndrome and different eosinophilia severity, it was fixed significant increase of IL-2 (9,18±0,08 pg/ml, p<0,05), IL-4 (7,42±0,09 pg/ml, p<0,05), and IL-5 (211,6±29,5 pg/ml, p<0,001) and decrease of IL-10 (1,98±0,05 pg/ml, p<0,05) level in patients with Churg-Strauss syndrome with severe eosinopilia compared with patients with Churg-Strauss syndrome and mild eosinophilia. Also, it was fixed significant higher IL-5 level in patients with Churg-Strauss syndrome and severe eosinophilia compared with patients with moderate eosnophilia (p<0,001) too.

The patients with systemic vasculitis and eosinophilia and with Churg-Strauss syndrome were divided in some subgroups depended on ANCA -presence.

In our series of patients, we found that ANCA positivity was correlated with renal involvement, especially with the histologic picture of necrotizing crescentic glomerulonephritis, and, to a lesser extent, with constitutional symptoms. Moreover, ANCA-positive patients had a significantly higher frequency of certain organ system clinical manifestations, such as pulmonary hemorrhage, purpura, and mononeuritis multiplex. In contrast, ANCA-negative patients had a higher frequency of heart and (less severe) lung disease.

Limited data have been reported on the correlation between ANCA positivity and the clinical features in CSS, even though it should be noted that most (if not all) reported cases of necrotizing crescentic glomerulonephritis in CSS involved ANCA-positive (usually MPO pANCA) patients, as in our cohort. Moreover, the results of studies of small series of patients have suggested that MPO ANCAs may be associated with the onset of glomerular disorder in CSS.

There were fixed some morphological peculiarities in patients with Churg-Strausss syndrome depending of eosinophilia severity, that is presented in pictures 1,2 and 3.

We have selected the three most informative results of skin-muscular samples biopsies patients with Churg-Strauss syndrome with different eosinophilia severity, that reflected in three figures.

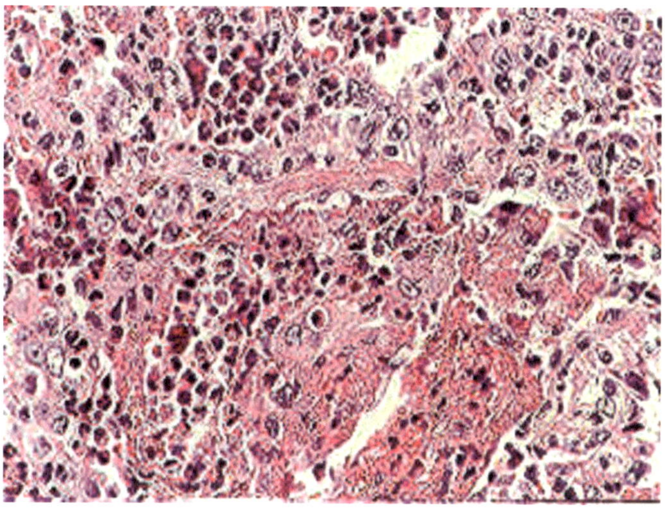

Fig. 1. Churg-Strauss syndrome: Tissue eosinophilia is a frequent finding in cutaneous lesions of Churg–Strauss syndrome. Hematoxylin, eosin × 300; clinical: light/mild eosinophilia

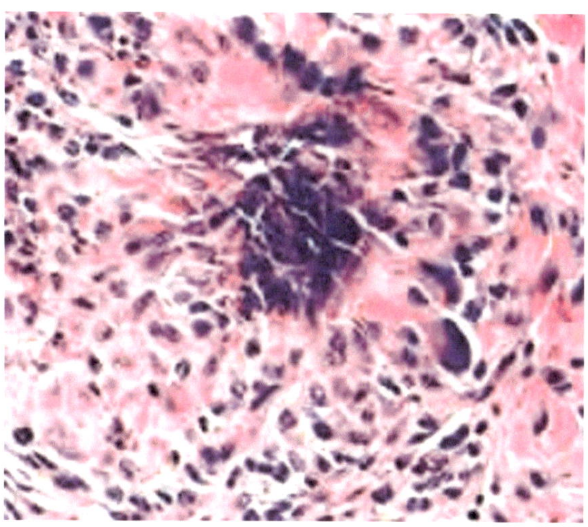

Fig. 2. Churg-Strauss syndrome: Skin biopsy which was indicative of small vessel vasculitis, showing the presence of an inflammatory infiltrate predominantly constituted by eosinophils and plasmocytes around blood vessels. Hematoxylin, eosin × 400; clinical: medium eosinophilia

The analysis of the founded morphological features, that were identified in patients with Churg-Strauss syndrome with different eosinophilia severity, shoved eosinophilc infiltration of the dermis in patients with Churg-Strauss syndrome and mild eosinophilia

(Fig.1); necrotizing changes in the center of granulomas, extensive infiltration of neutrophils, eosinophils of vessel wall until the formation of circular eosinophil infiltrates in the vessels of patients with Churg-Strauss syndrome and severe eosinophilia (Fig.3)

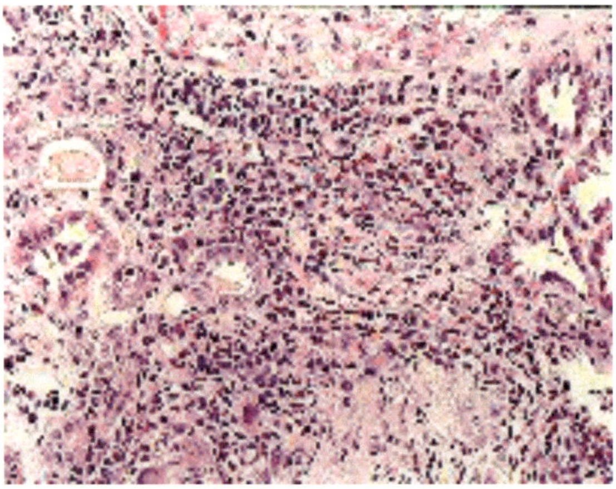

Fig. 3. Churg-Strauss syndrome: Skin-muscular biopsy which showing eosinophilic circular infiltration of the intermuscular arteriole. Hematoxylin, eosin × 400; clinical: severe eosinophilia

4. Conclusion

Substantial advances have been made in the understanding of immune mechanisms (especially eosinophils, circulating immune complexes, total IgE, antineutrophicytoplasmic antibodies, cytokines) implicated in Churg-Strauss syndrome and its management. While it definitively remains a systemic necrotizing small-sized vessel vasculitis, its membership in the ANCA-associated vasculitis group has become more controversial. More complex and numerous mechanisms are involved in Churg-Strauss syndrome (Hoffman and Langford, 2005; Pagnoux and Guillevin, 2010). Similarly, one of its earlier denominations, allergic granulomatous angiitis (Churg and Strauss, 1951), has become dated because not all patients have (eosinophilic) granulomas. Moreover, several disease subgroups have been identified, essentially based on clinical or biological findings (Walsh &August, 2010). There are a large number of works devoted to studying of the problem of rare disease - Churg-Strauss syndrome - especially its clinical and laboratory features, but it was firstly by us described clinical, immunological and morphological features of Churg-Strauss syndrome with different severity of eosinophilia in these patients.

It was fixed special clinical signs in patients with Churg-Strauss syndrome and severe eosinophilia such as: underproductive, complicated nasal breathing cough, erythematous rash, erythema multiforme, palpable spot haemorrhagic rush and haemorrhagic rash with confluence ability, hyperpyrexia, arthritis, lymphadenopathy, diarrhea and polyneuropathy. There were found some peculiarities of immunological markers in patients with Churg-Strauss syndrome and different eosinophilia severity, such as the highest eosinophils level in patients with Churg-Strauss syndrome and severe eosinophilia in comparison to the patients with mild eosinophilia ($p<0,001$) and moderate eosinophila ($p<0,05$), significantly lower absolute lymphocytes level in patients with Churg-Strauss and severe eosinophilia (p<0,05) in comparison to patients with mild eosinophilia; significantly lower proportional and absolute level of CD3 +lymphocytes (p<0,05), CD4 +lymphocytes (p<0,05), CD19 +lymphocytes (p<0,05), significantly intensively expressed early lymphocyte activation markers such as (CD25 +) (p<0,01), late lymphocyte activation markers such as (HLA DR +) (p<0,001) and significantly intensively expression of CD95+ (p<0,001) in patients with Churg-Struss syndrome and severe eosinophilia compared with patients with Churg-Strauss syndrome and mild eosinophilia. Other subgroups may be brought forth in the future, relying on more subtle molecular and genetic characteristics (IL-4, IL-5, IL-5RA gene polymorphism).

Therapeutic strategies also require further improvement. Treatment should be adapted as closely as possible to each patient's characteristics. New treatments (monoclonal antibodies) are needed to lower the rate of frequent, low-dose but long-term, corticosteroid-dependence that represents a major issue and the lingering disappointment in current therapeutic strategies for Churg-Strauss syndrome.

5. References

[1] Bhagirath, K.M., Paulson, K., Ahmadie, R. et al. (2009). Clinical utility of cardiac magnetic resonance imaging in Churg-Strauss syndrome: case report and review of the literature. *Rheumatol Int.* Vol. 29(4):445-9.

[2] Bibby, S., Healy, B., Steele, R. et al. (2010). Association between leukotriene receptor antagonist therapy and Churg-Strauss syndrome: an analysis of the FDA AERS database. *Thorax* Vol.65(2):132-8.

[3] Brito-Babapulle, F. (2003) The eosinophilias, including the idiopathic hypereosinophilic syndrome. Br J Haematol.Vol.121:203-223.

[4] Cohen, P., Pagnoux, C., Mahr, A. et al. (2007). Churg-Strauss syndrome with poor-prognosis factors: A prospective multicenter trial comparing glucocorticoids and six or twelve cyclophosphamide pulses in forty-eight patients. Arthritis Rheum. Vol.57(4):686-93.

[5] Elsner, J., Kapp,A. (2001). The chemokine network in eosinophil activation. Allergy Asthma Proc. Vol.22:139-148.

[6] Gleich, G. J. (2009). The hypereosinophilic syndromes: current concepts and treatments. British Journal of Haematol. Vol.145(3):271-285.

[7] Harrold, L.R., Andrade, S.E., Go, A.S. et al. (2005). Incidence of Churg-Strauss syndrome in asthma drug users: a population-based perspective. *J Rheumatol.* Vol.32(6):1076-80.

[8] Keogh, K.A., Specks. U. (2003). Churg-Strauss syndrome: clinical presentation, antineutrophil cytoplasmic antibodies, and leukotriene receptor antagonists. *Am J Med.* Vol.115: 284–90.

[9] Masi, A.T., Hunder, G.G., Lie, J.T. et al. (1990). The American College of Rheumatology 1990 criteria for the classification of Churg-Strauss syndrome (allergic granulomatosis and angiitis). *Arthritis Rheum.* Vol.33: 1094–100.

[10] Neumann, T., Manger, B., Schmid, M. et al. (2009). Cardiac involvement in Churg-Strauss syndrome: impact of endomyocarditis. *Medicine (Baltimore)* Vol.88(4):236-43.

[11] Pagnoux, C., Guilpain, P., Guillevin L. (2007). Churg-Strauss syndrome. *Curr Opin Rheumatol.* Vol.19(1):25-32.

[12] Pagnoux, C., Guillevin, L. (2010). Churg-Strauss syndrome: evidence for disease subtypes? *Curr Opin Rheumatol.* Vol.22(1):21-8.
[13] Pagnoux, C. (2010). Churg-Strauss syndrome: evolving concepts. Discovery Medicine, Vol.9(46):243-252.
[14] Ribi, C., Cohen, P., Pagnoux, C. et al. (2008). Treatment of Churg-Strauss syndrome without poor-prognosis factors: a multicenter, prospective, randomized, open-label study of seventy-two patients. Arthritis Rheum. Vol.58(2):586-94.
[15] Rothenberg, M.E. (1998). Eosinophilia. N Engl J Med. Vol.338:1592-1600.
[16] Sablé-Fourtassou, R., Cohen, P., Mahr, A. et al. (2005). Antineutrophil cytoplasmic antibodies and the Churg-Strauss syndrome. *Ann Intern Med.* Vol.143(9):632-8.
[17] Seo, P., Stone, J.H. (2007) Small-vessel and medium-vessel vasculitis. In: Arthritis Care & Research, Vol.57(8):1552-1559.
[18] Sinico, R.A., Bottero, P. (2009). Churg-Strauss angiitis. *Best Pract Res Clin Rheumatol.* Vol.23(3):355-66.
[19] Tefferi, A. (2005). Blood Eosinophilia: A New Paradigm in Disease Classification, Diagnosis, and Treatment. Mayo Clin Proc. Vol.80(1):75-83.
[20] Walsh, E.R., August, A. (2010). Eosinophils and allergic airway disease: there is more to the story. *Trends Immunol.* Vol.31(1): 39–44.
[21] Watts, R.A., Lane, S., Scott, D.G. (2005). What is known about the epidemiology of the vasculitides? *Best Pract Res Clin Rheumatol* Vol.19(2):191-207.
[22] Wieczorek, S., Holle, J.U., Epplen, J.T. (2010). Recent progress in the genetics of Wegener's granulomatosis and Churg-Strauss syndrome. *Curr Opin Rheumatol.* Vol.22(1):8-14.

14

Drug-Induced Vasculitis

Mislav Radić
Department of Rheumatology and Clinical Immunology, University Hospital Split
Croatia

1. Introduction

This chapter aims to draw attention to the features that distinguish drug-induced vasculitis from those of idiopathic autoimmune syndromes, first and foremost primary vasculitides. Development of a systemic drug-induced syndrome only develops in a minority of patients treated with a drug over a prolonged period of time, whereas cutaneous vasculitis occurs quite commonly. The most frequent symptoms as onset are arthralgia, myalgia and skin rash. Early withdrawal of the offending drug mostly leads to complete recovery while more advanced disease and late withdrawal of the drug may necessitate use of corticosteroid and/or immunosuppressive therapy. The recent discovery of anti-neutrophil cytoplasm antibodies (ANCA) in a large serological subset of drug-induced vasculitis caused by long-term antithyroid drug treatment has opened new avenues for differential diagnostics. Certain medications such as propylthiouracil can induce ANCA associated vasculitis. This chapter focuses on the data on causal drugs, possible pathogenesis, clinical description, diagnosis, treatment and prognosis of patients with drug-induced vasculitis. ANCA with specificity to more than one lysosomal antigen combined with presence of antibodies to histones and beta-2 glycoprotein 1 constitute a unique serological profile for drug-induced vasculitis.
The pathogenesis of drug-induced ANCA associated vasculitis might be multifactorial. The clinical manifestations are similar to those of primary ANCA associated vasculitis, but ANCA with multi-antigenicity may help to differentiate it from primary ANCA associated vasculitis. Rational use of laboratory marker profiles is likely to aid in distinguishing drug-induced from idiopathic syndromes. However, the use of ANCA and other autoantibodies as biomarkers of different phenotypes of drug-induced vasculitis is one of the focuses of this chapter.
To date, ANCA are important serological markers for certain small-vessel vasculitides, encompassing Wegener granulomatosis (WG), microscopic polyangiitis (MPA) and Churg-Strauss syndrome (CSS). By indirect immunofluorescence (IIF) technique, ANCAs are classified as a perinuclear pattern (P-ANCA) and a cytoplasmic pattern (C-ANCA). C-ANCA is caused almost exclusively by antibodies against proteinase 3 (PR3). In contrast, P-ANCA can be caused by antibodies reacting with a variety of different neutrophil granule constituents, including myeloperoxidase (MPO), lactoferrin, human leucocyte elastase (HLE) and others. Evidence is mounting that these specific antibodies are pathogenic in small-vessel vasculitis. However, the aetiology of ANCA associated vasculitis is largely unknown.
The diagnosis of drug-induced ANCA associated vasculitis is based on the temporal relationship between clinically evident vasculitis and administration of the offending drugs,

and excluding medical conditions that mimic vasculitis and other definable types of vasculitis. After the diagnosis of drug-induced ANCA associated vasculitis was made, the offending drugs should be withdrawn immediately, and appropriate immunosuppressive therapy should be administered only for patients with vital organ involvement. The duration of immunosuppressive therapy should be much shorter than that in primary ANCA associated vasculitis and long-term maintenance therapy might not be necessary. The prognosis of patients with drug-induced ANCA associated vasculitis is good as long as the offending drug is discontinued in time.

This chapter summarizes the causal drugs, possible pathogenesis, clinical description, diagnosis, treatment and prognosis of drug-induced ANCA associated vasculitis.

2. Drug-induced vasculitis

Drug-induced vasculitis usually attacks the skin and sometimes the subcutaneous part of the skin, but sometimes also the kidneys and the lungs. Clinical symptoms include arthralgias and myalgias but usually do not develop into overt arthritis or myositis, manifested as muscle weakness. End-stage kidney disease due to glomerular vasculitis may occur, but early removal of the offending drug most often leads to resolution of the glomerular inflammation. A few cases of drug-induced vasculitis presenting with a hemorrhagic syndrome due to lung capillaritis have been reported. Drug-induced vasculitis patients typically harbor ANCA directed to one or more neutrophil cytoplasm antigens, the most common antigens being the granule proteins MPO, HLE, cathepsin G, and lactoferrin. In one study from Boston (Choi, 2000), the levels of MPO-ANCA were found to be much higher in 30 patients with drug-induced MPO-ANCA vasculitis than those usually found in idiopathic vasculitides, and there was a strong association between presence of HLE-ANCA and lactoferrin-ANCA and exposure to the candidate drugs. A study from Denmark showed a strong association between heredity and development of drug-induced vasculitis during treatment with propylthiouracil in monozygotic triplets with Graves' disease. Two of these children that were treated with propylthiouracil got multispecific ANCA including HLE-ANCA, while the third triplet had no signs of drug-induced vasculitis and no ANCA during treatment with carbimazole.

To date, many studies have indicated that drug-induced vasculitis may be a complication of therapy with prior use of certain medications in some patients, and unreported and/or undiagnosed cases may be beyond our imagination. As shown in Table 1, the most often implicated drug in the published work is propylthiouracil, which may result from more frequent prescriptions in clinical practice. Clear evidence for an association with the development of drug-induced vasculitis has also been shown for the following drugs: hydralazine, anti-tumour necrosis factor-α (TNF-α) agents, sulfasalazine, D-penicillamine and minocycline, however, most of them were limited to case reports. Propylthiouracil is a common anti-thyroid drug widely used all over the world. In the published work, over a hundred cases of propylthiouracil-induced vasculitis have been reported. Further studies in pathogenesis, treatment and long-term outcomes of patients with propylthiouracil induced vasculitis provide useful information on understanding drug-induced vasculitis. It has been shown that propylthiouracil is implicated in 80–90% cases of vasculitis induced by anti-thyroid drugs, while cases related to others are less frequent such as methimazole, carbimazole and benzylthiouracil. The increasing use of so-called 'biologic' agents in medical practice has been accompanied by growing evidence on the toxicity profile of these

agents, including drug-induced vasculitis. Anti-TNF-α drugs, such as adalimumab, infliximab and etanercept, are now established therapy in the management of rheumatoid arthritis and several other chronic inflammatory diseases. Repeated treatment with these agents can lead to the development of autoantibodies, including antinuclear antibodies (ANA), anti-dsDNA and anti-cardiolipin antibodies, in up to 10% of patients. The autoantibody synthesis is associated with a greater cumulative dose of therapy. Although uncommon, some patients receiving anti-TNF-α agents were found to develop vasculitis.
Minocycline, a semi-synthetic lipophilic tetracycline, is the favoured antibiotic for the treatment of acne and rheumatic diseases. The use of minocycline over the past decade has led to numerous reports on drug-induced lupus. Interestingly, the laboratory features of minocycline-induced lupus include positive ANA and frequently positive p-ANCA (>67% of cases). In Marzo-Ortega's study, 7% of the minocycline-treated patients at some point in the past became ANCA positive, however, only a few cases indicated the occurrence of drug-induced vasculitis. Because there seems to be a wide serological overlap between drug-induced lupus and drug-induced vasculitis, it may be difficult to discriminate between the two categories. Also, it might raise suspicion that some patients may actually contract drug-induced vasculitis rather than drug-induced lupus. In addition, there are a few published reports indicating the association between treatment with other drugs and the occurrence of vasculitis, including allopurinol, cephotaxime, clozapine, levamisole, phenytoin and thioridazine. However, the causative relationship is much less certain. Leukotriene antagonists (LTA, such as montelukast and zafirlukast) have been implicated in the pathogenesis of CSS. Further studies showed that no significant association was observed between CSS and LTA after controlling for the use of other anti-asthma drugs. In a case-crossover study, it was suggested that the onset of CSS might be not associated with montelukast but a phenomenon possibly associated with a group of medications prescribed for long term control of severe asthma. Based on this evidence, the National Institutes of Health/US Food and Drug Administration panel concluded that no one class of LTA was associated with CSS and that LTA are safe. A possible clue to distinguish the patients with early CSS from those with idiopathic asthma is that the former patients tend to have severe upper airway disease, especially sinusitis, with radiographs showing paranasal abnormalities.

2.1 Epidemiology

There are no clear data on the prevalence of drug-induced vasculitis due to lack of prospective studies. Several cross-sectional studies reported that the prevalence of propylthiouracil induced vasculitis ranged from 20% to 64%. In some other study (Gao, 2004), ANCA was detected in 22.6% of patients treated with propylthiouracil, but only 6.5% patients had clinical evidence of drug-induced vasculitis. In Slot's study (Slot, 2005); ANCA and drug-induced vasculitis were present in 11% and 4% of patients treated with anti-thyroid drugs, respectively. However, in Choi's study (Choi, 2000), no patient in any of the active study drug groups (minocycline, for a 48-week trial; sulfasalazine, for a 37-week trial; penicillamine, for a 104- week trial) demonstrated ANCA seroconversion. Some researchers speculated that it might be due to a short observation period, and the prevalence of positive ANCA might be higher in patients with much long-standing therapy. Prospective, longitudinal studies with a larger cohort of patients are needed to establish the true prevalence of drug-induced vasculitis.

2.2 Pathogenesis

A variety of agents may produce a typical clinical picture together with a similar autoimmune profile, suggesting a common mechanism for drug-induced vasculitis. To date, the mechanism is far from fully understood and it might be multifactorial.

- Most drugs are low-molecular-weight substances, and require the formation of a complex to stimulate antibody formation and then to drive an immune response. One hypothesis (Jiang, 1994) proposed that activated neutrophils in the presence of hydrogen peroxidase released MPO from their granules, which converted the offending drugs such as prophythiouracil and hydralazine into cytotoxic products, then the drugs and their metabolites were immunogenic for T cells, which in turn activated B cells to produce ANCA.
- The offending drugs and their metabolites may accumulate within neutrophils, bind to MPO and modify its configuration, with subsequent intermolecular determinant spreading the autoimmune response to other autoantigens and turning neutrophil proteins (including elastase, lactoferrin and nuclear antigens) immunogenic.
- Some drugs like sulfasalazine could induce neutrophil apoptosis. Moreover, neutrophil apoptosis, in the absence of priming, is associated with translocation of ANCA antigens to the cell surface, which then induce the production of ANCA, and ANCA in turn is able to bind the membrane-bound antigens, causing a self-perpetuating constitutive activation by cross-linking PR3 or MPO and Fcγ receptors.

The oxidation activity of MPO could be inhibited by prophythiouracil and prophythiouracil -induced MPO-ANCA in a dose-dependent manner, which might also be involved in the pathogenesis of drug-induced vasculitis. The cytotoxic products of the offending drug, ANCA as well as cytotoxic neutral serine proteinases, degranulated from the activated neutrophils, could directly cause vascular damage. In other cases, the causal drugs (e.g. anti-TNF-α agents) may act as modulators of the normal immune system, rendering it permissive for self-directed responses. Rheumatoid arthritis is generally considered as a T-helper cell (Th) 1-mediated disease and TNF-α plays an important role in driving Th1-associated responses. Other forms of autoimmunity, for example, systemic lupus erythematosus and vasculitis (especially CSS and MPA), are characterized by a Th2 cytokine profile with prominent B-cell activation. Therefore, anti-TNF-α agents, administered in patients with rheumatoid arthritis, may shift the immune system from a Th1 to a Th2 profile thus upregulating antibody production. Alternatively, an increase in clinical or subclinical bacterial infections in the setting of TNF-α blockade might act as an immunostimulant and enable autoantibody production by inducing polyclonal B-cell activation. It is also speculated that drug-induced vasculitis might be genetic factors linked, because four out of six patients with minocycline-induced P-ANCA had human leucocyte antigen (HLA) DRB1*1104. The major histocompatibility complex (MHC) class II background may indicate that autoantibody production in these patients is driven by a genetically restricted T-cell response to epitopes from native or drug-modified MPO. Indeed, the ability of exogenous agents to induce vasculitis may be an opportunity, as a greater understanding of drug induced vasculitis is likely to provide insight into the nature of primary autoimmunity.

Several studies have demonstrated that the majority of patients with drug-induced ANCA were free from clinically evident vasculitis. These conditions provide a natural platform for the study of idiopathic autoimmune disease. The autoantibody response is pathogenic will depend on many factors including the characteristics of the autoantibodies such as epitope specificity, avidity, subclass and idiotype. A series of studies on prophythiouracil-induced vasculitis has demonstrated the following.

Antibiotics
Cephotaxime
Minocycline
Anti-thyroid drugs
Benzylthiouracil
Carbimazole
Methimazole
Prophythiouracil
Anti-tumor necrosis factor-α agents
Adalimumab
Etanercept
Infliximab
Psychoactive agents
Clozapine
Thioridazine
Miscellaneous drugs
Allopurinol
D-Penicillamine
Hydralazine
Levamisole
Phenytoin
Sulfasalazine

Table 1. Medications associated with drug-induced vasculitis

- Almost all the patients with overt clinical vasculitis had MPO-ANCA or PR3-ANCA, which indicated that anti-MPO and anti-PR3 antibodies, just like those in primary ANCA associated vasculitis, might also be associated with the occurrence of clinically active vasculitis induced by drugs.
- A higher MPO-ANCA level, over a threshold, might be necessary to induce clinically evident vasculitis.
- Patients with prophythiouracil-induced vasculitis tended to have higher titres and higher avidity of MPO-ANCA than those with prophythiouracil induced anti-MPO antibodies but without clinical vasculitis.
- Most patients with prophythiouracil-induced ANCA but without clinical vasculitis had polyclonal MPO-ANCA recognizing both linear and conformational epitopes of the heavy chain of MPO; however, some patients with nephritis had MPO-ANCA

recognizing only the linear sites. They supposed that this clonality of MPO-ANCA might be a risk factor to induce clinical vasculitis.

- Anti-endothelial cell antibodies (AECA) are implicated in the pathogenesis of vascular injury. It was found that the majority (10/11) of patients with active prophythiouracil-induced vasculitis had serum AECA and their serum AECA disappeared quickly in remission; more importantly, patients with prophythiouracil induced ANCA but without clinical vasculitis did not have AECA. These findings indicated that AECA indeed might play an important role in the pathogenesis of drug-induced vasculitis.

The studies on immunological characteristics of drug induced ANCA might provide useful information on the pathogenetic role of ANCA in primary vasculitis. Some studies have shown that although serum ANCA in patients with primary ANCA associated vasculitis usually recognized only one target antigen, either MPO or PR3, antibodies against multiple ANCA antigens, especially the antigens other than MPO and PR3, might be the characteristic of drug-induced ANCA. Compared with immunological characteristics of anti-MPO antibodies in sera from patients with primary ANCA associated vasculitis, prophythiouracil-induced anti-MPO antibodies usually had a higher titre but lower avidity. MPO-ANCA from patients with prophythiouracil-induced ANCA associated vasculitis might recognize more restricted epitopes of MPO, although the epitopes were overlapping between the two groups. In a study of ANCA immunoglobulin (Ig)G subclass distribution, the anti-MPO IgG3 subclass, which has a potent complement-activation capacity and a firmly binding ability to Fc receptors on mononuclear cells, was not detectable in sera from patients with prophythiouracil-induced vasculitis. Furthermore, the levels of IgG4 subclass of MPO-ANCA decreased dramatically after cessation of prophythiouracil, in contrast to primary ANCA associated vasculitis, and this indicated that the production of prophythiouracil-induced MPO-ANCA might be a result of chronic antigen (prophythiouracil) stimulation. The above studies provide substantial evidence that the mechanisms of ANCA production might be different between prophythiouracil-induced vasculitis and primary ANCA associated vasculitis.

2.3 Clinical manifestations

The clinical manifestations of drug-induced vasculitis are similar to those of primary vasculitides, which range from less specific syndromes (fever, malaise, arthralgia, myalgia, weight loss) to single tissue or organ involvement and life-threatening vasculitis. Some researchers suggested that more severe specific organ involvement might develop in patients with non-specific systemic syndrome when the casual drug was not withdrawn in time. The clinical characteristics of drug-induced vasculitis are more likely in the category of MPA and isolated glomerulonephritis (GN) in the published work. Kidney is the most common involved organ and the renal features vary widely, including haematuria, proteinuria and elevated serum creatinine. Intra-alveolar hemorrhage is the most commonly reported pulmonary manifestation with consequent cough, dyspnea and haemoptysis. Some patients may only have lung involvement such as acute respiratory distress syndrome and interstitial pneumonia and without renal injury. Contrary to idiopathic vasculitides, drug-induced vasculitis usually has a milder course, and fewer patients have rapidly progressive GN in drug-induced vasculitis. Rare clinical manifestations were also described in case reports such as sensorineural hearing loss, pericarditis, pyoderma gangrenosum, central nervous system vasculitis presenting as cognitive symptoms and cerebral pachyleptomeningitis.

2.4 Laboratory and histopathology findings

There is no unique clinically pathological or laboratory marker for discrimination between drug-induced vasculitis and other vasculitides. The laboratory abnormalities could indicate organ involvement. Anemia is common in patients with drug-induced vasculitis. Urine abnormalities have consisted of haematuria and proteinuria in patients with kidney vasculitis. Accurate assessment of disease activity within the lungs may be difficult because disease activity correlates poorly with pulmonary symptoms. A plain chest radiograph is a tool to monitor disease activity and high-resolution computed tomography (CT) scanning of the chest offers a more sensitive imaging technique. Although acute-phase reactants such as erythrocyte sedimentation rate (ESR) or C-reactive protein (CRP) are usually elevated in patients with drug-induced vasculitis on diagnosis, they are neither sufficiently sensitive nor specific in making the diagnosis. In some studies, ESR, which was associated with the Birmingham Vasculitis Activity Score, might be a better indicator for disease activity than the titres of ANCA. Laboratory markers, including selected autoimmune serological findings such as ANA, anti-dsDNA and rheumatoid factor among others are commonly used for excluding other diseases or diagnosing other types of vasculitides.

Because detection of ANCA might serve as a warning of the possibility of drug-induced vasculits, ANCA assays using combined IIF and antigen-specific enzyme-linked immunosorbent assays (ELISA) rather than relying on either test alone are recommended in all patients suspected of drug-induced vasculitis. Detection of IgG ANCA is a routine laboratory test, and the presence of high titre IgM MPO-ANCA has also been noted in some cases. Eighty to ninety percent of cases are positive for P-ANCA, and almost all the patients with drug-induced vasculitis had antibodies to MPO rather than PR3. It has been shown that autoantibodies against multiple ANCA antigens might be the characteristic of drug-induced ANCA. Merely ANCA directed to other specific target antigens such as lactoferrin and HLE among others (except MPO and PR3), were found in rare cases. ANCA was also detected in bronchoalveolar lavage fluid (BALF) from a patient with drug-induced interstitial pneumonia. Although ANCA is an important serological marker for certain small-vessel vasculitides, it might not be suitable for monitoring the disease activity of drug-induced vasculitis. After discontinuation of the offending drug, even after immunosuppressive therapy, serum ANCA may still remain positive in remission in the majority of patients with drug-induced vasculitis for up to 5 years, and an increasing of ANCA titres may also occur without overt clinical relapse. Some studies showed that although the levels of MPO-ANCA decreased slowly, other immunological characteristics of MPO-ANCA might change substantially. For example, the avidity of MPO-ANCA could decrease rapidly after withdrawal of medication, indicating that the avidity of anti-MPO antibodies might be a more sensitive serological biomarker to monitor disease activity.

Tissue biopsy is usually necessary to provide a definitive diagnosis of vasculitis and to exclude other diseases. Specimens may come from skin lesions, renal and lung biopsies. Skin lesions are characterized by leucocytoclasia and fibrinoid necrosis of the blood vessels. The renal biopsy is recommended in patients with kidney vasculitis in order to reveal the disease severity and to guide treatment. Typical pauci-immune necrotizing crescentic GN could be identified in patients with drug-induced vasculitis, but not necessarily. Interestingly, it was reported that three out of 14 and seven out of 10 patients with prophythiouracil-induced vasculits had immune complex GN in renal biopsy. Bronchoscopic examination and bronchoalveolar lavage (BAL) can be useful in patients with lung involvement. BAL typically shows neutrophilic alveolitis. Haemosiderin-laden macrophages may be found in BAL..

2.5 Risk for drug-induced vasculitis

In contrast to primary ANCA associated vasculitis, which occurs more often in the elderly, the demographic characteristics of patients with drug-induced vasculitis may reflect the features of the underlying diseases. For example, patients with drug-induced vasculits are younger and predominantly female, which might merely be a reflection of the greater prevalence of thyroid disease in young women. Furthermore, a preponderance of reported cases are from countries in Europe and Asia where the medical community, in sharp contrast to that in the USA, preferentially manages hyperthyroid states with thionamides rather than with radioactive iodine. Long-standing therapy using the offending drug might be a risk factor for developing clinically evident vasculitis. *In vitro*, some studies confirmed that in contrast to short-term treatment with the parent drugs, long-term therapy, which allowed for more extensive generation of the reactive intermediates, resulted in sensitization of T cells to the intermediates. Because the risk of drug-induced lupus was increasing in patients receiving a higher cumulative dose of minocycline and hydralazine, similar results might exist in drug-induced vasculitis; however, there is no data on the cumulative threshold dose of the causal drugs in drug-induced vasculitis.

2.6 How to make a proper diagnosis

Because primary ANCA associated vasculitis is associated with high morbidity and mortality, as well as potentially life-threatening toxicity from immunosuppressive therapy, identification of potentially reversible causes of specific drugs is very important. Failure to recognize the offending drug can lead to fatal organ damage. However, the diagnosis of drug-induced vasculits is complicated and difficult for several reasons, including: (a) physicians often do not recognize the syndrome as drug-induced (inappropriate diagnosis); (b) variable and often prolonged duration between the commencement of therapy and initial vasculitic symptoms; and (c) failure to evaluate appropriate laboratory and invasive tests. The awareness of drug-induced vasculitis by physicians is important in order to make prompt diagnosis and treatment and thus achieving favorable outcomes. It is essential that a comprehensive drug history should be obtained in patients with vasculitis. Clinicians should seek information on drug use for at least 6 months before presentation. The evaluation of pertinent laboratory data and prompt histological confirmation of the disease may aid in the diagnosis. Biopsies are strongly encouraged to confirm the presence of vasculitis3 and to determine the disease severity. Patients with drug-induced vasculitis should fulfilled the 1994 Chapel Hill Consensus Conference definition for ANCA associated vasculitis. We suggest that drug-induced vasculitis should be defined further by the following: (a) the signs and symptoms of vasculitis are temporally related to using the offending drug, and regressed with its discontinuation; (b) serum ANCA is positive, especially those with multi-antigenicity; and (c) medical conditions that mimic vasculitis are excluded, especially infections and malignancies, and other definable types of vasculitis. A low percentage of patients treated long term with a drug risk developing hypersensitivity reactions, some of which appear as vasculitis. There are laboratory markers that can help distinguish drug induced vasculitis from idiopathic autoimmune diseases, and thorough knowledge about such serological changes may help to differentiate drug-induced from idiopathic syndromes (summarized in Table 2).

	Drug-induced vasculitis	SLE	AAV
Antihistone abs.	Can be seen	Rare	Absent
AntidsDNA abs.	Absent	Common	Absent
ANCA	Common[a]	Rare	Common[b]
Antiphospholipid abs.	Common	Common	Rare
Immune complexes	Rare	Common	Absent

SLE, systemic lupus erythematosus; AAV, anti-neutrophil cytoplasmic antibodies-associated vasculitis.
[a] Multispecific.
[b] Single ANCA specificity.

Table 2. Laboratory marker differences between drug-induced vasculitis and idiopathic systemic lupus erythematosus and ANCA associated vasculitis

2.7 Treatment

There is no standard approach to the treatment of drug induced vasculitis. Because the pathogenesis is different between primary and drug-induced vasculitis, the cornerstone of treatment for primary ANCA associated vasculitis, including induction therapy and maintenance therapy with combined corticosteroid and cyclophosphamide, might not be suitable for patients with drug-induced vasculitis. Treatment should be based on individualized assessment in patients with drug-induced vasculitis. Because the offending drugs are involved in the pathogenesis, cessation of the casual drug immediately after diagnosis is essential and might be enough for those with limited to general systemic symptoms. In some case reports, organ involvement such as renal and pulmonary vasculitis could resolve only after discontinuation of the casual drug. However, in another case report, vasculitis worsened in the next 5 months after withdrawal of medication. Furthermore, in the published work it was reported that at least seven patients had died of prophythiouracil-induced vasculitis in spite of intensive immunosuppressive therapy. Therefore, treatment for patients with organ involvement should depend on the severity of clinical manifestations and histopathological lesions. For patients with severe and active organ involvement, intensive immunosuppressive therapy such as corticosteroid and/or immunosuppressive agents could improve organ function and prevent progression to severe, irreversible disease. As shown in Table 3, prednisone should be administered at 1 mg/kg per day for the first 4–8 weeks, followed by a gradual tapering within 6–12 months. Cyclophosphamide (0.6–1.0 g/ month i.v., or 1–2 mg/kg per day p.o.) or mycophenolate mofetil (1.5–2.0 g/day) could be administered for 6–12 months. In addition, patients with severe necrotizing crescentic GN and diffuse pulmonary alveolar hemorrhage should receive pulse methylprednisolone (7–15 mg/kg per day) for 3 days, and patients with life-threatening massive pulmonary hemorrhage may respond to plasmapheresis. It is well accepted that treatment for patients with primary ANCA associated vasculitis comprised both induction and maintenance therapy. However, for patients with drug-induced vasculitis, the duration of immunosuppressive therapy is still inconclusive. The duration of immunosuppressive therapy in patients with drug-induced vasculitis could be much shorter than that in primary ANCA associated vasculitis and that as long as the offending drug was withdrawn, maintenance therapy might not be necessary. Although ANCA detection may provide a clue to the diagnosis of drug-induced vasculitis, positive seroconversion alone may not be a sufficient reason to discontinue the offending drug, because only a small proportion of the patients with positive ANCA will actually develop clinically evident vasculitis. Physicians should carefully monitor those with drug-induced ANCA but without clinical vasculitis. Resolution of most symptoms has generally occurred within 1-4 weeks except for severe organ involvement. Nonspecific symptoms may resolve dramatically only after cessation of the casual drug. However complete resolution of vasculitis occurred in most of the reported cases, some patients do have persistent laboratory abnormalities (elevated serum creatinine, proteinuria) throughout a long-term follow up. As we mentioned before, if necrotizing crescentic GN was present, the patients were at high risk of developing chronic renal failure.

Management of causal agents	
Withdrawal	
Avoid re-challenges	
Consider avoiding similar drug classes	
Individualized therapy	
Non-specific symptoms	Withdrawal of causal agents alone
Organ involvement	Corticosteroid and/or immunosuppressive drugs
Severe organ involvement (e.g. necrotizing glomerulonephritis, focal segmental necrotizing glomerulonephritis, diffuse alveolar hemorrhage)	Methylprednisolone pulse therapy, followed by combined corticosteroid and immunosuppressive drugs
Massive pulmonary hemorrhage	Plasmapheresis
Special notes for patients with drug-induced vasculitis	
A shorter course of immunosuppressive therapy	
Long-term maintenance may not be necessary	
Monitoring of serum ANCA	
Surveillance for emergence of a chronic underlying vasculitis	

AAV, anti-neutrophil cytoplasmic antibodies-associated vasculitis; ANCA, anti-neutrophil cytoplasmic antibodies.

Table 3. Treatment strategy for patients with drug-induced vasculitis

3. Conclusion

The clinician needs to be aware of this risk and quickly stop the offending drug therapy if signs of drug-induced vasculitis develop. In conclusion, patients undergoing treatments with the drugs able to induce vasculitis should be monitored closely during long-term therapy. ANCA is a useful tool to diagnose discontinued immediately after diagnosis. Appropriate immunosuppressive therapy should be administered only for patients with vital organ involvement in order to prevent progression to severe, irreversible disease. The duration of immunosuppressive therapy should be much shorter than that of primary ANCA associated vasculitis and long-term maintenance therapy might not be necessary. Identification of predisposing factors to drug-induced vaculitis may provide insight into the pathogenesis of primary vasculitis. Finally the recommendations for clinicians are:

- Avoid use of the drugs able to induce drug-induces vasculitis in the long term, and patients using long-term treatment with these drugs should be monitored carefully.
- Discontinue the offending drug immediately upon diagnosis of drug-induced vasculitis.
- Individualized immunosuppressive therapy should be initiated according to the severity of organ involvement.
- Adequate documentation of the potentially serious drug-induced reaction in patients' medical records is necessary to avoid re-challenge.

4. References

Doyle, MK.; Cuellar, ML. (2003). Drug-induced vasculitis. *Expert Opin Drug Saf,* Vol.2, No.4, (July 2003), pp. 401–409, ISSN 1474-0338.

Merkel, PA. (2001). Drug-induced vasculitis. *Rheum Dis Clin North Am,* Vol.27, No.4, (November 2001), pp. 849–862, ISSN 1558-3163.

Choi, HK.; Slot, MC.; Pan, G.; Weissbach, CA.; Niles, JL.; Merkel, PA. (2000) Evaluation of antineutrophil cytoplasmic antibody seroconversion induced by minocycline, sulfasalazine, or penicillamine. *Arthritis Rheum,* Vol.43, No.2, (February 2000), pp. 2488–92, ISSN 0004-3591.

Gao, Y.; Zhao, MH.; Guo, XH.; Xin, G.; Gao, Y.; Wang, HY. (2004) The prevalence and target antigens of anti-thyroid drugs induced antineutrophil cytoplasmic antibodies (ANCA) in Chinese patients with hyperthyroidism. *Endoc Res,* Vol.30, No.2, (May 2004), pp. 205–13, ISSN 1532-4206.

Slot, MC.; Links, TP.; Stegeman, CA.; Tervaert, JW. (2005). Occurrence of antineutrophil cytoplasmic antibodies and associated vasculitis in patients with hyperthyroidism treated with anti-thyroid drugs: A long-term follow-up study. *Arthritis Rheum,* Vol.53, No.1, (February 2005), pp. 108–13, ISSN 0004-3591

Jiang, X.; Khursigara, G.; Rubin, RL. (1994). Transformation of lupusinducing drugs to cytotoxic products by activated neutrophils. *Science,* Vol.266,No.5186, (November 1994), pp. 810–13, ISSN 1095-9203.

von Schmiedeberg, S.; Goebel, C.; Gleichmann, E.; Uetrecht J. (1995). Neutrophils and drug metabolism. *Science,* Vol.268,No.5210, (April 1995), pp. 585–6, ISSN 1095-9203.

15

Drug Induced Small Vessel Vasculitis

Jorge Daza Barriga[1], Mónica Manga Conte[2] and Arturo Valera Agámez[3]
[1]*Universidad Libre – Barranquilla, Professor; Neurologist; Neurology Unit Chief, Hospital Universitario CARI ESE; Neuroscience Group Member Caribbean, Universidad Simón Bolivar,*
[2]*Internal Medicine, Visalia Medical Clinic and Kaweah Delta District Hospital, California,*
[3]*Universidad Libre - Barranquilla, Hospital Universitario CARI ESE, Internal Medicine,*
[1,3]*Colombia,*
[2]*USA*

1. Introduction

Vasculitis is the inflammation of a blood or lymph vessel (Merriam - Webster Online Dictionary, 2011). Vasculitis is a broad term used to include a group of syndromes characterized by inflammation, fibrinoid necrosis or formation of granulomas in the blood vessel walls. These can be localized or multifocal, and have different causes and manifestations, depending on the location, size, presence or absence of necrosis. The latter can affect different organs. The vasculitides can be classified as primary or secondary, and are usually a diagnostic challenge for the physician. An open mind and great deal of suspicion is required. Once vasculitis is suspected, a thorough and systematic approach is mandatory. Laboratory tests, imaging studies, and, on occasion, tissue biopsies will help achieve an accurate diagnosis. Its etiology is also diverse (González-Gay et al., 2005) and hence provides the patient with an efficient and appropriate treatment.

Recent advances in technology, with more complete serologic, histochemical, and detailed images, have helped in understanding and differentiating vasculitis from each other. This has resulted in a classification based on etiology, as well as the identification of possible prevention techniques, and strategic treatments.

Medications can induce different side effects, including vasculitis. There are two recognized presentations: Drug Induced Lupus (DIL), and Drug Induced Vasculitis (DIV). These are difficult to separate, and are usually superimposed. Among the latter, one of the most well recognized is Antineutrophil cytoplasmic antibody (ANCA) associated autoimmune disease induced by antithyroid drugs (Aloush V et al., 2006; Bonaci-Nikolic B et al, 2005; Wiik, 2005; Pillinger & Staud, 2006). It has been proposed that neutrophile myloperoxidase (MPO) reacts with propylthiouracil (PTU), transforming this in a sulfa form, which initiates a chain reaction with activation of T lymphocytes, and B lymphocytes that induces vascular inflammation (Aloush V et al., 2006, Pillinger & Staud, 2006). It is interesting to note that, despite the elimination of PTU, the patient may continue having ANCA, and relapses of the

disease (Bonaci-Nikolic B et al., 2005, Aloush V et al., 2006, Bonaci-Nikolic B et al., 2005, Pillinger & Staud, 2006, Choi HK et al., 2000).
This article will focus on the historic evolution of the recognition of vasculitides as an autoimmune entity. We will also describe its pathophysiology, clinical presentation and treatment; paying special attention to drug induced vasculitides. Medications can induce different reactions, from local to systemic ones, including vasculitis. The skin and subcutaneous tissue are common targets, producing rashes and skin discolorations, usually associated with pruritus, edema, and, on occasion, ulceration and necrosis. There might be concomitant arthralgias and myalgias. In these cases, the discontinuation of the medication is recommended, and immunosuppressive therapies are usually required.

2. Epidemiology of small vessel vasculitis

Vasculitides are rare entities, and trustable epidemiologic data is limited. An annual incidence of cutaneous forms in 38.6 cases per million people has been estimated. It is usually most common in women (50.4 cases per million), than in men (26 cases per million). In any case, these are approximations, and likely underestimated, because some of the presentations like leucopenia are considered separately (Watts RA et al., 1998, Watts RA et al., 2000, Tidman, M et al., 1998).
The first publications regarding drug induced vasculitis described reactions by sulfadiazine and hydralazine, and referred to a DIL (Hofman BJ, 1945; Alarcon D, 1967; Scott DGI, 2000). In 1953 it was demonstrated that 7% of patients that took hydralazine for the treatment of hypertension develop DIL. These patients present fever, arthralgias, arthritis, myalgias, and serositis involving the pleura and pericardium. It is more common after prolonged use and in patients with advanced age. Antinuclear antibodies (ANA) are usually positive with a homogenous pattern, and autoantibodies to the nucleosome subunit (H2AH2B)-DNA. These patients rarely develop double stranded DNA antibodies (anti-DNA), which usually happen in DIL by sulphasalazine. The latter patients are usually carriers of HLA DR 0301, which is a recognized predisposing factor for DIL (Bonaci-Nikolic B et al., 2005, Morrow JD et al., 1953, Yung & Richardson 1994).
There are different ANA that are responsible for DIL (Yung &Richardson, 1994; Burlingame & Rubin, 1996; Ayer LM, 1994). These can be directed against MPO, human leukocyte elastase (HLE), catepsin G, lactoferrin and azurocidine, but they all have in common that they affect the neutrophils and monocytes in the perinuclear area (Jennette JC, 2000).
Medications that cause DIL, may also induce DIV, and in both cases there might be compromise of small vessels, the skin, synovial tissues, kidneys and lungs. These further complicates the differentiation between the two (Aloush V et al., 2006, Bonaci-Nikolic B et al., 2005, ,Pillinger & Staud, 2006, Choi HK et al, 2000).
There are two major antigens for the ANCA: MPO and proteinase (PR3) (Zhao MH, 1995). The combination of PR3-ANCA with normal neutrophils fixed with acetone produces a typical cytoplasmic discoloration, and hence the term C-ANCA. The MPO-ANCA induces a perinuclear change known as P-ANCA (Westman K, et al, 2003).
Other drugs that cause DIL and DIV include, but are not limited to: carbamazepine, chlorpromazine, isoniazide, methimazole, alpha methyldopa, mynocicline, phenytoin, procainamide and quinidine (Ullman S. et al, 2004). Similar findings have been described with Etanercept.

ANCA are found also in other conditions, where its role it is not well understood (DeBant et al, 2005), for example: Ulcerative Colitis, Crohn's disease and HIV (Doyle & Cuellar, 2003; Mekel PA, 2001).

3. Historical evolution

The first descriptions were made by Claudio Galeno, when he concluded that some of the peripheral arterial aneurysms that he found were of iatrogenic nature (Litton & Resurh, 1978). These are well written is his book "De tumoribus pareter naturam". Later, in the XVI century Montpellier described vasculitis of infectious origin, specifically related to syphilis (Saporta A, 1624, Cited by Garrison & Morton, 1970). But it was only until the XIX century that vasculitis was recognized as a separate entity (Iglesias et al, 2002). In 1801, William Heberden started describing a vascular purpura (Heberden, 1931). His studies were confirmed and completed in 1837 by Schönlein (Schönlein JL, 1837) and in 1874 by Eduard Henoch (Henoch E, 1868). In 1862, Karl Von Rokitansky proposed that the origin of atherosclerosis is the result of the deposit of material that came from the blood, which subsequently induces arteritis or inflammation (Rokitansky K, 1852). He established that this inflammation started in the external layer or adventicia (Rokitansky K, 1852). The concept of vasculitis was consolidated after the pathological analysis by Rudolf Maier and Adolf Kussmaul (Kussmaul A, 1866). This was the first description and recognition of the polyarteritis nodosa. Around 1827, an association between purpura and abdominal pain was determined. The term Henoch-Schonlein purpura was given (Henoch E, 1868).

It was in the XX century that Osler described a form of vasculitis that included purpura and visceral involvement (Glanzman E, 1920). This was later named Systemic Lupus Erythematosus (SLE). Wegener's granulomatosis was described in 1931. But it was only until 1948 that Douglas Gaaidner proposed that Henoch-Scholein purpura (Klinge F, 1933), acute nephritis, rheumatic fever and polyarteritis nodosa had a common etiology and were associated to an antibody-antigen reaction that occurred at the blood vessel level. Subsequent descriptions of different cases of Wegener's granulomatosis, Churg Strauss syndrome, Kawasaki, Henoch Schonlein, Behcet's, RA, Takayasu's, temporal arteritis and SLE were done (Wegener F, 1990; Hunder GG et al, 1990).

The first descriptions of DIL were recorded in 1945 with the use of sulfadiazine (Hoffman BJ, 1945); and in 1953 with hydralazine (Alarcon Segovia D, 1967; Ullman S et al, 1974; Yung & Richardson, 1994). The presentation was similar to the one of Systemic Lupus Erythematosus: fever, arthritis, myalgias, and serositis with involvement of the pericardium and pleura (Yung & Richardson, 1994).

In 1970, it was determined that DIV and DIL were usually observed in people with HLA DR0301 (Mielke et al, 1993; Gunnarsson I, 2000).

It was in 1973 when it was established that immunosuppressive therapy improved the prognosis of patients with Wegener's granulomatosis (Fauci & Wolff, 1993).

Around 1990, the classification criterion of different vasculitis was established, as well as its therapeutic and diagnostic approach (Churg J, 1991). However, it was in 1994 when simple nomenclature was made. This classified the vasculitis in big vessel vasculitis (giant cell arteritis and Takayasu's); median vessel vasculitis (Polyarteritis nodosa); and small vessel vasculitis (Wegener's granulomatosis, Churg Strauss syndrome, microscopic Poliangeítis, Henoch Schonlein purpura, Vasculitis induced by Cryoglobulins) (Jannette et al, 1994).

Vessel size	Presence of Granuloma.	No Granuloma
Large	Temporal arteritis.	Polyarteritis Nodosa.
	Takayasu's arteritis.	
Medium		Kawasaki's disease
Small	Wegener's Granulomatosis	Microscopic Polyangitis
	Churg Strauss Syndrome	Henoch Schonlein purpura
		Cutaneous leukocytolastic

Table 1. Classification of vasculitis depending on the presence or not of granulomas, by Jennette et al 1994

4. Clinical presentation

Clinical manifestations vary as well as the organs affected. In general, it depends on the cause, localization, the size of the vessel affected, and the degree of ischemia. Symptoms commonly found are: purpura, erythema, urticaria, vesiculobullous lesions, superficial ulcers, splinter hemorrhages, scleritis, episcleritis, uveitis, neutrophilic granulomatous dermatitis, glomerulonephritis, gastric colic, pulmonary hemorrhage, constitutional symptoms. When the compromise is in the middle of medium-caliber vessels, we find subcutaneous nodules, deep ulcers, livedo reticularis, digital gangrene, mononeuritis, aneurysms, and ischemic lesions (Iglesias Gamarra A, et al, 2006).

As we have stated, the most common skin manifestations are: Urticaria, edema, petequias, exanthema, livedo reticularis, purpura, vesicles or ulcerations. The distribution varies, affecting the extremities, trunk or both (Iglesias Gamarra A, et al, 2006).

If there is damage of the muscular vessels, a myopathy may develop with myalgia, weakness and elevation of CK and LDH (Iglesias Gamarra A, et al, 2006).

It is common to see a prodromal presentation of non specific symptoms like general malaise, weight loss, fever and night sweats. Specific symptoms develop once a major organ is affected. For example, in Wegener's granulomatosis, there is compromise of the upper and lower airways and the kidneys. Similarly, the kidneys are affected in microscopic polyangitis. This results in hematuria, proteinuria and kidney failure. The lower airways affection may result in pulmonary hemorrhage, which is fatal if not recognized and treated in a timely manner (Iglesias Gamarra A, et al, 2006).

In Churg Strauss the clinical presentation is often mistaken as asthma exacerbations. Chest x rays show transitory pulmonary infiltrates, and eosinophils are very elevated in blood. There might appear concomitant cutaneous vasculitis, as well as gastrointestinal abnormalities with abdominal pain and symptoms that can be confused with irritable bowel syndrome (Iglesias Gamarra A. et al, 2006).

Polyarteritis nodosa is less frequent, but more severe and devastating. It causes ischemic infarcts of various organs, which can induce to hemorrhage, specially the in bowel, pancreas and gallbladder. Urinary tract compromise is seen in 50% of the patients, but it is uncommon to have severe kidney insufficiency (Jennette JC, 1994).

In general, the gold standard diagnostic test for vasculitis is tissue biopsy that demonstrates fibrinoid necrosis with vascular inflammation. Common sources are the nose, lungs, skin or kidneys. Serological tests are also important in helping define the type of vasculitis (Iglesias Gamarra A, et al, 2006; Jennette JC, 1994).

In drug induced vasculitis, small vessels are usually affected. The histopathological findings are similar to other types of vasculitis. And this is usually considered a diagnosis of exclusion. Non specific symptoms are present as described above, including fever, weight loss, arthralgias and myalgias. Skin changes are frequently seen, like purpuric lesions, vesicles and bullae, urticaria and splinter hemorrhages. More severe cases may present with glomerulonephritis, alveolar hemorrhage, uveitis and scleritis. The syndrome might resolve in weeks after the drug has been discontinued. However in rare cases it might become persistent, especially in those with ANCA positive. There are no specific laboratory findings, eosinophilia is present in 79% of cases, ESR and CRP are commonly elevated. Hence, biopsy is mandatory (Jennette JC, 1994).

5. Laboratory findings

1. Complete blood counts and erythrosedimentation rate: Anemia is a common finding, usually normocytic, normochromic. Platelets are usually elevated, as is ESR. White blood cell counts are of extreme importance, since leucopenia is usually the limiting factor with immunosupression.
2. Chemistries: To assess renal (BUN, creatinine, eGFR), hepatic (Liver function tests) and muscular (CK, aldolase, LDH) compromise.
3. Creatinine is used to evaluate kidney function. An urianalysis is required to diagnose glomerular involvement, in which case proteinuria and hematuria are found. Kidney function is also a prognosis factor.
4. Chest X rays, to look for lung involvement or pulmonary nodules.
5. Electromyography (EMG) to assess nuropathy and neuritis.
6. ANCA: Anti PR3 and anti MPO are present in 90% of the Wegener's granulomatosis.
7. Cryoglobulins and complement levels (C3 and C4).
8. Hepatitis B, and C, which might be the underlying cause of cryoglobulins.
9. Angiograms to evaluate vascular compromise in Takayasu's artritis.

6. Histopathology

There is an inflammatory response, manifested as a cellular infiltration with subsequent wall vessel damage. Inflammation results in leukocytosis, and may end in vascular necrosis. When the latter occurs and becomes chronic, granulomas are usually present.

Fibrinoid necrosis is characterized by replacement of the vascular wall by eosinophils, fibrinogen deposits, immunoglobulins. In general, there is leucocyte destruction, but lynfocites might also be affected.

This results in immunoproliferative vasculitis. All the above findings make biopsy necessary. The skin, respiratory tract (either superior or inferior) and kidneys are the most frequently biopsied. Approximately 20% of cases of cutaneous vasculitis represent an adverse drug eruption and most will represent so-called hypersensitivity vasculitis (CLA) and exhibit a superficial dermal, small-vessel neutrophilic vasculitis or lymphocytic vasculitis (Carlson & Chen, 2006; Carlson & Chen, 2007). Identification of tissue eosinophilia in these biopsies is a clue to a drug etiology (Bahrami S, 2006). Pharmacological classes involved in drug-induced vasculitis are: 1. an ANCA-associated group, such as propylthiouracil, hydralazine, allopurinol, minocycline, penicillamine, and phenytoin; 2. an ANCA-negative group, such as colony-stimulating factors, isotretinoin, and methotrexate

(Holder SM et al, 2002). Identifying the offending drug is the most important aspect of treatment as its discontinuation is followed by a rapid improvement in the vasculitis in many cases.

7. Small vessel vasculitis

Small vessel vasculitis comprises a heterogeneous group of diseases and syndromes. To facilitate its understanding, they are classified as follows:

1. Immune complex mediated:
   1.1 GoodPasture's.
   1.2 Leucocitoclastic angitis.
   1.3 Henoch Schonlein Purpura.
   1.4 Urticarial Crioglobulinemia.
2. ANCA associated vasculitis:
   2.1 Wegener's granulomatosis.
   2.2 Microscopic polyangitis.
   2.3 Churg Strauss.
   2.4 Kidney vasculitis.
   2.5 Secondary vasculitis.
3. Miscelaneous:
   3.1. Connective tissue disorders (Rheumatoid vasculitis, SLE, Sjogren and inflammatory myopathies).
   3.2 Paraneoplastic syndromes.
   3.3 Infections.
   3.4 Drug induced.

8. Drug induced vasculitis mechanism

As stated above, the mechanism with which a medication can induce a vasculitis varies, and different ones have been established. The presentation of the disease also differs depending not only on the type, but also on genetic factors, geographic regions, age, sex, and race.
Clinically it is difficult to differentiate between drug induced and small vessel vasculitis. Skin manifestations are the most common in DIV, which ranges from a maculopapular rash to a palpable purpura. There might be concomitant arthralgias, arhthritis, kidney and liver compromise, as well as central nervous system affection (Molina J et al ,2000).
The duration of the process is also variable. It may resolve in a few weeks after discontinuation of the culprit agent, or persist afterwards. This is especially true in ANCA positive cases.
Again, DIV is a diagnosis of exclusion, and can only be made once other types of vasculitis, infections and malignancy have been ruled out (Jennette & Falk, 1997). There is no diagnostic test available. Eosinophilia is present in 79% of the cases (Jennette & Falk, 1997; Calabrese LH et al, 1990). A biopsy is usually required, and the list of medications taken in the last 6 months reviewed.
Treatment includes the discontinuation of the medication and immunosuppressive agents.
Patients with idiopathic vasculitis, more commonly develop ANCA to one neutrophil antigen, whereas in DIV it is usual to find several (Calabrese LH et al, 1990, Savige J et al 2000).

When used, anti-TNF agents can induce DIV. Cases have been described of antibodies against double stranded DNA when infliximab is used (Buttman et al, 2005).
Procainamide and Hydralazine share a structure similar to the nucleosome, which can induce an immunogenic reaction. This results in the formation of antibodies similar to the ones found in SLE. These drugs can also cause a direct toxicity by its metabolics, which inhibit DNA methyltransferase and induces autoimmunity (Carlson et al, 2005).
Interferon is a naturally found protein in the human immune system. There are three known types: alpha, gamma and lambda. The production of interferon is induced by interleukins and TNF. Different types of cells produce interferon: T and B cells, macrophages, fibroblasts, endothelial cells and osteoblasts. They constitute and important mechanism of defense against viruses, stimulating macrophages and natural killer cells. In synthesis, interferon prevents the viral replication and induces the destruction of infected cells. It was in the 80's when using DNA recombinant technology that interferon was produced massively. This is commonly used in the treatment of certain cancers, hepatitis C and B, as well of multiple sclerosis among others. It is given as an intramuscular injection. Frequent adverse reactions include: flu like symptoms, fever, myalgia, general malaise, headaches, and rarely seizures. Depression is also observed (Wiik, A 2008; O'Sullivan et al 2006). Most of the side effects are reversible, once treatment is completed (O'Sullivan et al 2006, Coppola G, 2006). Autoimmune side effects are rare. The induction of antithyroglobulins, sarcoidosis, diabetes and arthritis has been described. Buttmann proposed three possible mechanisms (Coppola G, 2006, Buttmann et al, 2005):

1. Quimiotactic effect of the immune system cells.
2. Direct effect over immune cells.
3. Indirect effect over immune cells through induction of proinflammatory substances.

9. Therapeutic approach

The conventional treatment of systemic vasculitis was introduced by Wolfe and Fauci in the 1970's with the use of cyclophosphamide and steroids (Fauci & Wolff, 1973). This consists of a year of induction with cyclophosphamide and 4 weeks of pulse dose steroids. After the initial 4 weeks, the steroids are gradually tapered. However, the toxicity of oral cyclophosphamide is high, with a mortality rate ranging from 14 - 20%. Common side effects are Myelodisplastic syndromes (8%), Neoplasia (4.5%), severe infections (26%) (Hogan SL, 2005; Koldingsnes & Nossent H, 2002; Mukhtyar C, 2009).
Due to the above, new strategies have been proposed with the purpose of reducing the overall accumulation. Currently, the parenteral approach is more commonly used with a dose of 0.6 mg/m2 (Reinhold-Keller et al, 2000).
Mycophenolate mofetil (MMF) is an alternative. It is an immunosuppressive agent; inosine monophosphate dehydrogenase (IMPDH) 23 inhibitor (Huang Y, 2005). MMF is rapidly absorbed following oral administration and hydrolyzed to form MPA, which is the active metabolite. MPA is a potent, selective, uncompetitive, and reversible inhibitor of inosine monophosphate dehydrogenase (IMPDH), and therefore inhibits the de novo pathway of guanosine nucleotide synthesis without incorporation into DNA. Because T- and B-lymphocytes are critically dependent for their proliferation on de novo synthesis of purines, whereas other cell types can utilize salvage pathways, MPA has potent cytostatic effects on

lymphocytes. MPA inhibits proliferative responses of T- and B-lymphocytes to both mitogenic and allospecific stimulation. The addition of guanosine or deoxyguanosine reverses the cytostatic effects of MPA on lymphocytes. MPA also suppresses antibody formation by B-lymphocytes. MPA prevents the glycosylation of lymphocyte and monocyte glycoproteins that are involved in intercellular adhesion to endothelial cells and may inhibit recruitment of leukocytes into sites of inflammation. Once remission is achieved, maintaining it is a challenge (Joy M et al, 2005; Stassen P, 2005). The ultimate goal is to minimize the toxicity.

In drug induced vasculitis, the first step is the discontinuation of the medication. If there is potentially fatal compromise, steroids and cyclophosphamide should be given. Different approaches have been described. In the first one, cyclophosphomide is administered in monthly boluses for 6 months, then every 3 months for 2 years. The alternative is to give the monthly boluses for 6 months, and then use azathioprine daily for 2 years (Klemmer PJ et al, 2003). Methorexate might be used for maintenance, too.

10. Case presentation

We had the case of a 42 year old woman with a history of multiple sclerosis (MS) diagnosed 9 years ago. Three years after the diagnosis was established, she was initiated on Beta Interferon 1a. Two years later, she developed non pruritic, palpable purpura in her lower extremities with subsequent ulceration and edema. Biopsy was consistent with vasculitis (Daza JS, 2008). She was then treated with high dose steroids, with poor response, and then started on cyclophosphamide. Beta interferon was discontinued. Resolution of the lesions was obtained.

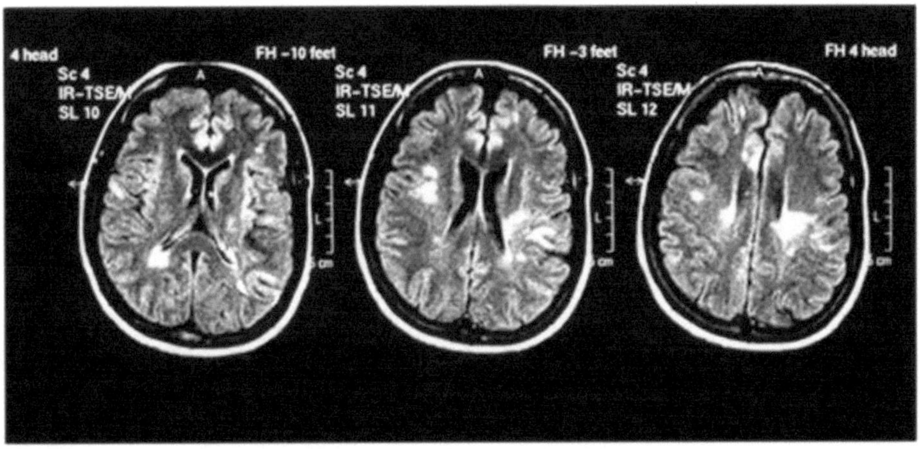

Fig. 1. MRI flash fair image: hyperdense lesions in the yuxtacortical area bilaterally, as well as in the semioval centre and periventricular matter.

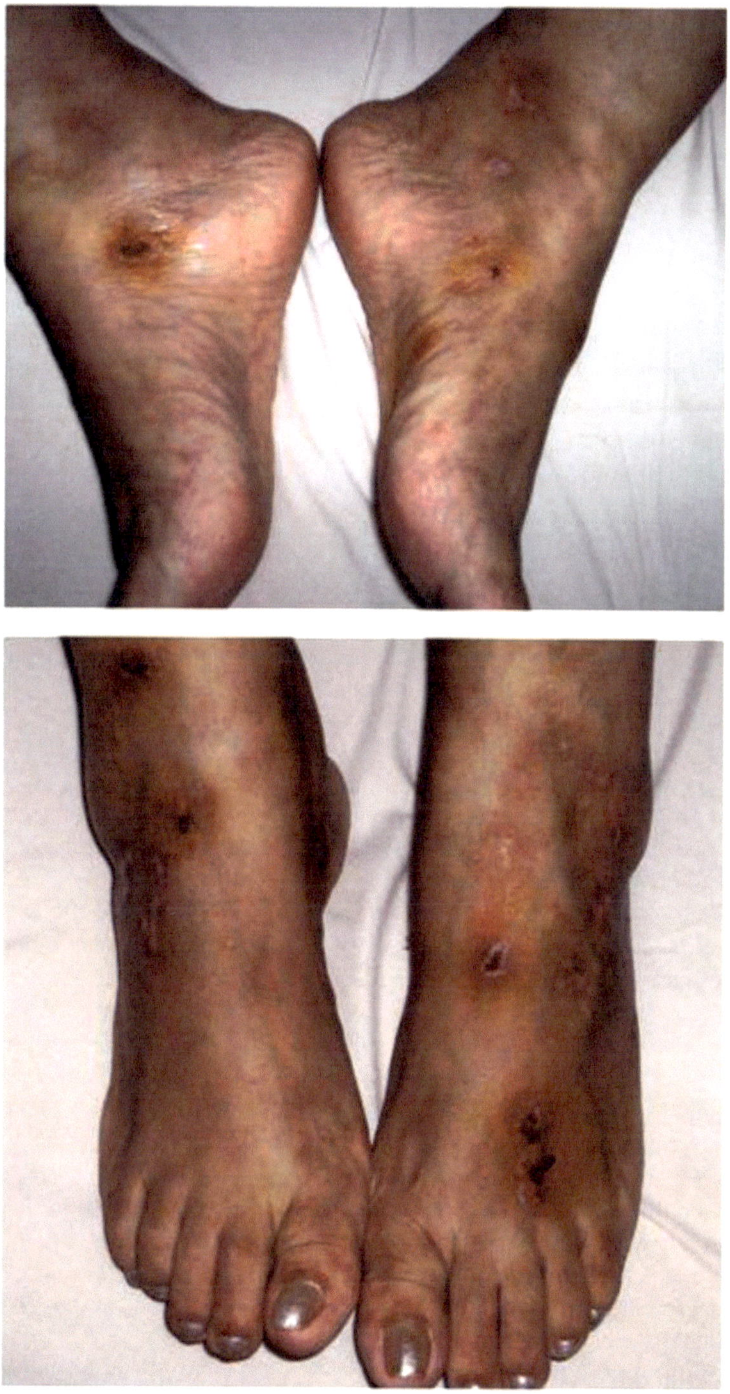

Fig. 2. and 3. In our clinical case lesions are seen in different stages of evolution, some necrotic and scarred other areas hyper pigmentation at the ankle and dorsum of the foot that correspond to areas of vasculitis

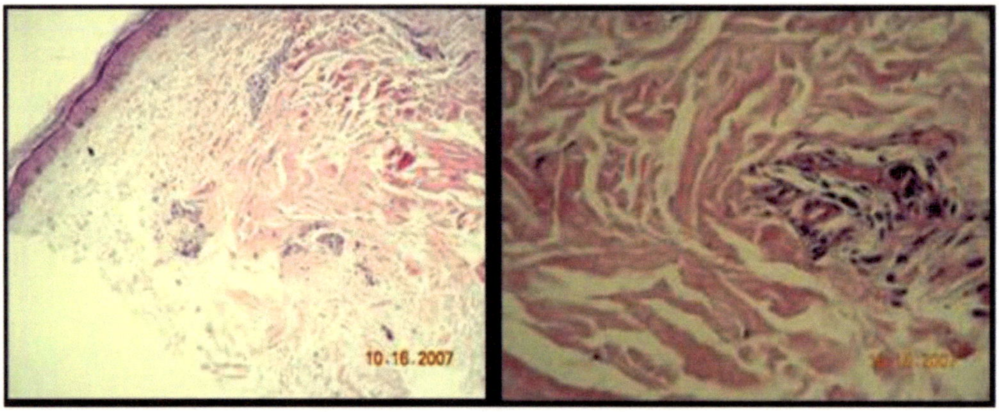

Fig. 4. Skin with preserved epidermis. Superficial and medial dermis with minimal edema. Small vessels with prominent endothelial cells; some of them obstructing the lumen. The wall vessels appears with fibrinoid exudates, neutrophils and debris. Above findings are compatible with small vessel vasculitis of the lower extremities.

The frequency of MS and vasculitis together is exceptional. This was first published in 1998. It has been hypothesized that these reactions are related to the presence of antibodies against interferon beta, which usually increase during the appearance of the lesions, and decrease with their resolution (Szilasiová J, 2003; Daza JS, 2008).

11. Conclusion

Vasculitis is a group of diseases characterized by vascular inflammation, which results in decrease of blood flow, and blood vessel wall damage. Any vessel may be affected, as well as one or several organs.

In drug induced vasculitis, small vessels are usually affected. Again this is a diagnosis of exclusion. The diagnosis is a clinical one, with the support of serologic and histological findings. The clinical manifestations are similar to the other vasculitis. The skin, subcutaneous tissue, kidneys and lungs are most commonly affected. C-ANCA antibodies are usually positive. Interferon is a protein naturally produced by the immune system as a response to viruses or malignant cells. Interferon beta is a biological product obtained by DNA recombination techniques, and is used for treatment of MS. Immune complications with this therapy are rare.

In the article, a patient treated for multiple sclerosis with interferon was presented. She developed vasculitis, which was later determined to be caused by Interferon, and was treated accordingly with the scheme depicted above.

The use of any medication opens the possibility to complications and reactions. It is the role of the physician to determine when the benefits outweigh the risks, and once the treatment has been established, close follow up is required.

Drug induced vasculitis, although rare, are not exceptional and should be included in the differential diagnosis of any vasculitis.

Research is needed, to learn which patients have higher possibilities to develop drug induced vasculitis, so screening methods can be designed to avoid such medications in susceptible individuals.

12. References

Alarcon Segovia D, Wakim KG, Worthington JW, et al (1967). Clinical and experimental studies on the hydralazine syndrome and its relationship to systemic lupus erythematosus. *Medicine* Vol. 46, pp 1-6. ISSN on line 1536- 5964

Aloush V, Litinsky I, Caspi D, Elkayam O (2006). Propylthiouracil-induced autoimmune syndromes: two distinct clinical presentations with different course and management. *Semin Arthritis Rheum* Vol.36, pp 4-9. ISSN 0049 0172

Ayer LM, Rubin RL, Dixon GH, et al (1994). Antibodies to HMG proteins in patients with drug-induced autoimmunity. *Arthritis & Rheum* Vol.37, pp 98-103. ISSN 1529 0131

Bonaci-Nikolic B, Nikolic MM, Andrejevic S, et al (2005). Antineutrophil cytoplasmic antibody (ANCA)- associated autoimmune diseases induced by antithyroid drugs: comparison with idiopathic ANCA vasculitides. *Arthritis Res Ther* Vol. 7:R1072-R1081. ISSN electronic 1478 6362

Burlingame RW, Rubin RL (1996). Autoantibody to the nucleosome subunit (H2AH2B) - DNA is an early and ubiquitous feature of lupus-like conditions. *Mol Biol Rep* Vol. 23, pp 159-166. ISSN electronic 0301-4851

Bahrami S, Malone JC, Webb KG, et al (2006). Tissue eosinophilia as an indicator of drug-induced cutaneous small-vessel vasculitis. *Arch Dermatology* Vol. 142 (2) pp 155-61. ISSN (electronic): 0096-5359

Buttmann M, Goebeler M, Toksoy A, Schmid S, Graf W, Berberich-Siebelt F, et al (2005). Subcutaneous interferon-beta injections in patients with multiple sclerosis initiate inflammatory skin reactions by local chemokine induction. *J Neuroimmunol* Vol. 168 pp 175-82. ISSN 0165 5728

Calabrese LH, Michel BA, Bloch DA, Arend WP, Edworthy SM, Fauci AS, et al (1990): The American College of Rheumatology 1990 criteria for the classification of hypersensitivity vasculitis. *Arthritis Rheum* Vol. 33 pp 1108 ISSN 1529 0131

Carlson JA, Ng BT, Chen KR (2005) cutaneous vasculitis update: diagnostic criteria, classification, epidemiology, etiology, pathogenesis, evaluation and prognosis. *Am J Dermatopathol.* Vol.27 (6) pp 504-28 ISSN on line 1533 0311

Carlson JA, Chen KR (2006). Cutaneous vasculitis update: small vessel neutrophilic vasculitis syndromes. *Am J Dermatopathol* Vol 28 (6) pp 486-506. ISSN on line 1533 0311

Carlson JA, Chen KR (2007). Cutaneous vasculitis update: neutrophilic muscular vessel and eosinophilic, granulomatous, and lymphocytic vasculitis syndromes. *Am J Dermatopathol* Vol. 29 (1) pp 32-43. ISSN on line 1533 0311

Churg J (1991). Nomenclature of vasculitic syndromes: a historical perspective. *Am J Kidney Dis* Vol. 18 pp 148-153 ISSN 0272 6386

Choi HK, Merckel PA, Niles JL (2000). Drug-associated antineutrophil cytoplasmatic autoantibody-positive vasculitis: prevalence among patients with high titers of antimyloperoxidase antibodies. *Arthritis Rheum* Vol. 43 (2) pp.405-413 ISSN 1529-0131

Coppola G, Lanzillo R, Florio C, Orefice G, Vivo P, Ascione S, et al (2006). Long-term clinical experience with weekly interferon beta-1a in relapsing multiple sclerosis. *Eur J Neurol* Vol. 13 pp 1014-1021 ISSN 1468-1331

Daza-Barriga JS (2008). Vasculitis de vasos pequeños asociada al uso de interferón beta-1a en la esclerosis múltiple. *Rev Neurol* Vol. 46 (11) pp 702-703. ISSN 1576-6578

DeBandt M, Sibilia J, Le Loe¨t X, et al (2005). Systemic lupus erythematosus induced by antitumour necrosis factor alpha therapy: a French national survey. *Arthritis Res Ther* Vol. 7:R545–R551 ISSN electronic 1478 6362

Doyle MK, Cuellar ML (2003). Drug-induced vasculitis. *Expert Opin Drug Saf* Vol. 2 pp 401–409 ISSN 1474 0338

Fauci AS, Wolff SM (1973). Wegener's granulomatosis: Studies in eighteen patients and a review of the literature. *Medicine (Baltimore)* Vol. 52 pp 535–61 ISSN 1536- 5964

Glanzmann E (1920). Die Konception der anaphylaktoiden Purpura. *Jahrb Kinderh Berl* Vol. 91 pp 391-431.

González-Gay, MA, Garcia-Porrua C, Pujol RM (2005). Clinical approach to cutaneous vasculitis. *Curr Op Rheumatol*, vol. 17, pp 56. ISSN 1040 8711

Gunnarsson I, Nordmark B, Bakri H, et al (2000). Development of lupus-related side effects in patients with early RA during sulphasalazine treatment. The role of IL-10 and HLA. *Rheumatology (Oxford)* Vol. 39 pp 886–893 ISSN on line 1462 0332

Heberden W (1801). Commentarii de Marlbaun. *Historia et curatione*. London, T. Payne.

Henoch E (1868). Zusammenhang von purpura and Intestinalstorungen. *Berl. Klin Wchnschr*, 5: 517

Hoffman BJ (1945). Sensitivity to sulfadiazine resembling acute disseminated lupus erythematosus. *Arch Dermatol Syphilol*; 51:190–192 ISSN 0022 202X

Hogan SL, Falk RJ, Chin H, Cai J, Jennette CE, Jennette JC, et al (2005). Predictors of relapse and treatment resistance in antineutrophil cytoplasmic antibody- associated small-vessel vasculitis. *Ann Intern Med.* Vol 143 pp 621–318. ISSN on line 1539 3704

Holder SM, Joy MS, Falk RJ (2002). Cutaneous and systemic manifestations of drug-induced vasculitis. *Ann Pharmacother* Vol. 36 (1) pp 130-47. ISSN on line 1060 0280

Huang Y, Liu Z, Huang H, Liu H, Li L (2005). Effects of mycophenolic acid on endothelial cells. *Int Immunopharmacol* Vol. 5 pp 1029–39. ISSN 1567 5769

Hunder GG, Arend WP, Bloch DA, Calabrese LH, Fauci AS, Fries JF, et al (1990). The American College of Rheumatology 1990 criteria for the classification of vasculitis: introduction. *Arthritis Rheum* Vol. 33 pp 1065-1067. ISSN on line 1529 0131

Iglesias Gamarra A, Restrepo Suarez JF, Valle R., Osorio E., et al (2002). Historia de las vasculitis. *Rev Col de Reumt.* Vol. 9 No. 2, pp. 87-121. ISSN 0121 5426

Iglesias Gamarra A; Cantillo Turbay J.; Restrepo Suárez J (2006). Análisis crítico de las clasificaciones de las vasculitis. *Rev Col de Reum Vol.* 13 (1), pp. 48-64 ISSN 0121 5426

Jennette JC, Falk RJ, Andrassy K, Bacon PA, Churg J, Gross WL, et al (1994). Nomenclature of systemic vasculitides: proposal of an international consensus conference. *Arthritis Rheum* Vol. 37 pp 187-192. ISSN on line 1529 0131

Jennette JC (1994). Pathogenic potential of anti-neutrophil cytoplasmic autoantibodies. *Lab Invest* Vol. 70 pp 135-137. ISSN 1530 0307

Jennette JC, Falk RJ (1997). Small-vessel vasculitis. *N Engl J Med* Vol. 337 pp 1512-23. ISSN 1533 4406

Jennette JC, Wilkman AS, Falk RJ (1998). Diagnostic predictive value of ANCA serology. *Kidney Int.* Vol. 53 pp 796-8 ISSN 1523 1755

Joy M, Hogan S, Jennette J, Falk R, Nachman P (2005). A pilot study using mycophenolate mofetil in relapsing or resistant ANCA small vessel vasculitis. *Nephrol Dial Transplant* Vol. 20(27), pp 25–32. 40. ISSN on line 1460 2385

Klemmer PJ, Chalermskulrat W, Reif MS, Hogan SL, Henke DC, Falk RJ (2003). Plasmapheresis therapy for diffuse alveolar hemorrhage in patients with small-vessel vasculitis. *Am J Kidney Dis* Vol. 42 pp 1149–53. ISSN 0272 6386

Klinge F (1933). Der Rheumatismus: pathologisch-anatomische und experimentell-pathologische Tatsachen und ihre Auswertung für das ärztliche Rheumaproblem. *Ergebn Allg Pathol Anat* Vol.27 pp 243-254.

Koldingsnes W, Nossent H (2002). Predictors of survival and organ damage in Wegener's granulomatosis. *Rheumatology (Oxford)* Vol. 41 pp 572–81. 9. ISSN 1462-0332

Kussmaul A, Maier R (1866). Ueber eine bisher nicht beschriebene eigenthümliche Arterienerkrankung (Periarteritis nodosa), die mit Morbus Brightii und rapid fortschreitender allgemeiner Muskellähmung einhergeht. *Deutsche Arch Klin Med* Vol. 1 pp. 484-518. ISSN 0003 4819

Litton DG & Resurh LM (1978). Galen on Abnormal Swellings. *J Hist Med Allied Sci* Vol 34 (4) pp 531-549 Online ISSN 1468-4373

Merkel PA (2001). Drug-induced vasculitis. *Rheum Dis Clin North Am*; 27:849–862. ISSN 0889-857X

Merriam - Webster Online Dictionary, 2011. Definition of vasculitis.

Mielke H, Wildhagen K, Mau W, et al (1993). Follow-up of patients with doublestranded DNA antibodies induced by sulfasalazine during treatment of inflammatory rheumatic diseases. *Scand J Rheumatol*; 22:299–301. ISSN electronic 1502 7732

Molina J, Alarcon D, Molina R J, Anaya J, Cardiel M (2000). *Fundamentos de Medicina, Reumatología*. CIB, pp 274-289. ISBN 958-9400-82-5.

Morrow JD, Schroeder HA, Perry HM Jr (1953). Studies on the control of hypertension by Hyphex. II. Toxic reactions and side effects. *Circulation*; 8:829–839

Mukhtyar C, Guillevin L, Cid MC, Dasgupta B, de Groot K, Gross W, et al (2009). EULAR Recommendations for the management of primary small and medium vessel vasculitis. *Ann Rheum Dis*; 68:310–7. ISSN on line 1468 2060

O'Sullivan SS, Cronin EM, Sweeney BJ, et al (2006). Panniculitis and lipoatrophy after subcutaneous injection of interferon beta-1b in a patient with multiple sclerosis. *J Neurol Neurosurg Psychiatry* Vol. 77 pp 1382-1383. ISSN electronic 1468 330X

Pillinger MH, Staud R (2006). Propylthiouracil and antineutrophil cytoplasmic antibody associated vasculitis: the detective finds a clue. *Semin Arthritis Rheum* Vol. 36 pp 1–3. ISSN 0049 0172

Reinhold-Keller E, Beuge N, Latza U, De Groot K, Rudert H, No¨ lle B, et al (2000). An interdisciplinary approach to the care of patients with Wegener's granulo- matosis: Long-term outcome in 155 patients. *Arthritis Rheum*; 43 pp 1021–32. ISSN 1529 0131

Rokitansky K (1852). Ueber einige der wichtigsten Krankheiten der Arterien. Denkschr Akad der Wisseensch. *Wien, Hof Staatsdrukerei*. Vol.4(1)

Savige J, Davies D, Falk RJ, Jennette JC, Wiik A (2000). Antineutrophil cytoplasmic antibodies and associated diseases: a review of the clinical and laboratory features. *Kidney Int* Vol. 57 pp 846-62

Saporta A. De tumoribus paeter naturam, (Ravaud, Lyons 1624). Cited by Garrison. F. H. and Morton, L.T.: *A medical bibliography;* 3rd ed. (Deutsch, London 1970). No. 2971, the manuscrip is from 1554.

Scott DGI, Watts *RA (2000).* Systemic vasculitis*:* Epidemiology, classification and environmental factors. *Ann Rheum Dis Vol. 59 pp. 161-3. ISSN on* line *1468 2060*

Schönlein JL. Allegemeine und specielle (1837). Pathologie and Therapie. *St. Gallen,* 1837; 2: 42

Stassen P, Cohen Tervaert J, Stegeman C (2007). Induction of remission in active anti-neutrophil cytoplasmic antibody-associated vasculitis with mycophenolate mofetil in patients who cannot be treated with cyclophosphamide. *Ann Rheum Dis* Vol. 66 pp 798–802. ISSN 1468 2060

Szilasiová J, Gdovinová Z, Jautová J, Baloghová J, Ficová M, Bohus P (2009). Cutaneous vasculitis associated with interferon beta-1b treatment for multiple sclerosis. *Clin Neuropharmacol.* Vol. 32(5) pp 301-3 ISSN on line 1537-162X

Tidman M, Olander R, Slavender C, et al (1998). Patients hospitalized because of small vessel vasculitis renal involvement in the period 1975 - 1995: organ involvement, anti-neutrophil cytoplasmic antibodies patterns, seasonal attack rates and fluctuation of annual frequencies. *J Intern Med, pp* 133 – 41. ISSN on line 1365 2796

Ullman S, Wiik A, Kobayasi T, et al (1974). Drug-induced lupus erythematosus syndrome. Immuno-pathological, electronmicroscopical and serological studies. *Acta Derm Venereol* Vol. 54 pp 387–390. ISSN 0001 5555

Watts RA, Jolliffe *VA,* Grattan *CE, et al (1998). Cutaneo*us vasculitis in a defined population-clinical and epidemiological associations. *J Rheumatol* Vol. 25 pp 920-4. ISSN on line 1499 2752

Watts RA, Lane SE, Bentham G, et al (2000). Epidemiology of systemic vasculitis: A ten-year study in the United Kingdom. *Artritis Rheum* Vol. 43 pp 422-7. ISSN on line 1529 0131

Wegener F (1990). Wegener's granulomatosis: thoughts and observations of a pathologist. *Eur Arch Otorhinolaryngol* Vol. 247 pp 133-142. ISSN on line 1434 4726

Westman K, et al (2003). High Proteinase 3–anti–neutrophil cytoplasmic antibody (ANCA) level measured by the capture enzyme-linked immunosorbent assay method is associated with decreased patient survival in ANCA-associated vasculitis with renal involvement. *J Am Soc Nephrol* Vol.14 pp 2926–2933. ISSN 1533 3450

Wiik A (2005). Clinical and laboratory characteristics of drug-induced vasculitic syndromes. *Arthritis Res Ther* Vol. 7 pp 191–192. ISSN On line 1478 6362

Wiik A (2008). Drug-induced vasculitis. *Current Opinion in Rheumatology* Vol. 20 pp 35–39 ISSN 1040 8711

Yung RL & Richardson BC (1994). Drug-induced lupus. *Rheum Dis Clin N Am* Vol. 20 pp 61–85. ISSN 1558 3163

Zhao MH, Jones SJ, Lockwood CM (1995). Bactericidal/permeability-increasing protein (BPI) is an important antigen for antigen-neutrophil cytoplasmic autoantibodies (ANCA) in vasculitis. *Clin Exp Immunol* Vol. 99 pp 49-56 ISSN 0749 0690

16

Hepatitis C Related Vasculitides

Reem H. A. Mohammed[1] and Hesham I El-Makhzangy[2]
[1]*Department of Rheumatology and Rehabilitation,*
[2]*Department of Tropical Medicine, Faculty of Medicine, Cairo University Hospitals,*
Egypt

1. Introduction

Vasculitides comprise a heterogeneous group of autoimmune diseases sharing the common histopathologic feature of inflammation and fibrinoid necrosis of the blood vessel walls. Vasculitis features a wide variety of clinical manifestations depending on the localization and the size of the vessels involved, type of inflammatory infiltrate, and associated conditions making the diagnosis of specific forms of vasculitis difficult. The classification of the vasculitis remains a matter of controversy. Some classification systems have focused on the size of the vessels, while others have been based on histologic findings, yet an overlap of vessels of various sizes may occur, also the type of inflammatory infiltrate may change over time. Epidemiologic factors including; age, gender and ethnic background, patterns of organ affection, histopathologic and serologic features represent potential considerations while establishing the diagnosis and classification of vasculitis. The etiologic factors associated with the triggering of vascular endothelial injury and inflammations are quite variable with an unrecognized clear etiology in almost 50% of the cases. (Pipitone and Salvarni, 2006)
The interest in infection related vasculitides has been boosted for the last two decades by the development of new molecular techniques. Currently, a causal relationship between hepatitis C virus (HCV) and vasculitis has been established. (Falk and Hoffman, 2007) Chronic hepatitis C viremia has been known to provoke a plethora of autoimmune syndromes, as well as nonspecific rheumatologic manifestations referred to as extra-hepatic manifestations of HCV. Such extra-hepatic syndromes have been reported in as much as 40-90% of the chronic HCV infected patients, with a variable clinicopathological and serological spectrum that ranges between nonspecific serological abnormalities to manifest clinical disease with subsequent affection of multiple organs and systems. Established associations include; mixed cryoglobulinaemia (MC), complete or incomplete MC syndrome, porphyria cutanea tarda, significant associations include; autoimmune hepatitis, B cell non Hodgkin's lymphoma, monoclonal gammopathies, possible association include; chronic polyarthritis, sicca syndrome, lung fibrosis, polyarteritis nodosa, poly/dermatomyositis, thyroiditis/thyroid cancer, diabetes mellitus, lichen planus, mooren corneal ulcers. (Kattab et al., 2010, Mohammed et al., 2010)

2. Natural history and epidemiology of hepatitis C virus infection

Hepatitis C virus infection is a major worldwide public health problem. The estimated global worldwide reservoir is almost 200 million or 3% of the global population. Hepatitis C virus is a retrovirus, member of the genus hepacivirus of the flaviviridae family enveloped with a 9.6 kb single-stranded RNA genome. Six different viral genotypes of HCV have been identified. The sero-prevalence of each of these genotypes varies according to geographic distribution; genotype 1 has a worldwide distribution, genotype 2 being more common in western Africa and genotype 3 in the northern Indian subcontinent, with a sero-prevalence rate of less than 1% in Western Europe and 2-3% in some Mediterranean areas. Regional geographic heterogeneity in the sero-prevalence rate can exist within the same country (in the USA, genotype 1 infection is significantly more prevalent in the northeastern, southeastern and middlewestern areas than in patients from the west and south). African-Americans are more likely to be infected with genotype 1 than Caucasians. Genotype 4 is predominant in the Middle East and Africa, genotype 4 is spreading in Western countries, especially among intravenous drug users. Genotype 5 is predominant in South Africa and genotype 6 in South-East Asia. Mixed cryoglobulinemia (MC), is considered the most highly associated and characteristic extrahepatic feature in HCV infection. (Mohammed et al., 2010) In HCV infected patients 30- 98% have cryoglobulinemia. Overt cryoglobulinaemic syndrome develops in 5-20% of patients. (Antonelli et al., 2009) The incidence of HCV infection in mixed cryoglobulinemia ranges from 40 to 90% and tests for viral genome concentrations in the cryoprecipitate might be as high as 1000 fold that of supernatant. (Ferri et al., 2002 a, Sansonno et al., 2007).

3. Mixed cryoglobulinemia

Mixed cryoglobulinemia (MC) is a chronic immune complex (IC) mediated systemic small vessel vasculitis, characterized by immune complex deposits (cryo-deposits) and frequent multiple organ involvement. A frequent synonym of this disease is "cryoglobulinemic vasculitis", a term that focuses on the typical histo-pathological alterations responsible for muco-cutaneous and visceral involvement. (Agnello, 1995) The term cryoglobulinemia refers to the presence of a single component (monoclonal) or more (polyclonal) immunoglobulins. These immunoglobulins typically precipitate at temperatures below 37°C giving rise to high molecular weight aggregates and re-dissolve on rewarming. Cryoglobulins are found in small quantities in normal serum and are present in variable concentrations in many pathological conditions, including myeloproliferative disorders, autoimmune disorders and several infectious diseases. They are classified on the basis of their Ig component into: Type I cryoglobulins (10-15% of cryoglobulins) is comprised simply of monoclonal immunoglobulins, typically IgM but less frequently IgG, IgA, or serum light chains. Individuals with Type I cryos typically have a paraproteinemia (e.g., myeloma, Waldenstrom's macroglobulinemia). Type II cryoglobulins (50-60% of cryoglobulins) occurs when a monoclonal Ig M recognizes and binds to polyclonal IgG's, accordingly, type II cryos are typically IgM-IgG complexes .Type III cryoglobulins (30-40% of cryoglobulins) are composed of polyclonal Ig M that binds to polyclonal IgG. Type II & III cryoglobulinemia are referred to as "Mixed Cryoglobulinemia", these are the types most commonly associated with hepatitis C. (Dammaco et al., 1997). The term essential cryoglobulinemia was used to describe cryoglobulinemia without identifiable underlying disease, currently it is clear that most of the patients with essential mixed cryoglobulinemia are chronically infected with HCV (Sansonno et al., 2007) **Table 1**

Cryoglobulins	Composition	Pathology	Clinical associations
Type I Cryoglobulins	Monoclonal Ig, (IgG, or IgM, or IgA) self-aggregation through Fc fragment of Ig	Histopathology of underlying disorder	Lympho-proliferative disorders: MM, WM, CLL, B-cell NHL
Type II MC	Monoclonal IgM (or IgG, or IgA) with RF activity (often cross-idiotype WA-m RF) + Polyclonal Ig (mainly IgG)	-leukocytoclastic vasculitis. + - B lymphocyte expansion.	- Infections (mainly HCV, HBV, HIV) - Autoimmune/lympho-proliferative disorders. - Rarely, essential
Type III MC	Polyclonal mixed Ig (IgG, IgA, IgM) + RF activity of one polyclonal component (usually IgM)	-leukocytoclastic vasculitis. + -B-lymphocyte expansion with tissue infiltrates.	- Autoimmune disorders. - Infections (HCV, HBV, HIV) - Rarely 'essential'
Type II-III Variant of MC	Oligoclonal IgM RF or Mixture of poly/ monoclonal IgM (often cross-idiotype WA-mRF)	-leukocytoclastic vasculitis. + -B-lymphocyte expansion with tissue infiltrates	- Infections (mainly HCV) - Autoimmune/lympho-proliferative disorders - Rarely 'essential'

MM;multiple myeloma, WM; Waldenstrom macroglobulinemia, CLL; chronic lymphocytic leukemia, B-NHL; B cell Non-Hodgkin's Lymphoma

Table 1. Classification of Cryoglobulins. (Ferri, 2008)

3.1 Etio-pathogenesis of mixed cryoglobulinemia with HCV infection

Combined Viral and host-related factors contribute to the pathogenesis of HCV-related MC and lymphoproliferative disorder.

3.1.1 HCV infection of hepatocytes

The HCV life cycle starts with virion attachment to its specific receptor on hepatocytes. Several candidate molecules have been suggested to play a role in the receptor complex, including tetraspanin CD81, the scavenger receptor BI (SR-BI), the adhesion molecules DC-SIGN and L-SIGN, the low-density lipoprotein (LDL) receptor and recently, the tight junction components claudins (mainly CLDN-1,CLDN-6 and CLDN-9) have been identified as additional key factors for HCV infection. The HCV RNA genome serves as a template for viral replication and as a viral mRNA for viral production. In addition, the HCV enzymes-NS2-3 and NS3-4A proteases, NS3 helicase and NS5BRdRp—are essential for HCV replication, and are therefore potential future therapeutic targets.The activity of liver disease associated with cryoglobulinemic vasculitis is usually mild suggesting the existence of a state of immune tolerance between virus and host. At the same time the virus provokes a state of persistent high viremia necessary for circulating immune complex formation, essential for the activation of vasculitic inflammatory reaction. (Racanelli et al., 2001)

3.1.2 HCV and B lymphocytes

It is believed that HCV infects B lymphocytes (BL) in the same way it infects hepatocytes due to the shared expression of CD81 receptors. HCV induces lowering of lymphocyte activation threshold leading to chronic lymphocyte stimulation and widespread autoantibody production. (Ferri et al., 2000) The proposed etio-pathogenic mechanisms in HCV- mixed cryoglobulinemia, involves the following:

3.1.2.1-HCV-viral iymphotropism

The characteristic genome variability and viral lymphotropism of HCV cause prolonged and sustained antigen stimulation of B cell compartment, mainly exerted by E2 protein (highly variable region 1 HVR1) that allows distinguishing different, but strictly virus related genomic variants called quasispecies (Zignego and Brechot, 1999) and expresses B cell immunodominant epitopes involved in viral neutralization. Viral E2 region is able to directly interact with B-lymphocytes through tetraspanin CD 81 lowering the lymphocytes activation threshold (Pileri et al., 1998) with subsequent clonal expansion of the rheumatoid factor (RF) IgM/k producing lymphocytes (Agnello et al., 1992). The idiotypic similarities shared by mRFs from different patients with ttype II MC syndrome that correspond with a restricted set of rearranged immunoglobulin (Ig) genes that encode mRFs (IGHV1-69, IGHV3-23, and IGKV3-20 are associated with the WA CRI, IGHV3-7), suggesting that a specific antigen contributes to development of type II mixed cryoglobulinemia. Persistent and prolonged stimulation of B lymphocytes induces genetic modifications that play a key role in the evolution of lymphoproliferative disorders (LPD), passing from a physiologic polyclonal activation to a mono-oligo-clonal expansion characteristic of MC until the frank monoclonality of B cell lymphoma. In HCV related non-Hodgkin's Lymphomas malignant monoclonal B cells produce an Ig M with rheumatoid factor activity and highly homologus to anti-E2 antibodies. (De Vita et al., 2000)

3.1.2.2 Impaired apoptosis of B lymphocytes

HCV-dependent gene translocation leads to Bcl-2 recombination, activation of this anti-apoptotic protoncogene protects B lymphocyte from apoptosis triggering sustained B lymphocyte proliferation, autoantibody production, and oligoclonal monotypic lymphoproliferations with cells expressing oligo or monoclonal IgM sharing rheumatoid activity (mixed cryoglobulins). Recent studies highlighted the existence of an elevated frequency of proto-oncogene bcl-2 rearrangement [t(14;18) translocation] with altered bcl-2/bax ratio in subjects affected by chronic HCV infection. High levels of Bcl-2 protein expression have been detected in bone-marrow and liver infiltrates of HCV infected patients with cryoglobulinemia upon histopatological analysis. (Zignego et al., 2002, Giannini et al., 2008)

3.1.2.3 B- Lymphocyte somatic hypermutations (SHM)

Sequence analysis of rearranged Ig heavy chain genes within hepatic lymphoid infiltrates of patients with type II MC syndrome confirmed the presence of monoclonal or oligoclonal B-cell populations with sustained clonal somatic hypermutations (SHM) generating intra-clonal diversity in infilterates. SHM enhances antibody affinity for a particular antigen by introducing nucleotide substitutions within the immunoglobulin variable (IgV) genes of germinal center (GC) B-cells. Genetic mutation arising from aberrant SHM has been proposed to contribute to B-cell NHL (e.g mutation in 5'-untranslated region of protooncogenes like PIM-1, PAX-5, RhoH/TTF, and c-myc). The bcl-6 (B cell lymphoma-6) proto-oncogene is a transcriptional repressor gene that prevents the terminal differentiation of mature B cells to plasma cells and promotes proliferation of B lymphocytes. Bcl-6 is recently recognized as another target of SHM in GC B- cells in patients with HCV infection. In vitro studies suggest that genetic mutations in HCV infected cells arise from induction of error prone DNA polymerase activity by HCV infection. (De Vita et al., 2002, Machida et al., 2004)

3.1.3 Cytokines and soluble factors

Cytokines play a central role in the immune response to viral agents. Increased intrahepatic levels of interleukin (IL)-2, IL-6 and IL-8 were demonstrated by RT-PCR in cirrhotic patients. **(Napoli et al., 1994)** In vitro studies showed that HCV, through the action of its NS5A protein, induces expression of Toll like receptors 4(TLR4), leading to enhanced IFN-β and IL-6 production and secretion. Members of the TNF-superfamily appear to play a relevant role in B cell expansion during chronic HCV infection. The two new members of the TNF-superfamily (B-lymphocyte stimulator-BLyS and APRIL- a proliferation inducing ligand) proved to play a crucial role in the control of humoral immunity. The binding of BLyS to its receptors (TACI and BLyS-R) induce strong B cells proliferation and extended survival via the strong activation of the antiapoptotic bcl-2 gene. Overexpression of BLyS in transgenic mice induced expansion and accumulation of mature B cells, high levels of serum IgG and IgM, and glomerulonephritis. BLyS, and its homologue APRIL, are now considered the main regulators of T-independent B-lymphocyte proliferation and autoimmunity. (Gross et al., 2000, Stein et al., 2002, Fabris et al., 2007, Sene et al., 2007)

3.1.4 HCV infection and T cell regulatory function (T reg)

The T-lymphocyte compartment was recently identified to acquire a distinct subset of lymphocytes with immune-regulatory properties named "regulatory T cells" (Treg). Treg. play a central role in modulating the immune response targeting infectious agents, in maintaining self-tolerance and lymphocyte homeostasis.(Sakaguchi, 2000) CD4+CD25+ T cells (T reg S) and "type 1 T regulatory cells" (Tr1) account for 5-10% of the CD4+ pool in normal subjects, they constitutively express CTLA-4 (CD152), and are anergic following in vitro TCR stimulation (partially reversed with high amounts of IL-2 and IL-15). The forkhead transcription factor Foxp3 is specifically expressed in CD4+CD25+ regulatory T cells and is required for their development and function. Several mutations within the Foxp3 gene alter CD4+CD25+ development, retroviral gene transfer of Foxp3 converts naive T cells toward a regulatory T cell phenotype similar to that of naturally occurring CD4+ regulatory T cells. "Type 1 T regulatory cells" (Tr1) are CD4+CD25-, which display a unique profile of cytokine production that is distinct from that of Th0, Th1 or Th2 cells and conversely to CD4+CD25+ they secrete high amounts of IL-10 and TGF-beta which in turn suppress naive and memory Th1 and Th2 responses, Such immune-dysregulation might contribute to chronic HCV viremia and cryoglobulin production. Patients with HCV-MC vasculitis were found to have a disturbed peripheral blood T cell repertoire, with a high frequency of T cell expansions. (Fontenot et al., 2003)

A role for C1q auto-antibodies has been reported in HCV infected patients. C1q receptor is overexpressed at sites of inflammation. C1q-R exacerbates inflammation by generating vasoactive peptides from the complement system and bradykinin from the contact system. HCV core protein interacts directly with the globular domain of C1q protein (gC1q-R).

Engagement of circulating HCV core protein with gC1q-R on the surface of B lymphocytes provides the virus with a direct means of affecting host immunity. Recently, there is also evidence of an important role of vascular cell adhesion molecule-1 (VCAM-1) a molecule exclusively involved in mononuclear cell recruitment, in the pathogenesis of severe forms of HCV-MC vasculitis. (Kittlesen et al., 2000, Kaplanski et al., 2005)

3.1.5 Paracrine/soluble factors

Other paracrine/soluble factors might be involved in the pathogenesis of HCV-related MC. The analysis of global protein pool (proteomic analysis) in sera and peripheral blood mononuclear cells (PBMC) samples represents a promising approach for identify new tumor markers, identification of post-translational modifications, protein-protein interactions, protein level expression, protein networks. (Leak et al., 2002) Figure 1

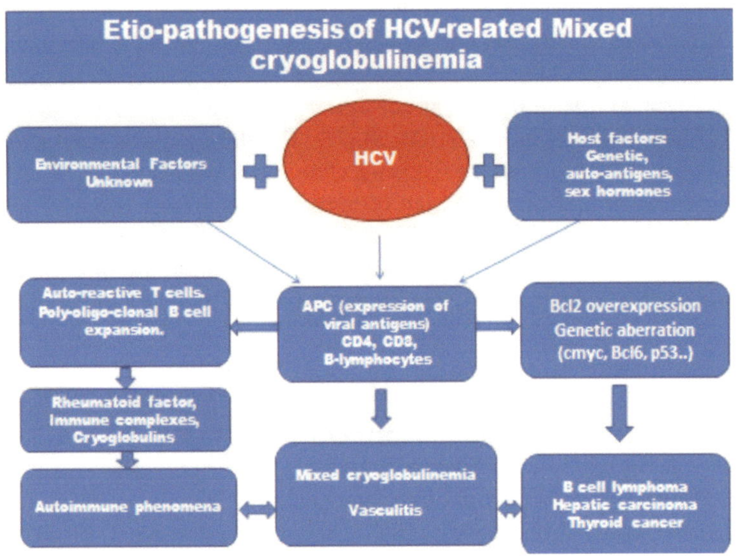

Fig. 1. Etiopathogenesis of HCV-Mixed Cryoglobulinemia

3.2 Mechanism of cryoglobulin production

The intrinsic mechanism by which HCV promotes cryoglobulin production remains unclear. It is postulated that upon initial antigenic stimulation, it is the interaction between HCV and lymphocytes that directly modulates B and T cell functions. Initial polyclonal activation and expansion of CD5þ cells (major source of IgM RF) occurs in type III mixed cryoglobulinemia. This is followed by the emergence of a single dominant clone of B lymphocytes with the production of monoclonal IgM RF. This clonal heterogeneity of IgM rheumatoid factor defines type II-type III variants which is considered a transitional stage in the switch between type III to type II MC. In HCV infection mixed cryoglobulins are predominantly type II cryoglobulins. (Sasso, 2000, Newkirk, 2002) Cryoglobulins interact with HCV forming immune complexes composed of HCV, anti-HCV polyclonal IgG and monoclonal IgM sharing Rheumatoid factor (RF) activity.

The presence of IgM RF in this megacomplex (cryoprecipitate complex) provides an obstacle to the incorporation of complement factor C3b into this complex. The incorporation of this C3b is important as it allows binding of the immune complex to CR1 erthrocyte surface receptor required for immune complex neutralization. Thus this immune complex escapes neutralization by erythrocyte. HCV induces abnormalities in the biogenesis of lysosomal enzymes impairing the capacity of monocytes to digest engulfed immune complexes a phenomena described as "phagocyte blockade". Failure of neutralization promotes the cryo-complex to circulate freely in an abundant form saturating the phagocyte ability to remove such immune complexes from the blood and creating a state of mixed cryoglobulinemia. This complex can easily deposit in tissues and promote inflammatory cascade. (Ferri et al., 2002 a, Sasso, 2000) The exact mechanisms leading to cryoprecipitation remain unclear. Different hypotheses have been proposed to explain this phenomenon, namely: (1) structural modification of the variable portions of Ig heavy (H) and light (L) chains; (2) a reduced concentration of sialic acid; (3) reduced amounts of galactose in the Fc portion of the Ig4; and (4) the presence of *N*-linked glycosylation sites in the CH3 domain as a result of somatic Ig mutations during autoimmune responses. (5) Specific interactions between the IgM cryoprecipitable rheumatoid factor (RF) and the Fc portion of IgG, the corresponding autoantigen. (6) Occupancy of the Fc portion of IgG by IgM molecules is probably a major factor in the functional properties of immune complexes (ICs). They are large ICs known to be poor acceptors of C3 and C4, and deplete complement rather than fix it. Precipitation of these cryocomplex in the small blood vessels leads to cryoglobulinemic vasculitis. (Curry et al., 2003, Ferri, 2008, Saadoun et al., 2007)

3.3 Pathology in cryoglobulinemic vasculitis

The classic pathology in cryoglobulinemic vasculitis is leukocytoclastic vasculitis, a form of immune mediated small vessel vasculitis with immune complexes deposit in the walls of small blood vessels. This is associated with activation of the complement cascade and the production of C5a (a neutrophil polymorph chemotactant). The resultant polymorph influx is associated with release of lysosomal enzymes, including elastases and collagenases, resulting in blood vessel wall damage, fibrin deposition and the release of red blood cells into the perivenular connective tissue (palpable purpura). Thrombosis with epidermal ischemic damage is not uncommon. High levels of circulating immune complexes which correlated with vasculitic lesions can be detected. Immunoglobulins and complement were identified in vitro, by immunofluorescence or immune-peroxidase techniques, visualized ultra-structurally as clumps of electron-dense material, usually within the basement membrane between endothelial cells and pericytes of post-capillary venules. Examination of apparently uninvolved skin from patients with leukocytoclastic vasculitis sometimes shows immunoglobulin and complement within the walls of dermal blood vessels. The findings of immunofluorescence studies vary according to the age of the lesion. Immunoglobulins have been described in up to 81% of patients in early lesions, C3 and Ig M predominate, in fully developed lesions there is predominance of fibrinogen and Ig G and in late lesions fibrinogen and C3. (Stone, 2009)

4. Cryoglobulinemic vasculitis, the disease

HCV-related mixed cryoglobulinemia represents a form of small vessel vasculitis which manifests by a variety of autoimmune manifestations referred to as cryoglobulinemic syndrome. The cryoglobulinemic syndrome typically presents by Meltzer triad which is a triad of purpura, weakness, arthralgia and/or arthritis, thereafter, a series of multisystem pathologies follow. Meltzer triad has been reported in 25-30% of patients with mixed cryoglobulinemia. Widespread vasculitis involving medium-small sized arteries, capillaries and venules with multiple organ involvement may develop in a small proportion of patients (Meltzer et al., 1996, Ferri et al., 2004, Ferri et al., 2006).

4.1 Frequency

4.1.1 United states

The prevalence of essential mixed cryoglobulinemia is reported as approximately 1:100,000. However, the exact prevalence of HCV related MC depends upon the geographic heterogenity of HCV infection.

4.1.2 International

The prevalence of mixed cryoglobulinemia is related to the endemic presence and geographic heterogeneity of HCV infection. The disease is more common in Southern Europe than in Northern Europe or Northern America. The incidence of HCV infection in mixed cryoglobulinemia in the Mediterranean Basin is 90%. A growing incidence of HCV-related MC is observed especially in developing countries. HCV is endemic in some countries of the middleeast. Egypt has an exceptionally high prevalence of HCV infection estimated to be between 10% and 15% of its' 75 million population. The annual infection rate is more than 70, 000 new cases of which at least 35, 000 would have chronic hepatitis C, with viral genotype 4 the predominant genotype being isolated in up to 91% of HCV infected persons in Egypt. In a recent research conducted on 306 Egyptian patients with chronic HCV infection the prevalence of MC amongst other extrahepatic manifestation was 0.7%.

4.2 Predisposing factors

4.2.1 Race

Mixed cryoglobulinemia doesn't appear to have any specific racial predilection.

4.2.2 Age

Reported age range between 30-70 years (mean age reported 42-52 years).

4.2.3 Hormonal factors

The female-to-male ratio in mixed cryoglobulinemia is 3:1, female sex is considered one of the risk factors for developing extra-hepatic manifestations. Recent studies revealed an association between female gender and the presence of certain manifestations including fibromyalgia, cryoglobulinemic syndrome, autoimmune hemolytic anemia and arthritis. (Mohammed et al., 2010, Stefanova Petrova et al., 2007)

4.2.4 Genetic factors

HLA-B8 and DR3 may be considered risk factors for HCV-related MC in addition to cirrhosis. Recent data suggest that the HLA- phenotype B8 and DR3 are associated with increased risk of developing mixed cryoglobulinemia in HCV infected patients with the strongest association being with HLA-B8. Patients exhibiting the B8-DR3 phenotype may carry the C4A deletion, which might contribute to the low C4 levels measured in a proportion of MC patients in addition to complement consumption by the disease process itself. Preliminary results on C4 allotyping in MC patients showed an increased frequency of C4AQ0 phenotype, thus suggesting a possible role of class III molecules in increasing the susceptibility to MC in HCV patients. (Ferri, 2008, Lenzi et al., 1998)

4.3 Criteria for the classification of mixed cryoglobulinemia

In 1989, the Italian group for the study of cryoglobulinemia has proposed preliminary criteria for the classification of MC. A revised version of these criteria including clinic-pathological and serological findings has been recently proposed, Criteria displayed in Table 2. (Ferri, 2008)

Criteria	Major	Minor
Serological	Mixed cryoglobulins Rheumatoid factor+ Low C4	Rheumatoid factor HCV + HBV +
Pathological	Leucocytoclastic vasculitis	Clonal B cell infiltrates (liver and/or bone marrow)
Clinical	Purpura	Chronic hepatitis Membrano-proliferative glomerulonephritis Peripheral neuropathy Skin ulcers

HCV+ or HBV+: markers of hepatitis C virus or hepatitis B virus infection (anti-HCV ±HCV RNA; HBV DNA or HBV surface antigen).
"Definite" mixed cryoglobulinaemia syndrome:
(a) Serum mixed cryoglobulins (±low C4) + purpura + leucocytoclastic vasculitis.
(b) Serum mixed cryoglobulins (±low C4) + 2 minor clinical symptoms + 2 minor serological/pathological findings.
"Incomplete" or "possible" mixed cryoglobulinaemia syndrome:
(a) Mixed cryoglobulins or low C4 + 1 minor clinical symptom + 1 minor serological ±pathological findings.
(b) Purpura and/or leucocytoclastic vasculitis + 1 minor clinical symptom + 1 minor serological ±pathological findings.
(c) Two minor clinical symptoms + 2 minor serological ± pathological findings.
"Essential" or "secondary" mixed cryoglobulinaemia:
Absence or presence of well known disorders (infectious, immunological, or neoplastic) at the time of the diagnosis.

Table 2. Classification Criteria for Mixed Cryoglobulinemia

4.4 Clinical picture of cryoglobulinemic vasculitis and related autoimmune syndromes

4.4.1 Skin involvement

Skin is the most commonly affected target organ in cryoglobulinemic vasculitis. The classical pattern in mixed cryoglobulinemia is cutaneous leukocytoclastic necrotizing vasculitis. (lee et al., 1998, Leon et al., 2002)

4.4.1.1 Purpura

The most commonly reported clinical feature of MC is palpable purpura. Palpable purpura manifests in as much as 70-90% of patients. Lesions are typically seen on the lower legs because of hydrostasis and blood vessel flow sludging, lesions might extend to the abdominal wall and less frequently to the trunk and upper limbs. The purpuric rash might acquire a petechial, papular, seldom necrotic aspect, and it can be compounded to erythematous maculae and dermal nodules. Lesions might be associated with other dermatological symptoms like upper malleolar ulcers as well as urticarial vasculitis. (Antonelli et al., 2009)

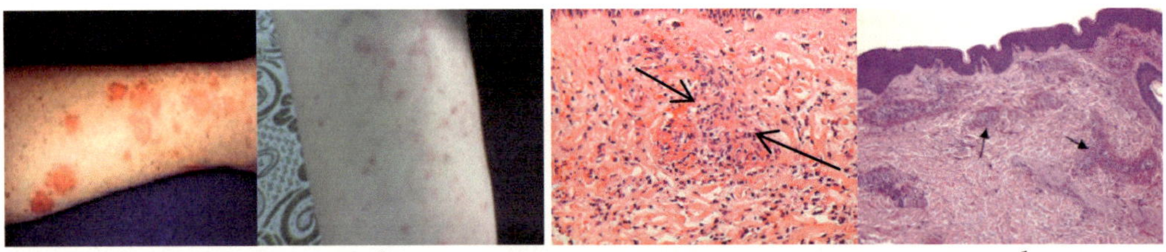

a b c d

Fig. 2. a- Cutaneous leukocytoclastic vasculitis in mixed cryoglobulinemia patient, b- Palpable purpura with cutaneous leukocytoclastic vascultitis in a female patient with cryoglobulinemic syndrome. c- Nuclear dust associated with a perivascular neutrophilic infiltrate. d- Leukocytoclastic vasculitis (black arrows point to small blood vessels in the subcutaneous tissue with perivascular leukocytes).

Histopathological examination: Skin biopsy is optimally performed by 24-48 hours after the appearance of the lesion. Biopsies should be obtained from non-ulcerated site. Light microscopic examination reveals that the cellular infilterate is composed of a combination of neutrophils and lymphocytes with a predominance of one cell type or another. Lymphocyte infilterates are seen in specimens from either new (<12 hours) or old (>48 hours) lesions. The typical histolopathologic features from cutaneous vasculitic lesions involve the disruption of blood vessels architecture by an inflammatory infilterate in and around the vessel walls. Endothelial swelling and proliferation, leukocytoclasis (characteristic degranulation of neutrophils with the production of nuclear dust), might be accompanied by extravasation of erythrocytes. The severity of the histo-pathological changes in the cutaneous lesions of leukocytoclastic vasculitis does not predict extra-cutaneous involvement. Direct immunofluorescence (if sufficient lesions exist, separate biopsies are recommended for histology and DIF). DIF helps to differentiate pauci-immune and immune complex mediated vasculitis. In DIF frozen sections are incubated with flourescein labeled anti human immunoglobulin (Ig) IgG, IgM, IgA and complement 3. The staining pattern of these immune-reactants provides insight into the diagnosis, the pathophysiology of the lesions and the autoantibody components of the immune complexes. (Stone, 2009, Antonelli et al., 2009)

Other cutaneous features of HCV-MC include; Ischemic necrosis (0-20%), Livedoid vasculitis (14%), cold-induced urticaria (10%), hyperkeratotic spicules in areas exposed to cold, scarring of tip of nose, pinnae, fingertips, and toes, raynaud's phenomenon, acrocyanosis which might evolve to digital ulceration might occur (Saadoun et al., 2007), and nail-fold capillary abnormalities. (Antonelli et al., 2009, Ferri, 2008)

4.4.2 Musculoskeletal involvement

Musculoskeletal complaints are present in as much as 70-80% of the cryoglobulinemic patients, with arthralgia in 40-80% of cases, frank arthritis occurs in less common < 10% of cases. Joint affection in MC is usually bilateral, symmetrical, non-deforming, affecting mainly large articulations, knees and hands, less commonly elbows and ankles with no radiographic evidences of joint destruction in HCV-MC related arthritis. RF activity is present in 70-80% of MC patients. Joint involvement can occur in the absence of RF seropositivity. (Lee et al., 1998, Mohammed et al., 2010) Antibodies to citrullinated C peptide (highly specific for rheumatoid arthritis) usually aren't significantly present. Myalgias, fibromyalgia, weakness and chronic fatigue are more frequent in cryoglobulin-positive than in cryoglobulin-negative HCV patients with recent evidences revealing higher prevalence of fibromyalgia and chronic fatigue syndrome with elevated fatigue score in HCV female patients. The elevated fatigue score is probably related to an increase in serum leptin levels which might interact with serotonin neurotransmission. Polymyositis is not uncommon. (Sene et al., 2006, Wener et al., 2004)

4.4.3 Neurological involvement

Neurological involvement in HCV-mixed cryoglobulinemia commonly presents by vasculitic peripheral neuropathy (subacute, chronic or acute on top of chronic). The pattern of affection ranges from pure sensory axonal neuropathy to mononeuritis multiplex. The most frequently described form is distal sensory or sensory motor polyneuropathy. Motor deficit is inconsistent, predominantly affecting the lower limbs appearing after sensory affection. The sensory involvement is usually bilateral commonly asymmetrical, with parasthesias and burning pain having characteristic nocturnal exacerbation. Polyneuropathies represent 40-70% of mixed cryoglobulinemic neuropathy, whereas mononeuritis multiplex represents 30-55% of cases. Nerve conduction studies show predominantly axonal neuropathy affecting mainly the sensory nerves. Nerve biopsies reveal axonal degeneration, differential fascicular loss of axons, signs of demyelination and small vessel vasculitis with mononuclear cell infilterate in the perivascular area, HCV-RNA was found in epineural cells by reverse transcriptase polymerase chain reaction (RT-PCR). (Authier et al., 2003) Central nervous system involvement in patients with HCV-associated vasculitis is rare. (Dawson et al., 1999) Clinical presentations might be in the form of transient ischemic attacks, stroke, progressive reversible ischemic neurological deficits, lacunar infarcts, pseudotumor cerebri or encephalopathic syndrome. Magnetic resonance imaging studies are consistent with ischemic injury, with either small lesions of the periventricular white matter and the cerebral trunk or extensive supra and infra-tentorial white matter lesions diagnostic of cerebral vasculitis predominantly small sized vessel vasculitis. Neurocognitive impairment and Guillian-Barre syndrome can exist. (Casato et al., 2005, Heckmann et al., 1992)

4.4.4 Renal Involvement in HCV-mixed cryoglobulinemia syndrome:

Renal involvement in HCV-infected patients occurs in 10-60% of cases (**figure 6**). The most commonly repoted form is cryoglobulinemic membranoproliferative glomerulonephritis. Less common forms of renal involvement include; non-cryoglobulinemic membranoproliferative glomerulonephritis, Ig A nephropathy, postinfectious glomerulonephritis, membranous nephropathy, thrombotic microangiopathies, focal and segmental glomerulosclerosis, fibrillary or immunotactoid glomerulopathy. Cryoglobulinemia is present in almost 100% of patients with HCV- nephropathy. Renal involvement in HCV-MC is an immune complex mediated nephropathy (deposition in the glomerulus of immune-complexes made by the HCV antigen, anti-HCV Ig G antibodies, and a rheumatoid factor, which is an IgM kappa), usually in the form of type I membrano-proliferative glomerulonephritis (MPGN). Such pattern of organ involvement severely affects the prognosis and survival of patients with HCV-mixed cryoglobulinemia. Renal disease in most cases, is a subsequent event to the cutaneous lesions (purpura), and might be associated with other extrahepatic manifestations like arthralgia and neuropathy. The commonest renal manifestation is asymptomatic proteinuria with microscopic hematuria, renal function is usually normal. In one quarter of patients there is nephritic syndrome, with macroscopic hematuria, proteinuria, hypertension, and increased serum creatinine. Hypertension develops in almost 80% of cases and often difficult to control. Occasionally, there is proteinuria in nephrotic range. The renal course of mixed cryoglobulinemia is variable; glomerular lesions usually have a more benign course than idiopathic membranoproliferative GN. Moderate renal insufficiency occurs in up to 50% of patients. Chronic renal failure develops years after the onset in approximately 10% of cases, oliguric or anuric renal failure develops in <5% of patients. There is hypo-complementemia in most of cases, but usually it is more marked for C4, with C3 slightly decreased or normal. (Garini et al., 2005, Kamar et al., 2006)

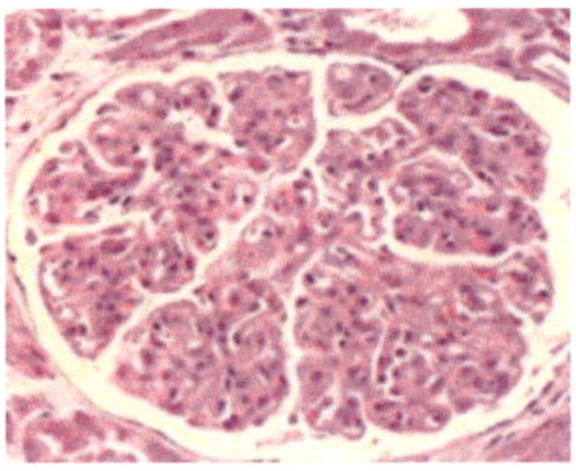

Fig. 3. Cryoglobulinemic glomerulonephritis with membranoproliferative and mesangial proliferative features. Strongly PAS-positive small cryoglobulin plugs are present within capillary loops. In the setting of subacute cryoglobulinemic glomerulonephritis, inflammatory cells can be present within the glomerulus. (periodic acid-Schiff stain original magnification x200)

Histopathological examination reveals glomerular hypercellularity predominantly by leukocytes and monocytes (different to idiopathic MPGN in which hypercellularity is mainly by mesangial and endothelial cells). Capillary walls show similar characteristics to those of idiopathic MPGN: double contours, "tram-tracking" aspect, duplication of the glomerular basement membrane and cells interposition in the subendothelial space (mainly monocytes). Usually there are nodular, eosinophilic, hyaline, homogeneous deposits occupying some glomerular capillary lumina: intraluminal thrombi; when present are highly suggestive of the disease. Crescents are not frequent. In few patients there is mesangial hypercellularity and sclerosis signifying chronicity with progressive organ damage. **Immunofluorescence:** There are parietal subendothelial deposits of IgG and IgM, usually accompanied by C3 and C4, with a variable intensity. Intraluminal thrombi are strongly positive for IgG and IgM demonstrating their origin in immune complexes. Staining for IgG and IgM may be present in mesangium, arterial walls, and arterioles. When there is a monoclonal component (in type II cryoglobulinemia) the monoclonal origin can be demonstrated (usually kappa light chain). **Electron microscopy:** Glomerular lesions are very similar to those found in type I MPGN, but in cryoglobulinemia deposits are characteristically: organized, fibrillary or microtubular, with a distinctive substructure; there is a combination of curved cylinders arranged in pairs and annular structures in the subendothelial space. The cells that interpose in the subendothelial space (between the original GBM and the new synthesized membrane, or between GBM and endothelial cell) are in their majority monocytes (in idiopathic MPGN, mesangial cells occupy this space). (Garini et al., 2004)

4.4.5 Sicca syndrome

Symptomatic xerophthalmia and xerostomia occurs in 10-53% of HCV infected patients, the classical definite picture of S jogren's syndrome is less commonly encountered in HCV-MC patients. In a recent study, serological screening of 1309 patients with Sjogren's syndrome for HCV seropositivity showed 156 patients (12%) to be seropositive for HCV. In HCV related sicca syndrome, xerostomia was found more abundant than xerophthalmia. **(8)** Sicca syndrome with HCV-MC represents a form of lymphocytic sialadenitis, the mechanism of damage to the salivary epithelial cells might be due to; either direct viral sialotropism (virus secreted in the saliva) or indirect immune mediated inflammatory process. Unlike patients with primary Sjogren's syndrome in patients with HCV-MC related Sjogren's syndrome, serological markers for MC are usually present including low complement 4, rheumatoid factor seropositivity and detectable mixed cryoglobulins. Salivary gland biopsy shows pericapillary and non-pericanalary lymphocytic infilterate with lack of glandular canal damage. In patients with HCV related sialadenitis the prevalence of anti-SSA and anti-SSB antibodies were nearly 20%. (Doeffoel- Hantz et al., 2005, Ramos-Casals et al., 2001)

4.4.6 Lung involvement

Pulmonary involvement is more common in cryoglobulinemic HCV-infected patients compared to non-cryoglobulinemic patients. Pulmonary involvement is mild and mostly in the form of interstitial lung disease. The disease is usually clinically inert, except for some patients who present with cough, moderate exertional dyspnea and a minimal decrease in pulmonary function tests. Pleural effusion and alveolitis with alveolar hemorrhage, hemoptysis, severe acute lung insult with acute respiratory distress might develop in HCV-MC. The condition is usually fatal and is mostly due to diffuse pulmonary vasculitis (autopsy disclosed pulmonary perivascular localization of IgG and IgM with immune complex materials containing IgM (kappa) and IgG occluding the pulmonary vessels in these patients (Ferri et al., 1997, Okutan et al., 2004, Suzuki et al., 2003).

4.4.7 Gastrointestinal tract involvement

Gastrointestinal involvement occurs in 2-22% of cases. Mesenteric vasculitis with abdominal pain, acute abdomen and even gastrointestinal bleeding might occur in HCV cryoglobulinemic vasculitis. Liver damage is common, over 50% of patients show signs of mild to moderate chronic hepatitis at diagnosis. Liver involvement is characterized by abnormally increased liver enzymes with or without echographic and/or histological features of chronic hepatitis, cirrhosis, or hepatocellular carcinoma. Late evolution into overt cirrhosis occurs in 25% of cases. Cryoglobulins are a prognostic indicator for increased risk of cirrhosis in patients with chronic hepatitis C. Splenomegaly might coexist. (Kayali et al., 2003, Remoroza and Bonkovsky, 2003)

4.4.8 Cardiovascular involvement

Patterns of cardiovascular involvement in HCV-MC include: mitral valvular damage with mitral regurge, coronary vasculitis complicated by myocardial infarction, pericarditis, congestive heart failure and hypertrophic cardiomyopathy. Arterial thrombosis reported in 1%. **(Antonelli et al., 2009)**

4.4.9 Ocular

Retinopathy with cotton-wool spots, hemorrhages and arteriolar occlusion on fundus examination can occur in HCV patients with cryoglobulinemia, but rather a frequent complication of interferon therapy than HCV related small vessel vasculitis, uveitis is rare. Mooren's ulcer is a rapidly progressive, painful ulceration of the cornea that might occur. The diagnosis of Mooren's ulcer is a diagnosis of exclusion. (Remoroza and Bonkovsky, 2003)

4.4.10 Endocrine system

Some endocrinological disorders are significantly more frequent in HCV-MC patients compared to the general population. The most common endocrinal disorders are the thyroid disorders including; autoimmune thyroiditis, subclinical hypothyroidism, thyroid cancer with high prevalence of anti-thyroperioxidase antibody and antithyroglobulin antibody. Hyperthyroidism is less frequent, generally as reversible complication of interferon treatment. Type 2 diabetes is another frequent endocrinal disorder in cryoglobulin-positive than in cryoglobulin-negative patients. The raised prevalence of type 2 diabetes in HCV-patients with mixed cryoglobulinemia is attributed to an immune-mediated mechanism **(127)**. Insulin resistance mediated by proinflammatory cytokines, rather than a deficit in insulin secretion, is propably the primary pathogenic mechanism involved in the development of type 2 diabetes in HCV infection. Erectile dysfunction is another disorder in male patients with HCV-MC attributable to hormonal and/or neuro-vascular alterations. (Antonelli et al., 2004 a&b, Ferri et al., 2002,b)

4.4.11 Hematological abnormalities

Anemia of chronic disease and thrombocytopenia are amongst the commonly reported hematololgical abnormalities in HCV-patients with cryoglobulinemia. The proposed pathological mechanisms in HCV related thrombocytopenia involved; platelet sequestration and destruction in the spleen, along with low thrombopoetin production and direct viral infection of the megakariocytes with immune mediated platelet destruction. (De Almeida et al., 2004, Doi et al., 2002, Giannini et al., 2002, Jiang et al., 2002). Autoimmune hemolytic anemia has been reported in female patients with cryoglobulinemic syndrome **(8),** Leukocytosis, an elevated erythrocyte sedimentation rate (ESR) and an elevated C-reactive protein level are common findings in most types of vasculitis. The auto-antibodies seen in patients with HCV infection resemble those seen in chronic viral infections - the autoantibody titers are low, frequently found during the clinical course of cryoglobulinemia, however, not essentially associated with typical autoimmune disease. Serological abnormalities in HCV-MC involve positive antinuclear antibodies (ANA), antismooth muscle antibodies (ASMA), anti-neutrophil cytoplasmic antibodies (ANCA), and anticardiolipin autoantibodies. The prevalence of ANA and ASMA ranges from 4.4% to 41% and 7% to 66% respectively usually with low titre ≤ 1/160. HCV core particles concentrated in the cryoprecipitate provoke an interaction between the cryoglobulins, endothelial cells and neutrophil granulocytes. A positive ANCA has been found in <5-10% of patients with HCV-associated mixed cryoglobulinemia with proteinase 3 and dihydrolipoamine dehydrogenase as the main anti-neutrophil cytoplasmic antigens in patients with HCV-MC. HCV patients with ANCA had a higher prevalence of skin involvement, anemia, abnormal liver function tests and elevated alpha feto-protein levels. Anti-cardiolipin antibodies occur in 3.3% to 22% of HCV patients, with higher frequency in patients with HCV-associated cryoglobulinemia yet insignificant being anti-b2-glicoprotein independent. (Cacoub et al., 1997, Lamprecht et al., 2003, Ordi-Ros et al., 2000, Yee et al., 2004, Wu et al., 2002)

4.4.12 Neoplastic disorders

Mixed cryoglobulinemia syndrome is considered as a pre-neopastic syndrome that features a cross road between virus related autoimmune syndromes and virus associated malignancies (B cell lymphoma, hepatocellular carcinoma). B-cell lymphoma is the most frequent neoplastic manifestation complicating mixed cryoglobulinemia that presents late in the course of the disease. **(Cacoub et al., 2000)** Neoplasia is attributed to sustained peripheral B-lymphocyte expansion with significantly persistent lymphoid infiltrates that remain unmodified for years in the liver and bone marrow of MC patients. Such infiltrates are considered as "early lymphomas", and are given the nomenoclature "monotypic lymphoproliferative disorder of undetermined significance (MLDUS)". Type II MC-related MLDUS has the highest incidence in the same geographic areas with high prevalence of HCV infection. The onset of malignant lymphoma is usually 5-10 years after disease diagnosis, with a reported incidence of less than 10% in some patients to as high as 40% in others. Overt lymphoid tumors develop in about 10% of cases. A sudden decrease or disappearance of serum cryoglobulins and RF with abnormally high levels of C4, are presenting symptoms of complicating B-cell malignancy. Other neoplastic manifestations, i.e. hepatocellular carcinoma or papillary thyroid cancer, are less frequently observed (Ferri et al., 2002, Matsuo et al., 2004, Quartuccio et al., 2007).

4.4.13 Other disease related features

Constitutional symptoms like fever, fatigue, anorexia, weight loss, amongst other immune mediated HCV related extra-hepatic manifestations including: Porphyria cutanea tarda, Lichen planus, pancreatitis, aplastic anaemia, systemic lupus erythematosus, CREST syndrome, and waldenstrom's macroglobulinemia might exist. (Ferri et al., 2002 a, Ferri et al., 2000)

5. HCV and polyarteritis nodosa PAN (medium sized vessel vasculitis)

Despite that polyarteritis nodosa is more commonly reported in patients with hepatitis B viremia, yet medium sized vessels inflammation can occur in patients with chronic HCV infection featuring a polyarthritis nodosa pattern of vasculitis. PAN can occur in cryoglobulinemic as well as non cryoglobulinemic HCV patients. HCV related PAN displays a more severe and acute clinical presentation with more frequent fever and weight loss, severe hypertension, gastrointestinal tract involvement, severe acute sensory-motor multifocal mononeuropathy, kidney and liver microaneurysms and elevated acute phase reactants levels. Cases of mesenteric vasculitis with stenosis and narrowing of the superior mesenteric vessels and reno-vascular micro-aneurysm with renal cortical infarcts have been described in HCV patients having purpuric eruptions, hypertension and abdominal pain. Such lesions resolved with antiviral therapy and prednisolone, supporting the possible etiopathogenic role of chronic HCV infection. Another case with vasculitic mucosal colonic ulceration with massive hematochezia, purpura, abdominal discomfort, pulmonary infilterate and acute renal failure was described in a female patient with chronic HCV infection and negative for cryoglobulinemia, colonic biopsy showed evidence of fibrinoid necrotizing arteritis diagnosing a case of HCV related PAN with no evidence of leukocytoclastic vasculitis. (Costedoat-Chalumeau et al., 2002, Elias et al., 1998, Saadoun et al., 2010a)

6. Diagnosis of HCV- mixed cryoglobulinemia

6.1 Cryoglobulin detection

The detection of serum cryoglobulins is fundamental for the diagnosis of mixed cryoglobulinemia. (Ferri et al., 2002 a, Ferri et al., 2008) Due to their thermal instability, the measurement of cryoglobulin level in the blood should be performed immediately after sampling. For a correct evaluation of serum cryoglobulins it is necessary to avoid false-negative results due to Ig cold precipitation at room temperature, blood sampling, clotting, and serum separation by centrifugation is carried out at 37°C and the cryocrit determination and cryoglobulin characterization at 4°C (after 7 days). Cryocrit determinations (percentage of packed cryoglobulins referred to total serum after centrifugation at +4°C) should be done on blood samples without anticoagulation to avoid false-positive results due to cryo-fibrinogen. The analysis of cryoprecipitates is generally carried out by means of immunoelectrophoresis or immunofixation, other more sensitive methodologies include; immunoblotting or two-dimensional polyacrylamide gel electrophoresis. Type II MC shows a microheterogeneous composition. Type II-III mixed cryoglobulinemia represents an intermediate, evolutive state from type III to type II. The absence of detectable serum cryoglobulins despite the presence of the clinical syndrome is described to be a transient phenomenon due to the wide variability of the percentage of cryoprecipitable immune-complex during the natural history of the disease or, less frequently, to a switching from 'benign' B-cell lymphoproliferation to malignant lymphoma. The levels of serum cryoglobulins usually do not correlate with the severity and prognosis of the disease. (Ferri et al., 2002 a, Ferri et al., 2000)

6.2 Laboratory tests

Laboratory workup includes complete blood cell count with evidences of anemia of chronic disease, thrombocytopenia or autoimmune hemolytic anemia. Erthrocyte sedimentation rate is almost always elevated in all types of vasculitis, but a normal ESR does not rule out systemic vasculitis. Blood urea nitrogen, creatinine for renal involvement, proteinuria and hematuria on urinalysis, a fresh-spun urine sample should be evaluated for red blood cell casts or dysmorphic red cells to diagnose glomerulonephritis. Up to 40 % of patients with chronic hepatitis C have normal serum ALT levels, even when tested on multiple occasions. (Ferri, 2008, Ghany et al., 2009)

6.3 Serological tests

For the diagnosis of HCV, hepatitis C antibody testing is crucial, regarding the response to treatment quantitative assessment of viral load HCV-RT-PCR as well as the viral genotyping are important prognostic markers. Sustained negative results for HCV-RT-PCR with treatment signifies a sustained viral response. Rheumatoid factor and serum anti-cyclic citrullinated C peptide antibodies (markers for rheumatoid arthritis)are useful diagnostic tools in arthritis patients. Complement 3 (C3) and complement 4 (C4) and CH50 are usually consumed in patients with renal disease. Anti-neutrophil cytoplasmic antibodies (P-ANCA might be found in patients with small to medium sized vessel vasculitis). Anti SSA and anti-SSB (in up to 20%) and thyroid specific antibodies (up t0 22.1%) are amongst associating serological abnormalities (Ghany et al., 2009, Ferri, 2008, Antonelli et al., 2009)

6.4 Imaging studies

Chest x ray and high resolution computerized tomography for diagnosis of pulmonary involvement, echocardiography and electrocardiogram (ECG) for cardiac disease, abdominal ultrasound for hepatic and renal disease. (Ferri, 2008)

6.5 Biopsy

Histopathological evidences of vasculitis remain the gold standard for the diagnosis of vasculitis. Biopsy from clinically involved sites (cutaneous lesions, nerve biopsy, renal biopsy) is a cornerstone in establishing the diagnosis. Bone marrow biopsy should be done to demonstrate polyclonal B cell proliferation and in suspected cases with lympho-proliferative disorders (Mukhtyar et al., 2009).

6.6 Differential diagnosis

A frequent clinico-pathological overlap exists between HCV-related cryoglobulinemic syndrome and some autoimmune diseases including; small and medium sized vessel vasculitides, infectious vasculitides (Bacterial vasculitis e.g., Neisserial, mycobacterial vasculitis e.g., Tuberculous, spirochetal vasculitis e.g., Syphilitic, rickettsial vasculitis e.g., Rocky Mountain Spotted Fever, fungal vasculitis e.g., Aspergillosis, viral vasculitis e.g., Herpes zoster, HIV), primary S-jogren's syndrome, secondary types of vasculitis (rheumatoid arthritis, systemic lupus erythematosus, seronegative arthritides), membranous glomerulonephritis, immune mediated thyroiditis, type II diabetes, autoimmune hepatitis, and myelo-proliferative disorders (lymphomas, leukemias and Plasma cell dyscrasias). (Ghany et al., 2009, Jennette et al., 1994)

7. Treatment of HCV related vasculitides

7.1 Treatment of HCV

Clinical improvement of HCV related vasculitides proved to correlate with virological response. Introducing anti-viral therapy namely interferon alpha with or without ribavirin remains the cornerstone in the management of HCV-MC. Antiviral therapy has been shown to reverse bone marrow monoclonal B-cell expansion in patients with HCV-MC. (Davis et al., 2002, Mukhtyar et al., 2009, NIDDK, 2010)

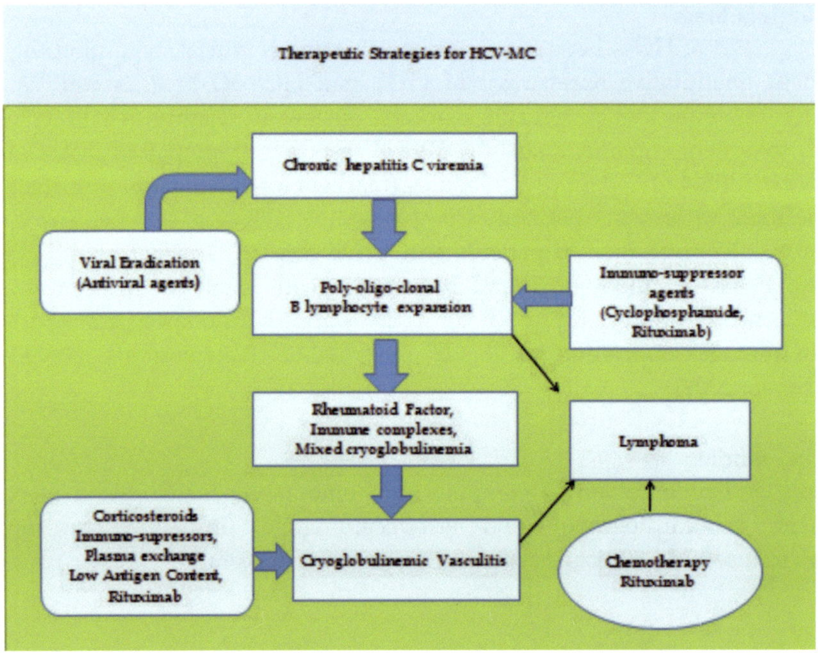

Fig. 4. Therapeutic strategies for hepatitis C mixed cryoglobulinemia.

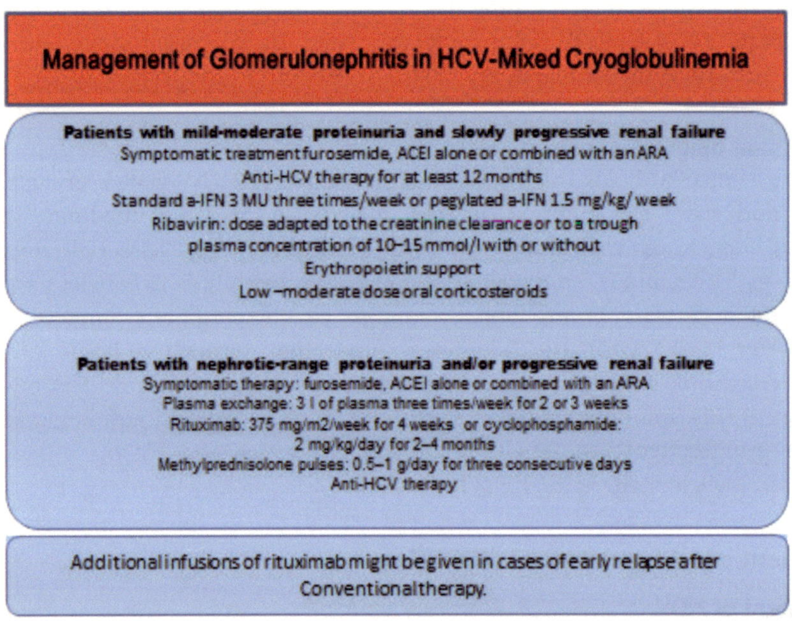

Fig. 5. Treatment of HCV cryoglobulinemic renal disease. The management of renal disease in HCV mixed cryoglobulinemia depends upon the severity of renal disease.The standard regimen is a combination of immunosuppressive drugs, antiviral agents in addition to symptomatic therapy. In refractory cases rituximab will be the drug of choice. (Alric et al., 2004, Kidney International, Guideline 5, 2008)

7.1.1 Interferon-alpha therapy

The standard initial therapy used to be recombinant interferon alfa-2b at a dose of 3 x 10^6 units administered subcutaneously 3 times per week for 6 weeks. Recombinant forms of alpha interferon are being currently replaced by pegylated interferon (peginterferon). Peginterferon is alpha interferon modified chemically by the addition of a large inert molecule of polyethylene glycol prolonging its half-life. Peg-Interferon being with better efficacy and easier administration replaced standard interferon both as monotherapy and as combination therapy for hepatitis C viremia. Peg-interferon is more active than standard interferon in inhibiting HCV and yields higher sustained response rates with equivalent side effects. Two forms of peg-interferon are available: peg-interferon alfa-2a and peg-interferon alfa-2b, roughly equivalent in efficacy and safety, with different dosing regimen. Peginterferon alfa-2a is given subcutaneously in a fixed dose of 180 micrograms (mcg) per week, while peginterferon alfa-2b is given subcutaneously weekly in a weight-based dose of 1.5 mcg per kilogram per week in the range of 75 to 150 mcg per week.

The goal of interferon treatment is suppression of active disease by achieving a sustained viral response (sustained decrease or negative HCV-RT PCR). **Table 4** Interferon alpha monotherapy is effective in purpuric skin lesions, thrombocytopenias, but less effective with neural or renal involvement. IFN-alpha monotherapy is associated with a relatively poor response and a high virologic relapse rate, detectable viremia with active liver disease can occur with normal alanine transferase. Higher initial doses and longer duration of therapy help to increase the interval before relapse and escalation of the dose might help to achieve response in some non-responders.

Peg-interferon therapy has bone marrow suppressive effects or cytopenias, therapy might be associated with immune mediated side effects including in about 2% of patients (particularly if high titers of antinuclear or antithyroid antibodies); peripheral sensory-motor neuropathy, nephropathy, retinopathy and micro-hemorrhages, thyroiditis, Sjogren's syndrome, rheumatoid like polyarthritis, psoriasis, fever, chills, headache, lethargy, somnolence, myalgia and fatigue, anorexia, hearing loss and tinnitus and serious CNS complications might occur during therapy. Rare side effects include; acute congestive heart failure, renal failure, vision loss, pulmonary fibrosis or pneumonitis, sepsis, acute myocardial infarction, stroke, suicide, and sepsis. Paradoxical worsening of hepatic disease provoking a form of autoimmune hepatitis that requires corticosteroid therapy is rare. Peginterferon therapy is contraindicated in severe depression or other neuropsychiatric syndromes, active substance or alcohol abuse, uncontrolled autoimmune disease (such as rheumatoid arthritis, lupus erythematosus, or psoriasis), bone marrow compromise, and inability to practice birth control measures. (Casato et al., 1997, Ferri et al., 1993, Iga et al., 2005, Lidove et al., 1999).

7.1.2 Ribavirin

Ribavirin is a broad spectrum antiviral nucleoside analog which acts through enhancement of host T-cell-mediated immunity against viral infection through switching the T-cell phenotype from type 2 to type 1, inhibition of the host enzyme inosine monophosphate dehydrogenase (IMPDH), direct inhibition of HCV, including NS5B-encoded RNAdependent RNA polymerase (RdRp) and being an RNA mutagen it drives a rapidly mutating RNA virus over the threshold to "error catastrophe". Ribavirin is an oral drug, given twice a day in 200-mg capsules for a total daily dose based upon body weight (1,000 mg< 75 kg or 165 pounds and 1,200 mg for those >75 kg). Combination of ribavirin and interferon increases the sustained response rate by 2- to 3-fold with rapid improvements in serum ALT levels and disappearance of detectable HCV RNA in up to 70 percent of patients. The optimal therapeutic dose of ribavirin and the optimal duration varies depending upon viral genotype (genotype I, rare genotypes 4, 5, 6 require the maximum therapeutic dose/body weight, and longer duration). Considering the variable responses to treatment, testing for HCV genotype is clinically useful before starting combination therapy. A response is considered "sustained" if HCV RNA remains undetectable for 6 months or more after stopping therapy.Some patients relapse by the end of treatment, the relapse rate is lower with combination therapy (55% sustained response with combination therapy for 48 weeks compared 35% with monotherapy)

Study	Patients (no)	TYPE OF STUDY	Treatment	Responses (%) (genotype unrelated)	Follow up
Calleja et al., 1999 (13)	**13**	**Prospective**	**IFN 3 MU × 3 per week + Riba 1200 mg/day × 1 year**	**65**	**22% relapse rate**
Zuckerman et al., 2000 (114)	**9**	**Prospective**	**IFN 3 MU × 3 per week + Riba 15 mg/kg/day × 6 months.**	**100**	**NA**
Donado et al., 1998 (28)	**17**	**Prospective**	**IFN 6 MU × 3 per week × 3 months, 3 MU × 3 per week × 3 months + Riba 15 mg/kg/day × 6 months**	**85**	**55% relapse rate within 1 year**
Mazzaro et al., 2003 (68)	**27**	**Prospective**	**IFN 3 MU × 3 per week + Riba 1200 mg/day × 1 year**	**CR+PR: 85**	**70% early relapse; 22% long-term clinical and virological response**

Table 5. Combined Treatment Interferon plus Ribavirin in HCV-related Cryoglobulinemia.CR = Complete remission; HCV = Hepatits C virus; NA = Not applicable; PR = Partial remission; Riba = Ribavirin.

Ribavirin therapy causes anemia, fatigue and irritability, itching, skin rash, nasal stuffiness, sinusitis, and cough, red cell hemolysis to a variable degree in almost all patients. Patients with a pre-existing hemolysis or anemia (hemoglobin < 11 grams or hematocrit < 33 percent) should not receive ribavirin. Similarly, patients who have significant coronary or cerebral vascular disease should not receive ribavirin, as the anemia caused by treatment can trigger significant ischemia. Fatal myocardial infarctions and strokes are amongst reported side effects during combination therapy with alpha interferon and ribavirin.

Ribavirin is excreted largely by the kidneys. Patients with renal disease can develop hemolysis that is severe and even life threatening. With serum creatinine above 2.0 mg per deciliter (dL) patients should not be treated with ribavirin. Ribavirin causes birth defects in animal studies and should not be used in women or men without contraception. Peg-interferon has direct antigrowth and anti-proliferative effects so it is contraindicated during pregnancy. Combination therapy should therefore be used with caution. Contraindications to ribavirin include marked anemia, renal dysfunction, and coronary artery or cerebrovascular disease, and inability to practice birth control. The newly emerging direct-acting antiviral (DAA) drugs are at the preclinical developmental stage and several are in clinical development. Initial clinical trials using some of these inhibitors, either alone or in combination with pegylated IFN-alpha and ribavirin, have yielded encouraging results. (Cacoub et al., 2002, Mazzaro et al., 2003, Pawlotsky, 2011) **Table 5.** Recently nucleotide polymorphism upstream of IL-28B gene has been found to be associated with response to PEG-IFN and ribavirin and spontaneous clearance of HCV infection in addition, genetic variants of inosine triphosphate (ITPA) have been correlated with protection against ribavirin induced hemolytic anemia (Fellay 2010)

7.2 Corticosteroids, standard Immunosuppression and plasma exchange therapy

The treatment of cryoglobulinemic vasculitis depends upon the severity of the acute manifestations and the extent of organ involvement. In asymptomatic MC monitoring without treatment is recommended. In patients with mild to moderate cryoglobulinemic symptoms (purpura, arthralgias, peripheral sensory neuropathy) first-line immnosuprression usually consists of low-dose corticosteroids. Patients with severe manifestations (cryoglobulinemic nephropathy, skin ulcers, sensory motor neuropathy, wide spread vasculitis) should promptly receive high-dose steroids and immunosuppressive therapy. Use of high dose intravenous corticosteroids might be useful for controlling life threatening organ involvement. Immunosuppressive drugs (e.g., Cyclophosphamide, Chlorambucil, and Azathioprine) can be used to suppress antibody and cryoglobulin production. The most effective and commonly used cytotoxic drug is Cyclophosphamide (750-1000mg intravenous pulse or orally at doses of 2 mg/kg per day). Recently; Mycophenolate Mofetil (1 g twice a day) is used as an alternative to Cyclophosphamide for the induction of remission in MC vasculitis. Mycophenolic Acid is more selective than Cyclophosphamide in inhibiting lymphocyte proliferation and functions, the drug was found to reduce viremia in HCV-infected renal or heart-transplant recipients due to its ability to inhibit inosine monophosphate dehydrogenase, the target enzyme inhibited by ribavirin. (Cacoub et al., 2005)

7.3 Plasma exchange

Plasma exchange therapy permits rapid control of life threatening symptoms of vasculitis by removal of circulating immune complexes with or without using high dose intravenous corticosteroids or immunosuppressive treatments, particularly in active cryoglobulinemic nephropathy. Oral cyclophosphamide (50-100 mg/day for 2-6 weeks) during the tapering of aphaeretic sessions can reinforce the beneficial effect of plasma exchange; and prevent the rebound phenomenon that may be observed after the aphaeresis discontinuation. Plasma The use of INF- alpha after each plasma exchange session doesn't modify the viral response (Hausfaster et al., 2002, Khattab et al., 2010, Morra, 2010)

7.4 Biologic agents

7.4.1 Anti-CD20 therapy -Rituximab

Rituximab is a humanized anti- CD-20 monoclonal antibody that was primarily successfully employed for the treatment of B-cell lymphomas and other chronic lymphoproliferative diseases. The drug has proven efficacy in autoimmune disorders including vasculitis and refractory systemic lupus with nephritis. Recently, rituximab showed efficacy in cases of HCV-mixed cryoglobulinemia. The drug was successfully used in combination with antiviral agents as well as monotherapy in HCV cryoglobulinemic vasculitis. Rituximab combined with Peg-IFN-α/ribavirin delete both virus-dependent and -independent B-cell clones. Antiviral therapy alone decreased the memory B cells; whereas in association with rituximab, naive B cells are the main depleted population. This fact accounts for the delayed B-cell reconstitution after rituximab plus Peg-IFN-α/ribavirin and stresses the synergistic action of rituximab and antiviral therapy at the immunologic level. Rituximab shortens the therapeutic interval required for achieving a complete clinical reponse. Clonal expansion of marginal zone-like IgM+ CD27+ B cells (VH1-69 clonal B) has been recently observed in certain HCV-MC patients. Rituximab with Peg-IFN and ribavirin exerts a synergistic effect on polclonal B lymphocyte expansion. Rituximab plus Peg-IFN-α/ribavirin was more efficient to suppress both memory and VH1-69 clonal B cells compared with Peg-IFN-α/ribavirin alone. (Zaga et al., 2003, Sansonno et al., 2003, Roccatello et al., 2008) A standard therapeutic dose of 375 mg/m2 weekly for 4 weeks is effective, well tolerated and induces a significant and rapid improvement of clinical signs (purpura, arthralgia, peripheral neuropathy) with a decline of cryocrit in most patients with mixed cryoglobulinemia even in cases resistant to IFN therapy.

Rituximab trials emphasized the benefit of the drug in inducing remission in cutaneous vasculitis, cryoglobulinemic nephropathy, cryoglobulinemic neuropathy and in underlying malignant lymphoproliferative disorder. Relapse of cryoglobulinemic vasculitis might occur. Complete clinical remission was associated with a significant reduction of RF activity and anti-HCV antibody titers. (Saadoun et al., 2008) An increase of viremia might be observed in responders, with insignificant variation of transaminases or deterioration of liver disease. Rituximab infusions proved effective on cryoglobulinemic vasculitis, with a Recent studies showed a relapse in 36.1% of patients within a few days to 19 months after the last rituximab infusion. Complete immunologic response was higher with the combination of rituximab plus Peg-IFN-α/ribavirin. Recently, rituximab treatment of a renal-transplant patient with de novo HCV-related type III cryoglobulinemic MPGN resulted in clearance of cryoglobulinemia, a decrease in proteinuria yet without a change in serum creatinine or HCV RNA. Rituximab, the drug can cause serum sickness, serum sickness like disease, neutropenia and increased risk of infections, pneumopathy, varicella zoster infection, erysipelas and as monotherapy increases HCV viremia. (Saadoun et al., 2010, Pereira et al., 2010) **Table 6**

Study	Patients (number with nephritis)	Rituximab dose	Other treatments	Remission overall (nephritis)	Remission purpura (neuropathy)	Side effects	HCV viral load	Relapse (number of cases)
Sansonno *et al.* *2003* (97)	20 (1)	375 mg/m^2 weekly × 4 weeks	S (low doses)	16/20 (1/1)	12/14 (6/12)	Septic fever (1)	↑ responders = nonresponders	4/16 (>7 months)
Zaja *et al.* 2003 (110)	15 (2)	375 mg/m^2 weekly × 4 weeks	S (<0.5 mg/ kg/day)	13/14 (1/2)	12/12 (5/5)	Retinal thrombosis (1)	↑ 2/8 ↑ 1/8 = 5/8	6 (3–6 months)
Roccatello *et al.* ,2004 (87)	6 (5)	375 mg/m^2 weekly × 4 weeks; 375 mg/m^2 monthly × 2 months		5/5	4/4 (5/6)	Transient bradycardia (2)	4 unchanged	2 (>12 months)
Quartuccio *et al.*, 2006 (83)	5 (5)	375 mg/m^2 weekly × 4 weeks	S (one case)	5/5 (5/5)	4/4 (1/2)	Transient neutropenia (1)	NR	3 (>5, >7 and >12 months)
Basse *et al.* 2005 (8)	7 (7) (post-kidney transplant)	375 mg/m^2 weekly × 2–4 weeks	CNI, MMF and S	7/7		Lethal infection (2, fungal and HSV)	NR	NR
Visentini *et al.* 2007 (106)	6 (2)	250 mg/m^2 weekly × 2 weeks	S	4/6 (1/2)	4/5 (2/2)	Lethal intestinal infarction	↓ 2/5 = 3/5	NR

Table 6. Rituximab treatment in Patients with HCV cryoglobulinemic vascultis.CNI = Calcineurin inhibitor; HCV = Hepatitis C virus; HSV = Herpes simplex virus; MMF = Mycophenolate mofetil; NR = Not reported; S = Steroids.↑: Increase; ↓: Decrease; =: No change.

7.5 Low antigen diet (LAC-diet)

LAC-diet is a particular dietetic treatment that can improve the clearance of circulating immune-complexes by restoring the activity of the reticulo-endothelial system, overloaded by large amounts of circulating cryoglobulins. LAC-diet can be used for controlling mild disease manifestations. (Ferri et al., 1989, Morra, 2010)

7.6 Symptomatic therapy

Controlling blood pressure: diuretics, renin–angiotensin system blockade, the treatment of hyperlipidemia, are of proven benefit in prognosis of renal disease. Colchicine, an anti-inflammatory agent has been proposed for MC patients with mild to moderate levels of the disease. (Khattab et al., 2010)

7.7 Treatment of HCV-related vasculitis relapses

Clinical relapses are usually associated with relapsing HCV viremia (detectable HCV-RT-PCR). The use of combination therapy for in escalating doses for longer duration (18-24 months) effective in limiting relapses particularly in cases with renal involvement or peripheral neuropathy. A relapsing cryoglobulinemic vasculitis without HCV viral relapse might occur and in such conditions the possibility of an underlying malignant lymphoma (B cell Non-Hodgkin's Lymphoma) should be considered. Relapses can be successfully treated with a second trial of combination antiviral therapy with immunosuppression or anti CD-20 monoclonal antibody rituximab. (Fois et al., 2003, Saadoun et al., 2010) New direct acting antiviral drug combinations are under trial, the evolution of these drugs might expand the therapeutic benefit of combination therapy in HCV infection as well as extrahepatic disease. (Franciscus, 2011)

8. Prognosis

The prognosis of HCV-MC depends upon the extent and severity of organ involvement and the response to treatment (viral load and clinical manifestations). The overall prognosis is worse in persons with concomitant renal disease or lympho-proliferative disease (B cell non Hodgkin lymphoma or malignant lymphoma). Mean survival is approximately 50% at 10 years after diagnosis. Survival rates reported among patients with cryoglobulinemic renal involvement varies from greater than 60% at 5 years of follow-up, up to 30% at 7 years of follow-up. Infection, cardiovascular disease and hepatic failue are amongst causes of morbidity. (Morra, 2010, Saadoun et al., 2010)

9. Conclusion

Mixed cryoglobulinemia represents a form of leukocytoclastic vasculitis, which is considered to be a relatively rare disorder. Given its clinical polymorphism, a correct diagnosis might be delayed in addition the actual prevalence of disease is probably underestimated. Establishing the diagnosis of HCV-MC requires careful patient evaluation, biopsy from involved sites is the gold standard for diagnosing leukocytoclastic vasculitis. Owing to its' complex etio-pathogenesis and clinical polymorphism, the treatment of mixed cryoglobulinemia and cryoglobulinemic vasculitis remains challenging. The initial therapeutic step must target hepatitis C viremia being the chronic trigger for sustained immune-stimulation and autoantibody production. The second therapeutic target is to control downstream B cell clonal expansion thereby controlling the autoimmune manifestations related to cryoglobulinemia (cryoglobulinemic vasculitis), and management of neoplastic complications. The prognosis of the disease depends largely upon the extent and severity of organ involvement and adequate therapeutic intervention.

10. References

[1] Agnello, V., Chung, R. T. and Kaplan, L. M. (1992) A role for hepatitis C virus infection in type II cryoglobulinemia. N Engl J Med, 1992; 327, 1490-5.

[2] Agnello V. (1995) The aetiology of mixed cryoglobulinaemia associated with hepatitis C virus infection. Scand J Immunol 1995;42:179–84.

[3] Alric L, Plaisier E, Thebault S, et al. (2004) Influence of antiviral therapy in hepatitis C virus-associated cryoglobulinemic MPGN. Am J Kidney Dis 2004;43:617-23.

[4] Antonelli A, Ferri C, Fallahi P, et al. (2004, a) Thyroid involvement in patients with overt HCV-related mixed cryoglobulinaemia. QJM 2004, 97:499-506.

[5] Antonelli A, Ferri C, Fallahi P, et al. (2004, b): Type 2 diabetes in hepatitis C-related mixed cryoglobulinaemia patients. Rheumatology (Oxford) 2004, 43:238-40.

[6] Antonelli A, Ferri C, Ferrari S M, et al., (2009). Serum levels of proinflammatory cytokines interleukin-1β, interleukin-6, and tumor necrosis factor α in mixed cryoglobulinemia. Arthritis & Rheumatism. December, 2009,Volume 60, Issue 12, pages 3841–3847.

[7] Authier FJ, Bassez G, Payan C et al. (2003) Detectio n of genomic viral RNA in nerve and muscle of patients with HCV neuropathy. Neurology 2003; 60:808–12.

[8] Basse G, Ribes D, Kamar N et al. (2005) Rituximab therapy for de novo mixed cryoglobulinemia in renal-transplant patients. Transplantation. 2005; 80, 1560-1564.

[9] Cacoub P, Musset L, Amoura Z, et al. (1997) Anticardiolipin, anti-beta2- glycoprotein I, and antinucleosome antibodies in hepatitis C virus infection and mixed cryoglobulinemia. Multivirc Group. J Rheumatol 1997; 24: 2139-2144.

[10] Cacoub P, Renou C, Rosenthal E, et al. (2000) Extrahepatic manifestations associated with hepatitis C virus infection. A prospective multicenter study of 321 patients. The GERMIVIC. Groupe d'Etude et de Recherche en Medecine Interne et Maladies Infectieuses sur le Virus de l'Hepatite C. Medicine (Baltimore). 2000; 79: 47-56.

[11] Cacoub P, Lidove O, Maisonobe T, et al. (2002) Interferon alpha and ribavirin treatment in patients with hepatitis C virus-related systemic vasculitis. Arthritis Rheum 2002;46:3317-26.b

[12] Cacoub P, Saadoun D, Limal N, et al., (2005). PEGylated interferon alfa-2b and ribavirin treatment in patients with hepatitis C virus-related systemic vasculitis. Arthritis Rheum, 2005; 52:911-5.

[13] Calleja JL, Albillos A, Moreno-Otero R et al. (1999) Sustained response to interferon-α or to interferon-α plus ribavirin in hepatitis C virus-associated symptomatic mixed cryoglobulinaemia. Aliment. Pharmacol. Ther. 13, 1179-1186 (1999).

[14] Casato M, Saadoun D, Marchetti A et al. (2005) Central nervous system involvement in hepatitis C virus cryoglobulinemia vasculitis: a multicenter case-control study

using magnetic resonance imaging and neuropsychological tests. J Rheumatol., 2005; 32:484–8.
[15] Costedoat-Chalumeau N, Cacoub P, Maisonobe T, et al. (2002) Renal microaneurysms in three cases of hepatitis C virus-related vasculitis. Rheumatology (2002) 41 (6): 708-710.
[16] Curry MP, Golden-Mason L, Doherty DG et al. (2003) Expansion of innate CD5pos B cells expressing high levels of CD81 in hepatitis C virus infected liver. J Hepatol 2003; 38:642–50.
[17] Dammacco F, Sansonno D. (1997) Mixed cryoglobulinemia as a model of systemic vasculitis. Clin Rev Allergy Immunol 1997; 15:97–119.
[18] Davis G L. (2002) HEPATITIS C THERAPY: The Liver in Health and Disease. AMERICAN LIVER FOUNDATION, 2002. Medline.
[19] Dawson TM and Starkebaum G. (1999) Isolated central nervous system vasculitis associated with hepatitis C infection. J Rheumatol 1999; 26:2273–6.
[20] De Almeida AJ, Campos-de-Magalhães M, de Melo Marçal OP, et al. (2004) Hepatitis C virus associated thrombocytopenia: a controlled prospective, virological study. Ann Hematol 2004; 83: 434-440.
[21] De Vita S, De Re V, Gasparotto D et al., (2000). Oligoclonal non-neoplastic B cell expansionis the key feature of type II mixed cryoglobulinemia: clinical and molecular findings do not support a bone marrow pathologic diagnosis of indolent B cell lymphoma. Arthritis Rheum 2000;43:94–102.Pipitone N and Salvarani C. (2006) Systemic Vasculitis: State of the Art and Emerging Concepts. Curr Opin Rheumatol. 2006;18(1):1-2.
[22] De Vita S, De Re V, Sansonno D, et al. (2002) Lack of HCV infection in malignant cells refutes the hypothesis of a direct transforming action of the virus in the pathogenesis of HCV-associated B-cell NHLs. Tumori. 2002; 88:400–406.
[23] Doffoel-Hantz V, Loustaud-Ratti V, Ramos-Casals M, et al. (2005) Evolution of Sjogren's syndrome associated with hepatitis C virus when hepatitis C is treated with interferon or the association of interferon and ribavirin. Rev Med Interne 2005; 26:88-94.
[24] Doi T, Homma H, Mezawa S, et al. (2002) Mechanisms for increment of platelet associated IgG and platelet surface IgG and their implications in immune thrombocytopenia associated with chronic viral liver disease. Hepatol Res 2002; 24: 23.
[25] Donada C, Crucitti A, Donadon V, et al. (1998) Interferon and ribavirin combination therapy in patients with chronic hepatitis C and mixed cryoglobulinemia. Blood 92, 2983-2984 (1998).
[26] Elias N; Sabo E; Naschitz JE; et al. (1998) Colonic ulcers in a patient with hepatitis C virus-associated polyarteritis nodosa. J Clin Gastroenterol. 1998; 26(3):212-5.
[27] Falk R J and Hoffman G S. (2007) Controversies in Small Vessel Vasculitis - Comparing the Rheumatology and Nephrology Views. Curr Opin Rheumatol. 2007;19(1):1-9.
[28] Fellay J, Thompson A J, Ge D, et al., 2010. ITPA gene variants protect against anemia in patients treated for chronic hepatitis C. Nature, 20220;464:405-8.

[29] Fabris M, Quartuccio L, Sacco S, et al. (2007) B-Lymphocyte stimulator (BLyS) up-regulation in mixed cryoglobulinaemia syndrome and hepatitis-C virus infection. Rheumatology (Oxford). 2007; 46:37–43.

[30] Ferri C. (2008) Mixed Cryoglobulinemia. Orphanet Journal of Rare Diseases 2008, 3:25. Review.

[31] Ferri C, Pietrogrande M, Cecchetti C, et al., (1989). Low-antigen-content diet in the treatment of mixed cryoglobulinemia patients. Am J Med, 1989. 87: 519-24.

[32] Ferri C, La civita L, Fazzi P et al. (1997) Interstitial lung fibrosis and rheumatic disorders in patients with hepatitis C infection. Br J Rheumatol 1997; 36:360-5.

[33] Ferri C, Pileri S, Zignego AL. (2000) Hepatitis C virus, B-cell disorders, and non-Hodgkin's lymphoma. In Infectious causes of cancer: targets for intervention. National Cancer Institute (NIH) Edited by: Goedert JJ. Totowa, NJ: The Humana Press Inc; 2000:349-368.

[34] Ferri C, Zignego AL, Pileri SA. (2002, a) Cryoglobulins (review). J Clin Pathol. 2002, 55:4-13.

[35] Ferri C, Bertozzi MA, Zignego AL (2002, b) Erectile dysfunction and hepatitis C virus infection. JAMA 2002, 288:698-9.

[36] Ferri C, Sebastiani M, Giuggioli D, et al. (2004) Zignego AL: Mixed cryoglobulinemia: demographic, clinical, and serological features, and survival in 231 patients. Sem Arthritis Rheum 2004, 33:355-74.

[37] Ferri C and Mascia MT: (2006) Cryoglobulinemic vasculitis: Review. Curr Opin Rheumatol 2006, 18:54-63.

[38] Fois E, Guimard Y, Sene D, et al. (2003) Rechute des vascularites systémiques liées au virus de l'hépatite C, sans rechute virologique: se méfier du lymphome. Rev Med Interne 2003; 24:93s.

[39] Fontenot, J. D., Gavin, M. A. & Rudensky, A. Y. (2003) Foxp3 programs the development and function of CD4+CD25+ regulatory T cells. Nat Immunol. 2003, 4, 330-6.

[40] Franciscus A. (2011) Hepatitis C Treatments in Current Clinical Development.Hepatitis C. Hepatitis C Advocate, Medline update, 5th april, 2011.

[41] Garini G, Allegri L, Vaglio A, et al. (2005) Hepatitis C virus-related cryoglobulinemia and glomerulonephritis: pathogenesis and therapeutic strategies. Ann Ital Med Int. 2005; 20:71-80.

[42] Ghany MG, Strader DB, Thomas DL, et al. (2009) Diagnosis, management, and treatment of hepatitis C: an update. Hepatology. 2009;49:1335–1374.

[43] Giannini E, Borro P, Botta F, et al. (2002) Serum thrombopoietin levels are linked to liver function in untreated patients with hepatitis C virus-related chronic hepatitis. J Hepatol 2002; 37: 572-577.

[44] Gross JA, Johnston J, Mudri S, et al. (2000). TACI and BCMA are receptors for a TNF homologue implicated in B-cell autoimmune disease. Nature. 2000 Apr 27;404(6781):995-9.

[45] Guideline 5: Diagnosis and management of kidney diseases associated with HCV infection Kidney International (2008) 73 (Suppl 109), S69-S77.

[46] Hausfater P, Cacoub P, Assogba U, et al. (2002) Plasma exchange and interferon-alpha pharmacokinetics in patients with hepatitis C virus-associated systemic vasculitis. Nephron, 2002;91:627-3.

[47] Heckmann JG, Kayser C, Heuss D, et al. (1992) Neurological manifestations of chronic hepatitis C. J Neurol 1999;246:486–91.

[48] Iga D, Tomimatsu M, Endo H, et al. (2005) Improvement of thrombocytopenia with disappearance of HCV RNA in patients treated by interferon-alpha therapy: possible etiology of HCV-associated immune thrombocytopenia. Eur J Haematol 2005; 75: 417-423.

[49] Jennette JC, Falk RJ, Andrassy K., et al (1994) Nomenclature of systemic vasculitides: The proposal of an international consensus conference. Arthritis Rheum 1994; 37:187-192.

[50] Jiang XH, Xie YT, Tan DM. (2004) Study on the influencing factors of thrombocytopenia in viral hepatitis. Zhonghua Ganzangbing Zazhi 2004; 12: 734-736.

[51] Kamar N, Rostaing L and Alric L. (2006) Treatment of hepatitis C-virus-related glomerulonephritis. Kidney International (2006) 69, 436–439.

[52] Kaplanski G, Maisonobe T, Marin V, et al. (2005) Vascular cell adhesion molecule-1 (VCAM-1) plays a central role in the pathogenesis of severe forms of vasculitis due to hepatitis C-associated mixed cryoglobulinemia. J Hepatol 2005, 42:334-340.

[53] Kayali Z, Buckwold VE, Zimmermann B, et al. (2002) Hepatitis C, cryoglobulinemia, and cirrhosis: a metaanalysis. Hepatology. 2002; 36:978-985.

[54] Khattab M, Eslam M, Allavian S M. (2010) Hepatitis C Virus as a Multifaceted Disease: A Simple and Updated Approach for Extrahepatic Manifestations of Hepatitis C Virus Infection. Hepat Mon. 2010; 10(4): 258-269.

[55] Kittlesen, D. J., Chianese-Bullock K A, Yao Z Q, et al. (2000) Interaction between complement receptor gC1qR and hepatitis C virus core protein inhibits T-lymphocyte proliferation. J. Clin. Invest. 2000, 106:1239–1249.

[56] Lamprecht P, Gutzeit O, Csernok E, et al. (2003) Prevalence of ANCA in mixed cryoglobulinemia and chronic hepatitis C virus infection. Clin Exp Rheumatol 2003; 21: S89-S94.

[57] Leak LV, Petricoin EF 3rd, Jones M, et al. (2002) Proteomic technologies to study diseases of the lymphatic vascular system. Ann N Y Acad Sci. 2002, 979, 211-28; discussion 229-34.

[58] Lee YH, Ji JD, Yeon JE, et al. (1998) Cryoglobulinaemia and rheumatic manifestations in patients with hepatitis C virus infection. Ann Rheum Dis.,1998;57:728–31.

[59] Lenzi M, Frisoni M, Mantovani V, et al. (1998) Mixed Cryoglobulinemia Haplotype HLA-B8-DR3 Confers Susceptibility to Hepatitis C Virus-Related. Blood, 1998: 91: 2062-2066.

[60] Leone N, Pellicano R, Ariata Maiocco I et al. (2002) Mixed cryoglobulinaemia and chronic hepatitis C virus infection: the rheumatic manifestations. J Med Virol 2002; 66:200–3.

[61] Lidove O, Cacoub P, Hausfater P, et al. (1999) Cryoglobulinemia and hepatitis C: worsening of peripheral neuropathy after interferon alpha treatment. Gastroenterol Clin Biol 1999, 23:403-6.
[62] Machida K, Cheng K T, Sung V M. et al. (2004) Hepatitis C virus induces a mutator phenotype: enhanced mutations of immunoglobulin and protooncogenes. Proc Natl Acad Sci., 2004, 101, 4262-7.
[63] Matsuo K, Kusano A, Sugumar A, et al. (2004) Effect of hepatitis C virus infection on the risk of non-Hodgkin's lymphoma: a meta-analysis of epidemiological studies. Cancer Sci 2004, 95:745-52.
[64] Mazzaro C, Zorat F, Comar C et al. (2003) Interferon plus ribavirin in patients with hepatitis C virus positive mixed cryoglobulinemia resistant to interferon. J. Rheumatol. 30, 1775-1781 (2003).
[65] Meltzer M, Franklin EC, Elias K, et al. (1996). Cryoglobulinemia--a clinical and laboratory study. II. Cryoglobulins with rheumatoid factor activity. Am J Med. Jun 1996; 40(6):837-56.
[66] Mohammed R H A, ElMakhzangy H I, Gamal A, et al., (2010). Prevalence of rheumatologic manifestations of chronic hepatitis C virus infection among Egyptians. Clin Rheumatol (2010) 29:1373–1380.
[67] Morra E. (2010) Cryoglobulinemia. American Society of Hematology, 2010. Medline.
[68] Mukhtyar C, Guillevin L, Cid M C, et al. (2009) EULAR recommendations for the management of primary small and medium vessel vasculitis for the European Vasculitis Study Group. Ann Rheum Dis., 2009; 68:310–317.
[69] Napoli J, Bishop GA, McCaughan GW. (1994) Increased intrahepatic messenger RNA expression of interleukins 2, 6 and 8 in hepatic cirrhosis.Gastroenterology. 1994 Sep; 107(3):789-98.
[70] National Digestive Diseases Information Clearing House. NIDDK, 2010Chronic Hepatitis C: Current Disease Management. 2010, Medline.
[71] Newkirk MM. (2002) Rheumatoid factors: host resistance or autoimmunity? Clin Immunol 2002; 104:1–32.
[72] Okutan O, Kartaloglu Z, Ilvan A, et al. (2004) Evaluation of high-resolution computed tomography and pulmonary function tests in patients with chronic hepatitis C virus infection. World J Gastroenterol 2004;10(3):381-384.
[73] Ordi-Ros J, Villarreal J, Monegal F, et al (2000) Anticardiolipin antibodies in patients with chronic hepatitis C virus infection: characterization in relation to antiphospholipid syndrome. Clin Diagn Lab Immunol 2000; 7:241-244.
[74] Pawlotsky J-M. (2011) Hepatitis C Virus Drug Pipeline Overview and Clinical Trial Design. Chapter 7, in Hepatitis C: Antiviral drugs discovery and development. Edited by: Seng-Lai Tan and Yupeng He. April, 2011. Caister Academic Press.
[75] Pereira P F, Lemos L B, Uehara S, et al. (2010) Long-term eYcacy of rituximab in hepatitis C virus-associated cryoglobulinemia. Rheumatol Int (2010) 30:1515–1518.
[76] Pileri P, Uematsu Y, Campagnoli S, et al., (1998). Binding of Hepatitis C virus to CD81. Science. 1998 Oct 30;282(5390):938-41.

[77] Pipitone N and Salvarani C. (2006) Systemic Vasculitis: State of the Art and Emerging Concepts. Curr Opin Rheumatol. 2006;18(1):1-2.

[78] Quartuccio L, Soardo G, Romano G, et al. (2006) Rituximab treatment for glomerulonephritis in HCV associated mixed cryoglobulinaemia: efficacy and safety in the absence of steroids. Rheumatology (Oxford), 2006;45(7):;45:842-846.

[79] Racanelli V, Sansonno D, Piccoli C, et al., (2001). Molecular characterization of B cell clonal expansions in the liver of chronically hepatitis C virus-infected patients. J Immunol. 2001 Jul 1; 167(1):21-9.

[80] Ramos-Casals M, García-Carrasco M, Cervera R, et al. (2001) Hepatitis c virus infection mimicking primary Sjogren's syndrome: a clinical and immunologic description of 35 cases. Medicine (Baltimore) 2001, 80:1-8.

[81] Remoroza R and Bonkovsky H.(2003) Extrahepatic manifestations of chronic Hepatitis C. The HCV Advocate Medical Writer's circle, HCV support project; August, 2003. Medline.

[82] Roccatello D, Baldovino S, Rossi D, et al. (2004) Longterm effects of anti-CD20 monoclonal antibody treatment of cryoglobulinaemic glomerulonephritis. Nephrol Dial Transplant. 2004;19(12):3054-3061.

[83] Roccatello D, Baldovino S, Rossi D, et al., (2008). Rituximab as a therapeutic tool on severe mixed cryoglobulinemia. Clin Rev Allergy Immunol. 2008 Feb;34(1):111-7. Review.

[84] Roncarolo MG, Bacchetta R, Bordignon C, et al. (2001) Type 1 regulatory T cells. Immunol Rev. 2001, 182, 68-79.

[85] Saadoun D, Boyer O, Trebeden-Negre H, et al. (2004) Predominance of type 1 (Th1) cytokine production in the liver of patients with HCV-associated mixed cryoglobulinemia vasculitis. J Hepatol. 2004;41:1031-7.

[86] Saadoun D, Bieche I, Maisonobe T et al. (2005) Involvement of chemokines and type 1cytokines in the pathogenesis of hepatitis C virus-associated mixed cryoglobulinemia vasculitis neuropathy. Arthritis Rheum 2005; 52:2917–25.

[87] Saadoun D, Landau D A, Calabrese L H et al. (2007) Hepatitis C-associated mixed cryoglobulinaemia: a crossroad between autoimmunity and lymphoproliferation. Rheumatology 2007; 46:1234–1242.

[88] Saadoun D, Rosenzwajg M, Landau D, et al. (2008) Restoration of peripheral immune homeostasis after rituximab in mixed cryoglobulinemia vasculitis. Blood. 2008;111(11): 5334-5341.

[89] Saadoun D, Terrier B, Semoun O, et al. (2010, a) HCV- associated polyarteritis nodosa. Arthritis Care Res (Hoboken). Oct, 2010. [Epub ahead of print]

[90] Saadoun D, Rigon M R, Sene D, et al. (2010) Rituximab plus Peg interferon-alpha/ribavirin compared with Peg interferon –alpha/ribavirin in hepatitis C related mixed cryoglobulinemia. Blood, 2010.116:326-334.

[91] Sakaguchi, S. (2000) Regulatory T cells: key controllers of immunologic self-tolerance. Cell. 2000, 101, 455-8.

[92] Sansonno D, De Re V, Lauletta G, et al. (2003) Monoclonal antibody treatment of mixed cryoglobulinemia resistant to interferon alpha with an anti-CD20. Blood. 2003; 101(10):3818-3826.
[93] Sansonno D, Carbone A, De Re V and Dammacco F. (2007) Hepatitis C virus infection, cryoglobulinaemia, and beyond. Rheumatology 2007;46:572–578.
[94] Sasso, E. H. (2000) The rheumatoid factor response in the etiology of mixed cryoglobulinemia associated with hepatitis virus infection. Ann Med Interne. 2000, 151, 30-40.
[95] Sene D, Ghillani-Dalbin P, Limal N et al. (2006) Anti-cyclic citrullinated peptide antibodies in hepatitis C virus associated rheumatological manifestations and Sjogren's syndrome. Ann Rheum Dis 2006; 65:394–7.
[96] Sene D, Limal N, Ghillani-Dalbin P, et al. (2007) Hepatitis C virus-associated B-cell proliferation—the role of serum B lymphocyte stimulator (BLyS/BAFF). Rheumatology (Oxford). 2007; 46:65–69.
[97] Stefanova-Petrova DV, Tzvetanska AH, Naumova EJ, et al. (2007) Chronic hepatitis C virus infection: prevalence of extrahepatic manifestations and its association with cryoglobulinemia in Bulgarian patients. Viral hepatitis. World Journal of Gastroentrol. 2007; 13(48):6518–6528.
[98] Stein JV, López-Fraga M, Elustondo FA., et al. (2002) APRIL modulates B and T cell immunity. J Clin Invest. 2002; 109, 1587-98.
[99] Stone J. (2009) Immune complex-mediated vasculitis. In Kelley's textbook of Rheumatology Eighth edition, Firestein G S, Budd R C, Harris E D, Mc Innes I B, Rudyy S and Sergent J S. 2009, p 1465-1473.
[100] Suzuki R, Morita H, Komukai D, et al. (2003) Mixed Cryoglobulinemia Due to Chronic Hepatitis C with Severe Pulmonary Involvement. Case report, Internal Medicine. 2003; 42: 1210–1214.
[101] Visentini M, Granata M, Veneziano ML et al. (2007) Efficacy of low-dose rituximab for mixed cryoglobulinemia. Clin. Immunol. 2007; 125, 30-33.
[102] Wener MH, Hutchinson K, Morishima C, et al. (2004) Absence of antibodies to cyclic citrullinated peptide in sera of patients with hepatitis C virus infection and cryoglobulinemia. Arthritis Rheum 2004; 50:2305–8.
[103] Wu YY, Hsu TC, Chen TY, et al. (2002) Proteinase 3 and dihydrolipoamide dehydrogenase (E3) are major autoantigens in hepatitis C virus (HCV) infection. Clin Exp Immunol 2002; 128: 347-352.
[104] Yee LJ, Kelleher P, Goldin RD, et al. (2004) Antinuclear antibodies (ANA) in chronic hepatitis C virus infection: correlates of positivity and clinical relevance. J Viral Hepat. 2004; 11: 459-464.
[105] Zaja F, De Vita S, Mazzaro C, et al. (2003,a) Efficacy and safety of rituximab in type II mixed cryoglobulinemia. Blood. 2003;101:3827-3834.
[106] Zaja F, Vianelli N, Sperotto A, et al. (2003 b) Anti-CD20 therapy for chronic lymphocytic leukemia associated autoimmune diseases. Leuk Lymphoma. 2003;44(11):1951-1955.
[107] Zignego A & Bréchot C. (1999) Extrahepatic manifestations of HCV infection: facts and controversies. J. Hepatol.1999; 31: 1152–1154.

[108] Zignego AL, Ferri C, Giannelli F et al. Prevalence of bcl-2 rearrangement in patients with hepatitis C virus-related mixed cryoglobulinemia with or without B-cell lymphomas. Ann Intern Med. 2002; 137:571-580.
[109] Zuckerman E, Keren D, Slobodin G et al. (2000) Treatment of refractory, symptomatic, hepatitis C virus related mixed cryoglobulinemia with ribavirin and interferon-α. J. Rheumatol. 27, 2172-2178 (2000).

Part 4

Selected Issues in Vasculitis

17

Audiovestibular Manifestations in Systemic Vasculitis: An Update

Juan Carlos Amor-Dorado[1] and Miguel Angel Gonzalez-Gay[2]
[1]Otolaryngology Division, Hospital Lucus Augusti, Lugo,
[2]Rheumatology Division, Hospital Universitario Marques de Valdecilla, IFIMAV, Santander,
Spain

1. Introduction

The term systemic vasculitis encompasses a group of diseases that were considered rare years ago. However, as knowledge of them has been expanded, there have become increasingly important in the differential diagnosis of patients with varied manifestations, not only rheumatological, but also with sensory and visceral affectation in diverse locations, extent and severity.

This is a heterogeneous group of diseases that often overlap each other, with various etiologies and clinical manifestations. The common feature among them is the inflammation of the lining of blood vessels, which causes ischemic events and tissue necrosis, as well as the occlusion of the lumen of vessels and, consequently, impaired function of the affected organ [1].

Any blood vessel can be affected by the vasculitic phenomenon. Moreover, the extent and site of affectation of the vessels varies depending on the type of vasculitis; in general, they tend to be irregular and segmental. In severe forms, lesions spread throughout the body. In mild forms, it can be located in a single region of the body; for example, limited to the skin in patients with cutaneous leukocytoclastic vasculitis. Others, however, cause lesions in several distant organs such as kidneys or lungs in patients with microscopic polyangiitis and Wegener's granulomatosis. Some types of vasculitis manifest with lesions in the same stage of development, as in the case of cutaneous lesions that appear with an outbreak of Henoch- Schönlein purpura. In others, such as polyarteritis nodosa, lesions that are at different stages of development in different organs. Some forms of vasculitis may have an acute course, mainly those with a predominantly skin involvement. In contrast, others such as Takayasu's arteritis have shown varying degrees of activity for over 20 years [1].

2. Audiovestibular manifestations in systemic vasculitis

The inner ear may be involved in organ-specific autoimmune diseases such as the autoimmune inner ear disease described by McCabe in 1979 and it may be the target organ in various non-organ specific systemic diseases. Among these, some are the result of direct autoimmune lesion and others of vascular damage which, in turn, can be primary or secondary to infections or collagen diseases. The systemic vasculitis forms belong to the group of diseases that have vascular damage as the main pathogenic factor [2, 3].

Vasculitis	Audiovestibular manifestations
Primary vasculitis	
Predominantly affecting large vessels	
Giant cell arteritis	Partially reversible asymmetric sensorineural hearing loss
	Sudden hearing loss and tinnitus
	Partially reversible vestibular hypofunction in caloric testing (canal paresis)
	BPPV (PSC more frequent than HSC)
Takayasu's arteritis	Sudden reversible hearing loss
Predominantly affecting medium vessels	
Classic Polyarteritis nodosa (PAN)	Sensorineural hearing loss or sudden hearing loss
	Vertigo, without vestibular function studies
Kawasaki disease	Reversible sensorineural hearing loss or conductive hearing loss
Predominantly affecting medium and small vessels	
Wegener's granulomatosis	Otitis media with effusion or chronic otitis media with conductive hearing loss or sudden hearing loss or sensorineural hearing loss in audiometric test and tinnitus
	Central and peripheral nystagmus with vertigo
Churg-Strauss syndrome	Otitis media with effusion or suppurative otitis media due to tympanic perforation and sensorineural hearing loss in audiometric test
Microscopic polyangiitis	Sensorineural hearing loss or sudden hearing loss
	Vertigo, without vestibular function studies

Secondary vasculitis	
Predominantly affecting medium and small vessels	
Rheumatoid arthritis	Conductive hearing loss or sudden hearing loss with sensorineural hearing loss in audiogram
Scleroderma	Symmetrical and bilateral sensorineural hearing loss with a flat curve in the audiogram
	Middle ear dysfunction manifested by a flattened tracing in tympanometry
	BPPV (HSC more frequent than PSC).
	Abnormal head thrust test, head-shaking nystagmus and positional nystagmus
Systemic lupus erythematosus	Conductive hearing loss or sudden hearing loss
Sjögren's syndrome	Conductive hearing loss or sudden sensorineural hearing loss
Ankylosing spondylitis	Symmetrical high frequency sensorineural hearing loss in audiogram
	Dysfunction of static postural control in CTSIB (conditions 5 and 6)
	Frequent BPPV and positional nystagmus
Behcet's disease	Sensorineural hearing loss or sudden hearing loss
	Central and peripheral (mixed) vestibular syndrome
Other vasculitis	
Cogan syndrome	Fluctuating sensorineural hearing loss with tinnitus
	and recurrent spontaneous vertigo
Relapsing polychondritis	Sensorineural hearing loss, tinnitus
	Peripheral vestibular syndrome

BPPV: benign paroxysmal positional vertigo; HSC: horizontal semicircular canal; PSC: posterior semicircular canal; PAN: panarteritis nudosa; CTSIB: Clinical Test for Sensory Interaction and Balance.

Table 1. Audiovestibular manifestations in systemic vasculitis

Interestingly, regardless of the etiology of the various diseases affecting the inner ear, pathological findings are identical. They include degeneration and destruction of the peripheral receptor; segmental and diffuse infiltration of lymphocytes, plasma cells, and macrophages; proliferation of fibrous tissue, and varying degrees of ossification of the inner ear [4].

Next, we discuss the studies to date that have disclosed an association of vasculitis involvement with auditory and vestibular manifestations. Table 1 presents an update of the different audiovestibular manifestations described according to the classification of vasculitis.

3. Primary vasculitis

Giant cell arteritis (GCA) is a multisystemic vasculitis of elderly people. It mainly involves large and medium-sized blood vessels with predisposition to the cranial arteries. GCA constitutes the most common systemic vasculitis in Western countries. Some cranial ischemic manifestations, in particular permanent visual loss, have been widely described in patients with this vasculitis. However, audiovestibular manifestations in GCA patients, such as hearing loss, vertigo, or tinnitus, have been less commonly reported. It is also characterized by granulomatous affectation of the aorta and its major branches, with a predisposition towards the cranial area, both in the arterial branches arising from the external carotid (explaining the topical headaches) and the internal carotid artery, leading to the feared blindness, either by affectation of the posterior ciliary arteries or the central retinal artery. GCA is often present with temporoparietal pulsating headaches, different from the usual, which often accompanied by polymyalgia rheumatica and, to a lesser extent, jaw claudication, amaurosis fugax, blindness, or stroke predominantly in the vertebrobasilar territory [5-8]. The definitive diagnosis is obtained by a temporal artery biopsy demonstrating disruption of the internal elastic lamina with lymphocytic inflammatory infiltration and multinucleated giant cells in 50% of cases [9].

The last 4 decades have witnessed a significant increase in the number of diagnosed cases of GCA. This increase has not only been found in areas where GCA is common [10] but also here the incidence was low [11-13]. This fact can be explained by a greater awareness of the disease. In our population in Lugo of individuals older than 50, the incidence of GCA adjusted for age and gender is 10/100 000 inhabitants/year, but it reaches 23/100 000 inhabitants/year in the group of patients between 70 and 79 [14,15].

In a prospective study of 44 patients with GCA and 10 with isolated polymyalgia rheumatica from our Lugo population, in 39 (89%) of the 44 GCA patients only exhibited abnormalities in the vestibular tests when these were performed in the first four days at the onset of diagnosis and parenterally corticosteroid therapy. Our data suggest that the vestibule is very sensitive to the ischemic effects of the GCA. Also, they suggest that the vestibular damage may be reversible in some cases. With respect to this, only 13 (30%) of the 44 after 3 months of treatment and 1 patient after 6 months of follow-up had persistent vestibular impairment, coinciding with the start of treatment with steroids. The most significant vestibular finding observed at 3 months was paretic horizontal nystagmus in the head shaking nystagmus test. Moreover, although in our study a Dix-Hallpike test was found to be positive in 7% of the control population, this test yielded positive results in 21% of the biopsy-negative GCA and 33% of biopsy-positive GCA patients. This finding in GCA patients seems to be extremely high. It may suggest that in some cases the benign paroxysmal positional vertigo (BPPV) may be related to a vasculitic inflammatory disorder. Furthermore, we found a close relationship between GCA and benign paroxysmal positional vertigo of the posterior semicircular canal in our population [16,17].

In our series, the audiometric tests at the time of diagnosis showed a remarkable auditory dysfunction in GCA patients. Another point to be considered from our study was the presence of a frequent asymmetrical auditory dysfunction that it is in keeping with the asymmetrical cranial manifestations reported in many patients with GCA. During follow-up improvement in auditory function was observed within the first 3 months after the onset of therapy. However, such an improvement was only found in 27% of the cases. In addition, despite corticosteroid therapy, further deterioration in auditory function after 3 months of treatment was detected in 3 patients. Moreover, no additional improvement in hearing function was observed after another 3 months of treatment. These data suggest that the possible improvement in hearing function may be achieved generally early during the first months after the onset of therapy [16]. In summary, our results support the presence of both auditory and vestibular dysfunction closely related to the vasculitic process in GCA patients.

Polymyalgia rheumatica is characterized by pain in the scapulae and proximal aspects of the shoulders, pelvis and proximal aspects of the lower extremities and the cervical region, together with morning stiffness of more than 1 h; it may be present in about 40% of patients with GCA [5]. However, polymyalgia rheumatica may be a separate entity [6] or the initial form of a GCA that does not initially show cranial condition data or other ischemic symptoms suggesting a GCA [18]. Therefore, the presence of audiovestibular abnormalities in one of our patients who initially showed only clinical symptoms of polymyalgia rheumatica was of particular importance. The patient did not initially present the ischemic vascular disease typical of GCA, but at follow-up showed the typical manifestations attributable to it. The presence of vestibular dysfunction may be an alarm sign to consider the possibility of having a "silent and subclinical" GCA in those patients presenting with PMR symptoms. In this regard, the presence of vestibular dysfunction, probably related to ischemic manifestations, may be considered as an early and reversible sign in the course of the disease. Thus, the knowledge of these manifestations as alert signs for a possible underlying GCA is of main importance in elderly people as early corticosteroid treatment reduces significantly the risk of blindness due to GCA. This fact is even more important in GCA whose presenting manifestation is PMR only, as in these cases low dose prednisone does not prevent the development of blindness. The presence of abnormal vestibular tests in patients presenting with PMR without cranial manifestations of GCA may be considered as a red flag to raise the suspicion of an underlying GCA [16].

Takayasu's arteritis is a chronic vasculitis of unknown etiology that affects the aorta, its major branches, the pulmonary artery and the coronary arteries; it causes headache, absence of arterial pulses, heart failure, renovascular hypertension and ocular and cerebral ischemia. In contrast to GCA, Takayasu's arteritis primarily affects young people, especially women between 15 and 25, more commonly in Asian or Central-American populations [19]. In this vasculitis affecting large vessels, a patient has been described who presented sudden deafness and decreased pulse in the radial artery. The hearing condition worsened upon withdrawal of parenterally administered steroids and improved when they were reintroduced [20]. Histopathological studies of the temporal bone are of great interest in patients with systemic vasculitis. Among them, those published for patients diagnosed with **polyarteritis nodosa (PAN)** should be highlighted. In a patient whose first manifestation of the disease was sudden unilateral deafness and vertigo, the temporal bone histopathological study showed bilateral cochlear condition in the form of loss of the organ of Corti in various portions of the cochlea, the absence of the tectorial membrane and atrophy of the stria vascularis, whereas no vestibular histopathological changes were observed [21]. In another patient with a diagnosis of PAN and unilateral profound hearing loss and vertigo, the histopathological study found vasculitis in the internal auditory artery, accompanied by ossification of the cochlea and the vestibular system as well as endolymphatic hydrops in the basal ramp of the cochlea [22]. The loss of sensory cells and neurons in the maculae of the semicircular canals, utricle and saccule has also been reported in PAN [23]. Most of the reported cases with a diagnosis of PAN met the criteria of the Chapel Hill Consensus Conference relative to microscopic polyangiitis. Recently, the possibility has been described of obtaining a recovery of hearing through a cochlear implant in a patient diagnosed with PAN by biopsy. This reinforces the impression that the lesion is located at the cochlear level. In this group of patients with PAN and profound bilateral hearing loss, this may be secondary to labyrinthine ischemia by a vascular phenomenon [24].

Kawasaki disease (KD) is a diffuse necrotizing vasculitis involving medium-sized vessels, with almost constant injury of the coronary arteries and large non-intraparenchymatous arteries. 85% of patients with KD are children under 5 in whom the disease occurs sporadically or in small outbreaks. It is predominant in males (1.5:1) and, although it is more frequent in Japan, the disease has been diagnosed in more than 40 countries [25]. In a study of 62 patients diagnosed with KD, sensorineural hearing loss was described in the acute phase of the disease in 30% and conductive hearing loss in 9%. On examination of auditory function after the acute phase, neurosensorial hearing loss persisted in 5.5% of patients, so the partially reversible character after treatment with steroids was confirmed [26].

Wegener's granulomatosis is defined as a granulomatous inflammation that affects the airways combined with necrotizing vasculitis of small and medium vessels together with glomerulonephritis and positive cANCA [27]. Furthermore to the known hearing loss secondary to obstruction of the Eustachian tube due to granulomas in the nasopharynx, a series of 21 patients described sudden hearing loss and tinnitus [28]. Bilateral sensorineural hearing loss was observed in 12 of 13 patients with auditory symptoms in a series of 19 patients diagnosed with Wegener's disease by biopsy [29]. Some patients also described vestibular manifestations such as vertigo and peripheral nystagmus [30].

Churg-Strauss allergic granulomatous vasculitis is characterized by granulomas in the upper airways, with eosinophilic infiltration and systemic vasculitis in medium and small vessels, along with a history of asthma, circulating eosinophilia and high concentrations of circulating IgE [27]. It has been described with otitis media with effusion, acute otitis media and progressive sensorineural hearing loss in 9.5% of patients, who improved or stabilized after administration of steroids and immunosuppressors [31].

Behcet's disease is a multisystemic, chronic and recurrent disease that almost always occurs with oral thrush and, in variable frequency, genital sores, uveitis, skin lesions and neurological, vascular and gastrointestinal manifestations with a pathological substrate of leukocytoclastic or lymphocytic vasculitis, preferably from capillaries and venules [32]. Auditory manifestations such as sudden deafness have been described, as well as vertigo during the course of the disease and in relapses [33,34]. Sensorineural hearing loss with a cochlear location was described in 30% of 62 patients diagnosed with Behcet's disease, and central vestibular syndrome in 40% [35].

Cogan's syndrome is characterized by fluctuating hearing loss, tinnitus, spontaneous sudden vertigo, and interstitial keratitis. A significant audiovestibular function has also been described. However, the reported damage is so severe that it does not seem to be the result of a true vasculitis, but rather of a primary labyrinthitis [36].

4. Secondary vasculitis

Rheumatoid arthritis is a chronic, multisystemic inflammatory disease characterised by persistent inflammatory synovitis, usually involving peripheral joints in a symmetrical manner, predominantly the wrists, the metacarpophalangeal and proximal interphalangeal joints of the hands, elbows and knees and metatarsal-phalangeal of feet. It is more common in women; although its etiology is unknown, there is a genetic predisposition, as shown by the tendency to familial aggregation, the high concordance with rheumatoid arthritis in monozygotic twins and the association with genes within the major histocompatibility complex, particularly with certain alleles that share a common sequence of amino acids within the hypervariable control region of the HLA-DRB1 chain, called shared epitope [37]. One study has described sudden hearing loss in patients with RA with an underlying vasculitic process affecting the eighth cranial nerve [38].

In the Lugo population, as in the Anglo-Saxon, an association of rheumatoid arthritis with HLA-DR4 alleles has been observed, in particular with HLA-DRB1*0401 and *0404. These alleles have also been shown as markers of vascular damage in patients with rheumatoid arthritis in Lugo, since patients with these alleles are at increased risk of endothelial vascular dysfunction [39] a marker of early stage of atherosclerosis and an increased risk of cardiovascular events [40].

Interestingly, in a series of 33 patients diagnosed with idiopathic sudden hearing loss in our Lugo population, we also observed an association of HLA-DR4 with increased susceptibility to the disease and a worse prognosis for recovery with steroid treatment [41]. Accordingly with this, an increased susceptibility to sensorineural hearing loss has been described in patients with rheumatoid arthritis with respect to a control group. Specifically, in a series of 194 patients diagnosed with rheumatoid arthritis, sensorineural hearing loss was also described in 39% [42]. The coincidence of findings involving HLA-DR4 alleles with increased severity of rheumatoid arthritis [37] and its association with increased risk of vascular damage in this disease [39,40] together with the finding of an increased risk of sudden deafness with worse functional outcome in people presenting HLA-DR4 may indicate that these alleles would be true markers of endothelial vascular damage regardless of the underlying disease [41].

Scleroderma or systemic sclerosis is included in the collagenosis group. Systemic sclerosis (SSc) is a disease characterized by excessive deposition of connective tissue and extracellular matrix proteins in different organs and tissues, and is more common in women. Its etiology is unknown, but it is known to involve disorders of collagen synthesis as well as vascular and immune system abnormalities. Two clinical forms have been established: the limited and the diffuse variants. The predominate features in the limited form are Raynaud's phenomenon, clinical data defined in the CREST syndrome (calcinosis, Raynaud's phenomenon, sclerodactyly, oesophageal disorders, and telangiectasia), increased risk of pulmonary hypertension and presence of positive antinuclear antibodies anticentromere B positive and distal skin condition in the extremities [43]. In the diffuse form, the predominate features are proximal skin condition and more intense injury to internal organs that leads to increased risk of pulmonary fibrosis and renal scleroderma crisis, typically associating with anti-SCL70 positive antibodies [43].

Recently, in the population of Lugo, we tried to assess the presence of audiovestibular damage in a homogenous cohort of patients with limited SSc and antibodies against CENB. We were able to observe abnormalities of audiometric and vestibular tests supporting the presence of audiovestibular damage in limited forms of SSc. We also examined the influence of disease duration on the development of audiovestibular abnormalities; however, we found no association between disease duration and the development of abnormalities of audiometric, vestibular, or postural tests. Nevertheless, we found a significantly increased frequency of patients with abnormal hearing loss in the audiogram (77%). Of interest, a high frequency loss in the audiogram was common in our series; the typical pattern of hearing impairment in our patients with limited SSc was a bilateral and symmetrical sensorineural hearing loss with a flat curve in the audiogram. Vasculitis leading to focal strial atrophy or malfunction of the hair cells of the organ of Corti, or both, has been proposed as responsible for sensorineural hearing loss in SSc. Besides sensorineural damage, we also found middle ear dysfunction, manifested by a flattened tracing in tympanometry in 20% of the patients with limited SSc, due to myringosclerosis confirmed by otomycroscopic examination.

Furthermore, our results confirm that the vestibule is also involved in SSc, even in limited forms of the disease. Patients with limited SSc had a significantly increased frequency of abnormal oculo-cephalic response or head thrust test (29%) and head-shaking nystagmus (26%), and a higher frequency of 3 or more abnormal positions when positional nystagmus was assessed by means of videonystagmography and videonystagmoscopy goggles [44]. The static postural study also yielded a significantly increased frequency of abnormal clinical test of sensory interaction and balance (CTSIB) in limited and diffuse SSc patients (46%) compared with controls (12%). Interestingly, vestibular loss was the main pattern of abnormal CTSIB in our patients. All these findings support the presence of a peripheral vestibular lesion, probably due to vascular involvement in patients with SSc.

In our series, almost a fifth of the patients with limited and diffuse SSc showed a benign paroxysmal positioning vertigo (BPPV) that was generally caused by the involvement of the horizontal semicircular canal (HSC). Interestingly, we observed the presence of abnormal caloric test in 43% of SSc patients with associated BPPV. These observations indicate that abnormalities found in our patients with SSc are not the result of an injury in a single semicircular canal of the inner ear. They also suggest that vascular disease in the setting of this connective tissue disease may be responsible for these findings, supporting an ischemic cause as responsible for the functional damage. However, an alternative cause for BPPV could be related to a possible intralabyrinthine autoimmune process [45].

In summary, we have described hearing and vestibular dysfunctions, as well as an abnormal postural control of static balance in systemic sclerosis, both in limited and in diffuse forms. The etiology is probably vasculitic, although a direct autoimmune mechanism in the inner ear cannot be ruled out. In this patient group studied, we highlight symmetrical and bilateral sensorineural hearing loss, vestibular hypofunction on caloric testing and an abnormal response in head shaking nystagmus test and oculocephalic maneuver (head thrust test), all these findings are typically related with peripheral vestibular dysfunction. Furthermore, we also describe a close association with benign paroxysmal positional vertigo (BPPV), predominantly of the horizontal canal [44,45].

Systemic lupus erythematosus (SLE) is the prototype of autoimmune disease, which primarily affects women between 15 and 50 and also causes secondary vasculitis [46]. Sensorineural hearing loss has been observed with relative frequency in this group of patients with SLE, and both autoimmune and vasculitic mechanisms have been involved in its pathogenesis [47].

Hearing loss and vertigo of probable ischemic origin have been described in **relapsing polychondritis**, an autoimmune disease that affects, unilaterally or bilaterally, the cartilage of the ear, nose and trachea. Its pathophysiology has been explained assuming the existence of a vasculitis of the labyrinthine artery and its branches [48].

Another disease involving audiovestibular manifestations and vasculitis is **Sjögren's syndrome**. This is a slowly progressing, chronic auto-immune disease, characterized by lymphocytic infiltration of exocrine glands, as well as hyper-reactivity and proliferation of B cells that end up producing xerostomia and dry eyes. It may be primary or secondary; in the latter case, it is accompanied by another auto-immune disease with systemic clinic, as occurs in 30% of patients. It mainly affects women between 40 and 50.

Like SLE, Sjögren's syndrome also causes secondary vasculitis [46]. Sensorineural hearing loss concomitant with cardiolipinic antibodies has been described in 14 of 30 patients with Sjögren's syndrome [49]. A sudden hearing loss has also been reported as initial and exceptional presentation in a case of Sjögren's syndrome [50].

Ankylosing spondylitis (AS) is a chronic inflammatory disease of unknown origin affecting up to 1% of the population. To further investigate hearing loss in AS we studied a series of 50 consecutive patients that fulfilled the modified New York diagnostic criteria for AS and 44 matched controls from the Lugo region of Northwest Spain. In this study, 29 (58%) of the patients with AS showed abnormal hearing loss in the audiogram compared to only 8 (18%) of the controls. Of interest, the audiogram shape disclosed a predominant pattern of symmetrical high frequency sensorineural hearing loss in AS patients (50%). In our study, individuals with severe extraspinal manifestations had an increased risk of having hypoacusia. Furthermore, the presence of hip involvement, anterior uveitis, and HLA-B27 in patients with AS appears to be a signal for sensorineural hearing loss (SNHL) that deserves further investigation. Besides sensorineural damage, in our series middle ear dysfunction, manifested by an abnormal tympanometry, was found in 8% of patients with a flattened tracing who was considered the most specific sign of abnormal tympanometry in AS patients. This finding could be explained by an increased rigidity of the tympanossicular system.

Furthermore, our results confirm that the vestibule is also involve in patients with AS. Patients with AS have a marginally increased frequency of abnormal head thrust test and a significantly increased frequency of abnormal head-shaking nystagmus in oculocephalic response study (vestibule-ocular reflex) and disclosed an abnormal vestibular function in caloric testing (canal paresis).

In our series from Lugo, we also founded a significantly increased frequency of abnormal CTSIB results in AS patients (36%). In this regard, increased frequency of abnormal postural control in CTSIB test was of vestibular origin, conditions 5 and 6 of the study, that correspond to a vestibular pattern of the study in patients with AS.

All our findings support the presence of a peripheral vestibular lesion in patients with AS. On the other hand, although the difference did not reach statistical significance, BPPV also was found more frequently in patients than in the controls. Therefore, these studies confirm the presence of inner ear compromise and audiovestibular dysfunction in patients with AS that may be the result of vascular involvement or due to a direct immune-mediated injury of the inner ear and it could provide justification for rheumatologists or physicians to screen for inner ear compromise in their AS population. [51,52].

5. Role of serological study

As for serological markers that could help diagnose diseases involving vascular damage, some studies suggest an etiopathogenic role of anti-endothelial cell antibodies (AECA). These could be regarded as markers of immune-mediated vascular damage in vasculitis, as well as sudden hearing loss, where some authors assign it a direct involvement in physiopathology [53,54]. However, in our population, we could not confirm the diagnostic or pathogenic role of AECA in patients diagnosed with GCA through temporal artery biopsy in whom vestibular dysfunction and sensorineural hearing loss had been confirmed [55].

As far as we know, there is no specific marker to support the diagnosis of immune-mediated inner ear disease. We must suspect it based on a combination of a compatible clinic together with the findings derived from conducting vestibular, hearing and laboratory tests for each disease.

6. Conclusions

The vasculitis forms are a heterogeneous group of diseases in which audiovestibular symptoms are relatively more common than was initially considered, both at the beginning of the vasculitis and in the evolution of the process. Studies confirm that the search for changes in auditory and vestibular tests shows both peripheral and central disorders. Furthermore, the audiovestibular dysfunction could be explained by an ischemic mechanism mediated by the inflammatory vasculitic phenomenon in primary vasculitis, but one cannot rule out the role of a direct autoimmune mechanism when the inner ear is involved in secondary vasculitis. In our population, BPPV was found more frequently when was studied in GCA, SS and AS. Moreover, patients with GCA showed more frequent findings of BPPV than SS and this more than AS. This finding may suggest that BPPV could be associated with more frequency when vasculitis was the main pathogenic factor mediated by ischemia. In SS and AS patients both autoimmune and vasculitic mechanisms could be involved in its pathogenesis.

7. References

[1] Lie JT. Vasculitis, 1815 to 1991: classification and diagnostic specificity (Dunlop Dottridge lecture). J Rheumatol. 1991; 19:19:83-89.

[2] McCabe BF. Autoimmune sensorineural hearing loss. Ann Otol Rhinol Laryngol. 1979;88:585-9.

[3] Garcia Berrocal JR, Ramirez-Camacho R. Immuneresponse and immunopathology of the inner ear: an update. J Laryngol Otol. 2000;114:101-7.

[4] Yoon TH, Paparella MM, Schachern PA. Systemic vasculitis: a temporal bone histopathologic study. Laryngoscope. 1989;99:600-609.

[5] Gonzalez-Gay MA, Barros S, Lopez-Diaz MJ, Garcia-Porrua C, Sanchez-Andrade A, Llorca J. Giant cell arteritis: disease patterns of clinical presentation in a series of 240 patients. Medicine (Baltimore). 2005;84:269-76.

[6] Gonzalez-Gay MA. Giant cell arteritis and polymyalgia rheumatica: two different but often overlapping conditions. Semin Arthritis Rheum. 2004;33:289-93.

[7] Gonzalez-Gay MA, García-Porma C, LlorcaJ, Hajeer AH, Branas F, Dababneh, A, et al. Visual manifestations of giant cell arteritis. Trends and clinical spectrum in 161 patients. Medicine (Baltimore). 2000;79:283-92.
[8] Gonzalez-Gay MA, Garcia-Porrua C, Vazquez-Caruncho M. Polymyalgia rheumatica in biopsy proven giant cell arteritis does not constitute a different subset but differs from isolated polymyalgia rheumatica. J Rheumatol. ;1998;25:1750-5.
[9] Gonzalez-Gay MA, Garcia-Porrua C, Llorca J, Gonzalez-Louzao C, Rodriguez-Ledo P. Biopsy-negative giant cell arteritis: clinical spectrum and predictive factors for positive temporal artery biopsy. Semin Arthritis Rheum. 2001;30:249-56.
[10] Machado EB, Michet CJ, Ballard DJ, Hunder GG, Beard CM, Chu, CP, et al. Trends in incidence and clinical presentation of temporal arteritis in Olmsted County, Minnesota, 1950-1985. Arthritis Rheum. 1988;31:745-9.
[11] Sonnenblick M, Nesher G, Friedlander Y, Rubinow A. Giant cell arteritis in Jerusalem: a 12-year epidemiological study. Br J Rheumatol. 1994;33:938-41.
[12] Gonzalez-Gay MA, Blanco R, Sanchez-Andrade A, Vazquez- Caruncho M. Giant cell arteritis in Lugo (Spain): a more frequent disease with less fewer classic features. J Rheumatol. 1997;24:2166-70.
[13] Gonzalez-Gay MA, Garcia-Porrua C, Rivas MJ, Rodriguez-Ledo P, Llorca J. Epidemiology of biopsy proven giant cell arteritis in northwestern Spain: trend over an 18 year period. Ann Rheum Dis. 2001;60:367-71.
[14] Gonzalez-Gay MA, Miranda-Filloy JA, Lopez-Diaz MJ, Perez- Alvarez R, Gonzalez-Juanatey C, Sanchez-Andrade, A, et al. Giant cell arteritis in northwestern Spain: a 25-year epidemiologic study. Medicine (Baltimore). 2007;86:61-8.
[15] Gonzalez-Gay MA, Garcia-Porrua C, Amor-Dorado JC. Arteritis de células gigantes y polimialgia reumática. In: Ramos Casals M, Garcia Carrasco M, Gomez de Salazar JR, Calvo Alen J, Font Franco J, editors. Enfermedades autoinmunes sistémicas y reumatológicas. Barcelona: Masson; 2005. p. 197-209.
[16] Amor-Dorado JC, Llorca J, Garcia-Porrua C, Costa C, Perez- Fernandez N, Gonzalez-Gay MA. Audiovestibular manifestations in giant cell arteritis: a prospective study. Medicine (Baltimore). 2003;82:13-26.
[17] Amor-Dorado JC, Llorca J, Costa-Ribas C, Garcia-Porrua C, Gonzalez-Gay MA. Giant cell arteritis: a new association with benign paroxysmal positional vertigo. Laryngoscope. 2004;114: 1420-1425.
[18] Gonzalez-Gay MA, Garcia-Porrua C, Amor-Dorado JC, Llorca J. Giant cell arteritis without clinically evident vascular involvement in a defined population. Arthritis Rheum. 2004;51:274-7.
[19] Hall S, Barr W, Lie JT, Stanson AW, Kazmier FL, Hunder GG. Takayasu's arteritis: A study of 32 North American patients. Medicine (Baltimore). 1985;64:89-99.
[20] Maruyoshi H, Toyama K, Kojima S, Kawano H, Ogata N, Miyamoto, S, et al. Sensorineural hearing loss combined with Takayasu's arteritis. Intern Med. 2005;44:124-8.
[21] Jenkins HA, Pollak AM, Fisch U. Polyarteritis nodosa as a cause of sudden deafness. A human temporal bone study. Am J Otolaryngol. 1981;2:99-107.
[22] Gussen P. Polyarteritis nodosa and deafness. A human temporal bone study. Arch Otorhinolaryngol. 1977;26:263-71.

[23] Adkins WY, Ward PH. Temporal bone showing polyarteritis nodosa, otosclerosis, and occult neuroma. Laryngoscope. 1986;96:645-52.
[24] Psillas G, Kyriafinis G, Danizilidis J. Polyarteritis nodosa and cochlear implantation. J Laryngol Otol. 2007;121:196-9.
[25] Dym L. Kawasaki disease. Curr Opin Rheumatol. 1993;5:41-5.
[26] Knott PD, Orloff LA, Harris JP, Novak RE, Burns JC, Kawasaki Disease Multicenter Hearing Loss Study Group. Sensorineural hearing loss and Kawasaki disease: a prospective study. Am J Otolaryngol. 2001;22:343-8.
[27] Gonzalez-Gay MA, Garcia-Porrua C, Guerrero J, Rodriguez-Ledo P, Llorca J. The epidemiology of the primary systemic vasculitides in northwest Spain: implications of the Chapel Hill Consensus Conference definitions. Arthritis Rheum. 2003;49: 388-393.
[28] Llompart X, Aumaitre O, Kemeny JL, Mom T, Gilain L. Early otorhinolaryngological manifestations of Wegener's granulomatosis. Analysis of 21 patients. Ann Otolaryngol Chir Cervicofac. 2002;119:330-6.
[29] Kempf HG. Ear involvement in Wegener's granulomatosis. Clin Otolaryngol. 1989;14:451-6.
[30] Bennett RW, Staker LV. Wegener's granulomatosis presenting as vertigo. West J Med. 1987;146:359-61.
[31] Bacciu A, Bacciu S, Mercante G, Ingegnoli F, Grasselli C, Vaglio, A, et al. Ear, nose and throat manifestations of Churg-Strauss syndrome. Acta Otolaryngol. 2006;126:503-9.
[32] Gonzalez-Gay MA, Garcia-Porrua C, Branas F, Lopez-Leizaro L, Olivieri I. Epidemiologic and clinical aspects of Behcet's disease in a defined area of Northwestern Spain, 1988-1997. J Rheumatol. 2000;27:703-
[33] Belkahia A, Ben Ayed H, Ben H'Mida M, Hamza M. Auditory and vestibular lesions in Behcet's disease. Ann Otolaryngol Chir Cervicofac. 1982;99:469-76.
[34] Narvaez J, Valverde-Garcia J, Alegre-Sancho JJ, Juanola X, Clavaguera MT, Roig-Escofet D. Sudden cochlear hearing loss in a patient with Behcet's disease. Rev Rheum (Engl ed). 1998;65:63-4.
[35] Kulahli I, Balci K, Koseoglu E, Yuce I, Cagli S, SenturkM. Audiovestibular disturbances in Behcet's patients: report of 62 cases. Hear Res. 2005;203:28-31.
[36] Schuknecht HF, Nadol Jr JB. Temporal bone pathology in a case of Cogan's syndrome. Laryngoscope. 1994;104:1135-42.
[37] Gonzalez-Gay MA, Garcia-Porrua C, Hajeer AH. Influence of human leukocyte antigen-DRB1 on the susceptibility and severity of rheumatoid arthritis. Semin Arthritis Rheum. 2002;31:355-60.
[38] Merrin PK, Macfarlane DG. Vestibulocochlear dysfunction in a patient with rheumatoid disease and vasculitis. Ann Rheum Dis. 1991;50:393-4.
[39] Gonzalez-Juanatey C, Testa A, Garcia-Castelo A, Garcia-Porrua C, Llorca J, Vidan, A, et al. HLA-DRB1 status affects endothelial function in treated patients with rheumatoid arthritis. Am J Med. 2003;114:647-52.
[40] Gonzalez-Gay MA, Gonzalez-Juanatey C, Lopez-Diaz MJ, Pineiro A, Garcia-Porrua C, Miranda-Filloy, JA, et al. HLA-DRB1 and persistent chronic inflammation

contribute to cardiovascular events and cardiovascular mortality in patients with rheumatoid arthritis. Arthritis Rheum. 2007;57:125-32.
[41] Amor-Dorado JC, Paco L, Martin J, Lopez-Nevot MA, GonzalezGay MA. Human leukocyte antigen-DQB1 and -DRB1 associations in patients with idiopathic sudden sensorineural hearing loss from a defined population of Northwest Spain. Acta Otolaryngol. 2005;125:1277-82.
[42] García Callejo FJ, Conill Tobías N, Munoz Fernandez N, De Paula Vernetta C, Alonso Castaneira I, Marco Algarra J. Hearing impairment in patients with rheumatoid arthritis. Acta Otorrinolaringol Esp. 2007;58:232-8.
[43] Arias-Nunez MC, Llorca J, Vazquez-Rodriguez TR, Gomez-Acebo I, Miranda-Filloy JA, Martin, J, et al. Systemic sclerosis in northwestern Spain: a 19-year epidemiologic study. Medicine (Baltimore). 2008;87:272-80.
[44] Amor-Dorado JC, Arias-Nuñez MC, Miranda-Filloy JA, Gonzalez- Juanatey C, Llorca J, Gonzalez-Gay MA. Audiovestibular manifestations in patients with limited systemic sclerosis and centromere protein-B (CENP-B) antibodies. Medicine (Baltimore). 2008;87:131-41.
[45] Amor-Dorado JC, Barreira-Fernandez MP, Arias-Nunez MC, Gomez-Acebo I, Llorca J, Gonzalez-Gay MA. Benign paroxysmal positional vertigo and clinical test of sensory interaction and balance in systemic sclerosis. Otol Neurotol. 2008;29: 1155-61.
[46] Gonzalez-Gay MA, García-Porrúa C. Systemic vasculitis in adults in northwestern Spain, 1988-1997, Clinical and epidemiologic aspects. Medicine (Baltimore). 1999;78:292-308.
[47] Andonopoulos AP, Naxakis S, Goumas P, Lygatsikas C. Sensorineural hearing disorders in systemic lupus erythematosus. A controlled study. Clin Exp Rheumatol. 1995;13:137-41.
[48] Schuknecht HF. Ear pathology in autoimmune disease. Adv Otorhinolaryngol. 1991;46:50-70.
[49] Tumiati B, Casoli P, Parmeggiani A. Hearing loss in the Sjogren syndrome. Ann Intern Med. 1997;126:450-3.
[50] García Berrocal JR, Arellano B, Vargas JA, Trinidad A, Ramírez Camacho R, Vergara J. Enfermedad inmunomediada del oído interno: Presentación de casos clínicos. Acta Otorrinolaringol Esp. 1997;48:565- 70.
[51] Amor-Dorado JC, Barreira-Fernández MP, Vázquez-Rodríguez TR, Miranda-Filloy JA, Llorca J, González-Gay MA. Benign paroxysmal positional vertigo and clinical test of sensory interaction and balance in ankylosing spondylitis. Otol Neurotol. 2011;32:278-83.
[52] Amor-Dorado JC, Barreira-Fernandez MP, Vazquez-Rodriguez TR, Gomez-Acebo I, Miranda-Filloy JA, Diaz de Teran T, Llorca J, Gonzalez-Gay MA. Audiovestibular manifestations in patients with ankylosing spondylitis. Medicine (Baltimore). 2011 ;90:99-109.
[53] Cadoni G, Fetoni AR, Agostino S, De Santis A, Manna R, Ottaviani, F, et al. Autoimmunity in sudden sensorineural hearing loss: possible role of anti-endothelial cell autoantibodies. Acta Otolaryngol Suppl. 2002;548:30-3.

[54] Ottaviani F, Cadoni G, Marinelli L, Fetoni AR, de Santis A, Romito, A, et al. Anti-endothelial autoantibodies in patients with sudden hearing loss. Laryngoscope. 1999;109:1084-7.

[55] Amor-Dorado JC, Garcia-Porrua C, Gonzalez-Gay MA. Antiendothelial cell antibodies and biopsy-proven temporal arteritis. Lupus. 2002;11:134.

18

Vasculitis of the Central Nervous System – A Rare Cause of Stroke

Małgorzata Wiszniewska[2] and Anna Członkowska[1]
[1]*Department of Neurology Institute of Psychiatry and Neurology Warsaw*
[2]*Specialist Hospital, Neurological Department, Piła*
Poland

1. Introduction

The term „vasculitis" encompasses a heterogenous group of multisystemic disorders characterized pathologically by inflammation and necrosis of the blood vessel wall [1]. The sequelae of vascular inflammation depend on the number, site and size of involved blood vessels. In vasculitis a disturbances of the blood vesels wall are focal. The segmental lesions lead, most common, to stenosis, occlusion and infarction. The lesions can also produce aneurysms, vessel wall rupture and haemorrhage. Almost all forms of vasculitis can involve the vessels feeding the brain parenchyma and cause stroke-like episodes [2, 3]. The clinical presentation of involvement the central nervous system (CNS) is very variable. Headaches and encephaloppathy are most typical. Meningeal signs, psychiatric syndromes, dementia, cranial nerve palsies, epileptic seizures alone or in combination with neuropathy/ polyneuropathy or muscle damage , multiorgan involvement and non-specific systemiec symptoms (fever, weight loss) are also well known symptoms. Vasculitis is an infrequent disorder: the overall annual incidence (excluding giant cell arteritis) is estimated to be 31-47 cases/milion, but exist very rare types of vasculitis such as Churg-Strauss where annual incidence amounts ony 1-5 cases/milion [1, 4]. For polyarteritis nodosa (PAN) an annual incidence of 1.6 per milion has been described [5]. Vasculitis is a rare cause of stroke, even in the young age groups: only 1 case among 515 consecutive intracerebral haemorrhage, 13 among 1904 consecutive transient ischaemic attacs (TIA), 8 out of 254 (3%) stroke patients aged under 50 years [6] and 10 out of 215 (5%) patients aged under 45 years [7]. Neurological symtoms and stroke may be the first manifestation of vasculitis or may complicate the clinical course of previously diagnosed case.

2. Classification of vasculitis

There have been several proposals for the classification of vasculitis [1, 8-11], but all have limitation. The simple division of vasculitis usually consider as primary and secondary [12]. According to the Chapel Hill Consensus Conferences (CHCC) the primary systemic vasculitides are classified into three main groups: the affecting predominantly large-sized vessels, medium- and small-sized vessels, respectively (table 1) [13].

Vessel size	Granulomatous	Nongranulomatous
Large	Giant cell arteritis Cranial arteritis Takayasu arteritis	
Medium		Polyarteritis nodosa Kawasaki disease Microscopic polyarteritis
Small (with ANCA)	Wegener granulomatosis Churg-Strauss syndrome	
Small (with immune complexes)		Cryoglobulinemic vasculitis Behcet syndrome

Table 1. Classification of primary vasculitides (according Berlit)

Blood examinations: Erytrocyte sedimentation rate (ESR), C-reactive protein (CRP), blood cell differentiation , liver enzymes, creatinine, glomerular filtration rate, coagulation tests with search for coagulopaties [especially anticardiolipin-antibodies (ACA), lupus anticoagulant (LA)], electrophoresis, creatinine kinase, lactate dehydrogenase (LDH), haptoglobulin, ferritine, angiotensin converting enzyme, immunofixation, quantitative evaluation of immunoglobulins, search for cryoglobulins, TSH, thyroid antibodies, rheuma factor, antinuclear antibodies (ANA), ds-DNA antibodies, histon antibodies, complement, anti-Ro (SS-A), anti -La (SS-B) antibodies, c- and p ANCA/MPO [myeloperoxidase [MPO]], anti-endothelial antibodies, drug screening, blood culture Serologic tests for syphilis, borreliosis, hepatitis B and C, HIV Urine examination including electrophoresis Cerebrospinal fluid (CSF): cell differentiation, isoelectric focussing, cultures, antigens, PCR [viruses, bacteria, mycosis]

Table 2. Laboratory tests which are performed in suspected vasculitis (according Berlit)

3. Diagnosis

If the diagnosis of vasculitis is suspected, a comprehensive medical history and physical examination should be very carefully carry out. Then appropriate laboratory tests and other ancillary procedures must be performed to asses organ damage [12, 14]. Laboratory findings suggestive of a systemic vasculitis include an acute inflammatory response like: raised erythrocyte sedimentation rate (ESR) and increased values of C-reactive protein (CRP). Anemia, thrombocytosis, elevated liver enzymes and low complement are frequent associated findings. Specific antibodies in the blood are evaluated in second order of laboratory tests in specialistic laboratories. It ought to exclude diseases which can also cause the lesions in the blood vesels mimic vasculitis – that's why should carry out serologic tests for syphilis, borreliosis, hepatitis B and C as well as HIV in such case. In primary angiitis of central nervous system (PACNS) serum findings usually are normal, but cerebrospinal fluid (CSF) studies reveal inflammatory findings - a mild lymphomonocytic pleocytosis or protein elevation. The disorders in CSF are present in more than 90% of patients, but they are non specific [15]. Table 2 contains laboratory tests which are carry out in patients with suspicion of vasculitis.

Imaging radiological techniques which demonstrate arterial vessels play significant role in securing the diagnosis of vasculitis, and also demonstrate the cerebral involvement [12, 14, 16, 17, 18]. Computed tomography (CT) and magnetic resonance imaging (MRI) detect multiple CNS vascular lesions when only one is clinically apparent. MRI is more sensitive than CT and good detect the lesions in the cerebral trunk which is not visible in CT. Multiple infarcts in different vascular territories and of different ages are suggestive of vasculitis [17] Normal MRI rather excludes intracranial vasculitis. On digital subtraction cerebral angiography (DSA), angio- CT, MR angiography (MRA), areas of stenosis, dilatation, occlusion, microaneurysm, and narrowing in multiple-vessel tributaries, collateral flow, and regionally prolonged circulation time are suggestive of vasculitis [16, 17, 18, 19]. MRA offers the possibility of directly evaluating small vessel vasculitis. Small vessel vasculitis is currently best demonstrated by changes seen in brain parenchyma on MRI, but high field strength (7T) [16, 17]. These findings are, however, non specific, as they can be seen in other conditions such as vasospasm related to subarachnoid haemorrhage, drugs or severe hypertension, diabetes with intracranial atheroma, embolus recanalization, radiation, infectious or carcinomatous leptomeningitis, sickle-cell disease, reversible angiopathies, dissection. Therefore it is very important to analyse the radiological findings in clinical context. MRI performed with and without contrast medium is the good investigation not only for detection but also for monitoring cerebral involvements [20]. Noteworthy is 18-fluorodeoxyglucose positron emission tomography as well as certain MRI techniques which allow the visualization of vessel wall inflammation when the lumen is still unaffected on angiography, but these are methods high specialistics and not commonly used [16, 17, 21].

Confirmatory evidence can be obtained from tissue biopsy of occupied organ but this is invasive method not always perform. Moreover the lesion in vasculitis is segmental, and it can not encounter on involvement vessel [12, 14]. Thut's why a normal tissue biopsy does not exclude vasculitis.

4. Treatment of vasculitis

There are few controlled studies on the treatment of vasculitis. Usually a combination of steroids and cytotoxic drugs is used, but there is considerable variation between centres on current therapeutic regimens [12]. Cytotoxics drugs are usually used if the response to steroids is poor, if there are too much steroid side effects, in diseases that respond better to cytotoxic agents and in severe cases [12, 18, 22].

We present pathological and clinical aspects of most importants primary vasculitides.

5. Primary vasculitis

5.1 Primary, large vessel vasculitis

Giant cell (temporal) arteritis (GCA)

GCA (Horton disease) is the most common of all the vasculitides. It is a chronic, granulomatous vasculitis of large- and medium sized arteries. Women are affected more frequently than men (3:1 to 5:1). Mean age at the beginning of the disorder is 65 years or more. The American College of Rheumatology (ACR) diagnostic criteria [23] include at least three of: 1. Age 50 years or more, 2. New developed headache, 3. Tenderness of the superficial temporal artery, 4. Elevated sedimentation rate, at least 55 mm/h, 5. Giant cell arteritis in a biopsy specimen from the temporal artery. The definitive diagnosis of GCA requires the pathologic demonstration of biopsy with the typical mononuclear, granulomatosus cell infiltration of all mural layers, usually with multinucleated giant cells (fig.1). The lesion of vessels involves most often superficial temporal artery, vertebral, ophthalmic and posterior ciliary arteries, seldom external and internal carotid arteries, while intracranial arteries are almost never involved [24]. The biopsy is the cornerstone of diagnosis and often remains positive for two to six weeks after the commencement of treatment but the best delivery is performance of biopsy as quick as possible but this procedure can not delay treatment. Besides biopsy may be negative in some patients with GCA, due to the presence of skip lesions or to sub-optimal biopsy. Therefore, patients with negative biopsy should be managed as having GCA if there is typical clinical and laboratory picture [25] . Duplex ultrasonography can detect the characteristic appearance of a hypoechoic "halo", occlusion and stenosis, but requires a high level of experience and training. Positron emission tomography scanning can pick up aortic and large vessel disease, and 3-tesla MRI has shown mural enhancement in inflamed temporal and others arteries. These new techniques can be useful for diagnosis and monitoring the disease, but currently are to expensive, not easy accessible, and not replace the temporal artery biopsy.

Clinicians should remember that jaw and tongue claudication, visual symptoms, constitutional symptoms (fever, weigh loss and tiredness) and acute phase response may go unrecognised especially if not accompanied by headache [26]. Abrupt and irreversible loss of vision due to anterior ischaemic optic neuritis is the most dramatic complication of GCA. Two-thirds of the patients had premonitory visual symptoms like blurring, diplopia or amaurosis fugax the week preceding visual loss [27]. Cervical and muscular pain can occur, usually in the early phase of the disease. Transient ischemic attack (TIA) and stroke are rare (about 7%) and often in the vertebrobasilar territory [28]. Very rare stroke is the first symptoms of GCA [29].

Steroids are the first line drugs in treatment of GCA. High-dose glucocorticosteroid should be initiated immediately when clinical suspicion of GCA is raised. In uncomplicated GCA prednisolone 40-60 mg (not less than 0.75 mg/kg) daily until resolution of symptoms and laboratory (most important decrease of ESR) abnormalities is recomended. In visual loss or history of amaurosis fugax as well as in stroke intravenous methylprednisolone 500mg to 1 g daily for three days before oral prednisolone should be given [25]. During steroids treatment it should to remember of bone and gastrointestinal protection applicating weekly bisphosphonate and calcium/vitamin D supplementation, and protein pump inhibitors (eg omeprazole, lanzoprazole). Prednisolone is continued in full dose during four weeks or until withdrawal of symptoms and lab abnormalities. Then dose is reduced by 10 mg every two weeks to 20 mg, then 2.5 mg every two to four weeks to 10 mg, and in the end by 1 mg every one to two months, provided there is no relapse. Sometimes the dose reduction is more rapid. In case relapsing disease it ought to use steroids again [25].

Primary angiitis of the CNS (PACNS)

PACNS is a rare form of vasculitis of unknown cause, which accounts for just 1% of the systemic vasculitides [30]. The mean age of onset is 50 years, and men are affected twice as

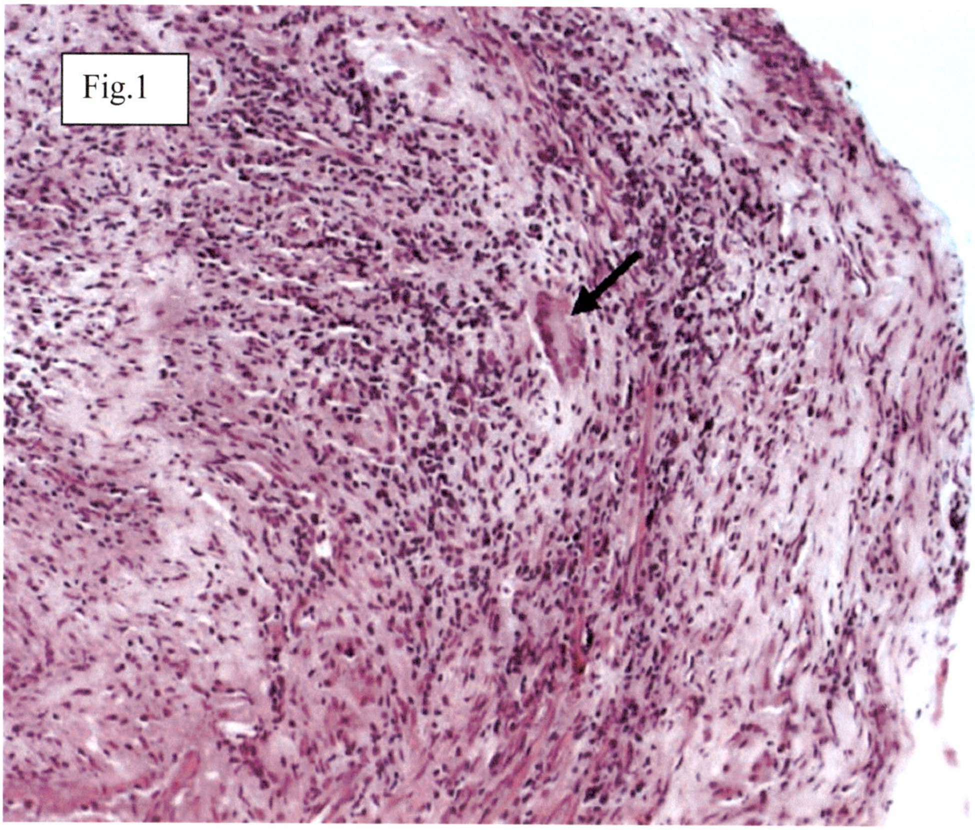

Fig. 1. GCA – biopsy of the wall of the superficial temporal artery (typical multinuclear large cell) (from collection of prof. J. Bogousslavsky)

often as women. It causes focal and diffuse neurological symptoms. Headache and encephalopathy are the most frequent initial symptoms. Stroke or focal symptoms develop in less than 20% of patients at the onset of the disease [30]. Serologic markers of inflammation are typically normal. Seizures have been reported in less than 25% of patients, fevers, weight loss, and night sweats have been reported in less than 20% of patients. Similarly, the erythrocyte sedimentation rate is elevated in less than 25% od patients. Substantial number of patients suspected of having PACNS will have signs and symptoms caused by vasospasm rather than true vasculitis of intracerebral vessels. Sometimes in difficult to distinguish these two disorders. PACNS typically affects middle-aged men, reversible vasoconstriction syndrome is primarily seen in women aged 20 to 40 years. Puerperous period, migraines, illicit drug use, and use of over-the counter cold medicines, is frequently conncted with vasoconstriction syndrome. Sometimes PACNS mimic cerebral tumors [31]

MRI should be the neuroimaging modality of choice for patients with suspected PACNS, and abnormality are present in 90% to 100% of patients. MRI may demonstrate ischemic and hemorrhagic lesions most common seen in the subcortical white matter, followed by the deep gray matter, the deep white matter, and the cereberal cortex. Infarcts may be seen in approximately 50% of cases; when present , infarcts are usually seen bilaterally in multiple-

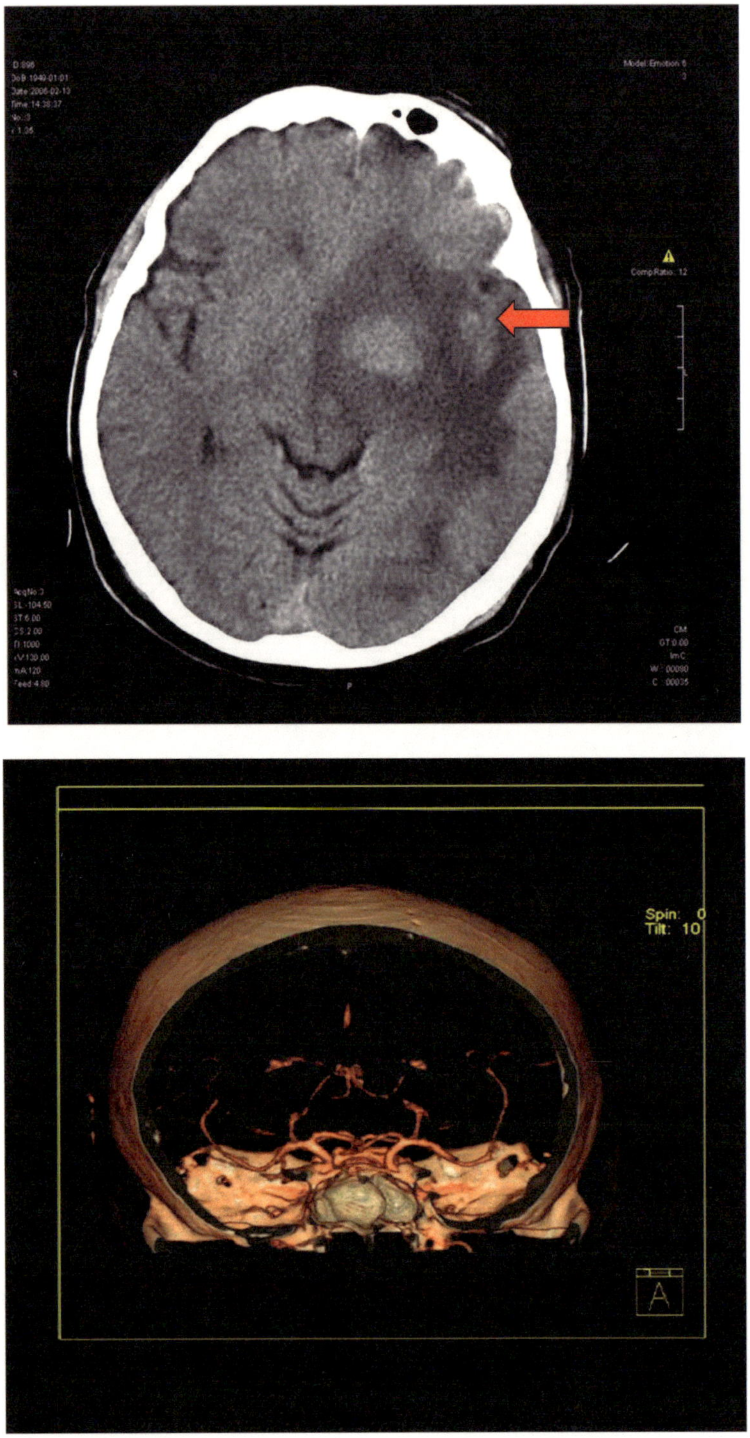

Fig. 2. CT and agio CT of the brain with lesion on left hemisphere, and typical segmental arterial stenosis in PACNS (owne case)

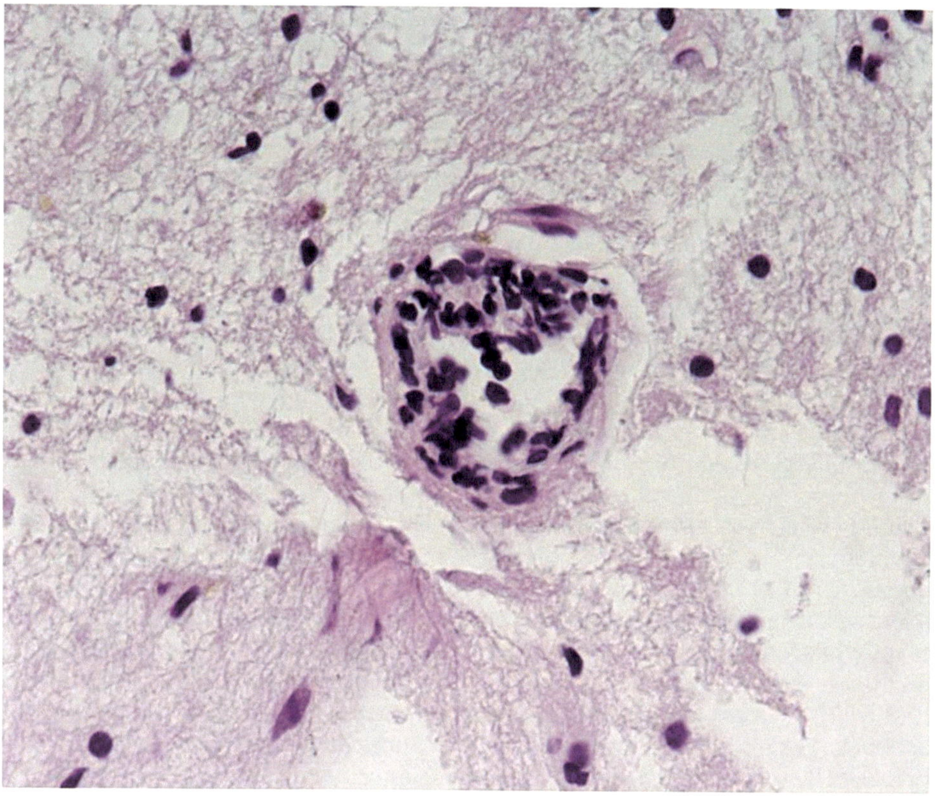

Fig. 3. Brain stereotactic biopsy from lesion in PACNS (lymphocytic cellular infiltrates of vessel wall) (own case)

vessel tributaries, affecting the cortex as well as the subcortex area. Both subarachnoid and intraparenchymal haemorrhages occur in approximately 10% of cases. Mass lesions mistaken for malignant neoplasms can be seen in as many as 15% of cases. Other common patterns include diffuse small-vesel changes of ischemic demyelination. Less common patterns include confluent white-matter lesions, which can be mistaken for multiple sclerosis [18, 30, 32]. Angiography sometimes demonstrates bilateral vessel stenoses or occlusion consistent with an angiitis (fig.2) [12, 18, 30, 32]. In cerebro-spinal fluid some findings have been reported [15, 32]. Pleocytosis and a protein elevation are frequent but not specific [15].

Criteria for the diagnosis of PANCS were suggested in 1987 by Calabrese and Mallek [33]: 1. Acquired neurological deficit unexplained after complete evaluation, 2. Diagnostic cerebral angiogram with narrowing of vessels, areas of dilation and/or beaded vessel appearance, displacement of vessels or vessel occlusions, 3. No evidence of systemic vasculitis or any other condition that could mimic the angiogram findings.

Definite diagnosis can give brain/leptomeningeal biopsy, which has a 53% sensitivity, and not rare it is negative [12, 30, 32, 34, 35]. Besides that brain biopsy remains the gold standard for the diagnosis of PACNS and stereotactic biopsy is generally only recommended for mass lesion. The brain biopsy is proposed all patients with a suspected diagnosis of PACNS before starting the plan of prolonged immunosuppressant treatment [30], but not always patients decide for this invasive procedure. The histological findings of PACNS consist of granulomatous inflammation, fibrinoid necrosis of vessel wall or exclusively lymphocytic cellular infiltrates (fig.3.). There was no correlation between the histological pattern and clinical manifestations or prognosis [18, 36].

No controlled therapy studies for CNS angiitis have been performed yet. In general, a combination of steroids and pulse cyclophosphamid (CYC) is recommended [18]. Birnbau propose treat patients with definite PACNS initially with oral CYC 2mg/kg/d and corticosteroid (usually in the form of prednisone 1mg/kg/d. if the patients has immediate life-threatening disease, it begin therapy with methyprednisolone 1g intravenously daily for 3 days. Thereafter, the patient is given oral prednisone 1mg/kg/d for 1 month, and the dose then is tapered slowly over 12 months [30]. During such high doses of prednisone, all patients should be received bisphosphonate, calcium and vitamin D, as well as pantoprazole, and supplementation of kalium periodically. Appropriate adjustments for CYC therapy, considering the patient's age, renal status, and other comorbidities, have been described elsewhere. In addition, all patients should be given Pneumocystis infection prophylaxix (eg trimethoprim and sulfamethoxazole 80mg/40mg, 1 tablet daily). Because the myelosuppresive effects of CYC are unpredictable it should be complete blood cell counts at least every 15 days imaging [30]. The therapy with CYC is management until induction of remission. After that is stoped and is continued by others immunosupresants like azathioprine or methotrexate. These agents are continued for 2 to 3 years [30]. The prognosis of PACNS is uncertain and careful; most patients dying within 1 year. Altered consciousness or mental state and diffuse cerebral dysfunction are associated with poor outcome, while focal symptoms are associated with better outcome [12, 18, 30, 37].

In this disease it should remember that a substantial number of patients suspected of having PACNS will have signs and symptoms caused by vasospasm rather than true vasculitis of intracerebral vessels. The vasoconstriction syndrome is reversible is primarly seen in women aged 20 to 40 years. A history of syndromes or provocative agents associated with vasospasm, including the puerperium period, migraines, illicit drug use, and use of over-the counter cold medicines, is frequently elicited. The most common presenting syndrome is of a thunderclap headache of sudden onset and sufficient severity to warrant diagnostic evaluation for subarachnoid hemorrhage. Focal symptoms can predominate with stroke or TIA as a presenting feature. Cerebrospinal fluid is normal. Prednisone with calcium channel blockers are used for treatment reversible vasoconstriction syndrome [30]. The prognosis in this disturbance is good.

Takayasu's arteritis

Takayasu's arteritis is a variant of giant cell arteritis affecting the aorta and its main branches to the limbs and the head. This disease is much more common in Asians than in Europeans and predominates in young female subjects. ACR diagnostic criteria include at least three of the following: 1. age at disease onset < 50 years, 2. Claudication of extremities especially upper limbs, 3. Decrease brachial artery pulse, 4. Blood pressure (systolic) difference > 10 mmHg between arms, 5. Bruit over subclavian arteries or abdominal aorta, 6. Arteriographic narrowing or occlusion of the aorta, its primary branches or large arteries (not due to arteriosclerosis, fibromuscular dysplasia or similar causes [38]. The disease starts with nonspecific systemic signs and symptoms such arthralgia, fever, fatigue, headaches, rashes and weight loss. In Takayasu's arteritis there are no specific laboratory abnormalities. An elevation of ESR or CRP and a mild anaemia are possible, but the acute phase response may be normal. Anti-endothelial antibodies (AEA) can bee present [18]. Main neurological symptoms are syncope and visual troubles. TIA or stroke are rare, and they are more often secondary to hypertension related to involvement of the renal arteries.

Digital subtraction angiography (DSA) is the gold standard for the demonstration of vessel stenoses or occlusion. MRI, and MRA, CT angiography, PET and high-resolution ultrasound are used more frequently for the investigation of Takayasu's arteritis [39].
Steroids are useful in therapy of the disease, and fifty percent of patients respond to them alone in early phase of the illness. The prognosis is relatively benign, 90% of patients being alive at 10 years [12]. In 20% of the patients the disease is monophasic and selflimited. Some patients need steroids plus CYC or low - dose methotrexate or azathioprine. Angiotensin II receptor antagonists are applied for treatment renovascular hypertension. Concomitant therapies include low-dose aspirin and statin even in normolipidemic patients [18]. Angioplasty and other vascular surgical procedures are used if it's necessary besides pharmacological treatment [40].

6. Primary, medium-sized vessel vasculitis

Periarteritis nodosa (PAN)

PAN is the systemic necrotizing vasculitis only of medium sized arteries without the involvement of smaller vessels. This disease may be associated with hepatitis virus infection. The diagnostic criteria of the ACR for the diagnosis of PAN include at least three of: 1. loss of weight > 4 kg, 2. livedo reticularis, 3. testicular pain, 4. myalgias, 5. mononeuritis or polyneuritis, 6. blood pressure elevation > 90 mmHg, 7. creatinine > 1,5 mg/dl, 8. hepatitis B or C virus antibodies, 9. pathologic arteriography (aneurysm, occlusion), 10. typical histology finding in biopsy of muscle with necrotizing granulomatous inflammation (fig. 4.) [12, 18, 41, 42].

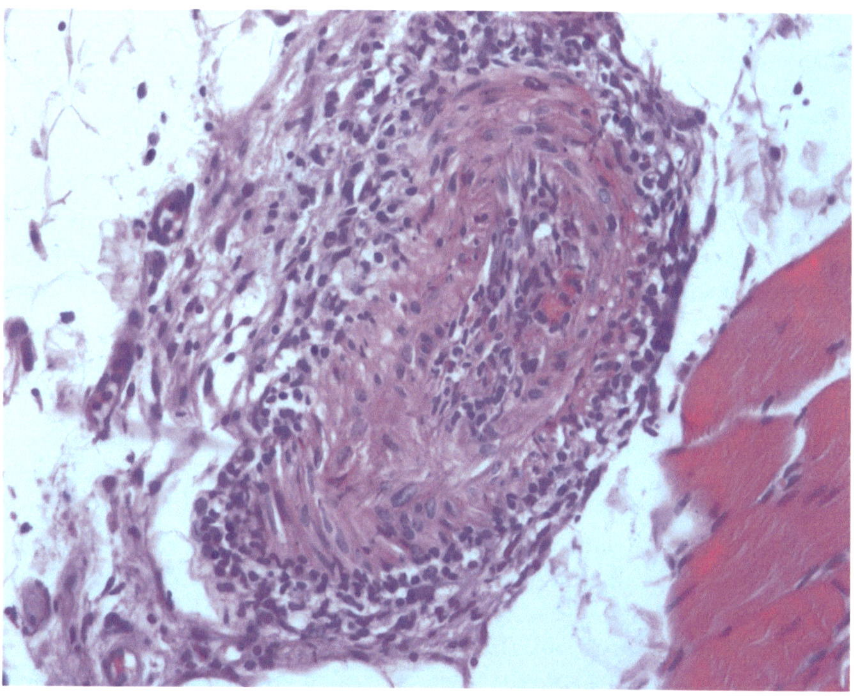

Fig. 4. Polyarteritis nodosa (PAN) - muscle biopsy with typical granulocyte infiltrates of small vessel wall with occlusion of vascular lumen (own case)

Twenty of patients with PAN had brain involvement in the monograph by Schmidley [15]. Ischemic stroke, hemorrhages and a progressive encephalopathy, seizures may occur. This disease is severe thats why it should be treated aggressively with steroids (pulses of methylprednisolone in severe forms) and cytotoxic drugs, mainly CYC. In emergency situations plasmapheresis may be tried [18]. Eighty percent of subjects who receive appropriate treatment are alive at 5 years [12].

Kawasaki disease

This is a rare medium-sized vessel vasculitis that causes stroke or encephalopathy in children. Its manifestations include fever, conjunctival infection, infected or fissured lips, infected pharynx or "strawberry tongue, erythema of palms or soles or oedema of hand or feet, polymorphous non-vesicular rash and cervical adenopathy. Treatment includes iv immunoglobulin and aspirin [12]

7. Primary small vessel vasculitis

Wegener's granulomatosis

This is rare small vessel (arteries and veins) arteritis frequently associated with autoantybodies: cANCA/PR3 and sometimes with MPO-ANCA [18]. Men are affected more frequent than women. The ACR criteria for classification of Wegener's granulomatosis include at least two of the following four: 1. necrotizing ulcerating inflammation of nose, sinuses, mouth, or pharynx, 2.irregular lung infiltrates, 3. nephritis, 4. granulomatous vascular and perivascular inflammation. In Wegener's granulomatosis a nonseptic meningitis with enhancement of the basal meninges and the development of an occlusive or communicating hydrocephalus are possible. Poyneuropathies, myelopathies and cerebrovascular symptoms frequently occur but stroke is a very rare complication [43, 44]. Nishino et al. and Fauci et al. descreibed neurologic invpolvement in Wegener's granulomatosis in 22 - 33.6% of patients [45, 46]. Prednisone or CYC are used for treatment 45, 46, 47]. During CYC treatment don't ought exceed a cumulative dose > 30g, and higher doses should be strictly avoided [47]. During CYC therapy are useful: antiemetics, bladder protection with NaCl infusions and uromitexane perfusor as well as ovarien protection. Alternative treatment option is methotrexate 20-25 mg per week [48] or rituximab [49]. Azathioprine can be effective in supporting therapy. The presence of ANCA at diagnosis, cardiac or renal involvement increase the risk of relapses.

Behcet's disease

This rare disease is chronic-relapsing vasculitis affecting predominantly the venous system. It is more prevalent in the Middle East, Far East and the Mediterranean. Diagnostic criteria for Behcet's disease include at least three of the major signs (oral ulcers, genital ulcers, ocular lesions, mainly uveitis, cutaneous involvement-erythema nodosum) or the combination of two major signs and one minor (gastrointestinal or central nervous system (CNS) or peripherial nervous system (PNS) involvement, arterial lesions,thrombophlebitis, arthritis and familiar history) [50]. The course of Behcet's disease is fluctuating. The diagnosis of Behcet's disease is entirely based on clinical grounds since no pathognomonic laboratory or histologic findings exist. CNS involvement occurs in about 30% of patients after an average of 5 years. The most common clinical syndromes are encephalitis, meningoencephalitis, and neuropathy as well as headaches, and brainstem symptoms. Cerebral oedema and cerebral stroke can also be present. Cerebral oedema is occurred in cerebral sinus thrombosis [18]. For the treatment of sinus thrombosis corticosteroids in combination with oral anticoagulation are recommended. Pulses of methylprednisolone of 1000mg (3 -5 days) followed by oral prenisolone (2 - 3 month) are used [51]. Occasionally may be used other immunosuppressive agents [52].

Churg -Strauss syndrome

Churg - Strauss syndrome is the rarest of the small-vessel vasulitides. Patients report in interview allergic diathesis and asthma. Pathologic hallmark of the disease are eosinophil-rich granulomas. p/ANCA/MPO are present in 40% of patients [53]. The criteria for the diagnosis of Churg-Strauss syndrome include at least four of: astma, history of allergy, eosinophilia (>10%), mono- or polyneuropathy, migratory or transitory pulmonary infiltrates and sinusitis [12]. Renal, lung, and central nervous system are involvement. 6-8% of patients present central nervous system symtoms Iike ischemic stroke, ischaemic optic neuropathy as well as intracerebral haemorrhage can occur in the disease [53, 54]. These patients may bee treated with prednisone alone, but sometimes combined therapy with CYC is needed. The remission rate is 80-90%. Patient survival varies between 60% and 97% at 5 years [56].

8. Summary

Vasculitis is a rare, miscellaneous, and potentially treatable cause of stroke. The diagnosis contain labourious tests, neuroradiological image (CT, MRI with arteriography option) and often requires invasive procedures, including brain-meningeal biopsy. Treatment of vasculitis has an empirical basis and most common it is immunosuppressive. Multicentre therapeutic trials are ongoing. A lot of organs are damaged in vasculitis. These sickness required a great physician acumen and carefulness, as well as cooperation with others specialists. Fast reconnaissance of disease and accustoming of proper treatment can bring big benefits patient.

9. References

[1] Watts RA, Scott DGI. Classification and epidemiology of vasculitis. Baillieres Clin Rhematol 1997; 11: 191-217.

[2] Sigal LH. The neurologic presentation of vasculitic and rheumatologic syndromes. A review. Medicine 1987; 66: 157-180.

[3] Futrell N, Millikan C. Frequency, etiology, and prevention of stroke In patients with systemie lapus erythematosus. Stroke 1989; 20: 583-591.

[4] Watts RA, Carruthers DM, Scott DGI. Epidemiology of systemie vasculitis-changing incidence Or definition. Semin Arthritis Rheum 1995; 25: 28-34.

[5] Selga D, Mohammad A, Sturfelt G, Segelmark M. Polyarteritis nodosa when applying the Chapel Hill nomenclature - a descriptive study on ten patients. Rheumatology 2006; 45: 1276-1281.

[6] Ferro JM, Crespo M. Young adults stroke: neuropsychological dysfunction and recovery. Stroke 1988; 19: 982-986.

[7] Ferro JM, Crespo M. Prognosis after transient ischemic attacks and ischemic stroke In Young adults. Stroke 1994; 25: 1611-1616.
[8] Bloch DA, Michel BA, Hunder GG, Mc Shane DJ, Arend WP et all. The American College of Rheumatology 1990 criteria for the classification of vasculitis. Patients and methods. Arthritis Rheum. 1990; 33: 1068-1073.
[9] Hunder GG, Bloch DA, Michel BA, Calabrese LH et all. The American Collage of Reumatology. 1990 criteria for the classification of vasculitis: introduction. Arthritis Rheum 1990; 33: 1065-1067.
[10] Jeanette JC, Falk RJ, Andrassy K, Bacon PA et all. Nomenclature of systemic vasculitides. Proposal of an international consensus conference. Arthritis Rheum 1994; 37: 187-192.
[11] Lie JT. Nomenclature and classificationof vasculitis : plus ca change, plus c'est la meme chose. Arthritis Rheum 1994; 37: 181-186.
[12] Ferro J M. Vasculitis of the central nervous system. J Neurol 1998; 245: 766 – 776.
[13] Jennette JC, Falk RF. Nosology of primary vasculitis. Curr Opin Rheumatol 2007; 19: 10-16.
[14] Berlit P. Diagnosis and differentia diagnosis of cerebral vasculitis. Nervenarzt 2004a; 75: 105-112.
[15] Schmidley JW. Central Nervous System Angiitis. Butterworth-Heinemann: Boston 2000.
[16] Saam T, Habs M, Cyran CC, Grimm J et al. New aspcts of MRI for diagnosis of large vessel vasculitis and primary angiitis of central nervous system. Radiologe 2010; 50: 861-71.
[17] Gomes LJ. The role of imaging in the diagnosis of central nervous system vasculitis. Curr Allergy Asthma Rep. 2010.; 10: 163-70.
[18] Berlit P. Diagnosis and treatment of cerebral vasculitis. Ther Adv Nerol Disord. 2010; 3: 29-42.
[19] Alhalabi M, Moore PM. Serial angiography in isolated angiitis of the central nervous system. Neurology 1994; 44: 1221-1226.
[20] Pipitone N, Salvarani C. Role of imaging in vasculitis and connective tissue disease. Best Pract Res Clin Rheumatol 2008; 22: 1075-1091.
[21] Both M, Ahmadi-Simab K, Reuter M, Dourvo SO, Fritzer E, Ullrich S et al. MRI and FDG-PET in the assessment of inflammatory aortic arch syndrome in complicated courses of giant cell arteritis. Ann Rheum Dis 2008; 67: 1030-1033.
[22] Marder W, Mc Cune WJ. Advances in immunosuppressive therapy. Semin Respir Crit Care Med. 2007; 28: 398-417.
[23] Hunder GG, Bloch DA, Michel BA, Stevens MB, Arend WP, Calabrese LH, Edworthy SM et al. The American College of Rheumatology. 1990 criteria for the classification of giant cell arteritis. Arthritis Rheum 1990; 33: 1122-1128.
[24] Wilkinson IMS, Russel RWR. Arteritis of the head and neck in giant cell arteritis. A pathological study to show the pattern of arterial involvement. Arch Neurol 1972; 27: 378-391.
[25] Dasqupta B and Giant Arteritis Guideline Development Group. Concise guidance: diagnosis and management of giant cell arteritis. Clinical Medicine 2010; 10: 381-6.
[26] Caselli RJ, Hunder GG, Whisnant JP. Neurologic disease in biopsy-proven giant cell arteritis. Neurology 1988; 38: 352-359.

[27] Font C, Cid MC, Collvinent B, Lopezsoto C, Grau JM. Clinical features in patients with permanent visual loss due to biopsy - proven giant cell arteritis. Br J Rheumatol 1997; 36: 251-254.
[28] Borg FA, Salter VIJ, Dasgupta B. Neuro-ophtalmic complications in giant cell arteritis.. Curr Allergy Asthma Rep 2008; 8: 323.
[29] Wiszniewska M, Devuyst G, Bogousslavsky J. Giant cell arteritis as a cause of first-ever stroke. Cerebrovasc Dis 2007; 24: 226-230.
[30] Birnbau. Primary angiitis of the Central Nervous System. Arch Neurol. 2009; 66: 704-709.
[31] Wiszniewska M, Szylberg T, Harat M. Primary central nervous system vasculitis imitating the brain tumor. Neurol Neurochir Pol 2008; 42: 358-61.
[32] Salvarani C, Brown Jr, Calamia KT, Christianson TJH, Huston J, Meschia JF et al. Primary central nervous system vasculitis: analysis of 101 patients. Ann Neurol 2007; 62: 442-451.
[33] Calabrese LH, Mallek JA. Primary angiitis of the CNS: report of 8 new cases, review of the literature, and proposal for diagnostic criteria. Medicine 1987; 67: 20-37.
[34] Lie JT. Primary (granulomatous) angiitis of the central nervous system: a clinicopathologic analysis of 15 new cases and review of the literaryre. Hum Pathol. 1992; 23: 164-171.
[35] Johns Hopkins Vasculitis Center. http://vasculitis .med,jhu.edu/typesof/cns.html. 2011. Central nervous system vasculitis.
[36] Salvarini C, Brown Jr, Calamia KT, Christianson TJH, Huston J, Meschia JF et al. Primary CNS vasculitis with spinal cord involvement. Neurology 2008; 70: 2394-2400.
[37] Hankey GJ. Isolated angiitis/angiopathy of the central nervous system. Cerebrovasc Dis 1991; 1: 2-5.
[38] Arend WP, Michel BA, Bloch DA, Hunder GG, Calabrese LH, Edworthy SM et al. The American College of Rheumatology. 1990 criteria for the classification of Takayasu arteritis. Arthritis Rheum 1990; 33: 1129-1134.
[39] Andrews J, Mason JC. Takayasu's arteritis - recent advances in imaging offer promise. Rheumatology 2007; 46: 6-15.
[40] Miyata T, Sato O, Koyama H, Shigematsu H, Tada Y. Long - term survival after surgical treatment of patients with Takayasu's arteritis. Circulation 2003; 108: 1474-1480.
[41] Watts R, Lane S, Hanslik T, Hauser T, Hellmich B, Koldingsnes W et al. Development and validation of a consensus methodology for the classification of the ANCA-associated vasculitides and polyarteritis nodosa for epidemiological studies. Ann Rheum Dis 2007; 66: 222-227.
[42] Khellaf M, Hamidou M, Pagnoux C, Michel M, Brisseau JM, Chevallier X et al. Vasculitis restricted to the lower limbs: a clinical and histopathological study. Ann Rheum Dis 2007; 66: 554-556.
[43] Nishino H, Rubino FA, De Remee RA, Swanson JW, Parisi JE. Neurological involvement in Wegener's granulomatosis: an analysuis of 324 consecutive patients at the Mayo Clinic. Ann Neurol 33:4-9.
[44] Savitz JM, Young MA, Ratan RR. Basilar artery occlusion in a young patient with Wegener's granulomatosis. Stroke 1994; 25: 214-216.

[45] Nishino H, Rubino FA, De Remee RA, Swanson JW, Parisi JE. Neurological involvement in Wegener's granulomatosis: an analysis of 324 consequtive patients at the Mayo Clinic. Ann Neurol 33: 4-9.

[46] Fauci AS, Haynes BF, Katz P, Wolff SM. Wegener's granulomatosis: prospective clinical and therapeutic experience with 85 patients for 21 years. Ann Intern Med 1983; 98: 76-85.

[47] Faurschou M, Sorensen IJ, Mellemkjaer L et al. Malignancies in Wegener's granulomatosis: incidence and relation to cyclophosphamide therapy in a cohort of 293 patients. J Rheumatol. 2008; 35: 100 - 105.

[48] Bosch X, Guilabert A, Espinosa G, Mirapeix E. Treatment of antineurophil cytoplasmic antibody - associated vasculitis: a systematic review. JAMA 2007; 298: 655-669.

[49] Keogh KA, Ytterberg SR, Fervenza FC, Carlson KA, Schroeder DR, Specks U. Rituximab for refractory Wegener's granulomatosis: report of a prospective, open-label pilot trial. AmJ Respr Crit Care Med 2006; 173: 180-187.

[50] Akman-Demir G, Serdaroglu P, Tasci B. Clinical patterns of neurological invement in Behcet's disease evaluation of 200 patients. The Neuro-Behcet Study Group. Brain 1999; 122: 2171-2182.

[51] Barnes CG. Treatment of Behcet's syndrome. Rheumatology. 2006; 45: 245-247.

[52] Hatemi G., Silman A, Bang D, Bodaghi B et al. EULAR recommendations for the management of Behcet disease. Ann Rheum Dis. 2008; 67: 1656-1662,

[53] Sable-Fourtassou R, Cohen P, Mahr A, Pagnoux C et al. Antineutrophil cytoplasmic antibodies and the Churg-Strauss syndrome. Ann Intern Mwd. 2005; 143: 632 - 638.

[54] Kattah JC, Chrousos GA, Katz PA, Mc Casland B, Kolsky MP. Anterior ischemic optic neuropathy in Churg-Strauss syndrome. Neurology 1994; 44: 2200-2202.

[55] Mukhtyar C, Flossmann O, Hellmich B, Bacon P et al. 2008 and on behalf of the European Vasculitis Group (EUVAS). Outcomes from studies, of antineutrophil cytoplasm antibody associated vasculitis: a systematic review by the European League Against Rheumatism systemic vasculitis task force. Ann Rheum Dis 2008; 67: 1004 - 1010

[56] Liou HH, Liu HM, Chiang IP, Yeh TS, Chen RC. Churg-Strauss syndrome presented as multiple intracebral, hemorrhage. Lupus 1997; 6: 279-282.

19

Vasculitis as a Cause of First-Ever Stroke

Malgorzata Wiszniewska[1] and Julien Bogousslavsky[2]
[1]*Małgorzata Wiszniewska - Neurological Department, Specialis Hospital Piła,*
[2]*Julien Bogousslavsky - Gendier Swiss Medical Network,*
Clinique Valmont, Glion/Montreux
[1]*Poland*
[2]*Switzerland*

1. Introduction

The term "vasculitis" includes a heterogeneous group of multisystemic disorders characterized pathologically by inflammation of blood vessels [1,2,3]. Inflammation can involve some, or all, of the thickness of the vessel wall. Immune complexes are a major component of vasculitis syndromes, and cellular mechanisms play a major pathogenic role in giant cell arteritis [4-12].

Arterial lesion can lead to stenosis, occlusion, and ischemic infarction [1,13]. The diagnosis of vasculitis is difficult in most cases because of the insidious nature of the disease and the fact that various parts of the circulation can be affected without definitive signs or symptoms [1, 13-15]. More often than not, the diagnosis of vasculitis is made indirectly [1,15,16]. It is an infrequent disorder and a rare cause of stroke, even in young age groups [1,17-19]. Corticosteroid therapy is the basic and most common treatment for this disease, irrespective of the antigen involved or the type of vasculitis syndrome [1,4,5,8,20,21].

The aim of this study was to use the Lausanne Stroke Registry (LSR) to evaluate how often vasculitis is a cause of first-ever stroke, and to determine the risk factors, clinical and radiological patterns, and early outcome for stroke with vasculitis.

2. Patients and methods

2.1 Patients

The patients studied were those enrolled in the LSR [22] between January 1, 1980, and December 31, 1998. All patients were admitted to the Department of Neurology for first-ever stroke and were evaluated by at least one neurologist with stroke subspecialty training and by other specialists, depending on the accompanying symptoms (often a rheumatologist).

All patients underwent a head CT or MRI, cardiac investigation (all by ECG, and, in most instances, by transthoracic or transesophageal echocardiography, with Holter ECG when needed), and Doppler investigation of the extracranial arteries. Serological or immunological testing was carried out when infection or immunological disease was suspected. Depending on need, patients also underwent cerebrospinal fluid (CSF) analysis and cerebral arteriography (including MRI angiography), while selected patients had a tissue biopsy. Patients with toxic vasculopathies were excluded due to the lack of clear-cut criteria for the differential diagnosis of pure vasculitis and drug-induced multiple vasospasm.

2.2 Methods

Vasculitis was recognized on the basis of a comprehensive medical history and physical examination and the presence of vascular lesions in the CT or MRI with abnormalities in appropriate laboratory blood tests, and positive auto-antibodies or positive serological tests or bacteriological culture (blood and/or CSF) for infections. The criteria of the American College of Rheumatology were used to establish the correct diagnosis of vasculitis [1,4,13,16,20,23-25]. The diagnosis was confirmed by a characteristic vessel wall inflammatory reaction, with irregularities in the intracranial vessels on angiography in some cases. In all patients, other causes of stroke were first excluded.

The functional status at 1 month after stroke onset (early outcome) was measured using a 5-point scale, with 1 indicating no disability and 5 death. A good outcome was defined as patients with no or mild disability (points 1 and 2), while a bad outcome was defined as patients with moderate or severe disability, or death (points 3-5).

2.3 Statistical methods

Frequencies were compared using Fisher's exact test for dichotomous factors or the chi-squared test when more than 2 categories were present. Age differences were compared using Wilcoxon's rank-sum test.

3. Results

Between January 1, 1980 and December 31, 1998, 27 of the 4,086 (0.7 %) patients in the LSR were found to have vasculitis, 15 (55.5 %) having primary vasculitis (PV) and 12 (44.5 %) secondary vasculitis (SV). The mean age of all stroke patients with vasculitis was 54.2 years, significantly lower than that of the 4,059 patients with stroke without vasculitis (mean age 63.5 years, p= 0.02). The frequency of vasculitis in men and women was similar, being 0.76% and 0.5%, respectively (p=0.43). The 27 patients consisted of 11 men and 4 women with PV (male/female ratio 2.75; mean age, 61.3 years, range 20-81) and 8 men and 4 women with SV (male/female ratio 2.0; mean age, 45.3 years, range 22-81). Risk factors were found in 17 of the 27 patients (63%), of whom 11 had hypertension (41% vs 49% of patients without vasculitis; p=0.2) and 8 (29.6%) were active smokers. Other risk factors, which were rare, were only seen in single patients (see Tables 1 and 2). The early outcome in patients with vasculitis was similar to that in patients without vasculitis, a good outcome being seen in 55.6% of patients with vasculitis and in 59% of patients without vasculitis (p=0.7).

Tables 1 and 2 show the main characteristics of the patients with vasculitis.

We would like to present GCA.

4. Discussion

Most authors have stated that vasculitis usually manifests as headache, meningeal signs, encephalopathy, psychiatric syndromes, dementia, cranial nerve palsies, and seizures, and only rarely as stroke [1,13,14,17]. There are also generally non-specific systemic symptoms, such as fever, fatigue and weight loss [19-21,25]. In our vasculitis patients, non-specific symptoms were most common, being present in 26 out of the 27 (96.3%). Meningeal signs were present in all 8 SV patients with infection. Headache-most typical sign for PACNS and GCA occurred in 15 patients (55%), but significant psychotic syndromes only in 2 (7.4%).

Characteristic	PACNS n = 6	GCA n = 6	PAN n = 3
Age, y (mean)	20▲, 26, 43, 54, 67, 75▲ (47.5)	72°, 75°, 78°, 81°, 81°, 81° (78)	45◊, 55◊, 68° (56)
Sex	2 F, 4 M	1 F, 5 M	1 F, 2 M
Risk factors, N° patients	2 ac smok, 1 ac smok + hCh	1 diabetes+HY, 4 HY	3 HY
Neurological disorders :		2 (with ataxia)	2 (1 with ataxia)
Hemiparesis	3		1
Aphasia	1		
Hemianopsia	2	4	
Cerebellar	6	6	
Headache	1	1	
Disturbances cons.	2		1
Epileptic seizure			
Meningeal signs	1	not	not
Ictus territory :			
Superficial	4 (MCA posterior reg)	3 (2 ACA super ant, 1 PCA reg)	
Subcortical			2 (1 hemorrhagic)
Brainstem/cerebellum	1	2	
Multiple	1 (superficial)	1	1 (deep)
Arteriography, N° patients	5: 3-intracranial vessels irregularities 1-intracranial vessels iirregularities + 50% stenosis of SA 1-sclerotic changes in both ICA▲	5: 3-arteriosclerotic changes in VAs 2-arteriosclerotic changes in ICA	2: normal view
Outcome, disability			
None		1	1
Mild	6	2	2
Moderate		2	
Severe		1	
Death			
Disease onset-to-stroke Latency	Inaugural (all patients)	2 mo (n=1), 1mo (n=4), inaugural (n=1)	6 y, 3 y, 2 mo
Coexisting symptoms	fever (n=3), fatige (n=3)	fatigue in all, polymyalgia (n=1) claudication of jaw (n=1), weight loss (n=2), fever (n=2), amblyopia on one eye (n=1)	polyneuropathy in all, weight loss (n=2) fever (n=1) renal failure (n=1)
Therapy, N patients	1-Dx+Antipl, 1-Antipl , 2-P, 1-P+CY,1-P+CY+FR	1-MP followed by P, 5-P	1-P, 1-MP followed byP, 1-MP followed by P+CY

PACNS=Primary angiitis of the central nervous system, GCA=Giant cell arteritis, PAN=Polyarteritis nodosa, ac smok=active smoking, F=female, M=male, HY=hypertension, hCh=hypercholesterolemia, MCA=medial cerebral artery, ACA=anterior cerebral artery, PCA=posterior cerebral artery, VAs=vertebral arteries, SA=subclavian artery, reg=region, super ant=superior anterior, cons=conciousness, , °=disease recognized before stroke, ▲=positive meningo-brain biopsy, y=years, mo=month, MP=methylprednisolone, P=prednisone, Dx=Dexamethason, CY=cyclophosphamide, FR=fraxiparin, Antipl=antiplatelet

Table 1a. Clinical and neuroradiologic features, disease onset-to stroke latency, and current therapy for 15 patients with primary vasculitis

Laboratory investigations	Type of Primary Vasculitis		
	PACNS n = 6	GCA n = 6	PAN n = 3
ESR mm/h	<10 (n=4), 35, 40	5, 11, 15, 60, 70, 120	6, 68, 90
CRP mg/l	<10 (n=5), 73	<10 (n=4), 30, 65	<10, 205, 253
Immunological abnormalities in blood and in CSF	ANA (1/320) IgG for EBV (n=1) IgG for: HS, EBV, Va (n=2)	IgG 21.17(n:8.2-17) with rise of IgG Kappa and Lambda (n=1) ANA(1/80) +Antinucleoprotein 22 +Anti-SSB 22 (n=1)	ANCA (1/320) and positive in CSF + ANA(1/80) + IgG rise (n=1) Anticentriole Ab(1/8) + ANA positive (n=1) Immune complexes C1q 24% positive (n=1)
Tissue biopsy (n patients)	2: granulomatous inflammations in a meningo-brain biopsy (fig.1)	6: mononuclear and granulomatosus with multinucleated giant cells in TA (fig.2)	3: focal segmental necrotizing vasculitis of small and medium sized arteries in liver and kidney (n=1) vasculitis signed and ischemic neuropathy in muscle-nerve biopsy (n=2)
CSF: (n patients) Protein mg/l Cytosis cells/ml blood-CSF barrier rupture	(n = 3) 7,920, 4,260, 295 93 x 10^3, 6.3, 1 (n = 3)	(n = 2) 410, 250 46 (32-polynuclear), 1 (none)	(n = 3) 1.380, 355, 895 32, 2, 2 (n = 3)

ESR=erythrocyte sedimentation, CRP=C reactive protein, E=erythrocytes, TA=temporal artery, CSF=cerebrospinal fluid, ANCA-perinuclear antineutrophil cytoplasmic antibodies, ANA=antinuclear antibodies, Ab=antibodies, EBV=Epstein-Baar virus, Va=varicella zoster, HS=herpes simplex

Table 1b. Laboratory features for 15 primary vasculitis - associated strokes

Our analysis confirmed the results of previous studies that vasculitis is a rare cause of stroke, since, out of the 4,086 patients with first-ever stroke, only 0.7% presented signs of vasculitis that could be a cause of the stroke. The mean age of the patients with vasculitis was significantly lower than that of stroke patients without vasculitis (54.2 vs 63.5 years, p=0.02). A good early outcome was seen at a similar frequency in patients with or without vasculitis (55.6% vs 59.0%). Ischemic stroke was more frequent than hemorrhagic stroke (96.3% vs 3.7%), but the group of patients with vasculitis was too small to allow a statistical conclusion to be drawn. The most common risk factor was hypertension, which occurred at a similar frequency in patients with or without vasculitis (41% vs 49%). The largest groups were patients with PACNS or Horton's disease (GCA), with 6 cases in each group.

Characteristic	SLE n=1	Behçet's Disease n=2	Sarcoidosis n=1	Syphilitic n=3	Zoster n=2	Tuberculotic n=2	Borreliosis n=1
Age, y (mean)	22°	23°, 28° (25.5)	47°	41, 54, 81 (58.7)	50°, 65 (57.5)	51, 52° (51.5)	30°
Sex: F, M	1 F	2 M	1 M	1 F, 2 M	1 F, 1 M	1 F, 1 M	1 M
Risk factors N° patients	Not available	Not available	+ ac smok	3 ac smok (at 2 HY)	2HY+ ac smok + diab	1 diab	Not available
Neurological disorders :							
Hemiparesis	+		+	2+apraxia	2	2 (1+hemianosy)	+
Aphasia				1+apraxia			+
Cerebellar		2					
Headache		2				1	
Disturbances consciousness		1	+ (confusion)	1§		1 (drowsiness)	1§
Ictus territory :							
Superficial	MCA reg			1 PCA		1MCA post +tc	
Subcortical				1 MCA	1	1+hydrocephalus	+
Deep hemispheric			internal capsule	1 ACA			
Brainstem		2					
Multiple					1		
Arteriography, N° patients	Not done	1: thrombosis in intracranial sinuses	Not done	Not done	Not done	1: intracranial irregularities	Not done
Meningeal signs	not	not	not	yes in all	yes in both	yes in both	yes
Coexisting symptoms	Erythema + fatigue	•Uveitis+art +genital ulcer + familiar history of leukaemia •oral and genital ulcers + cervical adenopathy + fever +splenomegaly	Light respiratory failure + fatigue	dilated left pupil in one fatigue in 3	•oph zoster, glaucoma + occlusion of central ret. A, fever •otic zoster, surdity and fever	fatigue (both)	fever + erythema on thorax
Disease onset-to- stroke latency	1 y	3 y, 1 mo	9 y	Not known	6 weeks, inaugural	6 mo, inaugural	1 y
Therapy	MP followed by P	P + Cyclosporin, P + FR	P + Antipl	Pen in all and in 2 + Antipl	Zoovirax +Antipl, Zoovirax + P + Antipl	P + antituberculotic in all	P + Ceftriaxon
Outcome disability:							
None		1					
Mild			+	2	1		+
Moderate	+	1		1	1	2	
Severe							
Death							

SLE=systemic lupus erythematosus, F=female, M=male, MCA=medial cerebral artery, PCA=posterior cerebral artery, ACA=anterior cerebral artery, reg=region, post=posterior, ac smok=active smoking, , diab=diabetes , tc=tuberculoma, §=psychiatric syndrome, °=disease recognized before stroke, mo = mouth, y=year, art=arthritis, oph=ophthalmic, MP=metylprednisolon, P=prednison, FR=fraxiparin, Antipl=antiplatelet

Table 2a. Clinical and radiologic features, disease onset-to-stroke latency, and therapy for 12 patients with secondary vasculitis associated strokes

Laboratory investigations	Type of secondary Vasculitis						
	SLE N = 1	Behcet's N = 2	Sarcoidosis N = 1	Syphilitic N = 3	Zoster N = 2	Tuberculotic N = 2	Borreliosis N = 1
ESR mm/h CRP mg/l	27 not done	13, 28 <10 (both)	21 not done	12, 16 not done	25, 28 not done	40, 8 not done	5 not done
Serological Bacterial	Not available Not available	•CMV 3 (N<1,2) •EBV + HS in IgG Not available	Va (1/160) Not available	VDRL, TPH, FTA-ABS (in all positive) Not available	Oreillons IgG (both) Not available	Tox, Va, EBV (1 case) positive culture CSF (1 case)	Anti-Borreliosis Ab: IgG, IgM Not
Immunological Abnormalities	ANA 1/2560 Anti DNA 1/8 (in blood)	Rise of β-2-microglob (3,331ng/ml in CSF and 2,828ng/ml in blood) (n=1)	Not observed	Not observed	ANA 1/640 homogenic (anti-SSa 47, anti-RNP 25, anti-Sm 22, Sc 170) (n=1)	Not observed	Not observed
CSF Protein mg/l Cytosis cells/mm3 blood-CSF barier rupture oligoclonal bands (local synthesis)	 220 $1x10^3$ not not	 460, 300 373, $62x10^3$ in one not	 440 17,3 not IgG, IgM	 285,545;2,280 15, 8, 30 in 3 cases IgG in one	 1,590, 470 77, 20 in one IgG in one	 957; 2,580 10; $1,408x10^3$ in 2 cases IgG in both	 5,130 560 not IgG
Tissue biopsy	not available	Necrosis and inflammatory in crotal and lymphadenitis non specific in neck (n=1)	Bronchic and lung: granulomatous inflammation and vascular hyperplasia	Not available	Not available	Not available	Not available

Table 2b. Laboratory features for the 12 secondary vasculitis-associated strokes

The most significant manifestations of PACNS are reported to be headache or disturbances of consciousness [13,26-28]. All of our patients had headache, but only one showed disturbances of consciousness. The diagnosis of PACNS was proved histologically in 2 of our patients with typical granulomatous inflammation in a meningo-brain biopsy (fig.1); only one of the two underwent arteriography, which showed no significant sclerotic changes without irregularities of the intracranial vessels. In another 4 patients, the diagnosis was confirmed arteriographically (1 besides typical arterial irregularities also showed stenosis of the subclavian artery). This suggests that vasculitis and arteriosclerotic changes can coexist, which conflicts with the opinion of Woolfenden et al [23]. Many authors consider arteriography as a standard approach for patients suspected of vasculitis involving the cerebral vessels [14,23,29]. However, Vollner et al. [28] found that angiography reveals abnormalities in less than a third of PACNS patients, and these are often nonspecific. Many authors have reported that a good outcome is seen in many patients treated with prednisolone, but some have also reported a monophasic clinical course, usually with a benign outcome and not requiring aggressive immunosuppressive therapy [28,29]. A recent study shows similar results, as the early outcome was good in all our patients, one of whom did not receive glucocorticosteroids.

Fig. 1

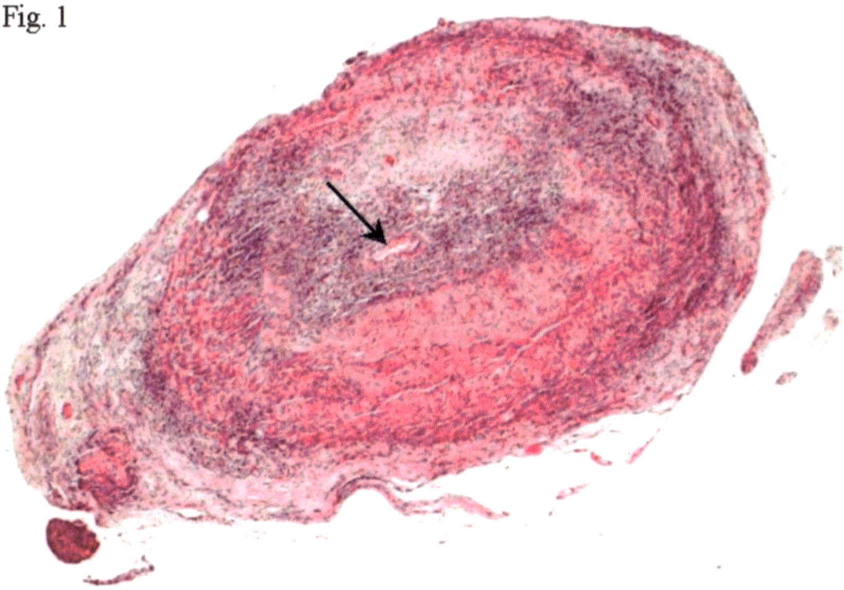

Fig. 1. PACNS – Primary angiitis of the central nervous system. Granulomatosus inflammation in meningo-brain biopsy.

In GCA, biopsy of the temporal artery is the principal means of making the diagnosis [1,2,4,12,13,30]. In all our patients, the diagnosis was confirmed histologically (fig.2). As in other reports [1,13], the outcome was good in most patients, but, in 1 patient, the early outcome was bad, despite intensive corticotherapy similar patient describing by Staunton et al [31]. The condition of our patient deteriorated 3 days after starting therapy with prednisolone. The MRI showed a new ischemic lesion, and arteriography and Doppler investigation demonstrated occlusion of the ICA. Both Conn et al [32] and Reichart et al [19] have referred to the use of glucocorticoid therapy as a possible "double-edged sword" and suggested that progression of occlusion of the vessels may occur after control of inflammation. All strokes in PAN [20,24] occurred while the illness was controlled by glucocorticosteroid therapy.

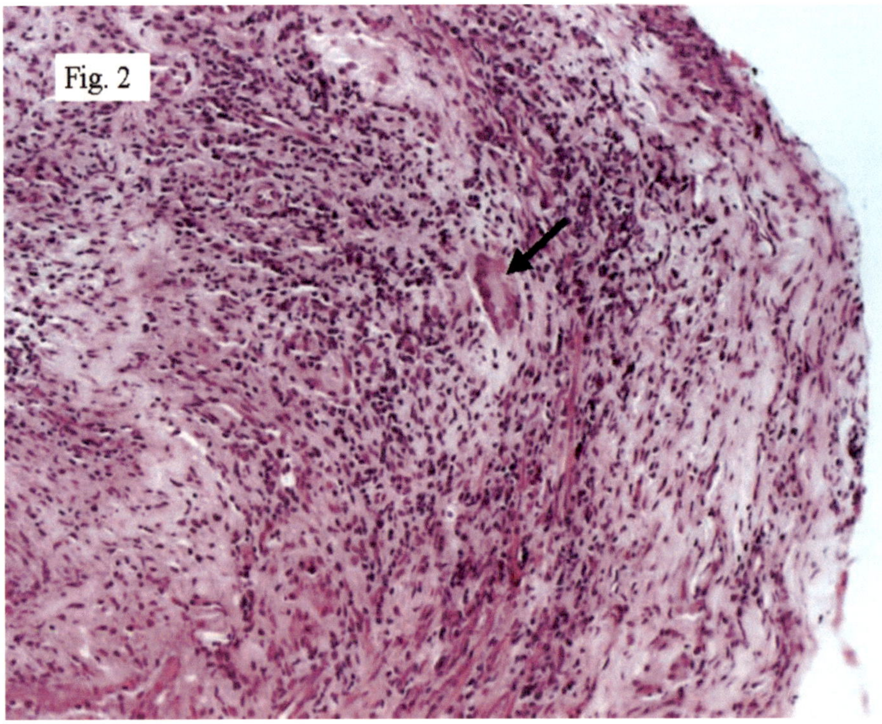

Fig. 2. GCA – Giant cell arteritis. Granulomatosus with multinucleated giant cells in the wall of temporal artery

Secondary vasculitis, which occurred in a very diverse group, was even rarer [1-4,8-10,13,33,34]. The patients with SLE, sarcoidosis, or Behçet's disease had recognized illness before the stroke and, when other causes of stroke were excluded, vasculitis was probably the cause of the cerebral ictus.

Some of our patients presented vasculitis connected with various infections. In all these patients, the history and clinical and meningeal signs was very helpful in establishing the diagnosis. The patients with lues led a style of living which could predispose to transmission of this disease, the patient with borreliosis had erythema one year previously, which was overlooked at the time, and patients with zoster vasculitis had suffered from ophthalmic and otic zoster. The diagnosis of infectious vasculitis should be based on suitable serologic or bacteriologic investigations [6,7,11,37,38]. All of these patients presented inflammatory changes in the CSF (see Table 2 b). The interval between stroke and the beginning of disease can be variable [7,38-40]. In the 3 lues cases, it was unknown and, in 1 tuberculosis patient, stroke disclosed the disease.

To the best of our knowledge, there are no published data on a casual relationship between various types of vasculitis and first-ever stroke. The only reports we have been able to find focused on the relationship between individual types of vasculitis and stroke and case reports [5,6,10,14,19,23,25,27-31,33-40]. The results of our study indicate that various types of vasculitis can also be responsible for the first-ever brain infarction in elderly patients. In all vasculitis patients, the CT and MRI showed only non-specific brain infarcts, but, in tuberculotic vasculitis, specific signs, such as tuberculoma or hydrocephalus [11,38], were also sometimes seen. The presence of classic segmental narrowing in the cerebral angiogram suggests vasculitis [11,12,14,16,23,26] but was not seen in some cases. In agreement with published data [19,28], the presence of atherosclerotic changes did not exclude vasculitis as a cause of stroke in our patients. In GCA, the literature states that the definitive diagnostic investigation is biopsy of an affected artery [1,4,12,30], but cerebral biopsy, which can establish the diagnosis of PACNS, is not recommended in all cases [12,14-16,23].

5. Conclusions

Our observations show that vasculitis is a rare cause of stroke. Vasculitis should be suspected in patients with first -ever stroke with previously recognized systemic autoimmune disease or presenting clinical and/or biological signs of autoimmune or infectious disease. The presence of atherosclerotic changes on the arteriogram does not exclude vasculitis. Recognition of vasculitis is often indirect after exclusion of other causes of stroke, while treatment depends on the disease type. Tissue biopsy is very helpful in establishing the diagnosis. Corticosteroid therapy does not protect patients against stroke.

6. Abstract

The aims of the study were to assess how frequently vasculitis is a cause of first-ever stroke and to assess risk factors, the clinical and radiological patterns in 4,086 patients from LSR. Methods: Vasculitis was recognized using the criteria of the American College of Rheumatology. Age differences were compared using Wilcoxon's rank-sum test, frequencies - Fisher's exact or the chi-squared test. Results: Vasculitis was found in 27 (0.7%) of stroke patients. The mean age of patients with vasculitis was significantly lower than patients without vasculitis (54.2 vs 63.5 years; p=0.02). 63% patients with vasculitis had various risk factors, the most common being hypertension, with a similar frequency (41%) to that seen in patients without vasculitis (49%). A good early outcome was seen in 55.6% of the patients with vasculitis, similar to patients without vasculitis (59%; p=0.7). Conclusion: Vasculitis is a rare cause of stroke. Corticosteroid therapy does not protect patients against stroke.

Key words: Vasculitis - Angiitis – Stroke

7. References

[1] Lahita R.G.: Vasculitis. In: Lahita R.G., Chiorazzi N., Reeves W.H.. Textbook of the autoimmune diseases. Philadelphia: Lippincott Williams & Wilkins PA, 2000:549-556.

[2]Watts RA, Scott DG: Classification and epidemiology of vasculitis. Baillieres Clin Rheumatol 1997;11:191-217
[3] Granger DM, Kubes P.: The microcirculation and inflammation: modulation of leukocyte endothelial cell adhesion. J Leukoc Biol 1994;55:662.
[4] Hunder GG, Bloch DA, Michel BA, Stevens MB, Arend WP, Calabrese LH, Edworthy SM, Fauci AS, Leavitt RY, Lie JT, Lightfoot RW Jr, Masi AT, Mc Shane DJ, Mills JA, Wallace SL, Zvaifler NJ: The American College of Rheumatology. 1990 criteria for the classification of giant cell arteritis. Arthritis Rheum 1990;33:122-1128.
[5] Quint L., Deny P, Guillevin L: Hepatitis C virus in patients with polyarteritis nodosa†: prevalence in 38 patients. Clin Exp Rheumatol 1991;9:253.
[6] Finkel TH, Torok TJ, Ferguson PJ.: Chronic parvovirus B19 infection and systemic necrotizing vasculitis: opportunistic infections or etiological agent. Lancet 1994;343:1255-1258.
[7] Mandell BF, Calabrese LH.: Infections and systemic vasculitis. Curr Opin Rheumatol 1998; 10:51-57.
[8] Lahita R.G.: Systemic lupus erythematosus. In: Lahita R.G., Chiorazzi N., Reeves W.H.. Textbook of the autoimmune diseases. Philadelphia: Lippincott Williams & Wilkins PA, 2000: 537-547.
[9] Lahita RG: The clinical presentation of SLE in the adult. In: Lahita RG, ed. Systemic lupus erythematosus. San Diego: Academic Press 1999:325-336.
[10] Sanches-Caballero FM, Marenco JL, Sanchez-Burson J, Rejon E, Aguilera JM, Jimenez MD: Cerebral infarct in systemic lupus erythematosus. Rev Neurol 1999; 29 (10): 985-90.
[11] Brutto O.H.: Infections and stroke. In: Ginsberg M.D., Bogousslavsky J.: Cerebrovascular disease. Blackwell Science, 1998 : 1628-1646.
[12] Hankey G.J.: Necrotizing and granulomatous angiitis of the CNS. In : Ginsberg M.D., Bogousslavsky J. : Cerebrovascular disease. Blackwell Science, 1998 : 1647-1683.
[13] Hinchey JA, Sila CA: Cerebrovascular complications of rheumatic disease. Rheumatic disease clinics of North America 1997; 23 (2): 293-316.
[14] Hankey GJ: Isolated angiitis/angiopathy of the central nervous system. Cerebrovasc Dis 1991; 1:2-15.
[15] Duna GF, Calabrese LH: Limitations of invasive modalities in the diagnosis of primary angiitis of the central nervous system. J Rheumatol 1995; 22: 662-667.
[16] Chu CT, Gray L, Goldstein LB, Hulette CM: Diagnosis of intracranial vasculitis: a multi-disciplinary approach. J Neuropathol Exp Neurol 1998 ; 57 (1): 30-8.
[17] Ferro JM, Crespo M: Young adults stroke: neuropsychological dysfunction and recovery. Stroke 1988; 19: 982-6.
[18] Ferro JM, Crespo M: Prognosis after transient ischemic attacks and ischemic stroke in young adults. Stroke 1994; 25: 1611-16.
[19] Reichart MD, Bogousslavsky J, Janzer RC: Early lacunar strokes complicating polyarteritis nodosa: thrombotic microangiopathy. Neurology 2000; 54 (4): 883-9.

[20] Goez CG: Polyarteritis nodosa. In Vinken PJ, Bruyn GW, Klawans HL, eds. Handbook of Clinical Neurology. Amsterdam: Elsevier Science Publishers B.V. 1980:295-311.
[21] Moore PM.: Neurological manifestations of vasculitis: update on immunopathogenic mechanisms and clinical features. Ann Neurol 1995; 37 (S1): S131-S141).
[22] Bogousslavsky J., van Melle G., Regli F.: The Lausanne Stroke Registry: analysis of 1000 consecutive patients with first stroke. Stroke 1988; 19: 1083-1092.
[23] Woolfenden A.R., Tong D.C., Marks M.P., Ali A.O., Albers G.W.: Angiographically defined primary angiitis of the CNS. Neurology 1998; 51: 183-188.
[24] Lightfoot RWJ, Michel AB, Bloch DA, et al: The American College of Rheumatology 1990 criteria for the classification of polyarteritis nodosa. Arthritis Rheum 1990; 33: 1088-1093.
[25] Provenzale JM, Allen NB: Neuroradiologic findings in polyarteritis nodosa. Am J Neuroradiol 1996, 17: 1119-1126.
[26] Biousse V, Bousser MG: Angiitis of the central nervous system in systemic diseases. Rev Med Interne 1998, 19 (6): 415-26.
[27] Calenbergh FV, van den Berg V, Wilms G: Benign isolated arteritis of the central nervous system. Clin Neurol Neurosurg 1986, 88: 267-273.
[28] Vollmer TL., Guarnaccia J., Harrington W, Pacia SV: Idiopathic granulomatous angiitis of the central nervous system. Diagnostic challenges. Archiv Neurol 1993, 50 (9): 925-30.
[29] Crane R, Kerr LD, Spiera H: Clinical analysis of isolated angiitis of the central nervous system: a report of 11 cases. Arch Intern Med 1991; 151: 2290-2294.
[30] Caselli RJ, Hunder GG, Whisnant JP: Neurologic disease in biopsy-proven giant cell (temporal) arteritis. Neurology 1988; 38:352-359.
[31] Staunton H, Stafford F, Leader M, O'Riordain D: Deterioration of giant cell arteritis with corticosteroid therapy. Archiv Neurol 2000; 57 (4): 581-4.
[32] Conn DL, Tompkins RB, Nichols ML : Glucocorticoids in the management of vasculitis : a double-edged sword ? J Rheumatol. 1988, 15 : 1181-1183.
[33] Brown MM, Thompson AJ, Wedzicha JA, Swash M: Sarcoidosis presenting with stroke. Stroke 1989, 20: 400-405
[34] Michotte A., Dequenne P, Jacobovitz D, Hildebrand J: Focal neurological deficit with sudden onset as the first manifestation of sarcoidosis†: a case report with MRI follow-up. Eur Neurol 1991, 31(6): 376-379.
[35] Canhao P, Ferro JM, Freitas JP: Manifestacoes neurologicas na doenca de Behcet. Acta Med Port 1992 ; 5: 369-371.
[36] Bousser MG, Bletry O, Launay M, Portier E, Guillard A, Castaigne P: Thromboses veineuses cerebrales au cours de la maladie de Behcet. Rev Neurol (Paris) 1980; 136: 753-762.
[37] Krist D., Wenkel H.: Bilateral papillary edema in cerebrospinal syphilis. Klinische Monatsblatter fur Augenheilkunde 2000; 216 (1): 54-56.
[38] Huang CR, Lui CC, Chang WN, Wu HS, Chen HJ: Neuroimages of disseminated neurotuberculosis: report of one case. Clin Imag. 1999; 23(4): 218-22.

[39] Nakane H, Okada Y, Ibayashi S, Sadoshima S, Fujishima M: Brain infarction caused by syphilitic aortic aneurysm. A case report. Angiology 1996; 47 (9): 911-917.
[40] Landi G, Villani F, Anzalone N: Variable angiographic findings in patients with stroke and neurosyphilis: Stroke 1990; 21: 333-338.

20

Acute Hemorrhagic Edema of Infancy

Hayrullah Alp
Selcuk University Meram Medical Faculty,
Department of Pediatrics
Turkey

1. Introduction

Acute hemorrhagic edema of infancy (AHEI) is a benign cutaneous small vessel leucocytoclastic vasculitis. The disease characterized by low-grade fever, acral inflammatory edema and large rosetta-, annular-, or targetoid-shaped ecchymotic purpura primarily over the face and extremities. The outbreak is frequently preceded by an immunization, drug intake or various infections. In spite of violent and alarming clinical presentation in a non-toxic infant, spontaneous recovery without any sequelaes occurs within a few weeks. Although some have suggested that AHEI is a purely cutaneous variant of Henoch-Schönlein purpura, most authors prefer to regard it as a separate clinical entity among the cutaneous small vessel vasculitic diseases of infancy.

2. Background

Although, AHEI was first described by Snow as a purely cutaneous variant of Henoch-Schönlein purpura in American literature in 1913 (Snow, 1913), it was well-recognised by Seidlmayer (Seidlmayer, 1936) and Finkelstein (Finkelstein, 1938) in European literature in 1930ies. Since then in Europe, many cases have been reported under different clinical terms, including Finkelstein disease and Seidmayer's 'cockade' purpura or syndrome. The name AHEI first appeared in Spanish written and used by Del Carril (Del Carril et al., 1936). Other names used for the disease include purpura en cocarde avec oedema, urticarial vasculitis of infancy, acute benign cutaneous leukocytoclastic vasculitis (Saraclar et al., 1990) of infancy and infantile post-infectious iris-like purpura and oedema. Already, more than 100 cases of AHEI have been published in medical literature worldwide. However, the current number of reported cases are being still unknown. This is probably because, the most papers on the subject being written different languages in the world and AHEI is called Henoch-Schönlein purpura in the United States. Although most of the prints were in case reports (Babic et al., 2008; Can et al., 2006; Di Lernia et al., 2004; Garty et al., 2002; Michael, 2006; Millard et al., 1999; Macea et al., 2003; Obeid et al., 2008; Serna et al., 1994, Silveira & Braganca, 2006), case series were also published (Alp et al., 2009; Caksen et al., 2002; Fiore et al., 2008; Gelmetti et al., 1985; Gonggryp & Todd, 1998; Ince et al., 1995; Karremann et al., 2009; Krause et al., 1996; Legrain et al., 1991; Poyrazoglu et al., 2003; Saraclar et al., 1990; Sites et al., 2008). Today, AHEI is considered as a separate entity, but not a variant of Henoch-Schönlein purpura, with clinical findings and prognosis.

3. Epidemiology

The exact incidence of AHEI is not well known because of rarity of the disease. So, multicenter epidemiologic studies are needed. Some authors believe that AHEI is often mistaken for other diseases and, therefore, its incidence may be more frequent. It is also probable that, using the synonyms for AHEI in the same population for different cases and to consider the disease as Henoch-Schönlein purpura may change the incidence.

3.1 Age

Usually, AHEI affects infants between 4 months and 2 years of age. However, cases at birth (Cunningham et al., 1996, 1999) and over 2 years of age (Alp et al., 2009; Dubin et al., 1990; Poyrazoglu et al., 2003; Slutsky et al., 2010), with classical features of AHEI, have been reported. Also, rare cases have been reported in older children up to 60 months of age (Alp et al., 2009; Fiore et al., 2008; Legrain et al., 1991). So, it can be suggested that AHEI can be diagnosed from newborn to 60 months of age. Actually, newly added reports of AHEI in English literature between 2008 and 2010 (Alp et al., 2009; Babic et al., 2008; Cicero, 2008; Ferraira et al., 2010; Fiore et al., 2008; Halıcıoglu et al., 2010; Jain & Patel, 2008; Javidi et al., 2008; Kumar et al., 2008; Karremann et al., 2009; Obeid et al., 2008; Slutsky et al., 2010; Sites et al., 2008) with the review by AlSufyani (AlSufyani, 2009) make the mean age approximately 16.56 months instead of 13.75 months reported by Alsufyani (Alsufyani, 2009). Indeed, there have been some reports of cases occurring beyond the age of 3 years; however, these cases have the features that overlap with those of Henoch-Schönlein purpura (Legrain et al., 1991; Shah et al., 2002).

3.2 Sex

Male predominance is clear in the literature. Case series are also support this data (Alp et al., 2009; Fiore et al., 2008; Ince et al., 1995; Legrain et al., 1991; Poyrazoglu et al., 2003; Saraclar et al., 1990). Also, AlSufyani suggests the male to female ratio approximately 4.64/1 (AlSufyani, 2009). However, adding the reported cases between 2008 and 2010 (Alp et al., 2009; Babic et al., 2008; Cicero, 2008; Ferraira et al., 2010; Fiore et al., 2008; Halıcıoglu et al., 2010; Jain & Patel, 2008; Javidi et al., 2008; Kumar et al., 2008; Karremann et al., 2009; Obeid et al., 2008; Slutsky et al., 2010; Sites et al., 2008) makes the male to female ratio approximately 4.34/1. Also, Fiore and colleagues reported the ratios of boys as %67 and girls as %33 in their systematic review (Fiore et al., 2008). But, they have reviewed 155 reports written in 6 languages, not only English literature.

3.3 Effect of seasons

AHEI, usually presents during the winter months. This may be associated with its potential etiology. However, some have presented in the spring, autumn (Fiore et al., 2008; Legrain et al., 1991; Poyrazoglu et al., 2003) and summer (Saraclar et al., 1990).

4. Etiology and pathogenesis

AHEI is probably an immune complex-mediated vasculitis and the pathophysiology is still not fully understood. The frequency of preceding infections and seasonal variation indicate an infective cause, but drugs and/or immunizations are also suspected. Legrain (Legrain et al., 1991) and AlSufyani (Alsufyani, 2009) reported these related causes up to %75 and %84.6 respectively. Obviously, it is difficult to attribute AHEI to an infection, drug or immunization as these are often present together; however, a few case reports have shown clearance of the first attack, as well as relapses, of AHEI after appropriate treatment of the associated infections (Dubin et al., 1990; Gonggryp & Todd, 1998; Ince et al., 1995; Morrison et al., 1999; Tomac et al., 1996). In addition, Cunningham and colleagues (Cunningham et al., 1996, 1999) have reported a newborn with the clinical findings of AHEI. Her mother had severe gastroenteritis 6 weeks prior to delivery and many lesions on the baby were faded and faint, suggesting that the process had evolved in utero. In conclusion, the authors hypothesized that there was a maternal-fetal transfer of the infectious agent or the immune complex triggering the skin lesions. This probably supports the role of infections and immune complexes in the pathogenesis of AHEI. Other infections described as prodromes that have been accused in the pathogenesis are upper respiratory tract infections (Alp et al., 2009; Babic et al., 2008; Blasini et al., 2007; Caksen et al., 2002; Dubin et al., 1990; Fiore et al., 2008; Gelmetti et al., 1985; Halıcıoglu et al., 2010; Ince et al., 1995; Karremann et al., 2009; Kumar et al., 2008; Lai-Cheong JE et al., 2007; McDougall et al., 2004; Michael, 2006; Millard et al., 1999; Paradisi et al., 2001; Poyrazoglu et al., 2003; Saraclar et al., 1990), pharyngitis (Gattorno et al., 1997; Gonggryp & Todd, 1998), tonsillitis (Legrain et al., 1991; Karremann et al., 2009), otitis (Caksen et al., 2002; Crowe et al., 1998; Karremann et al., 2009; Krause et al., 1996; Lantner et al., 1996; Macea et al., 2003), conjunctivitis (Legrain et al., 1991), neck abscess, bronchopneumonia (Alp et al., 2009; Saraclar et al., 1990), bronchitis (Karremann et al., 2009), pneumococcal bacteremia (Morrison et al., 1999), pulmoner tuberculosis (Gonggryp & Todd, 1998), cellulitis (Can et al., 2006), urinary tract infections (Saraclar et al., 1990) and gastroenteritis (Caksen et al., 2002; Chatproedprai & Wananukul, 2007; Fiore et al., 2008; Garty et al., 2002; Poyrazoglu et al., 2003; Silveira & Braganca, 2006).

Also, specific microorganisms have been isolated in the cases with AHEI, such as coxsackie B_4 virus (Krause et al., 1996), cytomegalovirus (Kuroda et al., 2002; Saraclar et al., 1990), rotavirus (Di Lernia et al., 2004), herpes simplex virus-1 (Garty et al., 2006), hepatitis A virus (Bozaykut et al., 2002) and parvovirus B19 (Erguven & Karaca Atakan, 2009). Escherichia coli grew in some of the children with urinary tract infections (Fiore et al., 2008) and campylobacter (Gonggryp & Todd, 1998) were isolated in some of the patients with diarrhea. Additionally, failure to convincingly relate AHEI to prodromal infectious caused by group A streptococcus or Mycoplasma pneumoniae is not surprising, considering that these agents mostly cause infections in children 5 years of age or older (Jaggi & Shulman, 2006; Principi & Esposito, 2002).

A wide range of medications have been reported such as anti-inflammatory and/or antipyretics including ibuprofen (Blasini et al., 2007), aspirin and paracetamol (da Silva Manzoni et al., 2004; Fiore et al., 2008; Karremann et al., 2009; Legrain et al., 1991; Poyrazoglu et al., 2003; Saraclar et al., 1990), antimicrobials including penicillins (Legrain et al., 1991; Saraclar et al., 1990), amoxicillin (Blasini et al., 2007; Gattorno et al., 1997), sultamisilin (Halıcıoglu et al., 2010), erythromycin (Krause et al., 1996), tobramycin (Blasini et al., 2007), trimethoprim-sulfomethoxazol (Poyrazoglu et al., 2003), cefaleksin (Crowe et al., 1998; da Silva Manzoni et al., 2004;), ceftriaxone (Can et al., 2006), ceftibuten (Fiore et al.,

2008) and other medications such as cough syrup (Dubin et al., 1990; Gonggryp & Todd, 1998) and probiotics (Fiore et al., 2008).

Vaccines have also been implicated in the pathogenesis of AHEI, including diphtheria-pertussis-tetanus (Krause et al., 1996; Saraclar et al., 1990), poliomavirus vaccine (Saraclar et al., 1990), hemophilus influenza conjugated (Krause et al., 1996), measles (Gonggryp & Todd, 1998; Saray et al., 2002), rubeola (Poyrazoglu et al., 2003), BCG (Lai-Cheong JE et al., 2007) and influenza A/H1N1 vaccine (Ferraira et al., 2010).

In the skin, postcapillary venules are the most commonly involved vessels. Leucocytoclastic vasculitis is the histological feature of AHEI that has been linked pathogenetically to immune complex deposition, complement activation and chemotaxis of neutrophils, with secondary damage to vessel walls due to the release of enzymes by activated neutrophils (Legrain et al., 1991, Saraclar et al., 1990). However, complement deficiency (Yavuz, 2000) or hypocomplementemia due to activation of the classical pathway of complement system (Watanabe & Sato, 2007) have not been showed in AHEI as they have been suggested. The location of vasculitic lesions to the extremities and especially the legs in children is thought to be related to increased hydrostatic pressure leading to immune complexes and fibrin deposition (Legrain & Taieb, 2000). Also, it has been suggested that proportionally larger had and face in infants corresponds to increased blood supply and susceptibility to facial purpura (Amitai et al, 1993).

5. Histopathology

Classically histological examination shows features of an intense dermal leucocytoclastic vasculitis involving small blood vessels in the dermis with (Acun et al., 2006; AlSufyani, 2009; Blasini et al., 2007; Braun-Falco & Dietrich Abeck, 2002; Caksen et al., 2002; Calıskan et al., 1995; Can et al., 2006; Chatproedprai & Wananukul, 2007; Colantonio et al., 1997; Crowe & Jonas, 1998; Cunningham et al., 1996, 1999; Bozaykut et al., 2002; da Silva Manzoni et al., 2004; Di Lernia et al., 2004; Dubin et al., 1990; Fiore et al., 2008; Fujimura et al., 2001; Garty et al., 2006; Gelmetti et al., 1985; Goraya & Kaur, 2002; Gonggryp & Todd, 1998; Gattorno et al., 1997; Javidi et al., 2008; Krause et al., 1996; Kuroda et al., 2002; Lakshmi & Srinivas, 2003; Lantner et al., 1996; Lee et al., 2006; Long & Helm, 1998; Macea et al., 2003; Michael, 2006; Millard et al., 1999; Morrison & Saulsbury, 1999; Paradisi et al., 2001; Poyrazoglu et al., 2003; Pride et al., 1995; Roh et al., 2004; Tomac et al., 1996; Saray et al., 2002; Scaramuzza et al., 1997; Serna et al., 1994; Shah et al., 2002; Silveira et al., 2006; Sites et al., 2008; Smitt et al., 2002, Watanabe & Sato, 2007; Wong & Harrington, 2004) (Fig. 1a, b) or without (Ince et al., 1995; Legrain et al., 1991; Saraclar et al., 1990) fibrinoid necrosis and erythrocyte extravasation. However, lymphohistiocytic perivascular infiltration with extravasation of erythrocytes and without fibrinoid necrosis was also reported by Legrain and colleagues (Legrain et al., 1991). The infiltrating inflammatory cells are predominantly neutrophils with less number of eosinophils (Krause et al., 1996; Macea et al., 2003; Millard et al., 1999; Saraclar et al., 1990).

6. Immunofluorescence study and immunologic characteristics

Immunofluorescence studies are usually negative (AlSufyani, 2009; Can et al., 2006; Cunningham et al., 1996; da Silva Manzoni et al., 2004; Gonggryp & Todd, 1998; Javidi et al.,

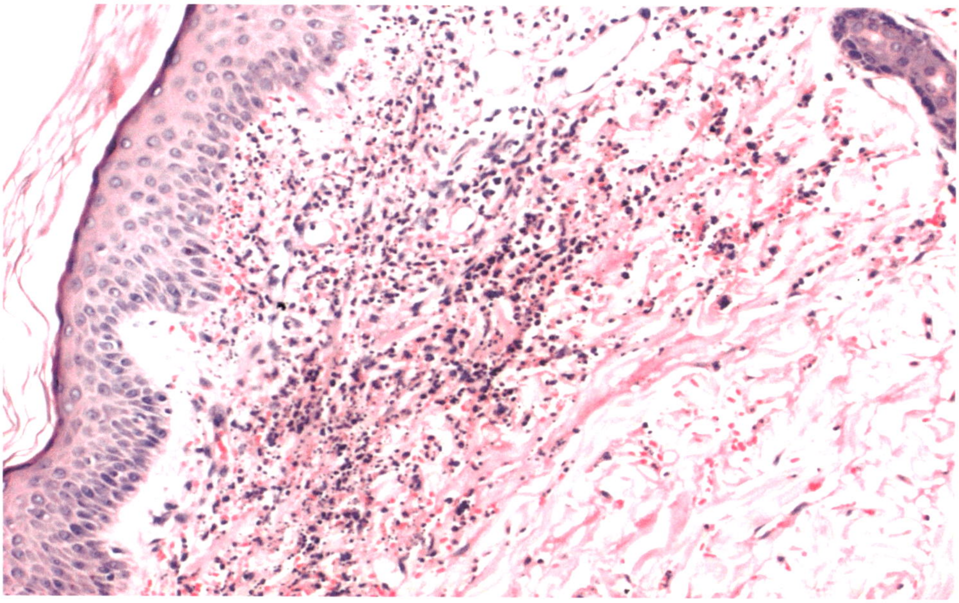

Fig. 1a. Hematoxylin and eosin-stained pathologic specimen from a purpuric skin lesion, showing perivascular leucocyte infiltration (x10).

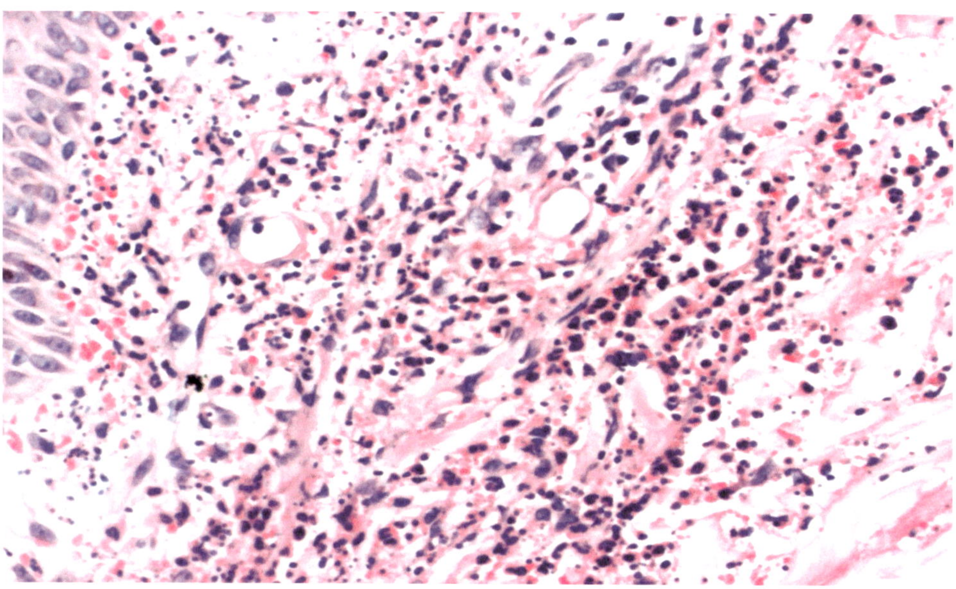

Fig. 1b. Extravasation of red blood cells, neutrophilic perivascular infiltration with leukocytoclasia, and fibrinoid necrosis (x40).

2008; Krause et al., 1996; Legrain et al., 1991; Paradisi et al., 2001; Serna et al., 1994). However; C_3, C_{1q}, fibrinogen, IgM, IgG, IgE and IgA were detected in the specimens with varying degrees of positivity (Amitai et al., 1993; Blasini et al., 2007; Caksen et al., 2002; Chatproedprai & Wananukul, 2007; Garty et al., 2006; Gattorno et al., 1997; Kuroda et al.,

2002; Legrain et al., 1991; Long & Helm, 1998; Michael, 2006; Paradisi et al., 2001; Roh et al., 2004; Tomac et al., 1996; Saraclar et al., 1990). In the study of Saraclar and colleagues, in the skin biopsy of 9 cases perivascular C_3, fibrinogen, IgM, IgG, IgE and IgA were detected 100%, 100%, 78%, 22%, 33% and 33% respectively (Saraclar et al., 1990). After the publication of their article they also examined an infant and in the lesional skin biopsy specimens of these 10 cases IgA, IgG, IgM, IgE and C_{1q} depositions were found in 30%, 20%, 80%, 30% and 100% respectively (Saraclar et al., 1992). So, based on these findings they suggested that the presence of C_{1q} and absence or infrequency of IgA deposition may help physicians to confirm AHEI rather than Henoch-Schönlein purpura. Additionally, Fiore et al. reported the deposition of IgA as 24% in their review (Fiore et al., 2008). Watanabe & Sato reported decreased levels of C_4, C_{1q} and CH50 in the serum of a 19-month-old boy with AHEI (Watanabe & Sato, 2007). So, they suggested that activation of the classical pathway of the complement might represent one of the pathogenic mechanisms underlying the development of AHEI. In summary, all of these immunohistologic and immunoserologic findings indicate that AHEI is an immunorelated disease.

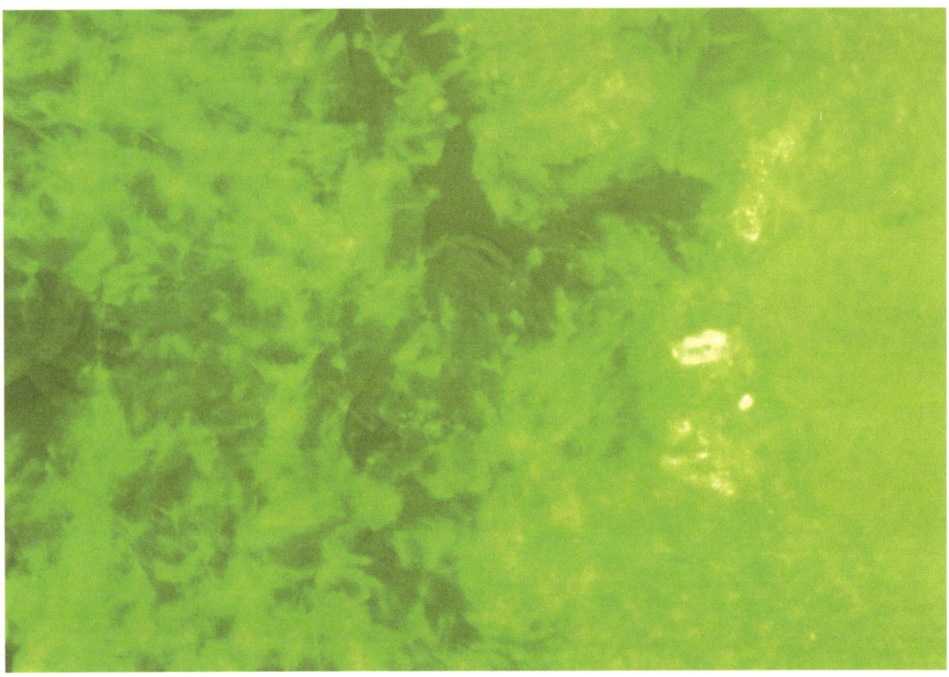

Fig. 2. Immunofluorescence study of epidermis with deposition of perivascular IgA.

7. Clinical features

The characteristic clinical features of AHEI are fever, purpura and edema. Additionally, the most striking feature is the contrast between the acuteness of the cutaneous signs and the good general condition of the child (Alp et al., 2009; Amitai et al., 1993; Dubin et al., 1990; Fiore et al., 2008; Ince et al., 1995; Lantner & Simon, 1996; Tomac et al., 1996; Saraclar et al., 1990). In the review of Fiore and colleagues, general appearance was reported as severely reduced in 1.0%, mildly reduced in 7.0% and very satisfactory in remaining 92% (Fiore et al.,

2008). Additionally, atypical presentations such as painful edema (Dubin et al., 1990; Gonggryp & Todd, 1998; Krause et al., 1996; Lantner & Simon, 1996; Millard et al., 1999; Morrison & Saulsbury, 1999; Shah et al., 2002), itching (AlSufyani, 2009; Caksen et al., 2002), irritability (Crowe & Jonas, 1998; Kuroda et al., 2002; Lantner & Simon, 1996) and decreased appetite (Lantner & Simon, 1996) may occur. Fever is typically low grade, but may range from mild to severe and also afebrile cases have been published in the literature (AlSufyani, 2009; Amitai et al., 1993; Dubin et al., 1990; Fiore et al., 2008; Gonggryp & Todd, 1998; Karreman et al., 2009; Krause et al., 1996; Saraclar et al., 1990; Scaramuzza et al., 1997; Serna et al., 1994). In the review of Fiore and colleagues fever of low grade was reported in 45% of the children (Fiore et al., 2008).

Purpura is the most dramatically presenting exanthema of AHEI and often appears in a cockade pattern in combined lesions (Legrain et al., 1991; Saraclar et al., 1990; Seildmayer, 1936). The erupsion usually starts with erythematous macules (Krause et al., 1996; Scaramuzza et al., 1997), papules (Lantner & Simon, 1996; McDougall et al., 2004; Tomac et al., 1996), or urticarial plaques (da Silva Manzoni et al., 2004; Legrain et al., 1991; Saraclar et al., 1990) that rapidly progress into annular (Lee et al., 2006; McDougall et al., 2004), rounded or oval (Alp et al., 2009), medallion-like (Karreman et al., 2009), cockade (Caksen et al., 2002), or targetoid-shaped purpuric lesions (Alp et al., 2009; Amitai et al., 1993; Caksen et al., 2002, Calıskan et al., 1995; Can et al., 2006; Crowe & Jonas, 1998; Cunningham et al., 1996; da Silva Manzoni et al., 2004; Di Lernia et al., 2004; Dubin et al., 1990; Fiore et al., 2008; Gelmetti et al., 1985; Gonggryp & Todd, 1998; Ince et al., 1995; Krause et al., 1996; Lantner & Simon, 1996; Lee et al., 2006; Legrain et al., 1991; Long & Helm, 1998; McDougall et al., 2004; Poyrazoglu et al., 2003; Saraclar et al., 1990; Scaramuzza et al., 1997; Serna et al., 1994; Silveira et al., 2006; Tomac et al., 1996; Watanabe & Sato, 2007) (Fig. 1a, b). However, other morphologies have been described, such as reticulated (Legrain et al., 1991), petechiael (Karreman et al., 2009), rosette-like (Paradisi et al., 2001), scalloped-border (Millard et al., 1999; Yu et al., 2007), tense hemorrhagic blistered or fluid containing lesions (either vesicles or bullae) (Al-Sheyyab et al., 1995; da Silva Manzoni et al., 2004; Gonggryp & Todd, 1998; Gattorno et al., 1997; Gattorno et al., 1999; Lai-Cheong et al., 2007; Lee et al., 2006; Legrain et al., 1991; Millard et al., 1999; Suehiro et al., 2007; Watanabe & Sato, 2007), arcuate and polycyclic (Di Lernia et al., 2004; Macea et al., 2003). Skin lesions may progress to 1 to 6 cm in diameter (Michael, 2006; Smitt et al., 2002). The rashes are usually sharped edged and the centre of the lesions may rarely have the colour of the normal skin (Legrain et al., 1991; Saraclar et al., 1990). Lesions usually occur in the face (mainly cheeks) (Alp et al., 2009; AlSufyani, 2009; Caksen et al., 2002; Fiore et al., 2008; Karreman et al., 2009; Krause et al., 1996; Legrain et al., 1991; Poyrazoglu et al., 2003; Saraclar et al., 1990), auricles (Fig. 2) and upper (Millard et al., 1999) (Fig. 3) or lower extremities (Alp et al., 2009; AlSufyani, 2009; Caksen et al., 2002; Fiore et al., 2008; Karreman et al., 2009; Krause et al., 1996; Legrain et al., 1991; Michael, 2006; Poyrazoglu et al., 2003; Saraclar et al., 1990) (Fig. 4) with relative sparing of the trunk (Fiore et al., 2008). Additionally, Fiore and colleagues reviewed that purpura had a relative frequency on the left side of the body (Fiore et al., 2008). Skin or mucous membranes are uncommonly involved in AHEI such as conjunctiva (McDougall et al., 2004; Poyrazoglu et al., 2003), buccal mucosa (Halıcıoglu et al., 2010; Roh et al., 2004), palate (Blasini et al., 2007; Chatproedprai & Wananukul, 2007; Gelmetti et al., 1985; Poyrazoglu et al., 2003), gums (Di Lernia et al., 2004), uvula, tongue, pharynx (Amitai et al., 1993; Di Lernia et al., 2004; Dubin et al., 1990; Krause et al., 1996; McDougall et al., 2005), calf

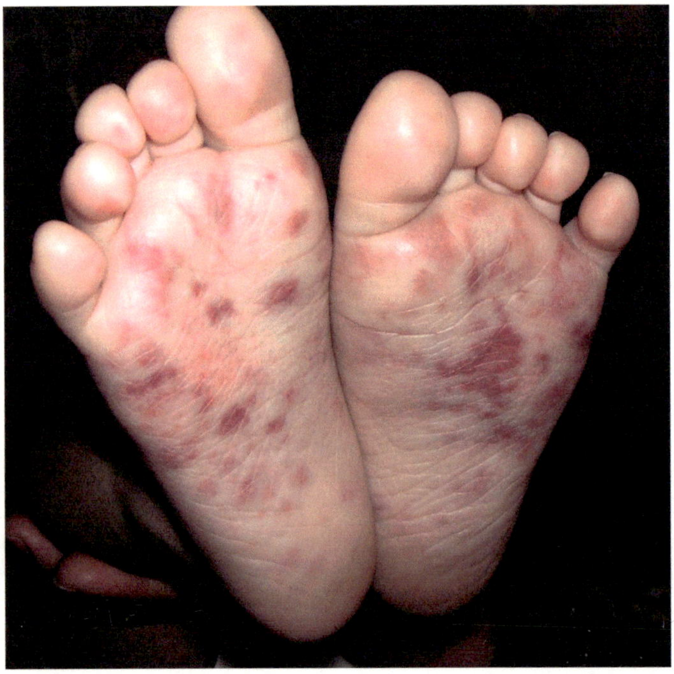

Fig. 3a. Purpuric involvement of the feet in a 30-month-old male patient with AHEI.

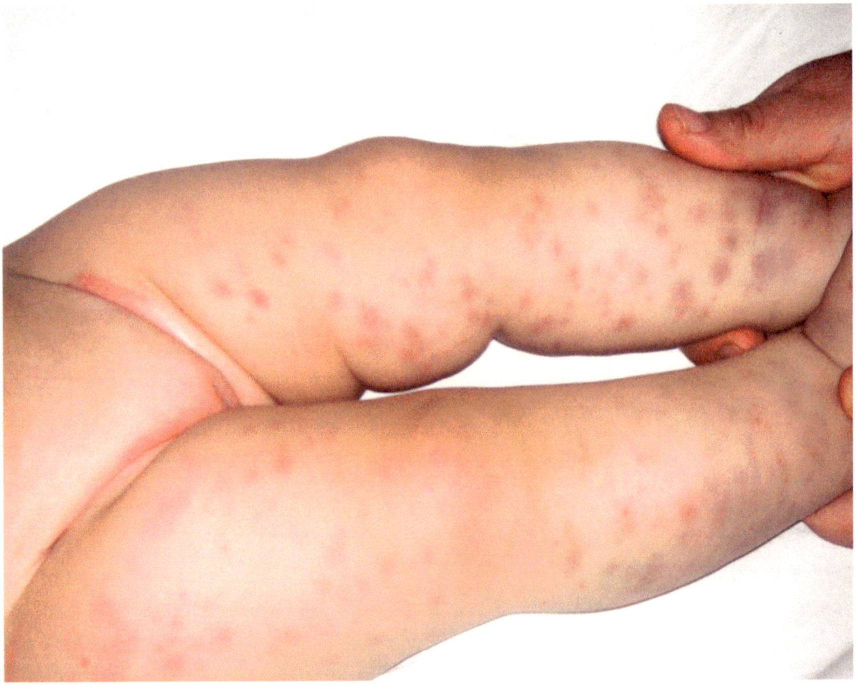

Fig. 3b. Ecchymotic and purpuric lesions with edema of the lower extremities in a 7-month-old girl.

(as hematoma) (Karreman et al., 2009), penis (Fiore et al., 2008; Poyrazoglu et al., 2003), scrotum (Dubin et al., 1990; Karreman et al., 2009; Poyrazoglu et al., 2003), buttocks (Amitai et al., 1993; da Silva Monzani et al., 2004; Legrain et al., 1991; Michael, 2006; Paradisi et al., 2001; Roh et al., 2004; Saraclar et al., 1990; Serna et al., 1994; Shah et al., 2002), joints (Al-Sheyyab et al., 1995; Gattorno et al., 1997) and perineum (Lantner & Simon, 1996). Extracutaneous manifestations rarely occur; however, renal involvement with microscopic hematuria, proteinuria and hypocomplementemia (Watanabe & Sato, 2007); transient and microscopic hematuria (Al-Sheyyab et al., 1995; Amitai et al., 1993; Gonggryp & Todd, 1998; Legrain et al., 1991; Millard et al., 1999); intusseption (Yu et al., 2007); bowel involvement as positive stool for occult blood (Al-Sheyyab et al., 1995; Di Lernia et al., 2004; Garty et al., 2002; Gonggryp & Todd, 1998; Yu et al., 2007) and abdominal pain with elevated transaminases (Obeid et al., 2008) associated with AHEI were reported. Proteinuria is usually transient (Legrain et al., 1991; Saraclar et al., 1990), but can be persistent (Millard et al., 1999). Hypertension is also rare and transient (Caksen et al., 2002) with no renal involvement. Cases of diarrhea, abdominal pain and vomiting have been reported (Di Lernia et al., 2004; Legrain et al., 1991), however these cases have shown an underlying cause, such as coxsackie virus (Legrain et al., 1991) and rotavirus (Di Lernia et al., 2004) growth in the stool.

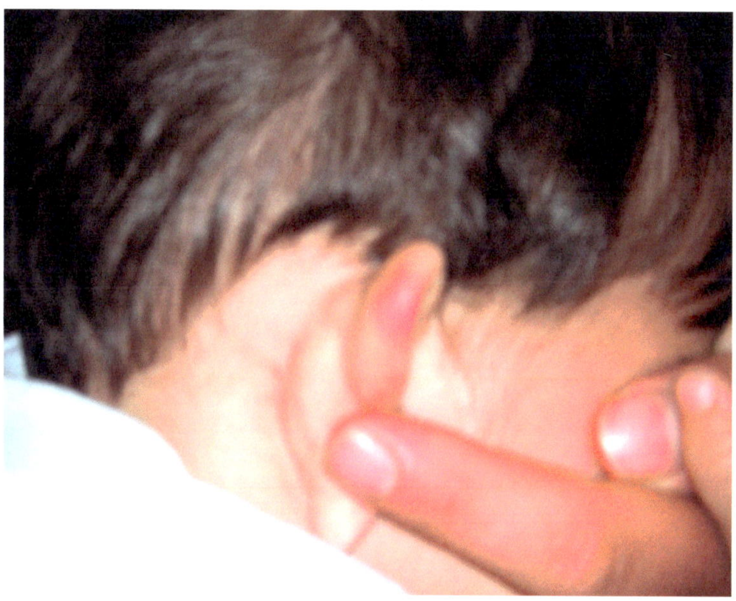

Fig. 4. Purpuric skin lesion on ear in a 11-month-old boy with AHEI.

Edema is classically asymmetrical nonpitting (mainly tender), usually affects the auricles, face and limbs (frequently dorsum of the hands and feet) (Alp et al., 2009; AlSufyani, 2009; Amitai et al., 1993; Caksen et al., 2002, Calıskan et al., 1995; Can et al., 2006; Crowe & Jonas, 1998; Cunningham et al., 1996; da Silva Manzoni et al., 2004; Di Lernia et al., 2004; Dubin et al., 1990; Fiore et al., 2008; Garty et al., 2006; Gonggryp & Todd, 1998; Ince et al., 1995; Krause et al., 1996; Lantner & Simon, 1996; Lee et al., 2006; Legrain et al., 1991; Long & Helm, 1998; McDougall et al., 2004; Michael, 2006; Millard et al., 1999; Paradisi et al., 2001;

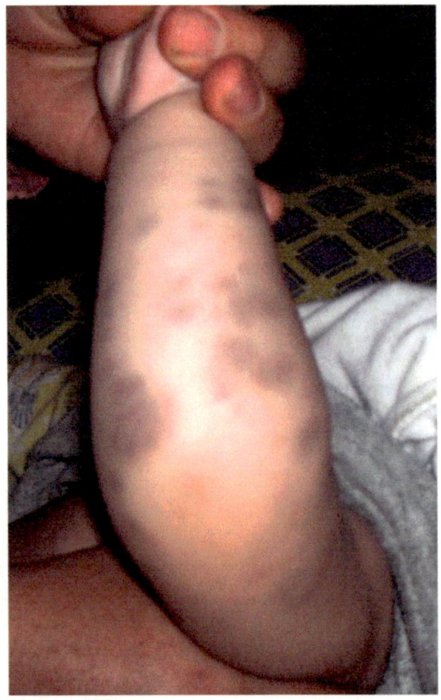

Fig. 5. Ecchymotic and purpuric lesions of upper extremities in a 10-month-old girl.

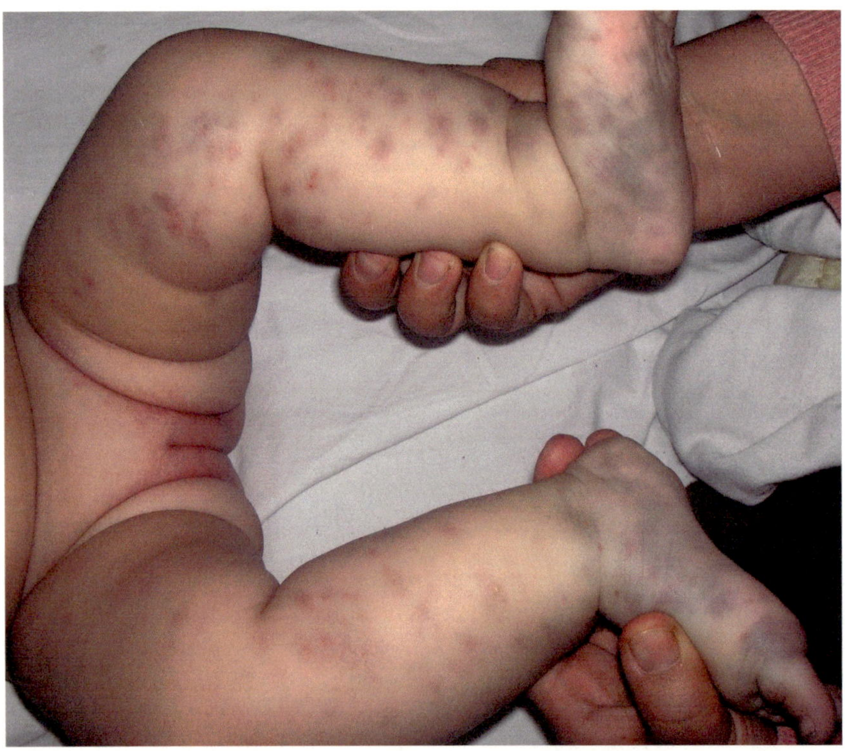

Fig. 6. Ecchymotic and purpuric lesions of the lower extremities in a 7-month-old girl.

Poyrazoglu et al., 2003; Saraclar et al., 1990; Scaramuzza et al., 1997; Serna et al., 1994; Silveira et al., 2006; Tomac et al., 1996; Watanabe & Sato, 2007). However, other parts of the body may be involved resembling nephrotic syndrome such as the eyelids (Caksen et al., 2002; Gonggryp & Todd, 1998; Karreman et al., 2009; Legrain et al., 1991; Paradisi et al., 2001; Saraclar et al., 1990), lips (McDougall et al., 2004), penis (Fiore et al., 2008; Poyrazoglu et al., 2003) and scrotum (Millard et al, 1999; Saraclar et al., 1990; Yu et al., 2007). Also, the edema can cause weight gain (Saraclar et al., 1990).

8. Laboratory findings

The laboratory investigations are nonspecific. Leukocytosis with lymphocytosis or eosinophilia (Alp et al., 2009; Amitai et al., 1993; Colantonio et al ., 1997; Cunningham et al., 1996; Fiore et al., 2008; Lantner & Simon, 1996; Legrain et al., 1991; Roh et al., 2004; Tomac et al., 1996; Saraclar et al., 1990; Scaramuzza et al., 1997; Watanabe & Sato, 2007), thrombocytosis (Di Lernia et al., 2004; Fiore et al., 2008; Garty et al., 2006; Halıcıoglu et al., 2010; Ince et al., 1995; Lantner & Simon, 1996; Legrain et al., 1991; Tomac et al., 1996) and increased erythrocytes sedimentation rate or C-reactive protein (Alp et al., 2009; AlSufyani, 2009; Blasini et al., 2007; Caksen et al., 2002; Can et al., 2006; Colantonio et al ., 1997; Di Lernia et al., 2004; Fiore et al., 2008; Garty et al., 2002; Halıcıoglu et al., 2010; Javidi et al., 2008; Kuroda et al., 2002; Lee et al., 2006; Macea et al., 2003; Millard et al., 1999; Paradisi et al., 2001; Poyrazoglu et al., 2003; Watanabe & Sato, 2007) are common findings.The coagulation tests are usually normal, but elevated fibrinogen (Di Lernia et al., 2004) was noted. Additionally, hypoalbunemia has been reported associated with intusseption (Yu et al., 2007). Urinalysis is frequently normal, however cases of proteinuria (Legrain et al., 1991; Saraclar et al., 1990; Watanabe & Sato, 2007) and microscopic hematuria (Al-Sheyyab et al., 1995; Amitai et al., 1993; Gonggryp & Todd, 1998; Legrain et al., 1991; Millard et al., 1999; Watanabe & Sato, 2007) have been reported. The stool is typically negative for blood, but positive stool for occult blood (Al-Sheyyab et al., 1995; Di Lernia et al., 2004; Garty et al., 2002; Gonggryp & Todd, 1998; Yu et al., 2007) have been documented. Antinuclear antibodies (ANAs), ASO titre, antideoxyribonucleic acid (anti DNA) antibodies and rheumatoid factor are always negative. However, elevated anti-DNAse B titer (Gonggryp & Todd, 1998) and IgG antineutrophil cytoplasmic antibody (Ozaltın et al., 2004) have been reported in two patients. Complement levels are normal in the patients, although cases with increased serum C_3 (Saraclar et al., 1990), decreased serum C_4 (Cunningham et al., 1996; Watanabe & Sato, 2007) and CH50 (Watanabe & Sato, 2007) levels have been mentioned. Classically, serum immunoglobulin levels are normal, however patients with increased levels of IgG (Legrain et al., 1991), IgM (Caksen et al., 2002; Di Lernia et al., 2004), IgE (Saraclar et al., 1990) and IgA (Di Lernia et al., 2004; Legrain et al., 1991) have been reported. Circulating immune complexes are normal, although some have reported positive findings (Saraclar et al., 1990; Scaramuzza et al., 1997). Additionally, Ozaltın and colleagues reported positivity of IgG ANCA in a patient with AHEI (Ozaltın et al., 2004). However, the importance of this finding has not been known. Generally, most of these uncommon laboratory findings are case reports and need future evaluations.

9. Diagnostic criteria and differential diagnosis

The diagnostic criteria can be proposed as follows (AlSufyani, 2009; Krause et al., 1996).

a. Between 4 months and 2 years of age.
b. Purpuric or ecchymotic target-like skin lesions with edema especially on the face, auricles and extremities with or without mucosal involvement.
c. Lack of systemic disease or visceral involvement.
d. Spontaneous recovery within 4-24 days.

Common laboratory investigations are follows.

a. Leukocytosis with lymphocytosis or eosinophilia.
b. Elevated erythrocytes sedimentation rate or C-reactive protein.
c. Leucocytoclastic vasculitis with or without fibrinoid necrosis involving small blood vessels in the dermis on histological examination.
d. Negative immunofluorescence studies are usual or rarely positivity of C_3, C_{1q}, fibrinogen, IgM, IgG, IgE and IgA in varying degrees can be detected.

AHEI and Henoch-Schönlein purpura (HSP) both fall within the spectrum of the leucocytoclastic vasculitis. Some authors believe that these two conditions are different disease entities (Cunningham et al., 1999; da Silva Manzoni et al., 2004; Gonggryp & Todd, 1998; Ince et al., 1995; Krause et al., 1996; Millard et al., 1999; Saraclar et al., 1990; Tomac et al., 1996) whereas others regard them as distinct but with some cases showing overlap (Legrain et al., 1991; Shah et al., 2002). Some of the points that differentiate these two entities are (Table 1); age of onset (3-7 years for HSP and 4 months-2 years for AHEI) (Legrain et al.,

	AHEI	**HSP**
Age	4-24 months	3-7 years
Sex	Slight male predominance in both diseases	
Prodromes	Respiratory infections, drug intake and immunization in both diseases	
Seasons	Usually winter months in both diseases	
Morphology of skin lesions	Purpuric, ecchymotic lesions	Papular, petechial and urticarial lesions
Location of skin lesions	Face, auricles and extremities with relative frequency on the left side of the body	Lower parth of the body
Edema	Constant and nonpitting, mainly tender	Inconsistent
Visseral involvement	Uncommon	Frequent
Duration of disease	1-3 weeks	One month or more
Relapses	Rare	Frequent
Histopathology	Leucocytoclastic vasculitis with frequent fibrinoid necrosis	Leucocytoclastic vasculitis
Immunofluorescence study	Perivascular C1q deposits	Perivascular IgA deposits

Table 1. Comparison of epidemiological, clinical and pathological findings of AHEI and HSP

1991; Saraclar et al., 1990; Tomac et al., 1996), morphology of skin lesions with location on the part of the body (papular, petechial, urticarial lesions located predominantly on the lower legs and gluteal regions in HSP and ecchymotic, cockade purpuric lesions mainly located on face and extremities in AHEI) (Legrain et al., 1991; Saraclar et al., 1990; Tomac et al., 1996), edema (not a clinical finding of HSP, but a classical finding of AHEI, commonly nonpitting with tender) (Legrain et al., 1991; Saraclar et al., 1990; Tomac et al., 1996), visceral involvement (frequently seen in HSP, but uncommon in AHEI) (Gelmetti et al., 1985; Legrain et al., 1991; Saraclar et al., 1990), duration of disease (one month or more in HSP, usually resolves between 1-3 weeks in AHEI) (Fiore et al., 2008; Legrain et al., 1991; Saraclar et al., 1990) and relapses (frequent in HSP, rare in AHEI, however there have been cases of AHEI showing multiple relapses) (Amitai et al., 1993; Dubin et al., 1990; Karreman et al., 2009; Legrain et al., 1991; Saraclar et al., 1990).

Also, duration of complete recovery in each attack is different between HSP (approximately 4 weeks) and AHEI (approximately 12 days) (Karreman et al., 2009; Legrain et al., 1991; Tomac et al., 1996). However, there have been cases of AHEI with long duration of attacks up to 24 days (Legrain et al., 1991). On laboratory, some authors suggested that these two diseases should be separated on the basis of the negative immunofluorescence studies of skin biopsies in the cases with AHEI (Millard et al., 1999; Saraclar et al., 1990). Although, as it was discussed in 'Immunofluorescence study and immunologic characteristics' some reported cases had positive direct immunofluorescence with any of C_3, C_{1q}, fibrinogen, IgM, IgG, IgE and IgA (Amitai et al., 1993; Blasini et al., 2007; Caksen et al., 2002; Chatproedprai & Wananukul, 2007; Garty et al., 2006; Gattorno et al., 1997; Kuroda et al., 2002; Legrain et al., 1991; Long & Helm, 1998; Michael, 2006; Paradisi et al., 2001; Roh et al., 2004; Tomac et al., 1996; Saraclar et al., 1990). However, Saraclar and colleagues suggested that presence of C_{1q} and absence or infrequency of IgA deposition may be helpful for physicians to confirm AHEI rather than HSP (Saraclar et al., 1992). Additionally, Goraya (Goraya et al., 2002) and Shah (Shah et al., 2002) reported that the observed immunohistologic differences between the two diseases are secondary to the immaturity of the IgA immune system at the ages of 12 and 24 months. In these age groups the IgA levels are at 19% and 25% of adult values, respectively. So, this might explain the observed clinical and immunologic differences between these two disorders.

The other differential diagnosis of AHEI includes meningococcemia, erythema multiforme, Kawasaki disease, purpura fulminans, eruptions of viral infections, drug-induced vasculitis, septic vasculitis, Sweet's syndrome (acute febrile neutrophilic dermatosis), dermatologic manifestations of hematologic diseases and child abuse (Caksen et al., 2002; Cunningham et al., 1996; Dubin et al., 1990; Ince et al., 1995; Legrain et al., 1991; Saraclar et al., 1990; Smitt et al., 2002). All these disorders can be differentiated from AHEI by results of history, physical examination and appropriate laboratory studies, including examination of skin biopsy specimen.

10. Treatment

There is no specific treatment for AHEI because of its natural course. Multiple treatments have been reported to be beneficial, such as topical hydrocortisone 1% cream twice daily (Long & Helm, 1998), systemic prednisone with a dose of 1.5-2 mg/kg/day (Dubin et al., 1990; Ince et al., 1995; Poyrazoglu et al., 2003), prednisolone with a dose of 0.5-1 mg/kg/day (AlSufyani, 2009; Blasini et al., 2007; da Silva Manzoni et al., 2004; Halıcıoglu et al., 2010; Roh et al., 2004), methylprednisolone with a dose of 1 mg/kg twice daily (Garty et al., 2006) and betamethasone with a dose of 1 mg/kg/day (Paradisi et al., 2001). Also, oral antihistamines such as hydroxyzine, diphenhydramine (Alp et al., 2009; Caksen et al., 2002; Ince et al., 1995; Poyrazoglu et al., 2003; Tomac et al., 1996), dapson (Gonggryp & Todd, 1998) and oral nonsteroidal anti-inflammatory drugs (Karremann et al., 2009, Poyrazoglu et al., 2003) have been suggested for management. Some authors believe that these treatments have a role in changing the course of the disease (Alp et al., 2009; Saraclar et al., 1990), but some do not (Krause et al., 1996; Legrain et al., 1991). Treatments with antimicrobials for a confirmed concurrent infection have been shown to be of some value during the course of AHEI (Caksen et al., 2002; Colantonio et al., 1997; Garty et al., 2002; Gonggryp & Todd, 1998; Ince et al., 1995; Karremann et al., 2009; Morrison & Saulsbury, 1999; Tomac et al., 1996).

11. Prognosis

AHEI is generally benign and self-limited. Spontaneous and complete resolution occurs within 4-24 days (Acun et al., 2006; Alp et al., 2009; AlSufyani, 2009; Blasini et al., 2007; Braun-Falco & Dietrich Abeck, 2002; Caksen et al., 2002; Calıskan et al., 1995; Can et al., 2006; Chatproedprai & Wananukul, 2007; Colantonio et al., 1997; Crowe & Jonas, 1998; Cunningham et al., 1996, 1999; Bozaykut et al., 2002; da Silva Manzoni et al., 2004; Di Lernia et al., 2004; Dubin et al., 1990; Fiore et al., 2008; Fujimura et al., 2001; Garty et al., 2006; Gelmetti et al., 1985; Goraya & Kaur, 2002; Gonggryp & Todd, 1998; Gattorno et al., 1997; Javidi et al., 2008; Karreman et al., 2009; Krause et al., 1996; Kuroda et al., 2002; Lakshmi & Srinivas, 2003; Lantner et al., 1996; Lee et al., 2006; Long & Helm, 1998; Macea et al., 2003; Michael, 2006; Millard et al., 1999; Morrison & Saulsbury, 1999; Paradisi et al., 2001; Poyrazoglu et al., 2003; Pride et al., 1995; Roh et al., 2004; Saraclar et al., 1990; Saray et al., 2002; Scaramuzza et al., 1997; Serna et al., 1994; Shah et al., 2002; Silveira et al., 2006; Sites et al., 2008; Smitt et al., 2002; Tomac et al., 1996; Watanabe & Sato, 2007; Wong & Harrington, 2004). Attacks have not been usually reported in the literature. This may because long-term follow-up is not available in most cases. However, attacks associated with AHEI have been reported in some cases and the duration of these attacks were not completely different from the duration of the main disease (Alp et al., 2009; Amitai et al., 1993; Dubin et al., 1990; Karreman et al., 2009). With either treatment or a conservative approach, AHEI usually resolves completely with no sequelae, but there have been reports of residual hyperpigmentation (Saraclar et al., 1990), slight atrophy (Macea et al., 2003) and depressed scars instead of cheeks (AlSufyani, 2009). Also, Smitt and colleagues stated that only necrotic areas may leave a scar (Smitt et al., 2002). On the other hand, AlSufyani suggested that scarring is genuine to the disease process itself and it is not clear whether earlier administration of either treatment would have prevented scarring (AlSufyani, 2009). Also, complications such as intussuseption (Yu et al., 2007) and torsion of testis (Gelmetti et al., 1985) have been reported.

12. Conclusion

Acute hemorrhagic edema of infancy is an uncommon cutaneous leukocytoclastic vasculitis. Various infections, drug use and vaccination are discussed as triggering factors more than

90 years after the first description of the disease. Also, the benign and self-limited course and excellent prognosis with mild to absent systemic involvement is well established. Today, it has been considered as a distinct entity either than a variant of Henoch-Schönlein purpura. Physicians might develop the skills necessary to consider the diagnosis of acute hemorrhagic edema of infancy when presented with a non-toxic infant having large targetoid purpuric lesions and edema in nonpitting character.

13. Acknowledgment

I give my thanks and gratitude to Prof. Ismail Reisli from Department of Pediatric Immunology for his suggestions about writing the text. I also thank to Assoc. Prof. Hatice Toy from Department of Pathology for the pictures of histopathology and immunofluorescence studies.

14. References

Acun, C., Ustundag, G., Sogut, A., Koca, R., & Numanoglu, G. (2006). Visual diagnosis: a child who had acute onset of unusual skin lesions and edema. *Pediatr Rev,* Vol. 27, No. 11, pp. 71-74, ISSN 0191-9601

Alp, H., Artac, H., Alp, E., & Reisli, I. (2009). Acute infantile hemorrhagic edema: a clinical perspective (report of seven cases). *Marmara Med J,* Vol. 22, No. 2, pp. 155-161, ISSN 10191941

Al-Sheyyab, M., El-Shanti, H., Ajlouni, S., Sawalha, D., & Daoud, A. (1995). The clinical spectrum of Henoch-Schönlein purpura in infants and young children. *Eur J Pediatr,* Vol. 154, No. 12, pp. 969-972, ISSN 0340-6199

AlSufyani MA. (2009). Acute hemorrhagic edema of infancy: unusual scarring and review of the English literature. *Int J Dermatol,* Vol. 48, pp. 617-622, ISSN 0011-9059

Amitai, Y., Gillis, D., Wasserman, D., & Kochman, RH. (1993). Henoch-Schönlein purpura in infants. *Pediatrics,* Vol. 92, No. 6, pp. 865-867, ISSN 0031-4005

Babic, S., Murat-Susic, S., Husar, K., Skerlev, M., & Rados, J. (2008). Acute hemorrhagic edema of infancy: a case report. *Acta Dermatovenerol Croat,* Vol. 16, No. 2, pp. 87-90, ISSN 1330-027X

Blasini, W., Saini, R., & Vincek, V. (2007). Acute hemorrhagic edema of infancy: a case report. *Dermatol Online J,* Vol. 13, No. 3, pp. 27, ISSN 1087-2108

Bozaykut, A., Atay, E., Atay, Z., Ipek, O., Akın, M., & Dursun, E. (2002). Acute infantile haemorrhagic oedema associated with hepatitis A. *Ann Trop Paediatr,* Vol. 22, No. 1, pp. 59-61, ISSN 0272-4936

Braun-Falco, M., & Dietrich Abeck, D. (2002). Acute infantile haemorrhagic oedema. *Lancet,* Vol. 360, No. 9328, pp. 210, ISSN 0140-6736

Caksen, H., Odabaş, D., Kosem, M., Arslan, S., Oner, AF., Atas, B., Akcay, G., & Ceylan, N. (2002). Report of eight infants with acute infantile hemorrhagic edema and review of the literature. *J Dermatol,* Vol. 29, No. 5, pp. 290-295, ISSN 0385-2407

Calıskan, S., Tasdan, Y., Kasapcopur, O., Sever, L., & Tunnessen, WW. (1995). Picture of the month. Acute hemorrhagic edema of infancy. *Arch Pediatr Adolesc Med,* Vol. 149, No. 11, pp. 1267-1268, ISSN 1072-4710

Can, B., Kavala, M., Turkoglu, Z., & Zemheri, E. (2006). Acute hemorrhagic edema of infancy: a case report. *Turk J Pediatr,* Vol. 48, No. 3, pp. 266-268, ISSN 0041-4301

Chatproedprai, S., & Wananukul, S. (2007). Acute hemorrhagic edema of infancy. *J Med Assoc Thai,* Vol. 90, No. 6, pp. 1205-1207, ISSN 0125-2208

Cicero, MX. (2008). The 2006-2007 PEMpix photo competition award winner: Mark Cicero, MD: Rash decisions: acute hemorrhagic edema of infancy in a 7-month-old boy. *Pediatr Emerg Care,* Vol. 24, No. 7, pp. 501-502, ISSN 0749-5161

Colantonio, G., Kinzlansky, V., Kahn, A., & Damilano, G. (1997). Pathological case of the month. *Arch Pediatr Adolesc Med,* Vol. 151, No. 5, pp. 523-524, ISSN 1072-4710

Crowe, MA., & Jonas, PP. (1998). Acute hemorrhagic edema of infancy. *Cutis,* Vol. 62, No. 2, pp. 65-66, ISSN 0011-4162

Cunningham, BB., Caro, WA., & Eramo, LR. (1996). Neonatal acute hemorrhagic edema of childhood: case report and review of the English-language literature. *Pediatr Dermatol,* Vol. 13, No. 1, pp. 39-44, ISSN 0736-8046

Cunningham, BB., Eramo, L., & Caro, W. (1999). Acute hemorrhagic edema of childhood present at birth. *Pediatr Dermatol,* Vol. 16, No. 1, pp. 68, ISSN 0736-8046

da Silva Manzoni, AP., Viecili, JB., de Andrade, CB., Kruse, RL., Bakos, L., & Cestari, TF. (2004). Acute hemorrhagic edema of infancy: a case report. *Int J Dermatol,* Vol. 43, No. 1, pp. 48-51, ISSN 0011-9059

Del Carrel, MJ., Diaz Bobillo, I., & Vidal, J. (1936). Edema hemoragico agudo en un lactante. *Prensa Med Arg,* Vol. 29, pp. 1719-1722

Di Lernia, V., Lombardi, M., & Scocco, GL. (2004). Infantile acute hemorrhagic edema and rotavirus infection. *Pediatr Dermatol,* Vol. 21, No. 5, pp. 548-550, ISSN 0736-8046

Dubin, BA., Bronson, DM., & Eng, AM. (1990). Acute hemorrhagic edema of childhood: an unusual variant of leucocytoclastic vasculitis. *J Am Acad Dermatol,* Vol. 23, No. 2, pp. 347-350, ISSN 0190-9622

Erguven, M., & Karaca Atakan, S. (2009). Infantile hemorrhagic edema due to parvovirus B19 infection. *J Child,* Vol. 9, No. 1, pp. 43-45, ISSN 1302-9940

Ferreira, O., Antunes, I., Cruz, MJ., Mota, A., Bettencourt, H., Canelhas, A., & Azevedo, F. (2010). Acute hemorrhagic edema of childhood after H1N1 immunization. *Cutan Ocul Toxicol,* Vol. 2, ISSN 1556-9527

Finkelstein, H. (1938). Lehrbuch der Sauglingskrankheiten. 4th ed. Amstefrdam , pp. 814-830

Fiore, E., Rizzi, M., Ragazzi, M., Vanoni, F., Bernasconi, M., Bianchetti, MG., & Simonetti, GD. (2008). Acute hemorrhagic edema of young children (cockade purpura and edema): A case series and systematic review. *J Am Acad Dermatol,* Vol. 59, No. 4, pp. 684-695, ISSN 0190-9622

Fujimura, T., Funayama, M., & Tagami, H. (2001). Acute hemorrhagic edema in a four-year-old Japanese boy. *J Dermatol,* Vol. 28, No. 5, pp. 279-281, ISSN 0385-2407

Garty, BZ., Ofer, I., & Finkelstein Y. (2002). Acute hemorrhagic edema of infancy. *Isr Med Assoc J,* Vol. 4, No. 3, pp. 228-229, ISSN 1565-1088

Garty, BZ., Pollak, U., Scheuerman, O., Marcus, N., & Hoffer, V. (2006). Acute hemorrhagic edema of infancy associated with herpes simplex type 1 stomatitis. *Pediatr Dermatol,* Vol. 23, No. 4, pp. 361-364, ISSN 0736-8046

Gattorno, M., Picco, P., Gambini, C., Buoncompagni, A., Castagnola, E., Pistoia, V., & Borrone, C. (1997). Erythema multiforme-like manifestations and arthritis in a 3-year-old child with leukocytoclastic vasculitis. *Clin Exp Rheumatol,* Vol. 15, No. 3, pp. 329-332, ISSN 0392-856X

Gattorno, M., Picco, P., Vignola, S., Di Rocco, M., & Buoncompagni, A. (1999). Brother and sister with different vasculitides. *Lancet,* Vol. 353, No. 9154, pp. 728, ISSN 0140-6736

Gelmetti, C., Barbagallo, C., Cerri, D., De Mattia, D., & Bonifazi, E. (1985). Acute haemorrhagic oedema of the skin in infants: clinical and pathogenetic observations in seven cases. *Pediatr Dermatol News,* Vol., 4, pp. 24-34

Gonggryp, LA., & Todd, G. (1998). Acute hemorrhagic edema of childhood (AHE). *Pediatr Dermatol,* Vol. 15, No. 2, pp. 91-96, ISSN 0736-8046

Goraya, JS., & Kaur, S. (2002). Acute infantile hemorrhagic edema and Henoch-Schonlein purpura: is IgA the missing link? *J Am Acad Dermatol,* Vol. 47, No. 5, pp. 801, ISSN 0190-9622

Halıcıoglu, O., Akman, SA., Sen, S., Sutcuoglu, S., Bayol, U., & Karci, H. (2010). Acute hemorrhagic edema of infancy: a case report. *Pediatr Dermatol,* Vol. 27, No. 2, pp. 214-215, ISSN 0736-8046

Ince, E., Mumcu, Y., Suskan, E., Yalcinkaya, F., Tumer, N., & Cin, S. (1995). Infantile acute hemorrhagic edema: a variant of leukocytoclastic vasculitis. *Pediatr Dermatol,* Vol. 12, No. 3, pp. 224-227, ISSN 0736-8046

Jaggi, P., & Shulman, ST. (2006). Group A streptococcal infections. *Pediatr Rev,* Vol. 27, No. 3, pp. 99-105, ISSN 0191-9601

Jain, G., & Patel, A. (2008). Acute hemorrhagic edema of infancy. *Indian Pediatr,* Vol. 45, No. 10, pp. 866-867, ISSN 0019-6061

Javidi, Z., Maleki, M., Mashayekhi, V., Tayebi-Maybodi, N., & Nahidi, Y. (2008). Acute hemorrhagic edema of infancy. *Arch Iranian Med,* Vol. 11, No. 1, pp. 103-106, ISSN 1029-2977

Karremann, M., Jordan, AJ., Bell, N., Witsch, M., & Durken, M. (2009). Acute hemorrhagic edema of infancy: report of 4 cases and review of the current literature. *Clin Pediatr (Phila),* Vol. 48, No. 3, pp. 323-326, ISSN 0009-9228

Krause, I., Lazarov, A., Rachmel, A., Grunwald, MM., Metzker, A., Garty, BZ., Halevy, S., & Nitzan, M. (1996). Acute hemorrhagic oedema of infancy, a benign variant of leucocytoclastic vasculitis. *Acta Pediatr,* Vol. 85, No. 1, pp. 114-117, ISSN 0803-5253

Kumar, R., Mittal, K., Rawal, M., & Kumar, S. (2008). Acute hemorrhagic edema of infancy. *Indian Pediatr,* Vol. 45, No. 12, pp. 1002-1003, ISSN 0019-6061

Kuroda, K., Yabunami, H., & Hisanaga, Y. (2002). Acute hemorrhagic oedema of infancy associated with cytomegalovirus infection. *Br J Dermatol,* Vol. 147, No. 6, pp. 1254-1257, ISSN 0007-0963

Lai-Cheong, JE., Banerjee, P., Hill, V., Kenny, P., & Ross, J. (2007). Bullous acute hemorrhagic oedema of infancy. *Clin Exp Dermatol,* Vol. 32, No. 4, pp. 467-468, ISSN 0307-6938

Lakshmi, C., & Srinivas, CR. (2003). Urticarial vasculitis of infancy (acute hemorrhagic edema). *Indian J Dermatol Venereol Leprol,* Vol. 69, No. 6, pp. 427, ISSN 0378-6323

Lantner, RR., & Simon, PR. (1996). Acute hemorrhagic edema of infancy. *Pediatr Emerg Care,* Vol. 12, No. 2, pp. 111-112, ISSN 0749-5161

Lee, HM., Kang, EY., Kim, HU., & Hwang, PH. (2006). Acute hemorrhagic edema in an infant mimicking Henoch-Schönlein purpura: a case study. *Korean J Pediatr,* Vol. 49, No. 12, pp. 1354-1357, ISSN 1738-1061

Legrain, V., Lejean, S., Taieb, A., Guillard, JM., Battin, J., & Maleville, J. (1991). Infantile acute hemorrhagic edema of the skin: study of ten cases. *J Am Acad Dermatol,* Vol. 24, No. 1, pp. 17-22, ISSN 0190-9622

Legrain, V., & Taieb, A. (2000). Acute hemorrhagic oedema of the skin in infancy, In: *Textbook of pediatric dermatology,* Harper, J., Oranje, A., & Prose, N., pp. 1569-1573, Blackwell Science Ltd, ISBN 0-86542-939-1, Malden

Long, D., & Helm, KF. (1998). Acute hemorrhagic edema of infancy: Finkelstein's disease. *Cutis,* Vol. 61, No. 5, pp. 283-284, ISSN 0011-4162

Macea, JM., Santi, CG., Sotto, MN., & Caputo, R. (2003). Multiple erhthematous plaques on a child. Acute hemorrhagic edema (AHE) of infancy. *Arch Dermatol,* Vol. 139, No. 4, pp. 531-536, ISSN 0340-3696

McDougall, CM., Ismail, SK., & Ormerod, A. (2004). Acute haemorrhagic oedema of infancy. *Arch Dis Child,* Vol. 90, No. 3, pp. 316, ISSN 0003-9888

Michael, DJ. (2006). Acute hemorrhagic edema of infancy. *Dermatol Online J,* Vol. 12, No. 5, pp. 10, ISSN 1087-2108

Millard, T., Harris, A., & MacDonald, D. (1999). Acute infantile hemorrhagic oedema. *J Am Acad Dermatol,* Vol. 41, No. 5, pp. 837-839, ISSN 0190-9622

Morrison, RR., & Saulsbury, FT. (1999). Acute hemorrhagic edema of infancy associated with pneumococcal bacteremia. *Pediatr İnfec Dis J,* Vol. 18, No. 9, pp. 832-833, ISSN 0891-3668

Obeid, M., Haley, J., Crews, J., Parhizgar, R., Johnson, L., & Camp, T. (2008). Acute hemorrhagic edema of infancy with abdominal pain and elevated transaminases. *Pediatr Dermatol,* Vol. 25, No. 6, pp. 640-641, ISSN 0736-8046

Ozaltın, F., Bakkaloglu, A., Ozen, S., Topaloglu, R., Kavak, U., Kalyoncu, M., & Besbas, N. (2004). The significance of IgA class of antineutrophil cytoplasmic antibodies (ANCA) in childhood Henoch-Schönlein purpura. *Clin Rheumatol,* Vol. 23, No. 5, pp. 426-429, ISSN 0770-3198

Paradisi, M., Annessi, G., & Corrado, A. (2001). Infantile acute hemorrhagic edema of the skin. *Cutis,* Vol. 68, No. 2, pp. 127-129, ISSN 0011-4162

Poyrazoglu, H., Per, H., Gunduz, Z., Dusunsel, R., Arslan, D., Narin, N., & Gumus, H. (2003). Acute hemorrhagic edema of infancy. *Pediatr Int,* Vol. 45, No. 6, pp. 697-700, ISSN 1328-8067

Pride, HB., Maroon, M., & Tyler, WB. (1995). Ecchymoses and edema in a 4-month-old boy. *Pediatr Dermatol,* Vol. 12, No. 4, 373-375, ISSN 0736-8046

Principi, N., & Esposito, S. (2002). Mycoplasma pneumoniae and Chlamydia pneumoniae cause lower respiratory tract disease in paediatric patients. *Curr Opin Infect Dis,* Vol. 15, No. 3, pp. 295-300, ISSN 0951-7375

Roh, MR., Chung, HJ., & Lee, JH. (2004). A case of acute hemorrhagic edema of infancy. *Yonsei Med J,* Vol. 45, No. 3, pp. 523-526, ISSN 0513-5796

Saraclar, Y., & Tinaztepe, K. (1992) Infantile acute hemorrhagic edema of the skin. *J Am Acad Dermatol,* Vol. 26, No. 2, pp. 275-276, ISSN 0190-9622

Saraclar, Y., Tinaztepe, K., Adalioglu, G., & Tuncer, A. (1990). Acute hemorrhagic edema of infancy (AHEI)-a variant of Henoch-Schönlein purpura or a distinct clinical entity? *J Allergy Clin Immunol,*Vol. 86, No. 4, pp. 473-483, ISSN 0091-6749

Saray, Y., Seckin, D., Sarifakioglu, E., Gulec, AT., & Demirhan B. (2002). Acute infantile hemorrhagic oedema: measles vaccination as possible triggering factor. *Acta Derm Venereol,* Vol. 82, No. 6, pp. 471-472, ISSN 0001-5555

Scaramuzza, A., Pezzarossa, E., Zambelloni, C., Lupi, A., Lazzari, GB., & Rossoni, R. (1997). Case of the month: a girl with oedema and purpuric eruption. Diagnosis: acute infantile haemorrhagic oedema of infancy. *Eur J Pediatr,* Vol. 156, No. 10, pp. 813-815, ISSN 0340-6199

Seidlmayer, H. (1936). Fruhinfantile postinfektiose Kokarde-Purpura. *Z Kinderheilk,* Vol. 61, No. 21, pp. 217-255

Serna, MJ., Leache, A., Sola, MA., Robledo, C., & Quintanilla, E. (1994). Target like lesions in an infant. Infantile acute hemorrhagic edema (AHE). *Arch Dermatol,* Vol. 130, No. 8, pp. 1058-1059, ISSN 0340-3696

Shah, D., Goraya, JS., Poddar, B., & Parmar, VR. (2002). Acute infantile hemorrhagic edema and Henoch-Schönlein purpura overlap in a child. *Pediatr Dermatol,* Vol. 19, No. 1, pp. 92-93, ISSN 0736-8046

Silveira, JCG., Quattrino, AL., Bragança, R., & Rochael, MC. (2006). Infantile acute hemorrhagic edema. *An Bras Dermatol,* Vol. 81, No. 5, pp. 285-287

Sites, LY., Woodmansee, CS., Wilkin, NK., Hanson, JW., Skinner, RB., & Shimek, CM. (2008). Acute hemorrhagic edema of infancy: case reports and areview of the literature. *Cutis,* Vol. 82, No. 5, pp. 320-324, ISSN 0011-4162

Slutsky, JB., Lee, K., Adams, CW., Jones, EC., & Hayman, RT. (2010). Acral petechiae and purpuric plaques in a 3-year-old girl—quiz case. Acute hemorrhagic edema of infancy (AHEI), or Finkelstein disease. *Arch Dermatol,* Vol. 146, No. 9, pp. 1037-1042, ISSN 0003-987X

Smitt, JH., Vermeer, MH., & Faber, WR. (2002). Acute hemorrhagic edema of infancy (AHEI). *Clin Dermatol,* Vol. 20, No. 1, 2-3, ISSN 0738-081X

Snow, IM. (1913). Purpura, urticaria and angioneurotic edema of the hands and feet in a nursing baby. J Am Med Assoc, Vol. 61, No. 1, pp. 18-19

Suehiro, RM., Soares, BS., Eisencraft, AP., Campos, LM., & Silva, CA. (2007). Acute hemorrhagic edema of childhood. *Turk J Pediatr,* Vol. 49, No. 2, pp. 189-192, ISSN 0041-4301

Tomac, N., Saraclar, Y., Turktas, I., & Kalaycı, O. (1996). Acute hemorrhagic oedema of infancy: a case report. *Clin Exp Dermatol,* Vol. 21, No. 3, pp. 217-219, ISSN 0307-6938

Watanabe, T., & Sato, Y. (2007). Renal involvement and hypocomplementemia in a patient with acute hemorrhagic edema of infancy. *Pediatr Nephrol,* Vol. 22, No. 11, pp. 1979-1981, ISSN 0931-041X

Wong, CT., & Harrington, JW. (2004). Infantile Henoch-Schönlein purpura. *Emerg Med Australas,* Vol. 16, No. 3, pp. 225-228, ISSN 1742-6731

Yavuz, H. (2000). Is acute hemorrhagic edema of infancy a complement deficiency state? *Pediatr Infection Dis J,* Vol. 19, No. 8, pp. 768-769, ISSN 0891-3668

Yu, JE., Mancini, AJ., & Miller, ML. (2007). Intusseption in an infant with acute hemorrhagic edema of infancy. *Pediatr Dermatol,* Vol. 24, No. 1, pp. 61-64, ISSN 0736-8046

21

The LAMP Story and What It Means for ANCA Positive Vasculitis in Nephrology

Hansjörg Rothe
Klinikum Coburg, III. Medical Department, Division of nephrology and hypertension
Germany

1. Introduction

From the nephrological point of view, the last couple of years have brought some major advances both in our understanding of ANCA positive vasculitis pathogenesis mechanisms and in treatment options. Recent discoveries of completely new antigens such as LAMP-2 meant a huge step forward, and the fact that this antigen is homologous to proteins of bacterial fimbria caused a shift in the focus regarding underlying pathomechanisms of ANCA vasculitis towards bacterial infections, mainly with Klebsiella or Escherichia species, playing a major role in triggering the disease. So nephrology has seen real progress in our understanding of glomerulonephritis disease mechanisms - not only regarding primary membranous glomerulonephritis (with the recent identification of the phospholipase A2 receptor being the underlying antigen) but also regarding secondary pauci-immune glomerulonephritis due to ANCA positive vasculitis.

At the same time, some important studies were successfully conducted. Especially the results of the RAVE and IMPROVE studies, will have an impact on nephrologists´ approaches to the treatment of patients suffering from this type of vasculitis.

The following chapter will focus on the new developments and briefly outline our already well established knowledge about ANCA positive vasculitis from a nephrological point of view.

2. Pathogenesis of ANCA positive vasculitis

There has been a long debate about the actual role of ANCA autoantibodies as causative agents of small vessel vasculitis . Although the correlation of ANCA titres with disease activity is not very strong [12], the fact that drug induced ANCA formation in patients treated with propylthiouracil, hydralazine or penicillamine can lead to exactly the same clinical picture of pauci-immune glomerulonephritis as "idiopathic" ANCA disease seams to indicate a causative role of the antibodies[3]. A well documented case report of a neonate with glomerulonephritis (GN) and pulmonary vasculitis due to Anti-MPO-antibodies that had passed the placental barrier from the maternal circulation[4] points in the same direction. The ability of these antibodies to cause GN when administered to mice intravenously has also been demonstrated[5].

The course of events leading to the inflammatory destruction of endothelial cells starts with activated neutrophils, which represents the flu-like initial phase of the disease. Cytokine activated neutrophils present antigens at their surface which attract IgG ANCA´ s binding to them, forming local immuncomplexes. Recent results show an essential involvement of the alternative complement pathway in these complexes - C3 and C5 rather than C4 are the main complement fragments involved. C5 knock out mice will not develop Anti-MPO antibody induced vasculitis[6], depletion of neutrophils also prevents the disease despite ANCA´s being administered, as demonstrated in an animal model[7]. T cells play a role in the pathogenesis, and so do B cells -indicated by the fact that anti-B cell agents such as rituximab are highly effective in therapy. Th17 cells are the major effector cells, while Th1, Th1 and regulatory T cells are also involved. Activated B cells produce the ANCA antibodies, and their number correlated with the disease activity. However, the actual role of B cells still needs to be elucidated.

While 70% of ANCA positive patients will show renal manifestations, there are about 10% of patients with the same clinical picture of pauci-immune GN who are ANCA negative. Conceivably other, as yet unknown antibodies might be involved in this patient subgroup. Similarly, the two classical antigens of proteinase 3 (c-ANCA´s) and myeloperoxidase (p-ANCA´s) are not the only ones, the lysosomal membrane protein lamp-2 which has a homologue protein in renal glomerular endothelial cells, is another important target of ANCA´s[8]. In fact this ANCA subtype is present in almost all patients with pauci-immune focal necrotizing glomerulonephritis. Most interestingly, lamp-2 is highly similar to certain bacterial fimbria proteins, as recently reported by Kain et al in Nature Medicine in 2008[9]. Some peptides of proteinase3 resemble epitopes of staphylococcus aureus antigens. Bacterial infections mainly with Klebsiella and Escherichia coli species may therefore trigger systemic ANCA associated vasculitis via a cross-reactivity mechanism.

3. The beginning of the LAMP story

In 1988, isolation and characterization of two human lysosomal membrane glycoproteins was reported by Carlsson et al. and the terms h-lamp-1 and h-lamp-2 introduced ("LAMP" being the acronym for lysosome associated membrane protein). The two major lysosomal membrane glycoproteins were described as major sialoglycoproteins carrying polylactosaminoglycan [10], with apparent molecular weights of 39.5 and 41.5 kDa, respectively. They were purified from chronic myelogenous leukemia cells. Already at this early stage it was noted that the apparent molecular weights differed between cell lines and that "this probably represents differences in the amount of polylactosaminoglycan expressed by each cell line". The first one of the glycoproteins was found to be very homologous to that of a mouse counterpart, m-lamp-1, it was therefore named human lamp-1 (h-lamp-1), while the other glycoprotein was called human lamp-2 (h-lamp-2). After cloning both proteins in the same year[11] , it became clear that major portions of both h-lamp-1 and h-lamp-2 reside on the luminal side of the lysosome and are heavily glycosylated by N-glycans: h-lamp-1 and h-lamp-2 were found to contain 19 and 16 potential N-glycosylation sites, respectively. Strong homology was noted and a common ancestor gene suggested. Diversion had to have happened at an early evolutionary stage however, since human lamp-1 has more similarity to lamp-1 from other species than to human lamp-2. Both LAMP`s are structural proteins without enzymatic activity. By means of in situ hybridization, the gene for human lamp-2 was localized to chromosome 12p133 and the h-lamp-1 gene to chromosome 13q34[12] . The authors argued that the fact of two genes on different chromosomes indicates that lamp-1 and lamp-2 diverged early in evolution and

probably have distinct functions which emerged as soon as eukaryotic cells acquired lysosomes as subcellular compartments. When mouse LAMP-2 had been cloned [13] it was found that mouse LAMP-2 and human LAMP-2 form one homology class (LAMP-2) that is separated from the LAMP-1 class of proteins. The localization of the polylactosaminoglycans [14] in the two lysosome membrane glycoproteins was analyzed, and in 1990 rat LAMP-2 was purified[15] and found to be present in all rat tissues examined, but at consistently lower concentrations than LAMP-1. The authors reported that their apparent molecular weights differed among the tissues, suggesting different glycosylation patterns. Later a soluble LAMP-2 was detected in rat liver[16]. When the exon structure of both protein classes was analyzed[17], it turned out that each of the nine exons encodes almost identical portions of the proteins. Since the amino acid sequence of human lamp-1 is more homologous to lamp-1 of other species than it is to human lamp-2, the two genes were most likely produced by duplication of a primordial gene, which took place early in evolution.
The old age, in evolutionary terms, of the LAMP-2 gene, is in fact not trivial but will shed some light on the pathogenetic role of this protein as the LAMP story unfolds. Homology with another protein outside the LAMP-2 class was already reported in 1993[18] , when glycoprotein II (GpII), a heterogenous glycoprotein isolated from the membranes of secretory chromaffin granules in the adrenal medulla was found to show a homology of greater than 70% of the sequence with LAMP-1 and -2. It became clear[19], that the LAMP-2 gene is in fact preserved from birds to mammals and all diversity due to alternative splicing from a single gene. In the following years a number of papers dealt with structural properties of the protein and its processing within the cell. So it was reported, that [20] clusters of O-glycans protect LAMP-2 from intralumenal lysosomal proteases - after removal of the asparagine-linked glycans from fully folded lysosomal membrane proteins by endoglycosidase H in cell culture, both LAMP-1 and LAMP-2 are rapidly degraded[21]. Tissue-specific expression of three different LAMP-2 variants due to alternative splicing was reported[22] in chicken. In cell culture it was found, that lamp-2, similar to lysosomal acid phosphatase (LAP), shuttles[23] in the endocytic membrane transport system of rat hepatocytes between lysosomes and the plasma membrane. After leaving the rough endoplasmic reticulum, newly synthesized lamp-2 is transported[24] to the trans-Golgi and then transferred to at least three compartments - the cell surface, cell peripheral early endosomes and perinuclear late endosomes, before it is finally delivered to the lysosomes. The extent of polylactosamine glycosylation of MDCK LAMP-2 is determined by its Golgi residence time[25]. Where the molecule will travel is governed by the COOH-terminal residue of its cytosolic tail[26]. Its plasma membrane variant was discussed as a possible tumour antigen; it was speculated, that LAMP-1 and -2 like several other glycoproteins[27] might be important in colon carcinoma adhesion and metastasis by functioning as its endogenous ligands - in fact there is evidence[28] suggesting an increase in their cell-surface expression in tumor cells, with some data indicating that the adhesion of some cancer cells to the extracellular matrix is partly mediated by interactions between LAMP´s and E-selectin and between Lamps and galectins (endogenous-galactoside-binding lectins). However, its physiological role and main pathophysiological importance remained unclear, until the next major discovery was made.

4. LAMP-2 as an additional autoantigenic ANCA target

While the association between the clinical picture of pauci-immune, necrotizing and crescentic glomerulonephritis (NCGN) with circulating antineutrophil cytoplasmic autoantibodies (ANCA) had been known for some time, only two of the actual targets had been identified until 1995: proteinase 3 (mainly associated with c-ANCA) and myeloperoxidase (mainly associated with p-ANCA). Then the group of Renate Kain et al. reported LAMP-2 to be another antigen targeted by ANCA, and they also found the link to the underlying disease mechanism when they identified gp130, a glycoprotein in the endothelial membranes of renal glomeruli, to be highly homologous to LAMP-2[29]. The same group later showed, that almost all patients with pauci-immune focal necrotizing glomerulonephritis have ANCA´s against LAMP-2, so that their prevalence is almost twice that of Anti-proteinase 3 and myeloperoxidase ANCA´s. They also demonstrated[30] the pathophysiological significance of these antibodies, since Anti-LAMP-2 ANCA´s injected into rats caused the same histological picture of pauci-immune focal necrotizing glomerulonephritis. In vitro, these antibodies cause apoptosis in microvascular endothelium. When studying the epitope, to which the ANCA´s commonly bound, it turned out that this part of the LAMP-2 protein had a 100% homology with to the bacterial adhesin FimH, a protein present in bacterial fimbria. The terminology of p- and c-ANCA refers to the distinct staining patterns due to the intracellular localization of the respective antigens. LAMP-2 is also localized in specific lysosomal fractions – together with Lamp-1 it is present in the specific-granule-enriched fraction and in the light-membrane fraction[31], but not in the azurophil granules. These further studies, fuelled by the increased interest in the LAMP´s as intracellular antigens, began to clarify their physiological role: Separation of secretory vesicles from plasma membranes disclosed that the light-membrane LAMP´s are present primarily in the secretory-vesicle-enriched fraction, and during phagocytosis both Lamp-1 and Lamp-2 become markedly concentrated around the ingested particle. Both appear on the cell surface when the secretory organelles are mobilized. This fact sparks the ongoing interest in Lamp-2 as a tumour marker, because - other than in the lysosomal membrane - Lamp-2 proteins are expressed at the plasma membrane of cells in a differentiation dependent and activation dependent manner[32]. Murine Lamp-2c expression is pronounced in mesenchyme early in development, in limb connective tissue, and in lung parenchyma, whereas m-Lamp-2a is prevalent in the liver, the pancreas, and in differentiating kidney epithelium, and becomes increasingly prominent in the epithelial lining of the digestive and the respiratory tract during development. Their expression pattern becomes more tissue and cell type specific as differentiation progresses. In adults, tumour cells undergoing dedifferentiation again have detectable amounts of LAMP-2 at their cell surface, where they might play a role in cell adhesion, metastasis or tumour progression, as a study about LAMP-1 in pancreatic carcinoma[33] suggests. Since morphogenesis often requires apoptotic removal of cells, an important role of phagolysosome activities and lysosomal proteins in these processes is evident.

5. Learning from rare genetic deficiencies: Danon´s disease and LAMP-2

The first time, when a rare genetic condition provided insight into the physiological role of LAMP-2, was when control platelets and those from an individual with Hermansky-Pudlak[34] syndrome were compared[35] regarding the presence of LAMP-2 expression: It turned out that LAMP-2, like CD63, is normally present not only in lysosomes but also in dense granules of platelets. Apart from oculocutaneous albinism, this autosomal recessive condition is characterised by platelet dense granule deficiency, prolonged bleeding time, a storage pool deficiency of platelets and lysosomal accumulation of ceroid lipofuscin. A major breakthrough in the understanding of the physiological role of LAMP-2 came with studies of knock-out lab animals and the discovery of Nishino, DiMauro et al. that the rare

condition of Danon´s[36] disease is due to LAMP-2 deficiency. It became evident, that a deficiency of this protein mainly impairs autophagy, i.e. the removal of aged cell material, lysosome biogenesis and cholesterol homoeostasis[37] - being a structural protein it has no enzymatic activity of its own, but a deficiency leads to partial mistargeting of a subset of lysosomal enzymes[38]. Lysosomal cholesterol transport[39], the ability of lysosomes to migrate by means of dynein-mediated transport and the fusion with autophagosomes and phagosomes depend on the LAMPs[40]. Therefore phagocytosis is also affected, and pathogenic Neisseria have been found to excrete a protease which selectively cleaves LAMP-1[41]. In the unicellular eukaryote Paramecium LAMP-2 was found to be required for phagosome maturation[42]. Since antigen presenting B-cells rely on normal lysosomal function, MHC class II antigen presentation to CD4 T-cells and the balance between endogenous and exogenous antigen presentation is impaired[43] in LAMP-2 deficiency.
The condition was first characterized by Moris J. Danon and Shin J.Oh in two patients as a 'lysosomal glycogen storage disease with normal acid maltase' in 1981[44]- the clinical picture involves hypertrophic cardiomyopathy (often associated with Wolff-Parkinson-White syndrome), myopathy and variable mental retardation. It was initially thought to be mainly X-linked, but as DiMauro et al. recall in their review[45], in 1993 they wrote that an "autosomal dominant inheritance cannot be ruled out". In the meantime more than 20 autosomal mutations of the LAMP-2 gene (chromosome 12) have been reported: in exon 7 resulting in the syndrome and with the patient requiring heart transplantation at 41years of age[46], in intron 6[47], in intron 8[48] with additional hepatopathy, in exon 5[49] and in exon 4 with several both male and female familiy members being affected[50]. Another missense mutation in the LAMP-2 gene caused a much milder clinical picture with exercise intolerance, persistent HyperCKemia and hypertrophic cardiomyopathy, but no mental retardation or severe heart failure[51]. Other genes have to be involved, suggested not only by the fact that the disease is always much more severe in male patients than in females, but also by marked phenotypic variation in unrelated patients with the same LAMP-2 gene mutation[52] - in a family with a mutation in exon 2 of the Lamp-2 gene[53], females developed isolated cardiomyopathy in adulthood, whereas males presented with cardiomyopathy, myopathy, and mental retardation before the age of 20 years. Intrafamilial variability of affected familiy members does occur[54]. Moreover, a case with quite the same clinical picture of Danon´s disease but normal LAMP-2 staining in the muscle biopsy has been reported[55]. In mice, LAMP-2 deficiency increases mortality between 20 and 40 days of age[56] , the surviving mice are fertile and have an almost normal life span. Only the additional knock-out of LAMP-1 and -2 results in a lethal phenotype at embryonic stage[57]. Many tissues including liver, pancreas, spleen, kidney and skeletal and heart muscle accumulate autophagic vacuoles. In hepatocytes, the autophagic degradation of long-lived proteins is severely impaired. Cardiac myocytes are ultrastructurally abnormal and heart contractility is severely reduced. The reason for this reduced contractility is not completely understood yet; calcium handling by the cardiomyocytes is normal[58]. Finally, when cases of Danon patients with oculocutaneous albinism were reported in 2006[59], it became clear that features of Danon and Hermansky-Pudlak syndromes may sometimes not be separable.

6. Conclusion

Recent years have seen a number of breakthroughs in our understanding of glomerulonephritis. The common theme in all of these cases is that disease entities, which used to be defined simply by histomorphological criteria or clinical pictures, could be traced down to the underlying causative agent. In ANCA positive vasculitis, as in polyarteriitis nodosa, hitherto unknown roles of infective agents that give rise to the disease-defining immunological responses were identified: while most polyarteriitis nodosa cases are related to the hepatitis B virus[60], fimbriated bacteria causing cross-reactions against lysosomal membrane proteins are involved in a majority of ANCA positive vasculitis cases.

The story of LAMP-1 and -2 (or CD107a and b, as they have also been referred to[61]) continues. More splice variants were detected, so a whole new nomenclature was introduced[62], the new class of LAMP-3 and the LIMP´s (lysosomal integral membrane proteins) entered the stage. Possible additional roles of LAMP-2 as a diagnostic marker need to be investigated further - conceivably it might play a role as a tumour marker as well as in screening of newborns for presymptomatic lysosomal storage disease: In a study LAMP-2 plasma concentrations were increased in >66% of patients with lysosomal storage disorders[63], and the increases coincided with increased LAMP-1 concentrations. Increased LAMP-1 and -2 levels have been associated with normal mast cell activation[64], increased LAMP-2 expression in peripheral leucocytes with coronary artery disease[65]. There seems to be the possibility of a non-genetic, acquired LAMP-2 deficiency in alcoholic acute pancreatitis or severe endotoxemia[66]. Whether all these associations, or the report of Anti-LAMP-2 ANCA´s in pyoderma gangrenosum[67], or indeed the slowing down of aging processes by restoration of chaperone-mediated autophagy in aging cells ("Live longer with LAMP-2 !" [68]) will gain clinical significance in the future, remains to be seen.

7. References

[1] Savige J, Davies D Falk RJ et al.: Antineutrophil cytoplasmic antibodies (ANCA) and associated diseases. Kidney Int 2000; 57: 846-862

[2] Savage CO, ANCA associated renal vasculitis. Kidney Int. 2001; 60:1614-1627

[3] Choi HK, Merkel PA, Walker AM, Niles IL: Drug associated antineutrophil cytoplasmic antibody positive vasculitis: Prevalence among patients with high titres of anti-myeloperoxidase antibodies. Arhtritis rheum. 2000;43: 405-413

[4] Schlieben DJ, Korbet SM, Kimura RE et al. Pulmonary renal syndrome in a newborn with placental transmission of ANCA´s. Am J Kidney Dis 2005; 45:758-761

[5] Xiao H, Heeringa P, Hu P et al. Antineutrophil cytoplasmic antibodies specific for myeloperoxidase cause glomerulonephritis and vasculitis in mice. J Clin Invest 2002; 110:955-963

[6] Savage CO. Pathogenesis of anti-neutrophil cytoplasmic autoantibody (ANCA)-associated vasculitis. Clin Exp Immunol. 2011 May;164 Suppl 1:23-6. doi: 10.1111/j.1365-2249.2011.04362.x.

[7] Xiao H, Heeringa P, Liu Z et al. The role of neutrophils in the induction of glomerulonephritis by anti-myeloperoxidase antibodies. Am J Pathol 2005; 167:39-45

[8] Kain R, Matsui K, Exner M, Binder S, Schaffner G, Sommer EM, Kerjaschki D. A novel class of autoantigens of anti-neutrophil cytoplasmic antibodies in necrotizing and crescentic glomerulonephritis: the lysosomal membrane glycoprotein h-lamp-2 in neutrophil granulocytes and a related membrane protein in glomerular endothelial cells. J Exp Med. 1995 Feb 1; 181(2):585-97.

[9] Kain R, Exner M, Brandes R, Ziebermayr R, Cunningham D, Alderson CA, Davidovits A, Raab I, Jahn R, Ashour O, Spitzauer S, Sunder-Plassmann G, Fukuda M, Klemm P,

Rees AJ, Kerjaschki D. Molecular mimicry in pauci-immune focal necrotizing glomerulonephritis. Nat Med. 2008 Oct;14(10):1088-96. Epub 2008 Oct 5.

[10] Isolation and characterization of human lysosomal membrane glycoproteins, h-lamp-1 and h-lamp-2. Major sialoglycoproteins carrying polylactosaminoglycan Carlsson SR, Roth J, Piller F, Fukuda M. J Biol Chem. 1988 Dec 15;263(35):18911-9

[11] Cloning of cDNAs encoding human lysosomal membrane glycoproteins, h-lamp-1 and h-lamp-2. Comparison of their deduced amino acid sequences Fukuda M, Viitala J, Matteson J, Carlsson SR. J Biol Chem. 1988 Dec 15;263(35):18920-8

[12] Two human lysosomal membrane glycoproteins, h-lamp-1 and h-lamp-2, are encoded by genes localized to chromosome 13q34 and chromosome Xq24-25, respectively Mattei MG, Matterson J, Chen JW, Williams MA, Fukuda M. J Biol Chem. 1990 May 5;265(13):7548-51

[13] The cDNA sequence of mouse LAMP-2. Evidence for two classes of lysosomal membrane glycoproteins Cha Y, Holland SM, August JT. J Biol Chem. 1990 Mar 25;265(9):5008-13

[14] The polylactosaminoglycans of human lysosomal membrane glycoproteins lamp-1 and lamp-2. Localization on the peptide backbones. Carlsson SR, Fukuda M. J Biol Chem. 1990 Nov 25;265(33):20488-95

[15] Purification, some properties, and tissue distribution of a major lysosome-associated membrane glycoprotein (r-lamp-2) of rat liver. Akasaki K, Yamaguchi Y, Furuno K, Tsuji H. J Biochem. 1991 Dec;110(6):922-7

[16] Purification and characterization of a soluble form of lysosome-associated membrane glycoprotein-2 (lamp-2) from rat liver lysosomal contents Akasaki K, Tsuji H. Biochem Mol Biol Int. 1998 Sep;46(1):197-206.

[17] The genes of major lysosomal membrane glycoproteins, lamp-1 and lamp-2. 5'-flanking sequence of lamp-2 gene and comparison of exon organization in two genes Sawada R, Jardine KA, Fukuda M. J Biol Chem. 1993 Apr 25;268(12):9014-22. Erratum in: J Biol Chem 1993 Jun 15;268(17):13010

[18] Characterization of glycoprotein II from bovine adrenal medullary chromaffin granules. Identification of components representing the secretory vesicle counterparts of the lysosomal-associated membrane glycoproteins (lamp-1 and lamp-2). Hieber AD, Christie DL. J Biol Chem. 1993 May 25;268(15):11073-8

[19] The family of LAMP-2 proteins arises by alternative splicing from a single gene: characterization of the avian LAMP-2 gene and identification of mammalian homologs of LAMP-2b and LAMP-2c Gough NR, Hatem CL, Fambrough DM. DNA Cell Biol. 1995 Oct;14(10):863-7

[20] Assignment of O-glycan attachment sites to the hinge-like regions of human lysosomal membrane glycoproteins lamp-1 and lamp-2 Carlsson SR, Lycksell PO, Fukuda M. Arch Biochem Biophys. 1993 Jul;304(1):65-73

[21] Asparagine-linked oligosaccharides protect Lamp-1 and Lamp-2 from intracellular proteolysis Kundra R, Kornfeld S. J Biol Chem. 1999 Oct 22;274(43):31039-46.

[22] Multiple mRNAs encode the avian lysosomal membrane protein LAMP-2, resulting in alternative transmembrane and cytoplasmic domains. Hatem CL, Gough NR, Fambrough DM. J Cell Sci. 1995 May;108 (Pt 5):2093-100

[23] Cycling of two endogenous lysosomal membrane proteins, lamp-2 and acid phosphatase, between the cell surface and lysosomes in cultured rat hepatocytes. Akasaki K, Fukuzawa M, Kinoshita H, Furuno K, Tsuji H. J Biochem. 1993 Oct;114(4):598-604

[24] Biosynthetic transport of a major lysosome-associated membrane glycoprotein 2, lamp-2: a significant fraction of newly synthesized lamp-2 is delivered to lysosomes by way of early endosomes Akasaki K, Michihara A, Fujiwara Y, Mibuka K, Tsuji H. J Biochem. 1996 Dec;120(6):1088-94.

[25] The extent of polylactosamine glycosylation of MDCK LAMP-2 is determined by its Golgi residence time Nabi IR, Dennis JW. Glycobiology. 1998 Sep;8(9):947-53.

[26] Different steady state subcellular distributions of the three splice variants of lysosome-associated membrane protein LAMP-2 are determined largely by the COOH-terminal amino acid residue. Gough NR, Fambrough DM. J Cell Biol. 1997 Jun 2;137(5):1161-9.

[27] Concomitant increases in galectin-1 and its glycoconjugate ligands (carcinoembryonic antigen, lamp-1, and lamp-2) in cultured human colon carcinoma cells by sodium butyrate Ohannesian DW, Lotan D, Lotan R. Cancer Res. 1994 Nov 15;54(22):5992-6000.

[28] Expression of Lamp-1 and Lamp-2 and their interactions with galectin-3 in human tumor cells. Sarafian V, Jadot M, Foidart JM, Letesson JJ, Van den Brûle F, Castronovo V, Wattiaux R, Coninck SW. Int J Cancer. 1998 Jan 5;75(1):105-11.

[29] A novel class of autoantigens of anti-neutrophil cytoplasmic antibodies in necrotizing and crescentic glomerulonephritis: the lysosomal membrane glycoprotein h-lamp-2 in neutrophil granulocytes and a related membrane protein in glomerular endothelial cells. Kain R, Matsui K, Exner M, Binder S, Schaffner G, Sommer EM, Kerjaschki D. J Exp Med. 1995 Feb 1;181(2):585-97

[30] Molecular mimicry in pauci-immune focal necrotizing glomerulonephritis. Nat Med. 2008 Oct ;14(10):1088-96. Epub 2008 Oct 5

[31] The lysosomal membrane glycoproteins Lamp-1 and Lamp-2 are present in mobilizable organelles, but are absent from the azurophil granules of human neutrophils. Dahlgren C, Carlsson SR, Karlsson A, Lundqvist H, Sjölin C. Biochem J. 1995 Oct 15;311 (Pt 2):667-74.

[32] Expression patterns of murine lysosome-associated membrane protein 2 (Lamp-2) transcripts during morphogenesis. Lichter-Konecki U, Moter SE, Krawisz BR, Schlotter M, Hipke C, Konecki DS. Differentiation. 1999 Jul;65(1):43-58.

[33] Influences of the lysosomal associated membrane proteins (Lamp-1, Lamp-2) and Mac-2 binding protein (Mac-2-BP) on the prognosis of pancreatic carcinoma Künzli BM, Berberat PO, Zhu ZW, Martignoni M, Kleeff J, Tempia-Caliera AA, Fukuda M, Zimmermann A, Friess H, Büchler MW. Cancer. 2002 Jan 1;94(1):228-39

[34] Matthew T. Hurford MT and Sebastiano C : Hermansky-Pudlak Syndrome: Report of a Case and Review of the Literature. Int J Clin Exp Pathol. 2008; 1(6): 550554.

[35] The lysosomal granule membrane protein, LAMP-2, is also present in platelet dense granule membranes. Israels SJ, McMillan EM, Robertson C, Singhory S, McNicol A. Thromb Haemost. 1996 Apr;75(4):623-9

[36] Primary LAMP-2 deficiency causes X-linked vacuolar cardiomyopathy and myopathy (Danon disease). Nishino I, Fu J, Tanji K, Yamada T, Shimojo S, Koori T, Mora M, Riggs JE, Oh SJ, Koga Y, Sue CM, Yamamoto A, Murakami N, Shanske S, Byrne E, Bonilla E, Nonaka I, DiMauro S, Hirano M. Nature. 2000 Aug 24;406(6798):906-10.

[37] Disturbed cholesterol traffic but normal proteolytic function in LAMP-1/LAMP-2 double-deficient fibroblasts Eskelinen EL, Schmidt CK, Neu S, Willenborg M, Fuertes G, Salvador N, Tanaka Y, Lüllmann-Rauch R, Hartmann D, Heeren J, von Figura K, Knecht E, Saftig P. Mol Biol Cell. 2004 Jul;15(7):3132-45. Epub 2004 Apr 30.

[38] Role of LAMP-2 in lysosome biogenesis and autophagy. Eskelinen EL, Illert AL, Tanaka Y, Schwarzmann G, Blanz J, Von Figura K, Saftig P. Mol Biol Cell. 2002 Sep;13(9):3355-68.

[39] Role for LAMP-2 in endosomal cholesterol transport. Schneede A, Schmidt CK, Hölttä-Vuori M, Heeren J, Willenborg M, Blanz J, Domanskyy M, Breiden B, Brodesser S, Landgrebe J, Sandhoff K, Ikonen E, Saftig P, Eskelinen EL. J Cell Mol Med. 2009 Nov 19.

[40] Saftig P, Beertsen W, Eskelinen EL: LAMP-2: a control step for phagosome and autophagosome maturation Autophagy. 2008 May 16;4(4):510-2. Epub 2008 Feb 13

[41] Binker MG, Cosen-Binker LI, Terebiznik MR, Mallo GV, McCaw SE, Eskelinen EL, Willenborg M, Brumell JH, Saftig P, Grinstein S, Gray-Owen SD: Arrested maturation of Neisseria-containing phagosomes in the absence of the lysosome-associated membrane proteins, LAMP-1 and LAMP-2 Cell Microbiol. 2007 Sep;9(9):2153-66. Epub 2007 May 15

[42] Phagosome maturation in unicellular eukaryote Paramecium: the presence of RILP, Rab7 and LAMP-2 homologues Wyroba E, Surmacz L, Osinska M, Wiejak J. Eur J Histochem. 2007 Jul-Sep;51(3):163-72.

[43] LAMP-2-deficient human B cells exhibit altered MHC class II presentation of exogenous antigens Crotzer VL, Glosson N, Zhou D, Nishino I, Blum JS. Immunology. 2010 Nov;131(3):318-30. doi: 10.1111/j.1365-2567.2010.03309.x

[44] Danon MJ, Oh SJ, DiMauro S, Manaligod JR, Eastwood A, Naidu S, Schliselfeld LH: Lysosomal glycogen storage disease with normal acid maltase. Neurology. 1981 Jan;31(1):51-7

[45] LAMP-2 deficiency (Danon disease) Di Mauro S, Tanji K, Hirano M. Acta Myol. 2007 Jul;26(1):79-82

[46] Danon's disease (X-linked vacuolar cardiomyopathy and myopathy): a case with a novel Lamp-2 gene mutation. Lacoste-Collin L, Garcia V, Uro-Coste E, Arné-Bes MC, Durand D, Levade T, Delisle MB. Neuromuscul Disord. 2002 Nov;12(9):882-5.

[47] Danon disease with typical early-onset cardiomyopathy in a male: focus on a novel LAMP-2 mutation. Bui YK, Renella P, Martinez-Agosto JA, Verity A, Madikians A, Alejos JC. Pediatr Transplant. 2008 Mar;12(2):246-50. Epub 2008 Feb 13.

[48] Danon disease: a novel Lamp-2 gene mutation in a family with four affected members. Tuñón T, Guerrero D, Urchaga A, Nishino I, Ayuso T, Matsuda Y, Caballero MC, Berjón J, Imizcoz MA. Neuromuscul Disord. 2008 Feb;18(2):167-74. Epub 2007 Dec 3.

[49] Novel LAMP-2 mutation in a family with Danon disease presenting with hypertrophic cardiomyopathy Dougu N, Joho S, Shan L, Shida T, Matsuki A, Uese K, Hirono K, Ichida F, Tanaka K, Nishino I, Inoue H. Circ J. 2009 Feb;73(2):376-80. Epub 2008 Dec 5. Review.

[50] Lobrinus JA, Schorderet DF, Payot M, Jeanrenaud X, Bottani A, Superti-Furga A, Schlaepfer J, Fromer M, Jeannet PY: Morphological, clinical and genetic aspects in a family with a novel LAMP-2 gene mutation (Danon disease) Neuromuscul Disord. 2005 Apr;15(4):293-8

[51] Asymptomatic hyperCKemia in a case of Danon disease due to a missense mutation in Lamp-2 gene. Musumeci O, Rodolico C, Nishino I, Di Guardo G, Migliorato A, Aguennouz M, Mazzeo A, Messina C, Vita G, Toscano A. Neuromuscul Disord. 2005 Jun;15(6):409-11. Epub 2005 Apr 19.

[52] Phenotypic heterogeneity in two unrelated Danon patients associated with the same LAMP-2 gene mutation Bertini E, Donati MA, Broda P, Cassandrini D, Petrini S,

Dionisi-Vici C, Ballerini L, Boldrini R, D'Amico A, Pasquini E, Minetti C, Santorelli FM, Bruno C. Neuropediatrics. 2005 Oct;36(5):309-13.
[53] Novel Lamp-2 gene mutation and successful treatment with heart transplantation in a large family with Danon disease. Echaniz-Laguna A, Mohr M, Epailly E, Nishino I, Charron P, Richard P, Guiraud-Chaumeil C, Tranchant C. Muscle Nerve. 2006 Mar;33(3):393-7.
[54] Danon disease: intrafamilial phenotypic variability related to a novel LAMP-2 mutation. Cottinet SL, Bergemer-Fouquet AM, Toutain A, Sabourdy F, Maakaroun-Vermesse Z, Levade T, Chantepie A, Labarthe F. J Inherit Metab Dis. 2011 Apr;34(2):515-22. Epub 2010 Dec 16.
[55] LAMP-2 positive vacuolar myopathy with dilated cardiomyopathy. Sugimoto S, Shiomi K, Yamamoto A, Nishino I, Nonaka I, Ohi T. Intern Med. 2007;46(11):757-60. Epub 2007 Jun 1.
[56] Accumulation of autophagic vacuoles and cardiomyopathy in LAMP-2-deficient mice. Tanaka Y, Guhde G, Suter A, Eskelinen EL, Hartmann D, Lüllmann-Rauch R, Janssen PM, Blanz J, von Figura K, Saftig P. Nature. 2000 Aug 24;406(6798):902-6.
[57] Roles of LAMP-1 and LAMP-2 in lysosome biogenesis and autophagy Eskelinen EL. Mol Aspects Med. 2006 Oct-Dec;27(5-6):495-502. Epub 2006 Sep 14. Review.
[58] LAMP-2 deficient mice show depressed cardiac contractile function without significant changes in calcium handling. Stypmann J, Janssen PM, Prestle J, Engelen MA, Kögler H, Lüllmann-Rauch R, Eckardt L, von Figura K, Landgrebe J, Mleczko A, Saftig P. Basic Res Cardiol. 2006 Jul;101(4):281-91. Epub 2006 Apr 8.
[59] Prall FR, Drack A, Taylor M, Ku L, Olson JL, Gregory D, Mestroni L, Mandava N. phthalmology. Ophthalmic manifestations of Danon disease . 2006 Jun;113(6):1010-3
[60] Frey FJ. :Polyarteritis Nodosa, a vanishing vasculitis since its main cause has been identified Ther Umsch. 2008 May;65(5):247-51
[61] Chang MH, Karageorgos LE, Meikle PJ: CD107a (LAMP-1) and CD107b (LAMP-2). J Biol Regul Homeost Agents. 2002 Apr-Jun;16(2):147-51.
[62] Unifying nomenclature for the isoforms of the lysosomal membrane protein LAMP-2. Eskelinen EL, Cuervo AM, Taylor MR, Nishino I, Blum JS, Dice JF, Sandoval IV, Lippincott-Schwartz J, August JT, Saftig P. Traffic. 2005 Nov;6(11):1058-61.
[63] Evaluation of the lysosome-associated membrane protein LAMP-2 as a marker for lysosomal storage disorders Hua CT, Hopwood JJ, Carlsson SR, Harris RJ, Meikle PJ. Clin Chem. 1998 Oct;44(10):2094-102.
[64] LAMP-1 and LAMP-2, but not LAMP-3, are reliable markers for activation-induced secretion of human mast cells. Grützkau A, Smorodchenko A, Lippert U, Kirchhof L, Artuc M, Henz BM. Cytometry A. 2004 Sep;61(1):62-8.
[65] LAMP-2 Gene Expression in Peripheral Leukocytes Is Increased in Patients With Coronary Artery Disease. Wu G, Huang J, Wei G, Liu L, Pang S, Yan B. Clin Cardiol. 2011 Apr;34(4):239-43. doi: 10.1002/clc.20870.
[66] Impaired autolysosome formation correlates with Lamp-2 depletion: role of apoptosis, autophagy, and necrosis in pancreatitis. Fortunato F, Bürgers H, Bergmann F, Rieger P, Büchler MW, Kroemer G, Werner J. Gastroenterology. 2009 Jul;137(1):350-60, 360.e1-5. Epub 2009 Apr 9.
[67] Hoffman MD: Pyoderma gangrenosum associated with c-ANCA (h-lamp-2) Int J Dermatol. 2001 Feb;40(2):135-7
[68] Live longer with LAMP-2 Saftig P, Eskelinen EL. Nat Med. 2008 Sep;14(9):909-10.

22

Quality of Life Issues in Vasculitis

Delesha Carpenter and Robert F. DeVellis
University of North Carolina at Chapel Hill
USA

1. Introduction

Over the past 40 years, the advent of more effective treatment regimens has transformed vasculitis from a frequently fatal, acute disease to a chronic condition with relapsing and remitting episodes with which patients can live for many years. Because vasculitis is now viewed as a chronic disease, the role of treatment has expanded from an almost exclusive focus on reducing mortality and inducing remission to include improving patient quality of life. In fact, most research studies with vasculitis patients, including clinical trials and observational studies, now measure patient quality of life to determine what factors hinder and facilitate optimal patient functioning and well-being.

The World Health Organization has defined quality of life as "individuals' perception of their position in life in the context of the culture and value systems in which they live and in relation to their goals, expectations, standards and concerns" (WHO, 1997, p. 1). Implicit in this definition is the fact that many layers of influence, ranging from intrapersonal beliefs to environmental factors, affect quality of life. In chronic disease populations, researchers often focus on patient health-related quality of life (HRQOL). Although HRQOL is more narrowly focused than quality of life, it is a still a complex concept that refers to the overall perceived well-being of an individual as well as his/her ability to function in daily life (Hays et al., 1993). There are many definitions of HRQOL, but most scholars agree that HRQOL includes both multidimensional and subjective components (Cella, 1994). The multidimensional component refers to the many dimensions (e.g. physical, functional, emotional, financial, and social) on which chronic disease can affect the patient's health and functioning. The subjective component suggests that patients, rather than health care providers, for example, are in the best position to report their HRQOL.

Although the HRQOL literature has primarily described how vasculitis negatively impacts patients' physical and mental health, there is also some evidence that patients experience positive impacts. Moreover, in addition to directly affecting the patient, vasculitis also has the potential to influence patients' relationships with spouses, family members, and friends. Garnering a holistic understanding of how vasculitis affects patients and their social networks is of interest because individuals having a chronic disease often seek support from others to help cope with disease-related stressors, which can lead to improved physical and mental health (Pennix et al., 1996).

This chapter not only describes how vasculitis positively and negatively impacts patients' HRQOL, but also, the impacts of vasculitis on members of patients' social networks. We first focus on patient HRQOL issues, including an examination of how vasculitis affects patients physically, functionally, psychologically, and financially. Next we describe how vasculitis impacts patients' social quality of life, including relationships with spouses, family, and friends. Last, we propose areas for future research and offer conclusions.

2. Patient quality of life issues

We identified 21 articles that have been published in English and primarily describe the HRQOL of vasculitis patients (Table 1). Taken together, these articles demonstrate that vasculitis negatively affects patients physically, functionally, psychologically, financially, and socially. Table 1 provides a brief overview of the articles, including the study design, subjects, and domains of quality of life assessed. In this section, we summarize the results of these studies by quality of life domain. Social quality of life is described in Section 3 "Impact on patients' relationships with social network members."

Study	Design	Subjects	Domains of quality of life assessed
Abdou et al., 2002	Cross-sectional	Granulomatosis with polyangiitis (GPA) (n= 701)	• Physical • Financial
Abularrage et al., 2008	Cross-sectional	Takayasu's arteritis (n= 158)	• Physical • Psychological • Functional • Financial • Social
Akar et al., 2008	Cross-sectional case-control	Takayasu's arteritis (n= 51)	• Physical • Functional • Psychological
Basu et al., 2010	Cross-sectional case-control	ANCA-associated vasculitis (n=74)	• Physical • Psychological
Bernabé et al., 2010	Cross-sectional	Behçet's disease (n= 362)	• Physical • Psychological
Boomsma et al., 2002	Cross-sectional case-control	Granulomatosis with polyangiitis (n =79)	• Functional • Psychological • Financial • Social
Carpenter et al., 2009	Cross-sectional	ANCA-associated vasculitis (n= 97)	• Physical • Functional • Psychological
Carpenter et al., 2011	Cross-sectional	Multiple vasculitis types (n=228)	• Physical • Functional • Psychological

Table 1. Summary of quality of life studies conducted with vasculitis patients

Study	Design	Subjects	Domains of quality of life assessed
Ertam et al., 2009	Cross-sectional case-control	Behçet's disease (n= 195)	• Physical • Functional • Psychological
Faurschou et al., 2010	Cross-sectional case-control	Granulomatosis with polyangiitis (n=68)	• Physical • Functional • Psychological
Hajj-Ali et al., 2011	Cross-sectional	Granulomatosis with polyangiitis	• Psychological
Hellmann et al., 2003	Cross-sectional	Giant cell arteritis (n= 145)	• Physical • Functional • Psychological
Herlyn et al., 1998	Longitudinal case-control	Multiple vasculitis types (n=303)	• Physical • Functional • Psychological
Hoffman et al., 1998	Cross-sectional	Granulomatosis with polyangiitis (n= 60)	• Physical • Functional • Psychological • Financial • Social
Koutantji et al., 2003	Cross-sectional	ANCA-associated vasculitis (n= 50)	• Physical • Functional • Psychological
Moses Alder et al., 2008	Cross-sectional case-control	Behçet's disease (n= 129)	• Physical • Functional
Mumcu et al., 2006	Cross-sectional case-control	Behçet's disease (n= 94)	• Physical • Functional • Psychological
Newall et al., 2005	Cross-sectional	ANCA-associated vasculitis (n= 30)	• Physical • Psychological
Reinhold-Keller et al., 2002	Cross-sectional	Granulomatosis with polyangiitis (n= 60)	• Physical • Functional • Psychological • Financial
Srouji et al., 2008	Cross-sectional	Churg-Strauss Syndrome (n= 25)	• Physical
Uguz et al., 2007	Cross-sectional	Behçet's disease (n= 50)	• Physical • Psychological • Social

Table 1. continued

2.1 Physical and functional quality of life

Of all the HRQOL domains, the physical domain has been best described for vasculitis populations. Physical quality of life can be directly affected by vasculitis symptoms, organ system damage, and treatment-related morbidities such as side effects and drug toxicity (Buhaescu et al., 2005; Exley & Bacon, 1996). Interestingly, physician-rated disease activity scores, such as the Birmingham Vasculitis Activity Score and the Vasculitis Damage Index (Flossmann et al., 2007), have been weakly correlated with patient HRQOL (Koutantji et al., 2003; Basu et al., 2010). This finding reinforces that quality of life cannot be reduced to biological effects of the disease and that accounting for other factors is important.

Physical HRQOL has commonly been assessed using scores from the four physical health subscales of the SF-36 (Ware & Kosinski, 2005). These include physical functioning, role limitations due to physical health, bodily pain, and general health. Although fatigue is sometimes categorized as a psychological quality of life issue, we include it here because it is a physical symptom of vasculitis that has been significantly correlated with the physical health component score (Ware & Kosinski, 2005). Thus, this section will describe fatigue, pain, and physical changes. Physical functioning and role limitations due to physical health are discussed in the functional quality of life section (Section 2.2).

2.1.1 Fatigue

Fatigue is a major problem affecting the quality of life of vasculitis patients. In studies using the SF-36, energy/vitality was one of the most consistently, negatively affected SF-36 subscales. Four studies have shown that over 75% of patients report problems with vasculitis-related fatigue (Abularrage et al., 2010; Bernabé et al., 2010; Hajj-Ali et al., 2011; Hoffman et al., 1998). More specifically, Basu and colleagues (2010) found that patients were more than twice as likely as controls to report mild/moderate and severe fatigue; and fatigue was a stronger predictor of worse physical health than disease activity.

Herlyn and colleagues (2010) found that fatigue and reduced energy levels were the most important patient-reported disease burden. One reason fatigue may be so important to vasculitis patients is that it can negatively impact other domains of quality of life by reducing the amount of energy patients have to engage in social activities and limiting patients' ability to fulfill important work- and home-related roles. Hajj-Ali and associates (2011) found that almost half of vasculitis patients believed that fatigue significantly limited their activities.

2.1.2 Pain

The results regarding pain have not been as consistently negative as those for fatigue. Although most studies have found that vasculitis patients report more bodily pain than national norms or healthy controls, two studies report results to the contrary. Specifically, Carpenter and colleagues (2009) and Faurschou and associates (2010) documented that bodily pain was not significantly different for vasculitis patients when compared with national norms or age and sex-matched controls, respectively. However, Carpenter et al. (2011) found that bodily pain was worse for relapsing patients than for those in remission. Thus, mixed results may partially be due to the proportion of patients in relapse versus remission in any given sample; the Faurschou et al. (2010) sample included only patients with inactive vasculitis. Also, both studies consisted primarily of Granulomatosis with polyangiitis (GPA; formerly Wegener's) patients, and pain may be a greater issue for other types of vasculitis.

Kountantji and associates (2003) have conducted more thorough analyses of how pain affects GPA patients. They found that patients in greater pain reported significantly worse quality of life when compared to patients who reported little or no pain. Also, patients in greater pain experienced more problems with depression, fatigue, and sleep. Moreover, patients with significant pain had more severe role limitations due to physical health than patients in less pain. Moses Alder and colleagues (2008) also found that Behçet's (BD) patients with arthritis reported more pain than patients without arthritis.

2.1.3 Physical changes

In addition to fatigue and pain, vasculitis symptoms and organ damage can negatively impact patient quality of life. Hearing loss, headaches, shortness of breath, and comprised kidney function are some examples of how vasculitis affects patients physically (Langford, 2005; Seo et al., 2005). In some cases, vasculitis can directly alter a patient's physical appearance by causing weight loss or nasal bridge collapse, otherwise known as saddle nose deformity. Patients may also experience skin problems, such as ulcers or purpura (i.e. a rash of purple spots). Readers who are interested in learning more about vasculitis and organ system damage are referred to articles by Seo and colleagues (2005) and Langford (2005).

Vasculitis medications can also cause changes to a patient's physical appearance. For example, patients who are treated with steroids often report weight gain and a condition called moon face, where the face swells into a rounded shape. Patients treated with immunosuppressive medications also report hair loss, hair growth, acne, and mouth sores. Although side effects like these are physical in nature, they can also take a toll on patients psychologically by adversely affecting their self-esteem. Thus, it is important to account for physical changes due to the disease itself as well as treatment-related effects when considering physical quality of life for vasculitis patients.

2.2 Functional quality of life

Functional quality of life is intimately related with physical quality of life and is commonly considered part of the physical domain. In this chapter, we dedicate a separate section to functional quality of life to specifically focus on how vasculitis affects patients' ability to engage in activities of daily living, such as bathing and completing household chores. Most studies have captured functional quality of life issues with the physical functioning subscale of the SF-36 (Ware & Kosinski, 2005). The physical functioning scale contains 10 items that ask how limited patients are in conducting a range of physical activities, from bending and kneeling to running and lifting heavy objects.

Overall, research using the SF-36 has shown that vasculitis patients have worse physical functioning when compared with healthy controls or national norms. In two cases, physical functioning was the most negatively affected of the eight SF-36 dimensions (Herlyn et al., 1998; Koutantji et al., 2005). Furthermore, the physical changes associated with vasculitis, including pain and fatigue, often led to increased role limitations. For example, patients often have to cut down the amount of time they spend on work or have to exert extra effort to engage in activities of daily living.

Other studies have provided more detail about the extent to which vasculitis negatively impacts patients' ability to engage in activities of daily living. For example, Hoffman and colleagues (1998) found that 56% of Granulomatosis with polyangiitis (GPA) patients reported moderately or severely compromised activities of daily living. Similarly, two-thirds of GPA patients reported that vasculitis had negatively affected their ability to perform everyday activities, with many patients noting that the disease had a stronger impact on their physical functioning at the time of diagnosis (Boomsma et al., 2002). Moreover, daily activities, like being able to shower, shave, chew, and walk without difficulty or losing balance, were all ranked among the top ten most important quality of life issues for patients living with giant cell arteritis (Hellmann et al., 2003), while patients with Behçet's disease noted negative changes to their ability to engage in usual activities and mobility (Ertam et al., 2010). Additionally, patients who were unemployed (Reinhold Keller et al., 2002), had active disease (Mumcu et al., 2006; Ertam et al., 2009), or were in more pain (Koutantji et al., 2003) were more likely to report greater physical role limitations.

2.3 Psychological quality of life

Most of the studies listed in Table 1 used the SF-36 (Ware & Kosinski, 2005) to measure psychological quality of life. The SF-36 contains four subscales, including social functioning, energy/vitality, role limitations due to emotional health, and mental health, which load on a summary mental health component score. Overall, SF-36 results reveal that vasculitis patients experience compromised psychological health. A more in-depth discussion of psychological aspects of vasculitis appears in an editorial by Koutantji and colleagues (2000). We save the discussion of social functioning issues until Section 3, which summarizes the impact of vasculitis on patients' relationships with social network members.

2.3.1 Depression and anxiety

It is common for patients living with chronic disease to experience feelings of depression and anxiety. Because depression is associated with many other negative sequelae, including worse treatment adherence (DiMatteo et al., 2000), it is important to assess the mental health of vasculitis patients. An examination of the mental health subscale results from studies that used the SF-36 shows that mental health is generally lower for vasculitis patients than either healthy controls or the general U.S. population. There are some exceptions to this as a few studies have found that vasculitis patients did not differ significantly from controls in terms of mental health (Basu et al., 2010; Koutantji et al., 2003). These mixed results may be due to differences in study populations. Because few studies have provided a more detailed description of depression and anxiety in vasculitis populations, little is known about what factors may moderate depression or which patients are most at risk. As we will describe below, preliminary results indicate that depression and anxiety are serious issues for patients that warrant further examination.

Depression and anxiety are problems for vasculitis patients regardless of the type of vasculitis with which they have been diagnosed. To illustrate, Hajj-Ali and colleagues (2011) discovered that the prevalence of depression in GPA patients was much higher than the general population; 23.6% and 7.6%, respectively. Other studies have documented that between 33% and 43% of GPA patients report disease-related depression, with 7% to 14% reporting depression associated with suicidal thoughts (Hoffman et al., 1998; Boomsma et al., 2002). Similarly, Bernabé and colleagues (2010) found that 60% of Behcet's patients noted problems with depression and anxiety, and Koutantji and associates (2003) documented that fully 43% of patients reported increased anxiety and 25.5% experienced increased depressive symptoms.

2.3.2 Other psychological impacts

Unfortunately, other than depression and anxiety, there is not much published information about how vasculitis impacts patients psychologically. In fact, some of the other psychological variables examined are conceptually related to depression and anxiety (e.g., happiness and stress, respectively) but are sufficiently distinct to warrant a separate discussion. Regarding happiness, 32% of GPA patients were unhappy because of their vasculitis (Boomsma et al., 2002), while 52% of Takayasu's arteritis (TA) patients reported being less happy overall (Abularrage et al., 2008). One study has documented that over half of GPA patients reported problems with stress (Abdou et al., 2002), suggesting that further examination of stress and vasculitis is justified. In addition, although positive effects of vasculitis are reported less frequently than negative effects, there appears to be a subset of patients who describe beneficial changes that result from a vasculitis diagnosis. Because vasculitis exacts a negative toll physically, functionally, and financially, the majority of these positive effects are seen in the psychological and social domains. For example, Abularrage and colleagues (2008) have found that 11% of TA patients reported an improvement in overall happiness and 12% reported an improvement in overall mood. No analysis was presented of differences between patients reporting positive effects versus those who reported negative or no effects; thus, we do not know whether other factors moderated the effect of vasculitis on patients' psychological responses.

We have unpublished qualitative survey data from a sample of 232 patients that offers some preliminary evidence as to why some patients report positive changes to their mood. In our study, patients commonly discussed how they reevaluated their lives and priorities after receiving a vasculitis diagnosis. Patients who recovered from a particularly bad relapse often described how they now appreciated every day and considered each moment precious. This reevaluation led patients to feel calmer and to not become stressed by minor inconveniences that used to bother them. Improvements in relationships with family members were also commonly reported, which may decrease patients' psychological distress.

2.4 Financial quality of life

Very few studies have explored the economic burden of vasculitis. Using hospital records from 1986-1990, Cotch (2000) estimated that the costs of vasculitis-related hospitalizations alone were $150 million per year in the United States. Although the author could not account for other direct medical costs, such as medication and physician visit expenses, and indirect costs due to changes in employment, it is reasonable to assume that vasculitis-related expenditures are substantial and negatively impact patients and their families (Herlyn et al., 2010). Five studies provide greater detail about the financial impact of vasculitis; they are summarized below.

Four studies have documented employment issues for Granulomatosis with polyangiitis (GPA) patients. In the first study, Hoffman and colleagues (1998) found that most patients (80%) were employed at the time of their vasculitis diagnosis; however, total household income was reduced by approximately 25%. Income reductions may have been due to patients' having to take at least 6 consecutive weeks of sick leave, receiving temporary disability status, or modifying their jobs. Similarly, Boomsma and associates (2002) found that GPA patients frequently missed work due to their disease, changed work duties, reduced work hours, and in rare cases (5%), had to resign from their jobs. Given these job-related changes, it is not surprising that 23% of patients reported a disease-related income reduction. A third study also found that patient financial quality of life was disrupted by vasculitis (Abdou et al., 2002). Specifically, 54% of patients reported losing 25% to 75% of their income, with almost half spending between $10,000 and $100,000 on their therapy and diagnosis. Additionally, 14% of patients reported having to retire due to their illness. In

addition, a study conducted by Reinhold-Keller and colleagues (2002), found that 27% of GPA patients were permanently unemployed as a result of their vasculitis and that women had a three-fold greater risk than men of losing their jobs. Patients who were employed reported missing a median of 14 days of work during the past year due to their vasculitis.
The fifth financial quality of life study involved Takayasu's arteritis (TA) patients (Abularrage et al., 2008). Almost half of those patients changed their work duties due to their TA. Additionally, approximately half of patients reported changing work hours and missing more than six consecutive weeks of work, while almost a third reported taking 6 consecutive months of sick leave from work. Moreover, TA caused almost a quarter of patients to resign from work and 15% to retire.

3. Impact on patients' relationships with social network members

Relatively little is known about the ways in which vasculitis impacts patients' relationships with spouses, family members, and friends. Many of the studies listed in Table 1 have measured social quality of life using the SF-36 (Ware & Kosinski, 2005), which includes two items about how the patient's physical health and emotional problems have interfered with his/her ability to engage in social activities. Overall, the results from these studies show that patient social functioning is compromised; however, the SF-36 social functioning items are so general that they offer limited utility in understanding *how* social relationships and activities have been affected. In this section, we will summarize existing research about the social impact of vasculitis as well as draw upon research from other disease populations to explain how a chronic, unpredictable illness like vasculitis can strain or enhance patients' relationships. We focus on the three studies that have documented social relationship issues in greater detail; Table 2 summarizes the results of these studies.

Relationship Effect	**Study**		
	Hoffman et al., 1998	Boomsma et al., 2002	Abularrage et al., 2008
Spouse/Partner			
No effect	25%	71%	44%
Improved relationship	56%	20%	36%
Worsened relationship	19%	9%	29%
Family			
No effect	40%	74%	35%
Improved relationship	47%	16%	41%
Worsened relationship	12%	10%	23%
Friends			
No effect	65%	70%	-
Improved relationship	14%	7%	-
Worsened relationship	21%	23%	-

Table 2. Percentage of patients reporting vasculitis-related effects on their relationship with their spouse/partner, family, and friends

3.1 Impact on spousal relationships

Chronic illness is a stressor that can affect the physical health and psychological well-being of patients as well as their spouses/partners (Baanders & Heijmans, 2007; Berg & Upchurch, 2007). Much of the stress that spouses experience may result from adapting to a new role as the patient's primary caregiver. For example, Marks and associates (2002) have shown that transitioning to a caregiving role increases depression in spouses of chronic disease patients. Vasculitis may be particularly mentally taxing for couples because spouses must be ready to act as a caregiver each time the patient experiences a relapse or disease flare-up. Because the severity of relapses varies considerably, the physical demands of caregiving for any particular relapse may range from minor to substantial, which requires additional adjustment on the part of the spouse. Moreover, patients often want to avoid being a burden on the caregiver, which can complicate interpersonal interactions as patients adapt to the sick role. These issues are discussed in greater detail by Koutantji and associates (2000).

Of the three studies that investigated the effect of vasculitis on spouse/partner relationships, two were conducted with Granulomatosis with polyangiitis (GPA) patients (Hoffman et al., 1998; Boomsma et al., 2002) and another was conducted with Takayasu's arteritis (TA) patients (Abularrage et al., 2008). The results from these studies reveal substantial variation in the extent to which vasculitis affects spousal relationships (Table 2). For example, in the two studies of GPA patients, the percentages of patients who reported that vasculitis did not affect their relationship with their spouse were 25% and 71%. The percentage of TA patients reporting no effect was in the middle (44%) of the previous two estimates. In all three studies, patients were more likely to report that vasculitis had improved, rather than worsened, their relationship with their partner. Unfortunately, greater detail about how relationships improved has not yet been reported. Based on some Qualitative data patients and their partners have shared with us, positive effects may include: 1) feeling closer to one another, 2) more equal distribution of household labor, and 3) making one's relationship a priority after experiencing a severe relapse (Carpenter et al., under review).

There is also little insight into how relationships with partners have worsened; however, both GPA studies found that about 70% of spouses were concerned about the long-term effects of vasculitis and its treatment and approximately one-third were concerned about how vasculitis will affect their financial security. Additionally, Hoffman noted that spouses sometimes had to alter their employment situation in order to care for the patient. Thus, it seems that emotional strain (e.g. worry and concern) as well as financial strain may take a toll on marriages. While these additional strains did not lead divorced GPA patients to believe vasculitis was the cause of their divorce (Hoffman et al.; 1998), 37% of TA patients believed their vasculitis was largely responsible for the termination of their relationship (Abullarage et al.; 2008). Although this has not been reported in the literature, qualitative data from our Accessing Social Support in Symptom Treatment (ASSIST) Study reveals that patients' sex lives are often negatively impacted. Moreover, patients often report partners' becoming frustrated with mood swings that are a side effect of certain vasculitis medications.

The negative impact of vasculitis on marriages may be markedly reduced if couples learn how to effectively manage and cope with vasculitis dyadically, as discussed by Lewis and colleagues (2006). Specifically, patients and their partners may minimize the negative effect of vasculitis on HRQOL through communal coping, developing a high level of dyadic efficacy, and effective communication (see Lewis et al. for a more thorough discussion of these topics). Effective dyadic coping may explain why spouses of vasculitis patients did not report a lower HRQOL when compared with the general U.S. population, even though the HRQOL of patients and spouses was moderately correlated, meaning that spouses were more likely to report reduced HRQOL if the patient did (Carpenter et al., 2009).

3.2 Impact on family relationships

As shown in Table 2, it was uncommon for patients to think that vasculitis negatively impacted relationships with family members. Although 74% of participants in the Boomsma et al. study believed that relationships with family were unaffected, between 40% and 50% of patients from the other two studies felt that their family relationships had improved. Again, details about how relationships had improved were not provided. It is likely that a serious life-threatening illness like vasculitis can cause patients to feel closer to their family, especially if they are emotionally and instrumentally supportive when the patient is experiencing a relapse. Indeed, qualitative data from the ASSIST Study supports this statement, with many patients reporting that they feel closer to family members, either through family members' increasing the frequency with which they interact with patients or telling the patient how concerned they are for the patient's well-being.

In all three studies, fewer than 25% of patients reported negative changes to family relationships. Between 5 and 10% of non-spousal family members of GPA patients changed their employment status in order to care for the patient, whereas 18% of family members of TA patients altered their work situation. Relationships are probably most at risk when a family member, like a child or parent, takes on a caregiving role, as those family members are under additional physical, mental, and financial strain.

3.3 Impact on friendships

Of the three relationships discussed in this chapter, friendships are the most likely to be negatively impacted by vasculitis. Although two studies in Table 2 document that approximately 20% of patients reported that vasculitis had worsened their friendships, a recent qualitative study has found that more than half of vasculitis patients experienced degradation in the quantity and quality of their friendships (Carpenter et al., under review). To be specific, 1 in 5 patients reported losing a friend as a result of their vasculitis diagnosis. Moreover, quality of friendships was compromised due to reduced social participation, with 25% of patients engaging in fewer social activities after their diagnosis. Reduced social participation was often attributed to friends' lack of understanding about vasculitis, vasculitis-related fatigue, lifestyle changes related to medication contraindications and infection precautions, as well as patient withdrawal.

Although previous research has found that between 7% and 14% of patients report that vasculitis led to improved friendships, more than 45% of patients reported positive friendship changes in the study by Carpenter and colleagues. Positive changes included becoming closer with friends and receiving social support. Supportive friends were described as those who showed some interest in vasculitis and its effects, understood and accepted that patients would not be able to engage in social activities at the same level as previous to illness onset, and were emotionally and instrumentally supportive. Many times, patients developed new friendships with other chronic disease patients. These relationships helped patients realize they were not alone and often became an avenue for sharing personal accounts of the disease as well as helpful disease-specific information that patients were unable to get elsewhere.

4. Limitations of existing research

Table 1 highlights several methodological limitations in the HRQOL literature that are worthy of greater discussion. First, all but one of the HRQOL studies was cross-sectional in nature. Without longitudinal data, we cannot determine how HRQOL changes over time, which may be particularly important for a relapsing, remitting disease like vasculitis. Furthermore, cross-sectional studies limit our ability to identify moderators or mediators of the effect of vasculitis on HRQOL. Disease status, or whether a patient is in relapse or remission, is likely one such moderator. Preliminary evidence demonstrates that: 1) remission status was the only significant predictor of better mental quality of life for Takayasu's arteritis patients (Abularrage et al., 2008) and, 2) relapsing patients reported lower quality of life for 7 of 8 SF-36 subscales when compared with patients in remission (Carpenter et al., 2011). Other potential moderators include number of comorbidities (Ertam et al., 2009), whether the patient is taking immunosuppressive medications (Faurschou et al., 2010), vasculitis type (Koutantji et al., 2003), and patient age (Faurschou et al., 2010). Additionally, patient coping (Koutantji et al., 2000) and social support (Carpenter et al., 2011) may mediate the relationship between vasculitis and HRQOL.
A second limitation concerns the measurement of health-related quality of life. For example, the majority (79%) of studies used generic measures of HRQOL, including the Short Form 36 (SF-36; Ware & Kosinski,), the World Health Organization's WHOQOL-100 (WHO, 1997), and the EQ-5D (EuroQol group, 1990). Only a few studies (26%) used disease-specific measures, such as the quality of life questionnaire developed specifically for vasculitis patients by Hoffman and colleagues (Hoffman et al., 1998). The rationale for these choices is not always clear. Measurement is the link between the concepts and variables researchers want to examine and the numbers they collect and analyze. Unless the correspondence between the measures and the concepts is high, the numbers may be subject to misinterpretation. Under some circumstances, for example, illness-specific concepts and variables may be of interest. For example, the uncertainty patients with relapsing/remitting illnesses face may expose them to forms of stress that may not be a part of other chronic illnesses with a less variable trajectory. When that is the case, using a less specific assessment tool may not fully capture the concept of interest to the researcher. On the other hand, when investigators wish to examine the same variables across different conditions, using illness-specific measures may impede their ability to do so. Another important measurement distinction that is often overlooked differentiates measures comprising indicators sharing a common cause from those sharing a common effect. As an example, most depression scales fit a common-cause model, with the response to each item being determined by the same subjective state experienced by the respondent. In contrast, comorbidity checklists typically aggregate variables that have a common effect (i.e., each contributes a quantum of poor health to a total) but that do not necessarily share a common cause (i.e., the various comorbid conditions may not share a common etiology). Certain measurement procedures are more readily applicable to the common-cause than to the common-effect situation and some psychometric procedures, such as the computation of internal-consistency reliability, are inappropriate for measures based on common effects (e.g., DeVellis, 2012). More generally, it is essential that sufficient attention is paid to

measurement issues to ensure that the information gathered accurately reflects the precise nature of the variables the investigators intend to quantify.

Third, although there are over 15 types of vasculitis, quality of life has been reported for only six different vasculitis types: ANCA-associated (Granulomatosis with polyangiitis, Churg-Strauss Syndrome, Microscopic polyangiitis), Takayasu's arteritis, giant cell arteritis, and Bechet's disease. GPA and Behçet's disease have received the most attention in the literature thus far. Because recruiting patients with a rare illness is often costly and logistically difficult, researchers' ability to describe HRQOL is limited, especially with rarer forms of vasculitis. Difficulties with recruitment are why many studies included fewer than 100 patients. Vasculitis researchers must strike a balance recruiting larger convenience samples versus using smaller randomly-selected samples.

Last, most research to date has focused on physical, functional, and psychological quality of life, with fewer studies investigating financial and social domains. To garner an understanding of how vasculitis affects patients' total well-being requires more data about non-physical consequences of the disease. Simply documenting the percentage of patients experiencing positive, negative, or no changes in these life domains is not enough to make concrete recommendations for how to enhance patient care. For example, more information about *how* social relationships have changed is needed to identify how family members can help patients manage the physical and emotional burden of vasculitis.

5. Future research directions

In attempting to summarize the vasculitis quality of life literature, we have identified several areas for future research. First, as noted in the previous section, we believe longitudinal studies are needed to help identify important moderators and mediators of the effect of vasculitis on patient quality of life. Longitudinal studies could be conducted in a cost-effective manner using web-based surveys. Carpenter and colleagues (2011) had a 98% retention rate for a 3-month, web-based longitudinal study of vasculitis patients. Although Internet-based studies are subject to selection bias, as the number of patients using the Internet continues to increase, selection bias will become less of an issue.

We also endorse mixed methods studies that qualitatively and quantitatively ascertain patients' quality of life. Qualitative studies would help illuminate how patients are positively affected by vasculitis and reveal quality of life domains that are untapped by existing measures. For example, even though we know that vasculitis and its treatment can affect patients' sex drive and fertility (Seo, 2007), no studies have documented how these issues are related to patients' psychological and social health. Telephone interviews may be the most feasible method for collecting in-depth qualitative data on these topics, though focus groups conducted at patient support groups or conferences may yield qualitative data on less sensitive topics, like positive effects of the disease.

Finally, greater attention to measurement issues would be beneficial. As mentioned earlier, measurement is a vital link between what investigators intend to learn and the actual data their studies produce. It is incumbent on investigators to explain why their measures have been chosen. Unfortunately, the only justification offered in some studies is that the instrument used was a "validated scale." In fact, neither reliability nor validity are properties of a scale per se, but of how a scale is used. Thus, a demonstration of a scale's validity in one instance does not guarantee it in a separate instance, especially if the two differ in important ways.

6. Conclusion

Although we have discussed several domains of HRQOL individually, they are inter-related. Physical health influences mental health, which is also affected by social functioning and the patients' financial situation. Together, these components make up the multidimensional construct of HRQOL. Between the years of 2000 and 2010, we have seen a marked increase in the number of studies that document quality of life issues for vasculitis patients. These studies show that vasculitis impairs patient quality of life in every domain but offer little insight into the mechanisms through which the disease affects patients psychologically and socially. The challenge for researchers is to build upon this base of studies and draw theoretical insights from research with other chronic diseases to identify areas where the negative impact of the disease can be reduced. During the coming years, we are confident that additional quality of life studies will better describe how vasculitis positively and negatively influences the quality of life of patients and their social network members. Additionally, we foresee that the field will shift from a focus on describing quality of life to developing non-medical interventions to improve quality of life.

7. References

Abdou, N.I.; Kullman, G.J.; Hoffman, G.S.; Sharp, G.C.; Specks, U.; McDonald, T.; Garrity, J.; Goeken, J.A.; Allen, N.B. (2002). Wegener's granulomatosis: survey of 701 patients in North America. Changes in outcome in the 1990s. *The Journal of Rheumatology*, Vol.29, No.2, pp. 309-316.

Abularrage, C.J.; Slidell, M.B.; Sidawy, A.N.; Kreishman, P.; Amdur, R.L.; Arora; S. (2008). Quality of life of patients with Takayasu's arteritis. *Journal of Vascular Surgery*, Vol.47, pp. 131-136.

Akar, S.; Can, G.; Binicier, O.; Aksu, K.; Akinci, B; Solmaz, D.; Birlik, M.; Keser, G.; Akkoc, N.; Onen, F. (2008). Quality of life in patients with Takayasu's arteritis is impaired and comparable with rheumatoid arthritis and ankylosing spondylitis patients. *Clinical Rheumatology*, Vol.27, pp. 859-865.

Baanders, A.N. & Heijmans, M. (2007). The impact of chronic diseases: the partner's perspective. *Family & Community Health*,Vol.30, pp. 305–417.

Basu, N.; Jones, G.; Fluck, N.; MacDonald, A.; Pang, D.; Dospinescu, P.; Reid, D.M.; Macfarlane, J.G. (2010). Fatigue: a principal contributor to impaired quality of life in ANCA-associated vasculitis. *Rheumatology*, Vol.49, pp. 1383-1390.

Berg, C.A. & Upchurch, R. (2007). A developmental-contextual model of couples coping with chronic illness across the adult lifespan. *Psychological Bulletin*, Vol.133, pp. 920–954.

Bernabé, E.; Marcenes, W.; Mather, J.; Phillips, C.; Fortune, F. (2010). Impact of Behçet's syndrome on health-related quality of life: influence of the type and number of symptoms. *Rheumatology*, Vol.49, No.11, pp. 2165-2171.

Boomsma, M.M.; Bijl, M.; Stegeman, C.A.; Kallenberg, C.G.; Hoffman, G.S.; Tervaert, J.W. (2002). Patients' perceptions of the effects of systemic lupus erythmatosus on health, function, income, and interpersonal relationships: a comparison with Wegener's granulomatosis. *Arthritis Care & Research*, Vol.47, No.2, pp. 196-201.

Buhaescu, I.; Covic, A.; Levy, J. (2005). Systemic vasculitis: Still a challenging disease. *American Journal of Kidney Diseases*, Vol.46, No.2, pp. 173-185.

Carpenter, D.M.; Thorpe, C.; Lewis, M.; DeVellis, R.; Hogan, S. (2009). Health-related quality of life for patients with vasculitis and their spouses. *Arthritis Care & Research*, Vol.61, No.2, pp. 259-265.

Carpenter, D.M.; Kadis, J.; DeVellis, R.; Hogan, S.; Jordan, J. (2011). The effect of medication-related support on the quality of life of patients with vasculitis in relapse and remission. *Journal of Rheumatology*, epub ahead of print; DOI: 10.3899 / jrheum. 100808.

Carpenter, D.M.; Meador, A.E.; Elstad, E.A., Hogan, S.L., DeVellis, R.F. (under review) The impact of vasculitis on patient social participation and friendships. Participation and friendships. Clinical and Experimental Rheumatology

Cella, D. (1994). Quality of life: Concepts and definitions. *Journal of Pain and Symptom Management*, Vol.9, No.3, pp. 186-192.

Cotch, M.F. (2000). The socioeconomic impact of vasculitis. *Current Opinion in Rheumatology*, Vol.12, pp. 20-23.

DeVellis, R. F. (2012). *Scale development: Theory and applications (Third Ed.)*. Thousand Oaks, CA: Sage Publications.

DiMatteo, M.R.; Lepper, H.S.; Croghan, T.W. (2000). Depression is a risk factor for noncompliance with medical treatment: a meta-analysis of the effects of anxiety and depression on patient adherence. *Archives of Internal Medicine*, Vol.160, pp. 2101–2107.

Ertam, I.; Kitapcioglu, G.; Aksu, K.; Keser, G.; Ozaksar, A.; Elbi, H.; Unal, I.; Alper, S. (2009). Quality of life and its relation with disease severity in Behçet's disease. *Clinical and Experimental Rheumatology*, Vol.27, pp. S18-S22.

Euro-Qol Group. (1990). EuroQol–a new facility for the measurement of health-related quality of life. The EuroQol Group. *Health Policy*,Vol.16, pp. 199-208.

Exley, A.R.; Bacon, P.A. (1996). Clinical disease activity in systemic vasculitis. *Current Opinion in Rheumatology*, Vol.8, pp. 12-18.

Faurshcou, M.; Sigaard, L.; Bjorner, J.B.; Baslund, B. (2010). Impaired health-related quality of life in patients treated for Wegener's granulomatosis. *Journal of Rheumatology*, Vol.37, No.10, pp. 2081-2085.

Flossmann, O.; Bacon, P.; de Groot, K.; Jayne, D.; Rasmussen, N.; Seo, P.; Westman, K.; Luqmani, R. (2007). Development of comprehensive disease assessment in systemic vasculitis. *Annals of the Rheumatic Diseases*, Vol.66, pp. 283-292.

Hajj-Ali, R.A.; Wilke, W.S.; Calabrese, D.O.; Hoffman, G.S.; Liu, X.; Clark, T.; Langford, C.A. (2011). A pilot study to assess the frequency of fibromyalgia, depression and sleep disorders in patients with Wegener granulomatosis. *Arthritis Care & Research*, Vol. 63, No. 6, pp. 827-833.; DOI 10.1002/acr.20442.

Hays, R.D.; Anderson, R.; Revicki, D. (1993). Psychometric considerations in evaluating health-related quality of life measures. *Quality of Life Research*, Vol.2, No.6, pp. 441-449.

Hellmann, D.B.; Ehlfelder, M.L.; Stone, J.H.; Jenckes, M.W.; Cid, M.C.; Guillevin, L.; Moreland, L.; Dellaripa, P.F.; Hoffman, G.S.; Merkel, P.A.; Spiera, R.; Brown, L.; Hernández-Rodriquez, J.; Rubin, H.R. (2003). *Arthritis Care & Research*, Vol.49, No.6, pp. 819-825.

Herlyn, K.; Reinhold-Keller, E.; Zeidler, A.; Raspe, H.; Gutfleisch, J.; Peter, H.H.; Gross, W.L. (1998) Health-related quality of life in primary systemic vasculitides. *Arthritis & Rheumatism*, Vol.41,p. S538.

Herlyn, K.; Hellmich, B.; Seo, P.; Merkel, P.A. (2010). Patient-reported outcome assessment in vasculitis may provide important data and a unique perspective. *Arthritis Care & Research*, Vol.62, No.11, pp. 1639-1645.

Hoffman, G.S.; Drucker, Y.; Cotch, M.F.; Locker, G.A.; Easley, K.; Kwoh, K. (1998). Wegener's granulomatosis: Patient-reported effects of disease on health, function, and income. *Arthritis & Rheumatism*, Vol.41, No.12, pp. 2257-2262.

Koutantji, M.; Pearch, S.; Harrold, E. (2000). Psychological aspects of vasculitis. Rheumatology; Vol.39, pp. 1173-1179.

Koutantji, M.; Harrold, E.; Lane, S.E.; Pearce, S.; Watts, R.A.; Scott, D.G. (2003). Investigation of quality of life, mood, pain, disability, and disease status in primary systemic vasculitis. *Arthritis Care & Research*, Vol.49, No.6, pp. 826-837.

Langford, C. A. (2005). Update on Wegener Granulomatosis. *Cleveland Clinic Journal of Medicine,* Vol.72,No.8, pp. 689-697.

Lewis, M.A.; Kalinowski, C.T.; Sterba, K.R.; Barrett, T.M.; DeVellis, R.F. (2006). Interpersonal processes and vasculitis management. *Arthritis Care & Research*, Vol.55, pp.670-675.

Marks, N.F.; Lambert, J.D.; Choi, H. (2002). Transitions to caregiving, gender, and psychological well-being: a prospective US national study. *Journal of Marriage & Family*, Vol.64, pp. 657–667.

Moses Alder, N.; Fisher, M.; Yazici, Y. (2008). Behçet's syndrome patients have high levels of functional disability, fatigue and pain as measured by a Multi-dimensional Health Assessment Questionnaire (MDHAQ). *Clinical and Experimental Rheumatology*, Vol.26, (Suppl. 50), pp. S110-S113.

Mumcu, G.; Inanc, N.; Ergun, T.; Ikiz, K.; Gunes, M.; Islek, U.; Yavuz, S.; Sur; H.; Atalay, T.; Direskeneli, H. (2006). Oral health related quality of life is affected by disease activity in Behçet's disease. *Oral Diseases*, Vol.12, pp. 145-151.

Newall, C.; Schinke, S.; Savage, C.O.; Hill, S.; Harper, L. (2005). Impairment of lung function, health status and functional capacity in patients with ANCA-associated vasculitis. *Rheumatology*, Vol.44, pp. 623-628.

Penninx, B.; Kriegsman, D.; van Eijk, J.; Boeke, A.; Deeg, D. (1996). Differential effect of social support on the course of chronic disease: a criteria-based literature study. *Families, Systems & Health*, Vol.14, pp. 223-244.

Reinhold-Keller, E.; Herlyn, K.; Wagner-Bastmeyer, R.; Gutfleisch, J.; Peter, H.H.; Gross, W.L. (2002). Effect of Wegener's Granulomatosis on work disability, need for medical care, and quality of life in patients younger than 40 years at diagnosis. *Arthritis Care & Research*, Vol.47, No.3, pp. 320-325.

Seo, P. (2007). Pregnancy and vasculitis. *Rheumatic Disease Clinics of North America*, Vol.33, pp. 299-317.

Seo, p.; Yuan-I, M.; Holbrook, J.T.; Hoffman, G.S.; Merkel, P.A.; Spiera, R.; Davis, J.C.; Ytterberg, S.R.; et al. (2005).Damage caused by Wegener's Granulomatosis and its treatment. *Arthritis & Rheumatism*, Vol.52, No.7, pp. 2168-2178.

Srouji, I.; Lund, V.; Andrews, P.; Edwards, C. (2008). Rhinologic symptoms and quality-of-life in patients with Churg-Strauss syndrome vasculitis. *American Journal of Rhinology*,Vol.22,No.4, pp.406-409.

Uguz, F.; Dursun, R.; Kaya, N.; Cilli, A. (2007). Quality of life in patients with Behçet's disease: the impact of major depression. *General Hospital Psychiatry*,Vol.29, pp.21-4.

Ware, J.E., Kosinski, M. (2005). *SF-36 physical & mental health summary scales: A manual for users of Version 1.* Lincoln, RI: QualityMetric Incorporated.

World Health Organization (1997). *WHOQOL: Measuring Quality of Life.* Available online at: http://www.who.int/mental_health/media/68.pdf.

23

Kawasaki Disease, Others Heart Injuries, Not Only Coronary Arteritis

Norberto Sotelo-Cruz
University of Sonora
Department of Medicine and Health Sciences
Hermosillo, Sonora,
Mexico

1. Introduction

1.1 Definition

Kawasaki disease to was described in 1967 by Tomisu Kawasaki (Kawasaki, 1967). it is manifested by an acute-course febrile syndrome associated with small-to-medium vessel vasculitis, which can lead to severe cardiovascular complications, including myocarditis, pericardial effusion, valve injuries, coronary aneurisms, and myocardial infarction, eventually involving many organs.

1.2 Epidemiology

Kawasaki disease (KD) is not well known worldwide; in Japan, in a recent survey (Nakamura, 2008), an increase was found of (151.0 to 184.0/100,000) in children aged <5 years; in other places, especially in Asiatic countries such as Korea (105/100.000), Taiwan (69.0/100,000), China (55/100,000), and in Hong Kong (39.0/100,000); in New Zealand, 8.1/100,000) were registered; in the U.S. (17.1/100.000), Canada (26.2/100,000); in Europe,(10/100.000) new cases are reported annually, while in Hispanic countries, 11 new cases are registered per year, and in Latin America, no exact figures are available, but it as been estimated that there are 3.0/100,000 cases (Yahi Lin, 2010 ;Martinez,2003 Nakamura, 2008).
In Mexico, the first case of KD was communicated by Rodríguez in 1977 (Rodríguez, 1977); from that date until June 2010, registries of case series published in medical journals in Mexico added up to 155 patients (Sotelo, 2011).

1.3 Etiology

The causal agent has not been identified 44 years after the original description; very diverse bacterial viral agents, as well as mites, have been considered, in addition to chemical substances, without fully convincing evidence; it has been suggested that the disease is related with superantigenic toxins due to their having found selective expansion of the cellular families T VB2 and VB8; however, this theory remains controversial. In a multicenter prospective study, no significant difference was shown in the prevalence of the toxin produced in toxin-producing strains in patients with KD and in control patients who

manifested fever due to other causes; with respect to this, on the other hand, an alternative hypothesis has been supported regarding that the immune response in KD is polyclonal, (antigen-driven, i.e., similar to a conventional antigen) rather than polyclonal (as found typically in superantigen-driven responses), and that an immunoglobulin A (IgA) plasma cell possesses a central role (Burns, 2004; Falcini, 2006; Nagata, 2009; Newburger, 2004).
In animal models, the properties of superantigenic proteins obtained from intestinal tract bacteria in 19 children with KD, have been studied it was observed that these had T-cell VB2 expansion properties *in vitro*; these superantigens could be involved in the genesis of this disease. During the past decade, *Staphylococcus aureus*, the *Streptococcus* virus for influenza, and the morbilivirus of the pramyxovirus family, bunyavirus, were investigated as a pathogenic agent for KD (Burns, 2004; Esper 2005; Falcini, 2006; Nagata, 2009; Rochol, 2004). Observations have also acquired importance concerning the participation of adenovirus and a new human coronavirus, denominated "New Haven Coronavirus" (Novel human coronavirus Nco-NH), identified in respiratory pathway secretions from a 6-month-old nursing infant with typical KD; in addition, KD was found positive in 8-11-year-old children utilizing the reverse polymerase transcriptase technique. Also reported has been the mycoplasma infection *pneumoniae*; in a recent publication, the participation is considered of nitric oxide and oxygen reactive species by the neutrophils in acute stages (Bruns, 2004; Esper, 2005; Falcini, 2006; Merlin, 2004; Nagata, 2009; Rochol, 2004; Yoshimura, 2009).
To date, no particular gene has been demonstrated to which the development of KD has been attributed; however, the relationship or association has been suggested of a polymorphic HLA-E histocompatibility antigen that could participate in the pathogenesis of the disease; it also has been considered that an imbalance between the Peroxisome proliferator-activated receptor gamma (PPAR-gamma) and low levels of High-molecular-weight (HMW) adiponectin in the disease can be of clinical importance for future development of premature atherosclerosis (Fukunaga, 2010; Lin, 2009).

2. Pathogenesis

Explain the disease's pathogenesis it is complex because of the various interactions among increased immunological components, immune system cells, in addition to vascular components; currently, it is to difficulty to explain the controversy regarding the imbalance the metalloproteins and the tissue inhibitors between KD and other febrile processes ; however, suggested that the complicated pathogenesis of this illness include this imbalance, there have been advances, which we will describe in the following text. (Newburger, 2004, Pinna, 2008, Sakata, 2010)
In the first observations relative to immunological perturbations, we include a marked stimulation in the cytokine cascade and in endothelial cell activation, this being the first step leading to coronary artery injuries, participating in the activation of CD68 endothelial cells, monocytes/macrocytes, and CD8 cytotoxic lymphocytes, and IgA plasma cell appear to be involved. The prominence of IgA plasma cells in the respiratory tract, as also occurs in fatal virus-associated respiratory infections, has suggested that the respiratory tract can be the entrance pathway for causal agents. In the genesis of arterial wall injury, the following intervene: Vascular endothelial growth factor (VEGF); Monocyte activator chemotactic factor (MACF) or Monocyte chemotactic protein-1 (MCP-1); Tumor necrosis factor-alpha

(TNF-α), and diverse interleukins that lead to the development of vasculitis (Neubauer 2004; Pinna, 2008,)
More recently, one study (sakata,2010), showed tahta the circulating matrix metalloproteins MMPs-9 levels are markedly increased in KD, while MMP-1 and tissue inhibitor metalloproteins (TIMPs), showed no significant changes as compared with control groups, previous reports demonstrate that MMP 1-2 and TIMP -2 were significantly higher in acute stage KD, than controls, those reports showed that the levels of MMPs/TIMPs were increased in other febrile patients, nevertheless there was no significant difference in the ratio of MMP/TIMP between febrile and no febrile patients. This features could play an important role in the vascular remodeling in this disease The expression of MMP-9 was detected in entire myocardium of a patient with acute KD, and staining revealed the presence of MMP-9 in Endothelial cells (EC), suggesting that the majority of individual monocytes, neutrophils, or myocardial cells express MMP-9. In the Sakata et al, the authors showed that MMP-9 mRNA expression in Human cells (HUEVECs) treated with plasma MMP-1, -2, and TIMP-2 levels were normal for KD. Plasma MMP-9 increased during the disease's acute phase; MMP-9 stained diffusely in coronary arterial lesions and MMP-9 mRNA levels were higher in HUEVECs treated with plasma in acute and convalescent disease phases. Interleukin (IL)-1B, IL-6, and TNF-alpha stimulated MMP-9 expression. The authors conclude that ECs are a source of MMP-9 in vascular lesions, and that KD is regulated by cytokines IL-1B, IL-6, TNF-alpha, and interferon gamma.
In a recent study conducted to clarify the role of peripheral CD8T cells in KD, researchers investigated these cells' activation, proliferation, and effector function, compared with healthy/febrile controls. Patients with KD showed a striking increase in early activator markers CD69 CD8T cells and in maturation subsets, but HLA-DR CD8T cells, which represent late activation, did not increase. The cell division reflected by Ki67, CD8T increased in KD and in febrile controls; however, the effector cells were lower in acute than in convalescent KD. The CD8T cells denoting cytolytic activity were lower in KD (Ehara, 2010; Sakata, 2010).

3. Arterial injury

In the evolution of the arterial injury, there is a series of changes that can involve not only the coronary arteries, but also other arteries, such as those of the muscles, the mesentery arteries, the femoral arteries, the iliac, the renal, the axillary, and the brachial arteries; in the different stages of the disease, in the median layer, edema, muscle cell disassociation, and subendothelial edema are observed, and later, mononuclear infiltration, internal elastic lamina destruction, fibroblastic proliferation, metalloprotein matrix-related remodeling, active inflammation, fibrous scar, and arterial remodeling or revascularization; the progressive stenosis results from the remodeling and the neoangiogenesis ; the intimal is markedly thickened and consists of linearly arranged micro vessels, an layer that is rich in smooth muscle cells, an fibrous layers many factors are expressed in aneuriysms. (Lau, 2008; Sakata, Newburger,2004; 2010; Tai-Lin, 2008)

4. Myocarditis

From 1978, it was communicated that myocarditis can present during the acute phase of KD and that it can be transitory; 20 years later, it was affirmed that up to 50% of patients with

KD can present myocarditis (Fujiwara, 1978; Rowley, 1998). The mechanism of injury is not yet clear, whether it is considered as secondary to the action of several cytokines, TNF, Interferon, or Interleukins 1 and 6, which can contribute to myocyte contractility dysfunction

On the other hand, there is evidence of myocarditis identified by serialized biopsies of myocardia in patients without coronary aneurysms (Takahashi, 1989; Yutani, 1981; Yonesaka, 1992). Findings from the histological viewpoint have been diverse, and among these are found the following: hypertrophy; myocyte degeneration; fibrosis; infiltration of lymphocytes and plasma cells, and disarray of myocardial fibers and, in adults after KD, we find the description of kariomyocyte dropout and diffuse fibrosis not in the watershed distribution of the epicardial coronary arteries; it has been supposed that the fibrosis is due to ischemic damage because of microinfarcts or kariomyocyte inflammatory damage. Mycocarditis in KD is characterized by inflammatory cell infiltration from the coronary arteries to the myocardiac instersticium, and necrosis of the myocardium is infrequently observed (Yoshikawa, 2006); on the other hand, diffuse myocarditis followed by myocardial fibrosis can lead to diastolic dysfunction, and in the acute phase of KD, measurement of ventricular flow has revealed an abnormal relaxation and has been associated with increased levels of type B naturiuretic peptide.

By other hand Myocarditis is recognized as a component on the half of KD patients, thought the left ventricular dysfunction ; Ajami, et al, evaluated myocardial function in patient during acute phase of illnees using the myocardial performance index also known as a Tei index, and they assessed the Tei index, the ejection fraction, shortening fraction and valvular regurgitation, pericardial effusion or coronary arterial involvement, they compared the changes in acute phase compared with pos-treatment data, confirming left ventricular dysfunction these index measures combined systolic and diastolic function is a simple sensitive and accurate tool for estimating myocardial function (Ajami 2010;Kurotobi, 2005). The pathogenesis of these myocardiac injuries and their consequences in the long term with respect to the heart are little understood to date and should not be underestimated; thus, it is necessary to establish methodological follow-up patterns in these patients. The possibility has also been set forth of reclassifying the clinical signs and other findings regarding left ventricle dysfunction in KD (Gordon, 2009; Dahdah, 2009).

5. Valvulitis

During the acute phase of KD, approximately 2% of children develop valvulitis followed by scarring of the valves leaflets, most commonly in the mitral valve, leading to valvular incompetence and the need for valve replacement in a subset of patients (Gordon, 2009; Pinna,2008; Sotelo, 2011).

6. Myocardial infarct

This is the main cause of death and occurs in 1.4 to 2.8% of patients; this can be caused by thrombosis or rupture of aneurisms, which lead to acute infarct; histopathologically, changes are observed in the cytoplasm, loss of transversal striae and of the nuclear membrane, neutrophil, lymphocyte, and macrophage infiltrate in the dead cell zone, with a formation of collagen that will confer later scarring (Schoen and Mitchell, 2008; Newbauer, 2004; Shimizu, 2009)

7. Other manifestations

In the heart, the development of progressive dilation of the aortic root with aortic valvular regurgitation has been observed. Pericardial effusion with ventricular dysfunction has also been observed (MacMorrow, 2001).

8. Ages at presentation

KD is more frequent in children <5 years of age in 76% of the cases, observing a maximum peak at between 2 and 5 years; in infants <1 year of age, special characteristics are present, with a higher number of atypical cases and also more complications. In adolescents, it presents with a lesser frequency; recently, a series of cases has been described in adult patients that, until now, has been limited to one hundred cases, in the majority of which the disease appears, to a greater degree, follow an atypical course, such as has been described in children, the existence of Incomplete KD in adults, suggest that the study algorithm proposed by multidisciplinary committee on experts to diagnose of this disease in children could be useful in adults . On the other hand, in patients with HIV, it is more feasible to find patients affected with KD in adults (Gommar-Menesson, 2010; Seve, 2011).
The children at greatest risk of complications and of having a deficient treatment response are those aged <1 year. With respect to gender, masculine predominates at a ratio of 1.7:1 (Cimaz, 2009; Newburger, 2004).

8.1 Season of the year

KD can present in isolated fashion, but in areas of greatest prevalence, epidemic outbreaks are registered, and it is the months of spring and fall that have the greatest number of cases, coinciding with the times of greatest incidence of viral diseases (Lin, 2010; Newburger, 2004).

9. Clinical manifestations

Currently, the most important elements for diagnosis are based on the clinical findings; included among these are fever >4 day, at the age < 5 years, associated with skin rash, oropharyngeal and lip erythema conjunctival injection, edema of the hands and feet, erythema of palms and soles, and, in the convalescent phase, these signs comprise the principal criteria for being able to make a diagnosis of KD of day 4 of the illness (Newburger, 2004). Periungual desquamation is a sign that presents at between 10 and 21 days of disease evolution, although additional clinical signs can also be observed, such as hepatomegaly, ictericia, abdominal pain, vesicular colic pain (gall bladder), vomiting, diarrhea, dysuria, the arthralgias, and interphalangeal articular pain; other less frequent clinical data have been described, but it is urgent to have among these the deep, transverse grooves across the nail (Beau's lines). These changes appear 1 or 2 months after disease initiation; striated leukonychia, which consists generally of two smooth bands that are parallel to the lunula of the nails, apparently are associated with Periungual edema and can be observed ca. day 9 of disease evolution (Berard, 2008; Imaz, 2009; Yeo, 2009).
Another sign observed in children <1 years of age is reddening of the Bacillus Calmette-Guérlin (BCG) scar, which is considered to be related with a cross-reaction (Shina, 2005) of the thermal shock protein HPS 65 and its human homologue, HPS; on the other hand, the

hydrotropic biliary vesicle, colonic edema, and pulmonary nodules are rare manifestations, but should be considered when there is abdominal pain in acute- state and persistent respiratory manifestations (Freeman, 2003; Kim, 2008; Newbauer, 2004; Rigante, 2010) (Table 1).

In cases of suspicion of KD that are catalogued as atypical, we should bear in mind the following data that are useful in the diagnosis: fever for >9 days; skin exanthema for some time, and the three basic disease signs, including leukocytosis with neutrophilia, elevation of transaminases, and albumin <3.5 g/dl, and thrombocytosis. There is also a scoring system, designed by Harada, for predicting coronary aneurisms, comprising the following parameters: masculine gender; age <1 year; leukocytes >12,000 × mm^3; reactive C protein >3 mg/dl; hematocrit >35; platelets >350, 000 mm^3, and albumin >3.5 g; a patient is considered to be at risk if he/she scores 4 or more points between day 1 and day 9.

There are serious difficulties involved in establishing the diagnosis in breast-feeding infants and in children aged <1 year, because the patients do not express the characteristic pain; it is, therefore, important to possess laboratory support in determining creatine kinase with the MB fraction, in addition to the Electrocardiogram (EKG) to observe test segment, Vf, Q, and T waves, echocardiogram, and myocardial perfusion and magnetic resonance gammagrams (Bao-thing, 2010; Javadzagean, 2009; Newburger, 2004; Shulman, 2003).

Basic signs
Persistent fever for >5 days
The presence of four or more signs of the disease
Conjunctival bulbar injection without exudates
Changes in lips and oral cavity
Erythema, cracking of lips, strawberry tongue, diffuse oral injection, and pharyngeal mucosa
Erythema of palms, soles, edema of hands, feet, leukonychia striata in nails at day 9
Polymorphous exanthema
Cervical lymphoadenopathy (>1.5 cm in diameter), unilateral or bilateral
Periungual peeling of fingers, toes, in weeks 2 and 3, transversal grooves in fingernails (Beau's lines) in week 4.

Other Clinical Features
Cardiovascular System: Precordial murmur, congestive heart failure, **myocarditis**, pericarditis, pericardial effusion, valvular regurgitation, coronary artery abnormalities.
Aneurysms of medium-size non coronary arteries.
Skin: Raynaud's phenomenon, peripheral gangrene, desquamating rash in groin, erythema, induration at Bacillus Calmette-Guérin (BCG) inoculation site.
Musculoskeletal System: Arthralgias, arthritis.
Gastrointestinal Tract: Diarrhea, vomiting, abdominal pain, hepatic dysfunction, hydops of gallbladder, colonic edema.
Central Nervous System: Irritability, sensorineural hearing loss, aseptic meningitis.
Genitourinary system: Meatitis, uretritis.

(Berard, 2008; Kim, 2008; Newburger, 2004; Shina, 2005; Sotelo, 2011).

Table 1. Basic signs and other findings that can present in Kawasaki disease.

10. Laboratory tests and others

There are no specific laboratory studies, although leukocytosis, an increase in globular sedimentation speed, and a discrete elevation of bilirubins in 10% of patients tend to be observed during the first 2weeks, as well as a moderate increase of transaminases in 40% of cases; in the general urine test, elevated leukocytes can be observed in 4 to 6 of every 10 patients, and thrombosis with a 3- to 6-week duration. In addition, with positive C-reactive protein in concentrations >6 mg/l, other studies have been recommended that suggest vasculitis, such as the following: Antinuclear antibodies (ANA); Anti-neutrophil cytoplasmic antibodies (ANCA), and endothelial anti-cellular antibodies, which have not demonstrated full usefulness and that can lead to confusion; in determination of Creatinine phospho kinase (CPK), MB fractions are useful for patients with very severe clinical pictures and with risk points that suggest greater susceptibility for presenting myocardial infarct. Methods have also been developed, such as determination of tryptophase and kynurenine in plasma by the liquid chromatography method, finding higher levels in patients with KD; this is a method that, once validated, could have an application as a useful laboratory diagnostic index; also, in patients with atypical clinical situations, it has been suggested that determination of natiuretic peptides is a good marker of evolution to myocardial infarct, and it has been recommended that this could be added to the diagnostic tests (Card, 2009; Dahdah, 2009; Kurotobi, 2005; Javadzagean, 2009; Newburger, 2004; Shulman, 2003; Zhan, 2009).

It has been found recently that early neutropenia indicates that circulating neutrophils on day 10 of illness evolution can play an important role in following the sequence of the formation of coronary artery injuries (Onouchi, 2009).

More recently, the measurement has been proposed of CD69 CD8T in peripheral blood as a marker to determine disease progression, treatment response, and convalescence in KD (Ehara, 2010).

On the other hand, studies have been conducted in order to identify whether there are genetic markers related with risks of complications in children with KD, and polymorphisms found in the *HLA-E* gene have been associated with the possibility of the development of coronary aneurysms; on the other hand, alterations in the extracellular matrix associated with Pro-collagen type III (PIIINP) and metalloproteins identified with biomarkers in 35 adolescents and young adults who had KD have shown an association between high levels of PIIINP and the severity of the coronary injuries; nonetheless, more confirmatory studies are required in this respect (Lin MT, 2008; Lin YJ, 2009). Unfortunately, many of these procedures are not within the reach of the poorest countries (Sotelo, 2007, 2011).

10.1 Thoracic x-rays

These can show pneumonic infiltrate in 15% of cases, especially in patients who present cough and respiratory difficulty, although there are radiologic changes that can be caused by pneumonitis, hemorrhages, and vasculitis-related pulmonary nodules (Freeman, 2003).

10.2 Electrocardiogram (EKG)

EKG can be normal in the first disease phases, or can show changes such as tachycardia, PR-QT prolongation, and abnormal Q waves (data of the infarct).

10.3 Echocardiography

This is a study conducted in the physician's office that is perhaps the most important in the diagnosis and it is necessary in the acute phase and within the first 15 days, independently of adequate treatment, and is especially required in children with an atypical or incomplete clinical situation who manifest fever and at least four basic disease signs. This procedure is also necessary to demonstrate left ventricular function in patients with myocarditis and shortening of the fraction of the left ventricle with (<0.28)-decreased values; however, fraction shortening increased significantly after treatment; also is utilized Tei index for measures combined systolic and diastolic function and estimating myocardial disfunction as an evidence of myocarditis, these has been demonstrated by means of other methods, for example, utilizing Galio citrate and scanner (planar or single-photon-emission [SPE]-CT) and Tc labeled with blood cell scans. By these methods and by echocardiography, it has been observed that there is improvement in the myocarditis after treatment. This situation probably is related with the fact that myocarditis has been considered as a transitory event, without its being studied more profoundly (MacMorrow, 2001; Newburger, 2004; Yoshikawa, 2006).

10.4 Perfusion gammagrams

To demonstrate coronary injuries, there are procedures that are also utilized that permit greater precision in the identification of these coronary lesions; among these procedures are found myocardial perfusion gammagrams and coronariographies; it is also possible to request coronary Angiography by magnetic resonance (MRA), which provides images equivalent to those of coronary angiography. In addition, there as also been information on flow in dilated arteries. Another procedure such as Electron beam computed tomography (EBT) is employed to estimate the characteristics of the myocardium and is useful for detecting progressive myocardial ischemia. Spiral CT (Multislice Spiral Computed Tomography) EBT is a non-invasive resource that is comparable with coronary angiography for visualizing arterial stenosis in children with KD; lately, there has been a recommendation for the use of Dual CT (DSCT) as a resource of greater usefulness than the color Doppler echocardiogram for the detection of coronary abnormalities. Notwithstanding this, of recent date technological innovations in echocardiography have also been described that allow to evaluate treatment response to GGIV, assessing the cardiac walls. Some of these procedures could in the future constitute the diagnostic and follow-up standards in KD (Abe, 2010; Bao-Ting, 2010; Endoh, 2004; Magroverni, 2004).

11. Treatment

Early identification of this disease and initiating treatment with gammaglobulin and aspirin during the course of week 1 has demonstrated that this avoids the development of coronary injuries and diverse cardiovascular injuries that, in the acute as well as in later disease stages, place the patient's life at risk (Mueller, 2009; Newbauer, 2004).

The most utilized treatment is the application of Intravenous gammaglobulin (GGIV) at a dose of 2 per kg in a sole dose for a 12- infusion; this is the most accepted treatment and has allowed to the reduction of prevalence of aneurysms to <5% and a mortality of 2% to 0.3%, although the GGIV scheme is at a dosage of 400 mg × kg × day for 5 days, plus aspirin at 80 to 100 mg × kg × day. According to response, the GGIV dose can be repeated, or corticoids can be added, especially in refractory cases (Cha, 2008; Chung, 2009; Falcini, 2006; Hung, 2009; Miura, 2008; Newbauer, 2004; Ogata, 2009; Okada, 2009; Sano, 2010; Tremoulet, 2008).

Other therapeutic agents have been recommended, such as cyclophosphamide, cyclosporine, and Ulinastatin in a limited number of cases (Newbauer, 2004).
Infliximab is a product based on monoclonal antibodies against Tumor necrosis factor-alpha (TNF-α), and it has been employed successfully in cases of resistance to gammaglobulin. (Burns,2008)
Abciximab is another monoclonal antibody that inhibits the platelet glycoprotein receptor IIb/IIIa, favoring the more rapid resolution of the aneurysms; however, these drugs require greater clinical experience (Burns, 2008; Williams, 2002; Tremoulet, 2008).
Concerning recommendation for treatment of KD during the past 3 years, it as been mentioned that the greatest effectiveness in cases of relapse or resistance is obtained on utilizing pulses of methylprednisolone in addition to GG.
In cases of recurrence of fever or resistance to GGIV, this combination has even been recommended as initial therapy (Cha, 2008; Chung, 2009; Miura, 2008; Ogata, 2009; Okada, 2009; Sha, 2008).
Cardiovascular sequelae of KD in the adult in Japan. A systematical follow-up all the patients who were diagnosed with this disease with observation periods of >15 years; The Committee of Experts of the American Heart Association has designed a follow-up model that includes stratification in five levels (I toV),Table 2 (Newburger,2004), the latter including coronary changes, size of the aneurysms, and the obstruction, and they also provided pharmacological recommendations and the procedures and diagnostic studies, both invasive and non-invasive, that should be performed, in addition to the surgical options (Gordon, 2009; Newburger, 2004). Included an indication that there should be long-term follow-up for patients who had echocardiogram-indicated coronary ectasias in an acute episode and who presented for development of aneurysms, independently of the internal diameters of these, but with special emphasis on patients who presented giant aneurysms of >8 mm, and also subjects who additionally had other cardiovascular risk factors, such as obesity and hypertriglyceridemia.
The complications most frequently observed in adults as sequelae of KD are the following: angor pectoris; ventricular tachycardia ventricular with left cardiac failure, secondary to calcified aneurysms, myocardial infarct, arrhythmias, and sudden death (Gordon JB, 2009).

Risk Level I – *Patients with no coronary artery changes on echocardiography at any stage of the illness*
No antiplatelet therapy is needed beyond the initial 6 to 8 weeks after the onset of illness.
No restriction of physical activity is necessary after 6 to 8 weeks.
Because the degree of future risk for ischemic heart disease in this category of patients is still undetermined, periodic assessment and counseling about known cardiovascular risk factors every 5 years is suggested.
Coronary angiography is not recommended.
Risk Level II – *Patients with transient coronary artery ectasia or dilatation (disappearing within the initial 6 to 8 weeks after the onset of illness)*
No antiplatelet therapy is needed beyond the initial 6 to 8 weeks after the onset of illness.
No restriction of physical activity is necessary after 6 to 8 weeks.
Risk assessment and counseling is recommended at 3- to 5-year intervals.
Coronary angiography is not recommended.

Risk Level III – *Patients with isolated (solitary) small to medium (>3 mm but <6 mm, orzscore between 3 and 7) coronary artery aneurysm in ≥ 1 coronary arteries on echocardiography or angiography*
Long-term antiplatelet therapy with aspirin should be administered, at least until the aneurysms regress.
Physical activity without restriction in infants and children in the first decade of life is permitted after the initial 6 to 8 weeks. Stress tests with myocardial perfusion evaluation may be useful in the second decade to guide recommendations for physical activity. Participation in competitive collision or high-impact sports is discouraged in children receiving antiplatelet therapy.
Annual follow-up by a pediatric cardiologist with echocardiogram and ECG is recommended. Stress tests with myocardial perfusion imaging is recommended every 2 years in patients >10 years old.
Coronary angiography is indicated if myocardial ischemia is demonstrated by stress tests with imaging.
Risk Level IV—Patients with ≥ 1 large coronary artery aneurysm (≥ 6 mm), including giant aneurysms, and patients in whom a coronary artery contains multiple (segmented) or complex aneurysms without obstruction
Long-term antiplatelet therapy is recommended. Adjunctive therapy with warfarin with a target INR of 2.0:2.5 is recommended for patients with giant aneurysms. Daily subcutaneous injections of low-molecular-weight heparin merits consideration as an alternative to warfarin for infants and toddlers, in whom blood drawing for INR testing is difficult. Low-molecular-weight heparin also may be used as a bridge during the initial phase of warfarin therapy or during the reintroduction of warfarin after the interruption of therapy for the purpose of elective surgery; therapeutic levels are assessed by measuring antifactor Xa levels. Some experts recommend a combination of aspirin and clopidogrel for patients with multiple or complex aneurysms.
Recommendations about physical activity should be guided by annual stress tests with myocardial perfusion evaluation. Collision or high-impact sports should be discouraged because of the risk of bleeding. Participation in noncontact dynamic or recreational sports is encouraged if no evidence exists of stress-induced myocardial ischemia.
Cardiology evaluation with echocardiogram and ECG should be done at 6-month intervals. Stress tests with myocardial perfusion evaluation should be performed annually. The patient should be monitored for known risk factors of atherosclerosis and his or her family should be counseled accordingly.
Cardiac catheterization with selective coronary angiography should be performed 6 to 12 months after recovery from the acute illness, or sooner if clinically indicated, to delineate the complex coronary artery anatomy. Follow-up angiography may be indicated if noninvasive studies suggest myocardial ischemia. In addition, elective cardiac catheterization in the absence of noninvasive evidence of myocardial ischemia may be useful to rule out subclinical major coronary artery obstructions in some situations, such as when the patient experiences atypical chest pain, the ability to perform dynamic stress testing is limited by age, unique activity restrictions or insurability recommendations are needed, or the anatomy or size of the aneurysm cannot be clearly defined by echocardiography for decisions regarding anticoagulation.
For females of childbearing age, reproductive counseling is strongly recommended.

***Risk Level V** – Patients with coronary artery obstruction confirmed by angiography*
Long-term antiplatelet therapy with or without adjunctive therapy with warfarin anticoagulation is recommended (see Risk Level IV)
ß-Adrenergic-blocking drugs should be considered to reduce myocardial oxygen consumption.
Recommendations about dynamic physical activities should be based on the patient's response to stress testing. Collision or high-impact sports should be discouraged because of the risk of bleeding. Patients should avoid a sedentary lifestyle.
Cardiology evaluation with an echocardiogram and ECG should be obtained at 6-month intervals. Stress tests with myocardial perfusion evaluation should be performed annually. The patient should be monitored for known risk factors of atherosclerosis and his or her family should be counseled accordingly.
Cardiac catheterization with selective coronary angiography is recommended to address the therapeutic options of bypass grafting or catheter intervention and to identify the extent of collateral perfusion. Repeat cardiac catheterization may be indicated when new onset or worsening myocardial ischemia is suggested by noninvasive diagnostic testing or clinical presentation. If the patient has undergone surgical revascularization or a catheter intervention, then repeat cardiac catheterization may be indicated to evaluate the efficacy of the treatment.
For females of childbearing age, reproductive counseling is strongly recommended.

Table 2. Risk Stratification according American Heart association (Newburger, 2004).

12. Conclusion

In view of the growing number of patients with KD who have been identified in different parts of the world, it is necessary for Pediatricians, Pediatric Cardiologists, Pediatric Cardiologist Internists, and Cardiologists for adults to carry out correct follow-ups, taking into consideration that patients can develop vascular injuries with different types of atherosclerosis, coronary aneurysms, with valve incompetence due to scarring of the leaflets or progressive aortic root dilation, and it is important not to underestimates the myocardial lesions, and the biochemical markers of this inflammatory process during acute phase, including moreover. diffuse fibrosis or local scarring in regions of myocardial, ischemia or infarct (Takahasi, 1989; Dahdah, 2009).

KD-associated inflammatory damage can potentially affect all of the components of the cardiovascular system and even other bodily areas as a consequence of vasculitis; thus, systematic follow-up is necessary until adult age in all children who have had this disease, even when his/her manifestations have not been severe, and especially in these children who manifested myocarditis without coronary artery injuries, because to date we do not know the characteristics and long-term consequences of this particular problem. On the other hand, some reports note an up to 12% frequency for myocarditis. The treatment for sequelae in coronary arteries is infrequent in pediatric ages and in the adult, and will depend on the damage established and the patient's evolution at the long term; the decision for the choice of the most adequate procedure (intervention with percutaneous catheter or surgery for bypass placement or specific procedures for valvular problems) will be determined by Cardiologists and Cardiovascular Surgeons (Careaga-Reyna, 2008; Crystal, 2009; Fukazawa, 2010; Gil-Veloz, 2009; Huerta-García, 2009; Kato, 1996; Mueller, 2009; Simizu, 2010; Sudo, 2010; Sotelo, 2011,Vizcaino, 1991).

13. References

Abe, O. et al (2010). Quantitative evaluation of coronary artery wall echogenicity by integrated backscatter analysis in Kawasaki Disease. Journal of the *American Society of Echocardiography*, Vol.23,No.9, pp.938-942 ISSN 0894-7317

Ajami, G.et al(2010). Evaluation of myocardial function using Tei index in pateients with Kawasaki Disease. Cardiology in the Young, Vol.20, pp.44-48. ISSN 1047-9511.

Bao-ting, CH. et al (2010). Diagnostic value of dual-source CT in Kawasaki disease. *Chinese Medical Journal*, Vol. 123, No.6, pp.670-674 ISSN 0366-6999

Berard, R. et al (2008). Leukonykia striata in Kawasaki disease. *Journal of Pediatrics* 2008, Vol.152, pp.889 ISSN 0022-3476

Burns, CJ. et al (2008). Infliximab treatment of intravenous immunoglobulin-resistant Kawasaki disease. *Journal of Pediatrics*, Vo.153, (December) pp,833-888 ISSN 0031-4005

Burns CJ, and Glode. (2004). Kawasaki syndrome. *The Lancet*, Vol. 364 pp. 533-544 ISBN 0140-6736

Careaga-Reyna, G. et al (2008). Revascularizaci6n miocárdica en una paciente pediátrica con enfermedad de Kawasaki. *Rev Mex Cardiol* Vol.19, No.3, pp.152-155 ISSN 0188-2198

Cervantes-Salazar, JL. y Col. (2006) Enfermedad de Kawasaki, conceptos sobre la cirugía de revascularizaci6n coronaria en edad pediátrica. *Archivos de Cardiolologia de México*, Vol. 76, pp 75-79, ISSN 1405-9940

Cimaz, R. and Sundel, (2009) Atypical and incomplete Kawasaki disease. Best Practice and Research. *Clinical Rheumatology* Vol.23, pp. 689-697, ISSN 1478-6362

Crystal, MA. et al (2009) Coronary artery dilatation after Kawasaki disease for children within the normal range. *International Journal of Cardiology* Vol.136 pp.27-32 ISSN 0167-5273 ...

Cha, S. et al (2008). Risk factors for failure of initial intravenous immunoglobulin treatment in Kawasaki disease. *Journal of Korean Medical Sciences*. Vol.23, pp.718-722, ISSN 1011-8934

Chung, AS. et al (2009) Advances in the use of biological agents for treatment of systemic vasculitis. *Current Opinion in Rheumatology*, Vol. 21, pp.3-9, ISSN 1040-8711

Dahdah, N. et al. (2009) Natruretic peptide as an adjunctive diagnostic test in the acute phase of Kawasaki disease. Pediatric Cardiology, Vol.30, pp.810-817 ISSN 0172-0643

Dahdah, N. (2010). Not just coronary arteritis, Kawasaki disease is a myocarditis, too. *Journal American College of Cardiology*, Vol.55, No.14,pp.150 ISSN 0735-1097

Ehara, H. et al (2010). Early activation does not translate into effector differentiation of peripheral CD8T cells during acute phase of Kawasaki disease. *Cellular Immunology* Vol.265, pp.57-64 ISSN 0008-8749

Endoh, H. et al (2004). Usefulness of electron beam computed tomography for quantitative estimation of myocardial ischemia in patients. *Pediatrics International*, Vol.46, pp.704-710 ISSN 1328-8067

Esper, F. et al (2005). Association between novel human coronavirus and Kawasaki disease. *The Journal of Infectious Disease*, Vol. 19, pp. 499-502 ISSN 0022-1899

Falcini, F. (2006). Kawasaki disease. Current Opinion Rheumatology, Vol. 18, pp. 33-38 ISSN 1040-8711

Freeman, A. et al (2003). Inflammatory pulmonary nodules in Kawasaki disease. *Pediatric Pulmonology*, Vol. 36, pp.102-106 ISSN 8755-6863

Fukazawa, R. (2010) Long term prognosis of Kawasaki disease: increased cardiovascular risk. *Current Opinion in Pediatrics*, Vol.22,pp. 587-592 ISSN 1040-8037

Fukunawa, H. et al (2010). Imbalance of peroxisome proliferator actívate receptor gamma and adiponectin predisposes Kawasaki disease patients to developed atherosclerosis. *Pediatrics International*, Vol.52, pp.795-800 ISSN 1328-8067

Gil-Veloz, M. y Cols (2009). Enfermedad de Kawasaki. Comportamiento clínico y complicaciones cardiovasculares en niños atendidos en un hospital de tercer nivel. *Archivos de Cardiología de México*, Vol. 79, No 1, pp 11-79, ISSN 1405-9940

Gommard-Mennesson, E. et al (2010). Kawasaki disease in adults. Report of 10 cases. *Medicine* Vol.89, No.3, pp.149-158 ISSN 1080-9775

Gordon, JB. (2009). When children with Kawasaki disease grow up. *Journal American College of Cardiology*, Vol.54, No.21, pp.1911-1920 ISSN 0735-1097

Javadzadegan, H. et al (2009). Acute myocardial infraction as the first manifestation of the incomplete Kawasaki disease in a young male. *Cardiology Young*, Vol.19, No. 6,(December),pp. 635-637, ISSN 1047-9511.

Kato, H. et al (1996). Long term consequences of Kawasaki disease a 10 to 21 years follow up study of 594 patients. *Circulation*, Vol.89, pp.919-922 ISSN 0009-7322

Kawasaki, T. and Kosaki, (1967). Febrile oculo-orocutaneous acrodesquematous syndrome with or without acute none. supurative cervical lymphadenitis in infancy and childhood: clinical observations of 50 cases. *Allergy*, Vol. 16.pp.178-222 ISSN 0105-4538

Kim, MY, and Ho Noh, (2008). A case of Kawasaki disease with colonic edema. *Journal of Korean Medicine Science*, Vol.23, pp.723-726 ISSN 1011-8934

Lau, AC. et al (2008). Breakdown in an animal model of Kawasaki disease. *Arthritis and Rheumatism*, Vol.58, No.3, pp.854-863 ISSN 0004-3591

Leung, YD. et al (2002). Prevalence of superantigen-secreting bacteria in patients with Kawasaki syndrome. *Journal of Pediatrics*, Vol. 140,pp.742-746 ISSN 0022-3476

Lin, YJ. et al (2009). HLA-E gene polymorphism associated with susceptibility to Kawasaki disease and formation of coronary aneurisms. *Arthritis and Rheumatism*, Vol.60, No.2,pp.604-610 ISSN 0004-3591

Lin, YT. et al (2010). Repeated systematic surveillance disease in Ontario from 1995-2006. *Pediatrics International*, Vol.52, pp.699-706 ISSN 1328-8067

Lin, TM. et al (2008). Abnormal matrix remodelling in adolescent and young adults with Kawasaki disease late after onset. *Clinical Chemistry*, Vol. 54, No.11, pp. 1815-1822 ISSN 0009-9147

McMorrow, TAM. et al (2001). How many echocardiograms are necessary for follow-up evaluation of patients with Kawasaki disease? *American Journal of Cardiology*, Vol.88, pp.328-330,ISSN 0002-9149

Martinez, RM. Et al (2003). Incidencia y cracterísticas clínicas de la enfermedad de Kawasaki .Anales de Pediatría de Barcelona, Vol. 59, No.4,pp 323-327 ISSN 1695-4033

Mavrogeni, S. et al (2004). Magnetic resonance angiography is equivalent to X-ray coronary angiography for the evaluation of coronary arteries in Kawasaki disease. *Journal American College of Cardiology*, Vol. 43, pp. 649-652 ISSN 0735-1097

Merlin, E. et al (2004). Kawasaki syndrome and mycoplasma pneumoniae infection. *Archives of Pediatrics*. Vol.11 pp.972-973 ISSN 0929-693X

Miura, M. et al (2008). Effects of methylprednisolone pulse on cytokine levels in Kawasaki disease patients unresponsive to intravenous immunoglobulin. *European Journal of Pediatrics* Vol.167, pp. 1119-1123 ISSN 0340-6199

Mueller, F. et al (2009). Long term follow-up of acute changes in coronary artery diameter caused by Kawasaki disease: risk factors for development of stenotic lesions. *Clinical Research Cardiology*, Vol. 98, pp. 501-507 ISSN 1861-0684

Muta, H, et al (2004). Older age is a risk factor for the development of cardiovascular sequelae in Kawasaki disease. *Pediatrics*, Vol. 114, pp. 751-754 ISSN 0031-4005

Nagata, S. et al (2009). Heat shock proteins and super antigenic properties of bacteria from the gastrointestinal tract of patients with Kawasaki disease. *Immunology*, Vol.128, pp. 511-520 ISSN 0953-4954

Nakamura Y, et al (2008). Yashiro M, Uehara R, Oki I, Kayaba K, Yanagawa H. Increasing incidence of Kawasaki disease in Japan: nationwide survey. *Pediatrics International* Vol.50,PP.287-290 ISSN 1328-8067

Newburger, JW. et al (2004). Committee on Rheumatic fever, endocarditis and Kawasaki Disease, Council on Cardiovascular Disease in the Young, American Heart Association. Diagnosis, treatment, and long term management of Kawasaki disease: a statement for health professionals from the Committee on Rheumatic Fever, Endocarditis and Kawasaki Disease, Council on Cardiovascular Disease in the Young. *American Heart Association. Circulation*, Vol. 110, pp.2747-2771 ISSN 0009-7322

Ogata, S. et al (2009). Clinical score and transcript abundance patterns identify Kawasaki disease patients who may benefit from addition of methylprednisolone. *Pediatric Research*, Vol.66, No.5, pp. 577-584, ISSN 0031-3998

Okada, K. et al (2009). Pulse methylprednisolone with gammaglobulin as an initial treatment for acute Kawasaki disease. *European Journal of Pediatrics*, Vol.168, pp. 181-185, ISSN 0340-6199

Onouchi, Z. et al (2009). Neutropenia in the acute phase of Kawasaki disease and prevention of coronary artery aneurysm. *Pediatrics International*, Vol.51, pp.448-452, ISSN 1328-8067

Pinna, SG. et al (2008). Kawasaki disease: an overview. Current Opinion in Infectious Disease, Vol.21, pp.263-270 ISSN 0951-7375

Rigante, D. et al (2010). Incomplete Kawasaki disease syndrome followed by systemic juvenile-onset idiopathic arthritis mimicking Kawasaki syndrome. *Rheumatology International*, Vol. 30,pp.535-539 ISSN 0172-8172

Rochol, C. et al. (2004). Adenoviral infections in children: the impact of rapid diagnosis. Pediatrics, Vol. 113, pp. 51-56 ISSN 0031-4005

Rodríguez-Suárez S. (1977) Síndrome linfomucocutáneo. *Boletín Medico del Hospital Infantil de México*, Vol. 34,pp.53-57 ISSN 1665-1146

Sano, S. et al (2010). Dynamics of endogenous glucocorticoid secretion and its metabolism in Kawasaki disease. *Steroids,* Vol 75, pp 848-852, ISSN 0039-128X

Schoen JF and Mitchell RN.(2008) Corazón en Robbins Patologia Humana.Eds, Kumar, Abba, Fausto, Mitchell..Ed, pp.393-434 Elsevier 8^{a}. 978-84-8086-332-2 Madrid España.

Seve, P and Lega (2011). Kawasaki disease in adult patients. *Revueu de Medicine Interne,* Vol.32, No.1, pp.17-25 ISSN 0248-8663

Shimizu, M. et al (2010). Arteries within the artery of coronary artery in an adult patient with acute coronary syndrome. *Internal Medicine,* Vol. 49,pp. 659-663 ISSN 0918-2918

Sakata, K. et al (2010). Matrix metalloproteinase-9 vascular lesions and endothelial regulation in Kawasaki disease. *Circulation Journal,* Vol. 74,pp.1670-1675 ISSN 0009-7322

Shinha, R, and Balakumar (2005). BCG reactivation: a useful diagnostic tool even for incomplete Kawasaki disease. *Archives Disease Children,* Vol. 90,pp.891 ISSN 1468-2052

Sohn, MH. et al (2003). Circulating interleukin 17 is increased in the acute stage of Kawasaki disease. *Scandinavian Journal of Rheumatology,* Vol. 32,pp.364-366 ISSN 0300-9742

Sotelo, N. and González (2007). Kawasaki disease: a rare pediatric pathology in Mexico. A report of twenty cases from the Hospital Infantil del Estado de Sonora. *Archivos de Cardiología de México,* Vol.77, No. 4, pp.299-307 ISSN 1405-9940

Sotelo, N. (2011). Incidencia y evolución de la enfermedad de Kawasaki en México. Salud (i) Ciencia, Vol. 18, No.2, pp.151-156 ISSN1667-8982

Sudo, D. et al (2010). Case control study of giant coronary aneurysmas due to Kawasaki disease: the 19th nationwide survey. *Pediatrics International,* Vol. 52,pp,790-794 1328-8067

Suzuki, H. et al (2010). Marker of T-cell activation is elevated in refractory Kawasaki disease. *Pediatrics International,* Vol.52, pp. 785-789 ISSN 1328-8067

Takahasi, M. (1989). Myocarditis in Kawasaki syndrome: a minor villain. *Circulation,* Vol.79,pp.1398-1400 ISSN 0009-7322

Tremoulet, AH. et al (2008). Resistance to intravenous immunoglobulin in children with Kawasaki disease. *Journal of Pediatrics* , Vol.153, No.1, pp.177-121 ISSN 0031-4005

Vizcaíno-Alarcón A. et al (1991). Enfermedad de Kawasaki en niños mexicanos. *Boletín Medico del Hospital Infantil de México,* Vol. 48, pp.398-408 ISSN 1665-1146

Williams, RV. et al (2002). Does Abciximab enhance regression of coronary aneurysm resulting from Kawasaki disease. *Pediatrics,* Vol. 109: E 4. 0031-4005.

Yeo, Y. et al (2009). Incomplete Kawasaki disease in patients younger than 1 year of age: a possible inherent risk factor. *European Journal of Pediatrics,* Vol.168,pp.157-162 ISSN 0340-6199

Yoshimura, K. et al (2009) Increased nitric oxide production by neutrophils in early stage of Kawasaki disease. *European Journal of Pediatrics,* Vol.168, pp.1037-1041 0340-6199

Yoshikawa H, et al (2006). Four cases of Kawasaki disease complicated with myocarditis. *Circulation Journal,* Vol.79,pp. 202-205 ISSN 0009-7322

Yonesaka. S. et al (1992). Histopathological study on Kawasaki disease with special reference to the relation between the myocardial sequelae and regional wall motion abnormalities of the left ventricle. *Japan Circulation Journal,* Vol.56, pp. 352-358, ISSN 0047-1828

Yutani, C. et al (1981). Cardiac biopsy of Kawasaki disease. *Archives Pathology Laboratory Medicine,* Vol. 105, pp. 470-473, ISSN 0003-9985

Zang, X. et al (2009). Simultaneous determination of tryptophan and kynurenine in plasma samples of children with Kawasaki disease by high-performance liquid chromatography with programmed wavelength ultraviolet detection. *Journal Chromatography B,* Vol. 877,pp.1687-1682 ISSN 1570-0232